KU-713-914

J. C. Tamraz, Y. G. Comair

Atlas of Regional Anatomy of the Brain Using MRI

Springer

Berlin
Heidelberg
New York
Barcelona
Hong Kong
London
Milan
Paris
Singapore
Tokyo

J. C. Tamraz, Y. G. Comair

Atlas of Regional Anatomy of the Brain Using MRI

With Functional Correlations

Foreword by Hans Otto Lüders

With 458 Figures in 817 Separate Illustrations

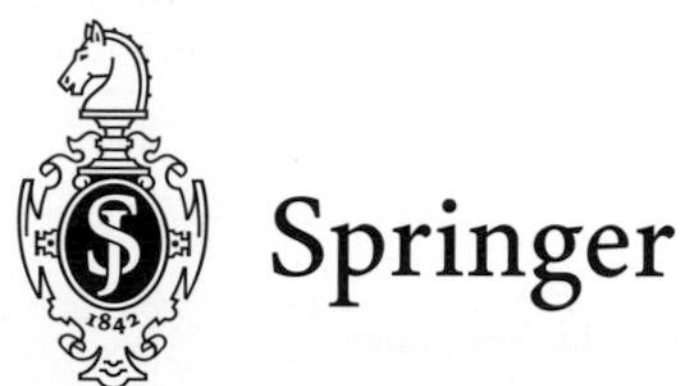

Springer

Jean C. Tamraz, MD, PhD
Professor and Chairman
Department of Neuroradiology
Hotel-Dieu de France Hospital
Saint-Joseph University
Beirut, Lebanon

Youssef G. Comair, MD, FRCSC
Professor and Chief
Division of Neurosurgery
American University of Beirut
Consultant Neurosurgeon
The Cleveland Clinic Foundation
44122 Cleveland, Ohio, USA

ISBN 3-540-64099-1 Springer-Verlag Berlin Heidelberg New York

Library of Congress Cataloging-in-Publication Data
Tamraz, J. C. (Jean Chucri), 1954-
Atlas of regional anatomy of the brain using MRI : with functional correlations / J.C. Tamraz and Y.G. Comair.
p. ; cm.
Includes bibliographical references and index.
ISBN
1. Brain--Anatomy--Atlases. 2. Brain--Magnetic resonance imaging--Atlases. I. Comair, Y. G. (Youssef G.)
[DNLM: 1. Brain--anatomy & histology--Atlases. 2. Magnetic Resonance Imaging--Atlases. WL 17 T159a 2000]
QM455.T35 2000
611'.81'0222--dc21 99-044535

Printed in Germany

Cover-Design: Studio Calamar

Typesetting: Verlagsservice Teichmann, Mauer

SPIN: 105 664 64 21/3135 – 5 4 3 2 1 0 – Printed on acid-free paper

Foreword

The anatomical dissections of Mundini dei Luzzi in 1316, mark the beginning of an era extending over more than 5 centuries in which the study of the brain was limited, almost exclusively, to description of its gross anatomy derived from the inspection of gross anatomical specimens. In the 19th century, new techniques like histology and electrical stimulation were developed allowing the first correlation studies of cortical anatomy and brain function. Shortly thereafter, the development of recording techniques of evoked potentials and spontaneous brain waves (EEG) further enhanced our understanding of brain function as a function of its anatomical correlation. One major limitation of all these studies was that at that time no technique was available to define the anatomy of the brain without its direct visualization. In other words, precise anatomo-functional correlation studies were only possible in experimental studies in animals, the unusual setting of human craniotomies and by careful clinico-pathological studies. These last studies also shed some light on the functions of structures that had been affected by a pathological process, and in the late 19th century and early 20th century, research efforts of clinical neuroscientists focused on anatomo-functional correlation studies making brain anatomy one of their pillars. However, soon these research techniques reached a limit and, progressively research efforts focused on pathogenesis, therapeutics and the development of clinical diagnostic techniques. Clinicians soon realized that precise knowledge of brain anatomy was not necessarily an essential clinical tool and brain anatomy classes in neuroscience curricula became only of secondary importance.

However, technological advances that had its beginnings in the early 1950's eventually lead to a reversal of this trend. A pioneer role in this development was played by the French school lead of Talairach and Bancaud. Taking advantage of newly developed imaging techniques, Talairach realized that angiography could be used effectively to define "non-invasively" the sulcal anatomy of the brain. This led to the development of the "Talairach Atlas", which even today, can be applied practically. Equally important, however, was the collaboration of Talairach with Bancaud that established functional correlations of the anatomical studies of Talairach. These pioneer studies of Talairach and Bancaud certainly led to significant contributions of our understanding of human anatomy and its physiological correlates. Unfortunately, the studies had only a limited impact in the general clinical neurosciences since they were only applicable to a very selected number of patients.

Recent neuroimaging developments, particularly high resolution MRI, provided the tools necessary to make detailed brain anatony available to all neuroscientist on a routine basis. This availability, and the expanded understanding of human anatomo-neurophysiological correlates, has led to a resurgence of the interest of clinical neurophysiologist in gross human brain anatomy and its functional correlates.

Tamraz and Comair's book on regional anatomy of the human brain using MRI, is certainly a welcome addition that fulfills our growing need for books correlating anatomy, function and MRI. There are two facts that make this book particularly appealing for clinicians. Both authors are busy clinicians who, on a daily basis, apply the information provided in the book to their clinical practice. This assures that all the information provided has immediate clinical relevance. In addition, the book is greatly influenced by Professor Tamraz and Professor Comair's exposure to the Paris and Montreal's schools, respectively, both stressing brain anatomy and its relationship to neurophysiology. The immediate clinical practicality of the book and the stress on correlating anatomy and function, make this book a unique and valuable contribution to the clinical neuroscience community, and should become a standard textbook for trainees in the clinical neurosciences. The clinical neurosciences will greatly profit from the practical approach to gross neuroanatomy, neuroimaging and correlative neurophysiology offered in this book.

HANS O. LÜDERS
Chairman and Professor
Department of Neurology
The Cleveland Clinic Foundation

Preface

To Claire, Caroline and Eve
JC T

To Liliane, Andréa and Marc Elie
YG C

Imaging of the human nervous system has traditionally attracted clinicians interested specifically in the fields of neurology, neurosurgery and radiology. However, interest has suddenly widened to include neurophysiologists, computer scientists, biophysicists and developers of biomedical technology. Several factors are responsible for this phenomenon. We believe that the most important is the development of magnetic resonance imaging (MR).

Angiography and ventriculography visualized brain cavities and computer tomography offered uni-dimensional views of structures. With MR, however, structures came to life. Suddenly patients could walk out of the machine with an atlas-like image of their brain. This advance revived the interest in correlating morphology with function.

Progress in reformatting techniques has facilitated the study of morphology. Details of the sulcal and gyral anatomy of the brain and its individual variations can be seen thanks to surface- and volume-rendering techniques that have allowed us to extract the brain out of its envelopes. The functional areas can therefore be readily identified by the trained eye. The core brain structures are visually dissected given the high contrast between gray and white matter.

Activation studies have traditionally been performed by expensive, labor-intensive techniques that do not visualize the details of morphology. Functional MR has the capability of combining morphology and function in a process similar to the mapping performed in the operating room by pioneering neurosurgeons who identified eloquent cortical areas.

In less than two decades a remarkable evolution in brain science has occurred and impacted on the diagnosis, natural history and treatment of disease processes. MR is presently a tool used for diagnosis and treatment.

The purpose of this book is to facilitate the study of brain anatomy by formulating a methodological analysis of functionally oriented morphology. Since the study of the human cortex has not received much attention in radiological or neurosurgical atlases, we have devoted a large part of this work to the study of the surface anatomy of the brain. Following an introductory chapter on the gyral and sulcal development and organization, functional areas are studied separately in four chapters, each devoted to essential cortical function. Primary motor cortex, speech, limbic system and vision are discussed individually. In addition to the standard sectioning methods, imaging of functional areas relied on extensive use of 3-D rendering and the introduction of innovative oblique sections displaying the temporalization process of the cerebral surface and core brain structures. These oblique cuts have the advantage of displaying in few images important cortical areas such as the primary motor-sensory cortex, the speech-related perisylvian areas and the amygdalar-hippocampal memory structures.

In order to appreciate the temporal evolution of brain imaging the first chapter reviews the progression in visual depiction of brain structures from rudimentary to cross-sectional and finally to realistic and precise illustrations, reminiscent of the progress in neuroimaging. This introduction is followed by an overview of the major referential brain systems and a proposal for a sylvian reference plane that is, in our view, the most natural way of studying brain structures in cross section.

The final chapters include three new MR atlases. The first comprises coronal sections acquired perpendicular to the proposed sylvian orientation. This is followed by two oblique approaches acquired along the forniceal plane and the ventricular plane.

The study of brain anatomy stands as a linking factor in the multidisciplinary effort to understand brain function. We hope that this book can contribute towards this crucial task.

Jean C. Tamraz — Youssef G. Comair

Acknowledgments

It is obvious that this volume could not have been finished without the published findings and morphological, functional and imaging materials derived from collaborative works developed over the past 20 years by highly specialized teams in Paris, Montreal and Cleveland.

I am deeply indebted to my mentors in Paris for their invaluable teaching and encouragement. They had a profound influence on my academic course in neuroanatomy and neuroradiology: Professors André Delmas, Chairman of Anatomy at the Institut d'Anatomie; Emmanuel A. Cabanis, Head of Neuroradiology at the Centre Hospitalier National d'Ophtalmologie des Quinze-Vingts who trained me in neuroradiology; and Roger Saban, Honorary Professor at the Museum National d'Histoire Naturelle, who introduced me to the fields of comparative anatomy and anthropology. The anatomical material included is part of a previous work developed under the leadership of E.A. Cabanis at the Institut d'Anatomie, and the primate brains and teratologic specimens are derived from the historical collections obtained from the Laboratory of Comparative Anatomy of the Museum in Paris. I would also like to express my deep gratitude to Professor Alex Coblentz, Director of the Centre Universitaire Scientifique et Biomédical des Saints-Pères, for his major support and counseling, and to Professors Georges Salamon, Ugo Salvolini, Henri Duvernoy, Marie-Germaine Bousser and Olivier Lyon-Caen who greatly contributed to our training in the fields of neuroimaging, neuroanatomy and clinical neurological sciences. Finally, I am extremely grateful for the collaborative work of Dr. Claire Outin-Tamraz at Trad Hospital, who provided us with part of the MR material to complete this book, and I have also benefited in the last few years from discussions at Hôtel-Dieu de France with my colleagues in the Departments of Neuroscience and Imaging. JCT

Essential contributions to human brain morphology, function and structural organization were made by successive generations of functional neurosurgeons. I was fortunate enough to train at the Montreal Neurological Institute, where some of these essential advances were made. It was a pleasure to train under Professor André Olivier, a master neurosurgeon and anatomist. Long before MR allowed us to see sulcal and gyral anatomy in vivo, Professor Olivier's teaching of stereoangiography made these structures visible and allowed us to comprehend the complex three-dimensional anatomy of the structures and the various pathologies that were subsequently dealt with in the operating room. The unique milieu of the Montreal Neurological Institute and the close collaboration between neuroradiology and neurosurgery was a model followed in this book. The content of this book stems from a desire to apply brain anatomy to our clinical practice. At the Cleveland Clinic Foundation, I was priviledged to be associated with Professor Hans Lüders. Our frequent discussions and his profound knowledge of applied electrophysiology and functional localization encouraged us to go ahead with this project. Finally, I am particularly indebted to my colleagues in the epilepsy and neuroradiology programs in Montreal and Cleveland, in particular, Professors Romeo Ethier, Denis Melanson and Paul Ruggieri. YGC

The authors express their sincere gratitude to the publisher, Springer-Verlag, especially Dr. Ute Heilmann and her co-workers, Mrs. Wilma Mc Hugh, Dr. Catherine Ovitt and Mr. Kurt Teichmann, for their help and unfailing patience during the preparation and publication of this atlas.

Contents

1 Historical Review of Cross-Sectional Anatomy of the Brain

It took nearly four centuries to obtain an accurate anatomic representation of the brain. Radiological imaging has undergone a similarly slow but progressive refinement.

The restrictions of the middle ages sharply contrast with the scientific explosion which characterized the Renaissance. Anatomical dissections were prohibited by religious and political authorities which prevented the advancement of medical knowledge. The earliest known anatomical dissections were performed by Mundino dei Luzzi in 1316 and reported by his student Gui de Chauliac in "Anathomia" (1363), one of the earliest dissection manuals.

Avicenna is credited with the first representation of the brain in 1000 A.D. The brain was described as being composed of three compartments or ventricles: the sites of common sense, judgment and memory. This was described by Magnus Hundt (1501) in an anthology on knowledge.

Almost ten years earlier, Leonardo da Vinci had performed numerous brain dissections. He was credited with the first sagittal sections showing the lateral ventricles and the optic chiasm (Fig. 1.1). Unfortunately, the illustrations were kept secret until their discovery towards the end of the fourteenth century. Da Vinci disputed the concept of the three cerebral compartments.

In 1523, Giacomo Berengario di Carpi, professor of surgery in Bologna, published the first anatomy textbook "Isagoge Breves". The brain was primitively represented as similar to intestinal loops ("venter superius"). However the lateral ventricles as well as the choroid plexus were clearly identified (Fig. 1.2).

The earliest axial brain representation was performed by Johannes Eichmann (Dryander), a German anatomist, in 1536. However his representation suffered from lack of perspective as the cut shown included the left lateral view of the head. The ventricles were well demonstrated and the convolutions again resembled intestinal loops (Figs. 1.3, 1.4). The critical role of anatomic dissection is demonstrated by the attempt to distinguish the brain covering from deeper structures, which are presented as anatomical sections. A detailed representation of the skull was also presented (Fig. 1.5).

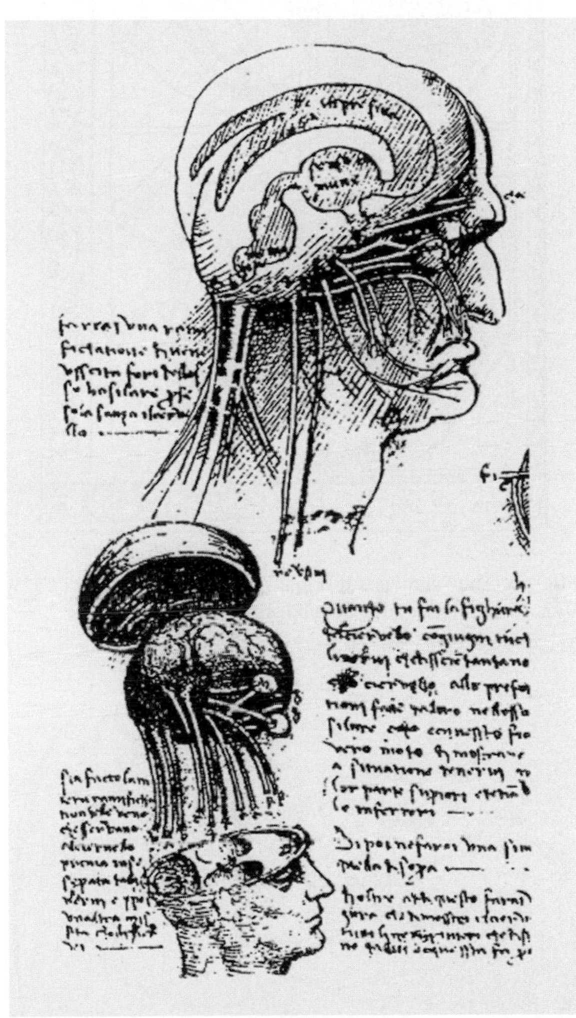

Fig. 1.1. The cerebral ventricles (Leonardo da Vinci 1490; Staatliche Kunstsammlung, Museum Weimar)

Seven years later, Andre Vesalius, professor of anatomy and surgery at Padua University described for the first time (1543) a realistic horizontal brain section in his work "De Humani Corporis Fabrica", which represented the first textbook of anatomy

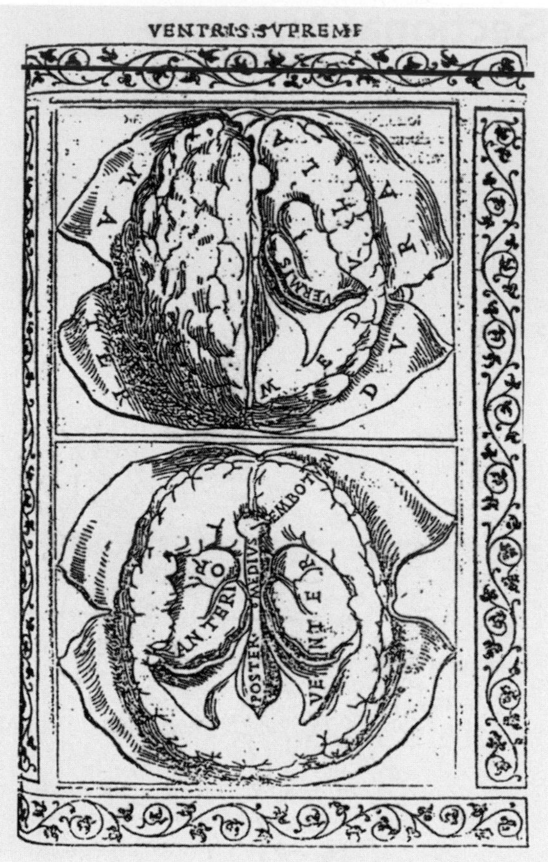

Fig. 1.2. The "ventris supremis" (Berengario di Carpi 1523; Bibl. Interuniversitaire de médecine, Paris)

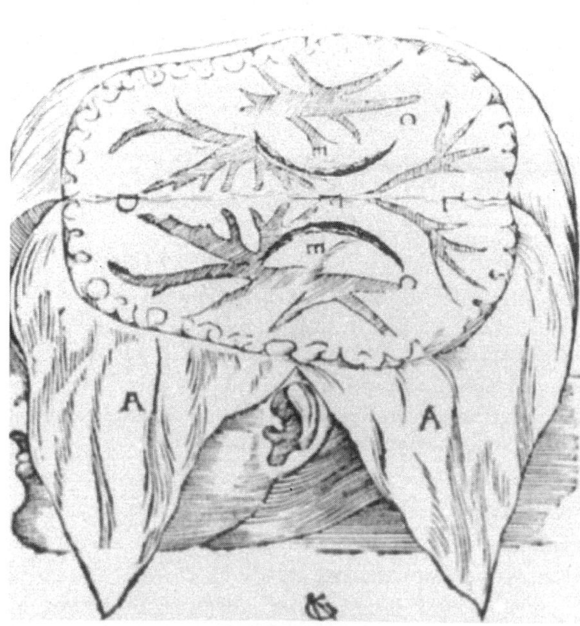

Fig. 1.3. Trial to obtain a horizontal cut of the head and brain through the lateral ventricles shown in perspective (Johannes Dryander 1536; Bibl. Museum National d'Histoire Naturelle, Paris)

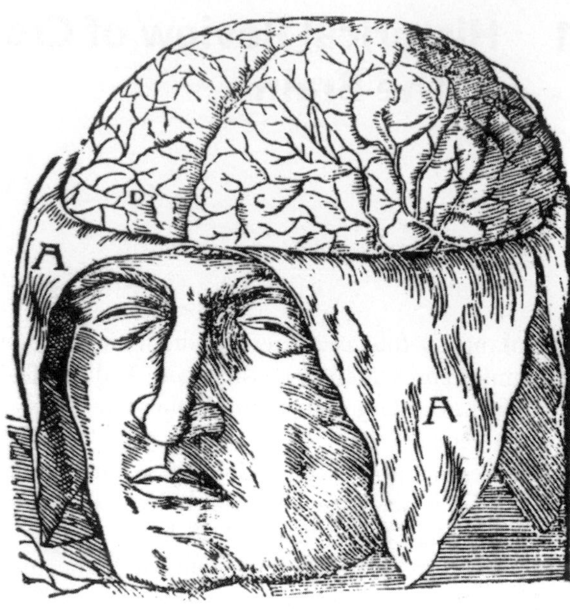

Fig. 1.4. Representation of brain convolutions (Johannes Dryander 1541; Bibl. Museum National d'Histoire Naturelle, Paris)

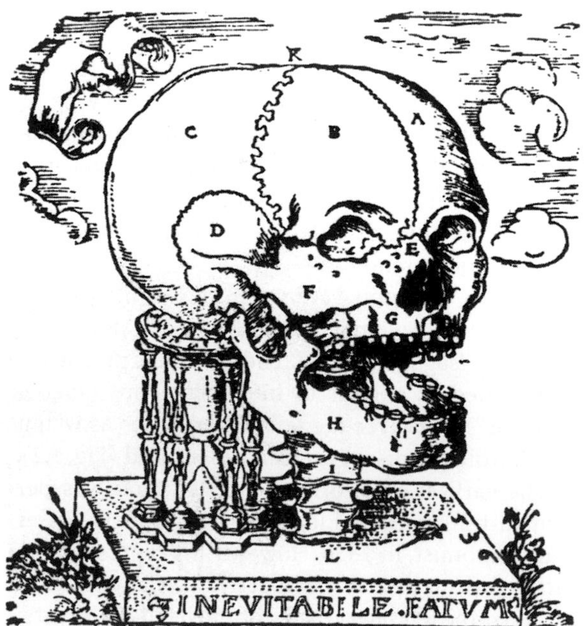

Fig. 1.5. Representation of the cranium in "Anatomia Capitis" (Johannes Dryander 1536; Bibl. Museum National d'Histoire Naturelle, Paris)

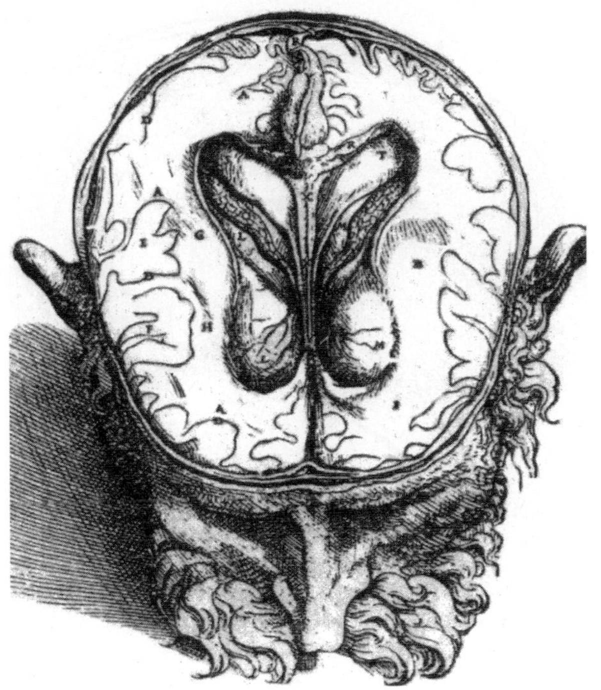

Fig. 1.6. First accurate representation of the brain and the ventricles cut in the horizontal plane in "De Humani Corporis Fabrica" (Andre Vesalius 1543; Bibl. Museum National d'Histoire Naturelle, Paris)

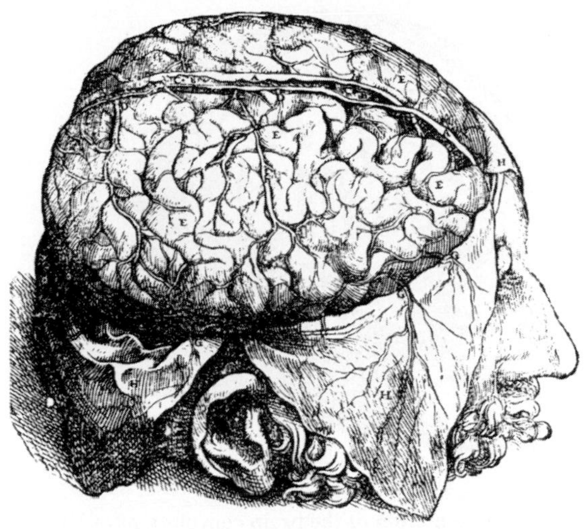

Fig. 1.7. The brain convolutions, in "De Humani Corporis Fabrica" (Andre Vesalius 1543; Bibl. Museum National d'Histoire Naturelle, Paris)

combining text and 323 illustrations. These sections were executed by Jean Stéphane Caillé under Vesalius' supervision and considerably enhanced the text. Indeed it was the first such combination of iconography and text. Vesalius distinguished between white and gray matter. His horizontal sections were universally adopted with some alterations for more than two centuries (Fig. 1.6). Vesalius pointed out the repeated errors of Galen, which emphasized the importance of autopsy material (Fig. 1.7), and refuted the existence of the rete mirabile, a key concept in Galenic theory.

Contemporaneously, Sylvius Jacques Dubois (1478–1555), a rival of Vesalius, was contributing to anatomical knowledge as evidenced by the nomenclature of major brain structures: e.g., sylvian fissure, sylvian artery, and the aqueduct of Sylvius.

The modern approach to brain dissection was described by Varole from Bologna in an innovative work on the optic nerve published in Padua in 1572. The method consisted in removing the brain from the skull and turning it upside down to emphasize the ventral aspect. Nevertheless, the brain convolutions remained poorly depicted in the work of Varole (Fig. 1.8), as well as in the contribution of Jules Casserius (1627) (Fig. 1.9).

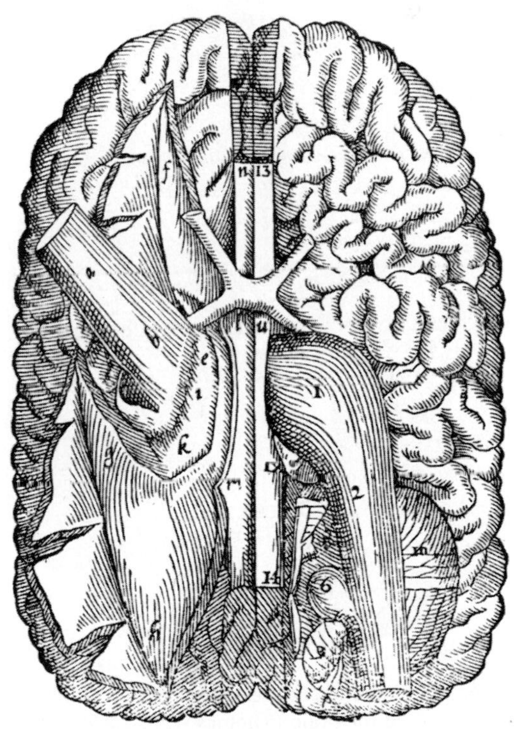

Fig. 1.8. View of the inferior aspect of the brain and the optic pathways (Constantini Varoli 1591; Bibl. Museum National d'Histoire Naturelle, Paris)

Building on previous work, Vesling, in a popular anatomy textbook published in 1647, demonstrated the periventricular structures including the choroid plexus, corpus callosum and hippocampus.

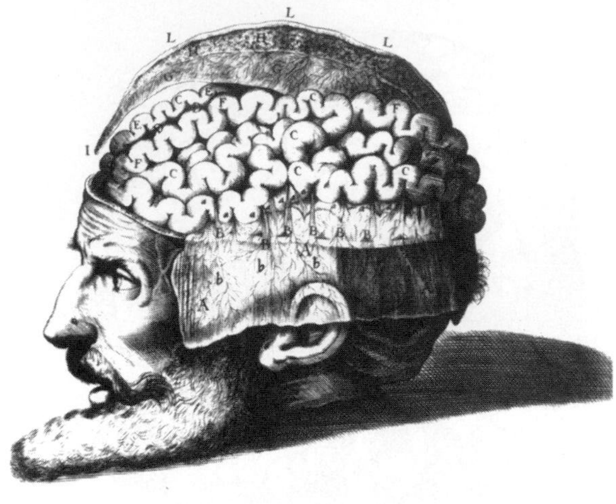

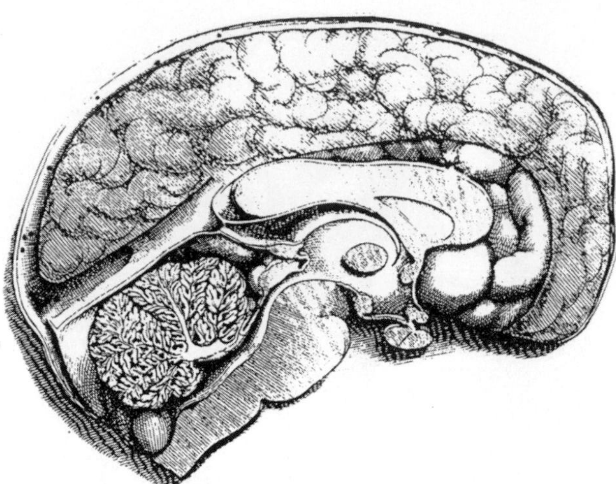

Fig. 1.11. First real sagittal cut of the isolated brain (Nicolas Stenon 1669; Bibl. Museum National d'Histoire Naturelle, Paris)

Fig. 1.9. Representation of the brain convolutions of "intestinal" type (Julius Casserius 1627; Bibl. Museum National d'Histoire Naturelle, Paris)

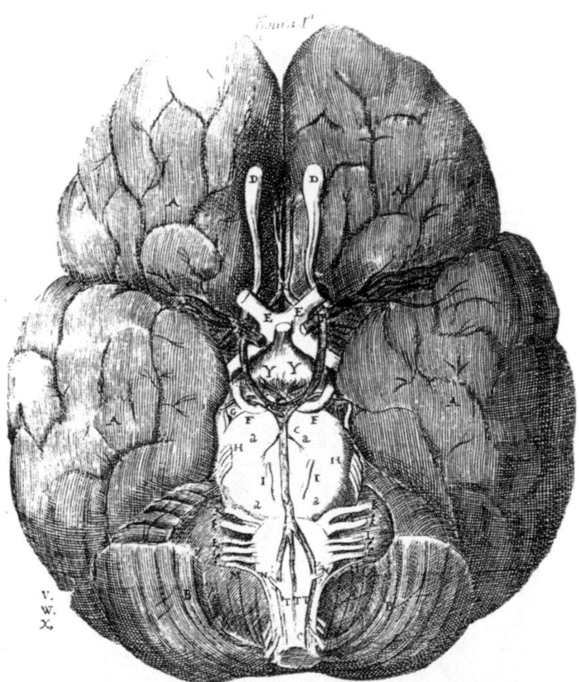

Fig. 1.10. Representation of the arterial circle of Willis at the inferior aspect of the brain (Thomas Willis 1680)

Neuroanatomy took a gigantic leap forward in 1664 when Thomas Willis published the first textbook exclusively dedicated to brain anatomy. He effectively used comparative anatomy to demonstrate the differences between the sheep and the human brain. However, his major contribution was his careful depiction of the vascular supply of the brain (Fig. 1.10), assisted by Edmund King. He was also credited for the demonstration of motor centers in the brain.

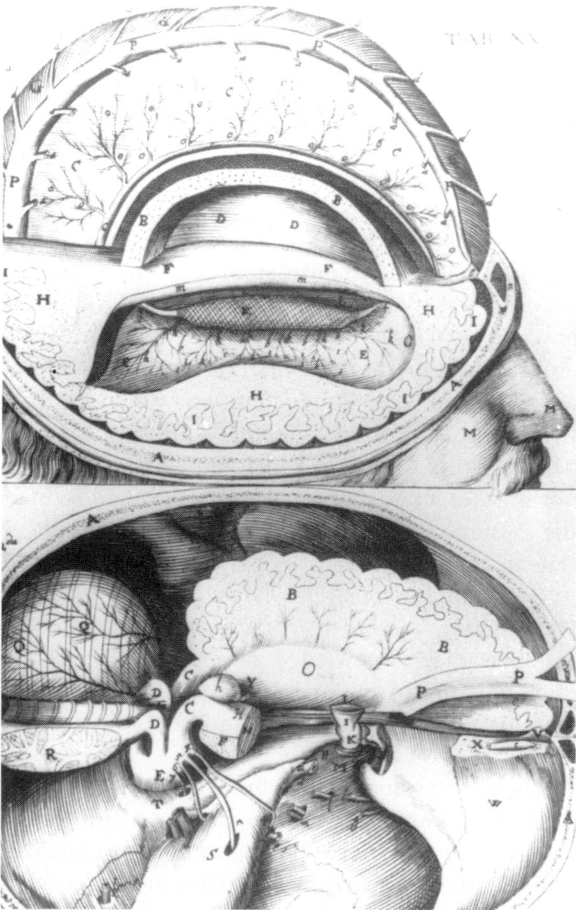

Fig. 1.12. First representations of the head and brain cut in profile (N. Highmorous 1651)

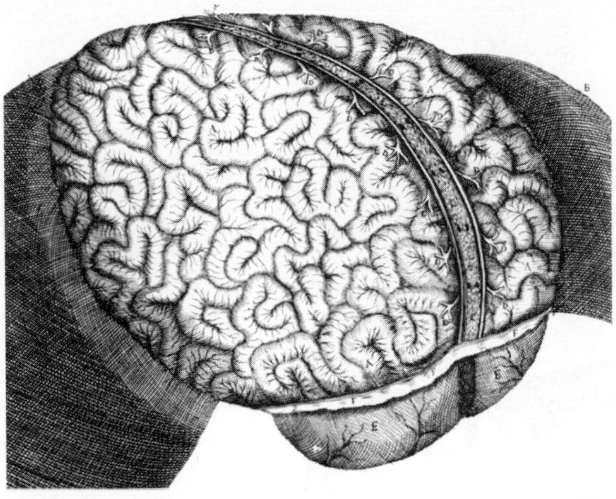

Fig. 1.13. Representation of brain convolutions still showing an "intestinal" type (Raymond Vieussens 1684; Bibl. Museum National d'Histoire Naturelle, Paris)

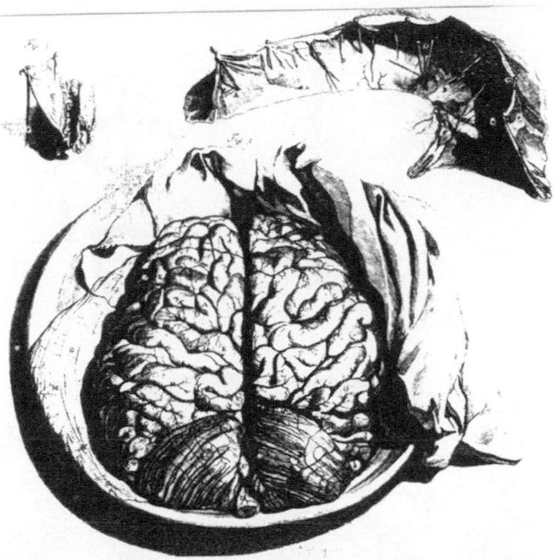

Fig. 1.14. The meninges and the cerebral hemispheres showing a fairly good representation of the convolutions (Godefroid Bidloo 1685; Bibl. Museum National d'Histoire Naturelle, Paris)

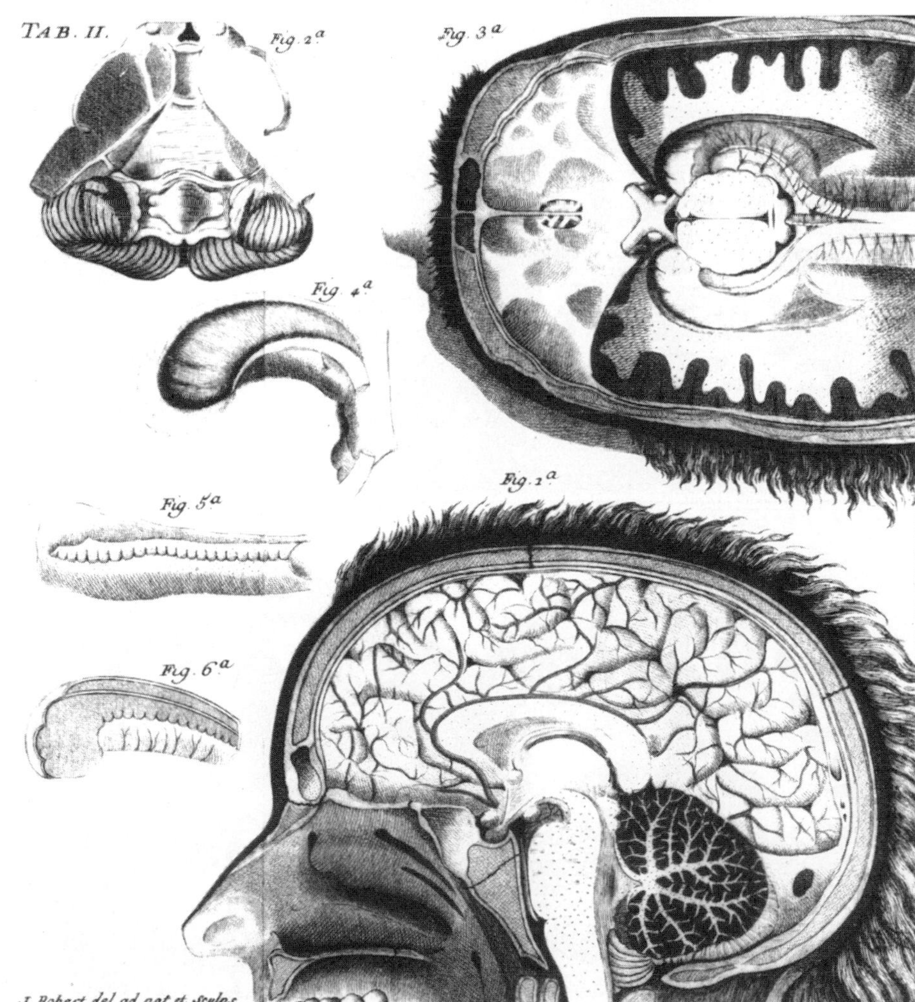

Fig. 1.15. First representation of the head and brain cut in the three planes. Midsagittal and horizontal cuts are shown. The hippocampus and dentate gyrus are represented (Pierre Tarin 1750; Bibl. Museum National d'Histoire Naturelle, Paris)

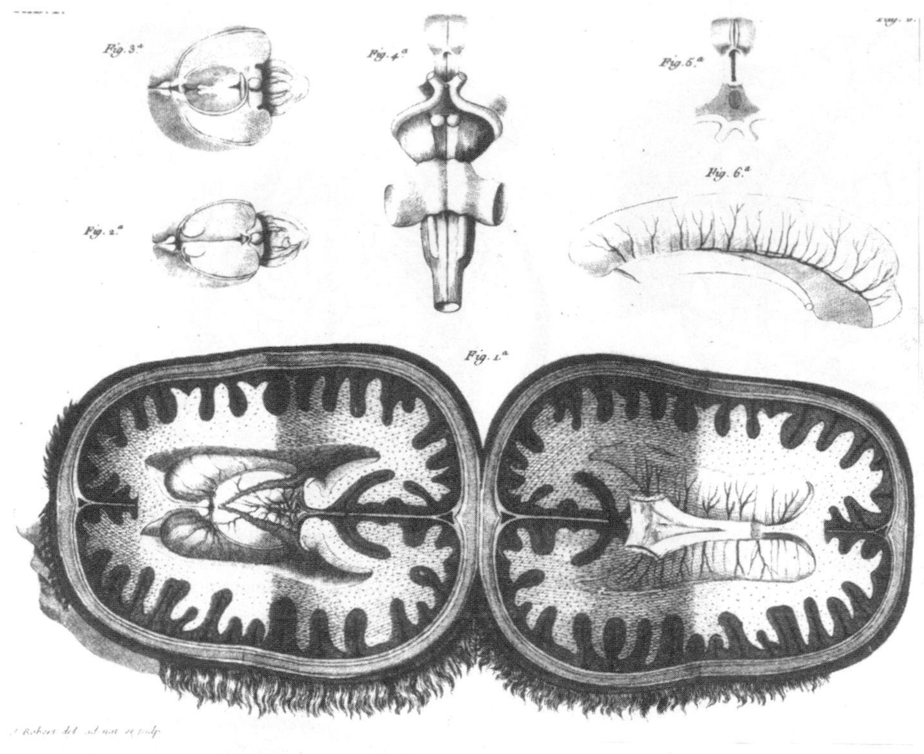

Fig. 1.16. Horizontal cuts of the brain through the ventricular levels (Pierre Tarin 1750; Bibl. Museum National d'Histoire Naturelle, Paris)

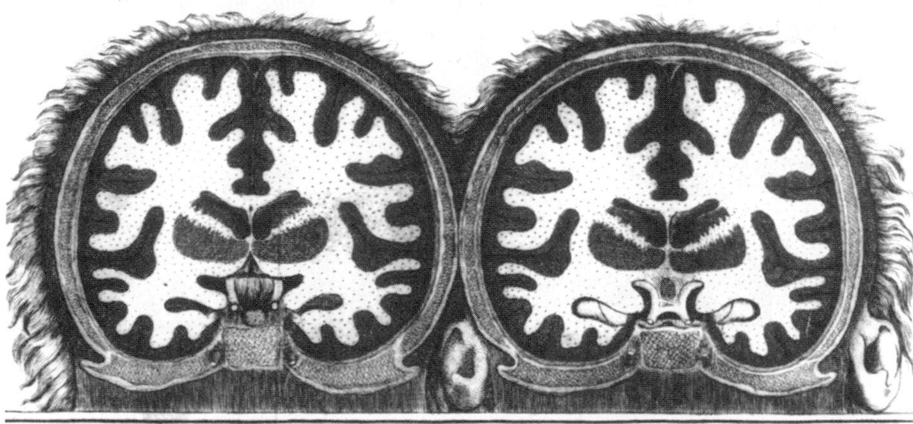

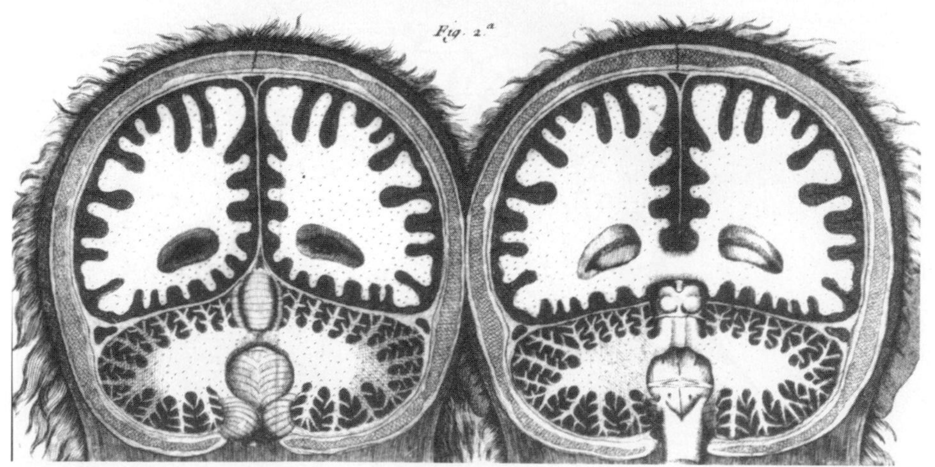

Fig. 1.17. Coronal cuts of the brain through the basal ganglia and the cerebellum (Pierre Tarin 1750; Bibl. Museum National d'Histoire Naturelle, Paris)

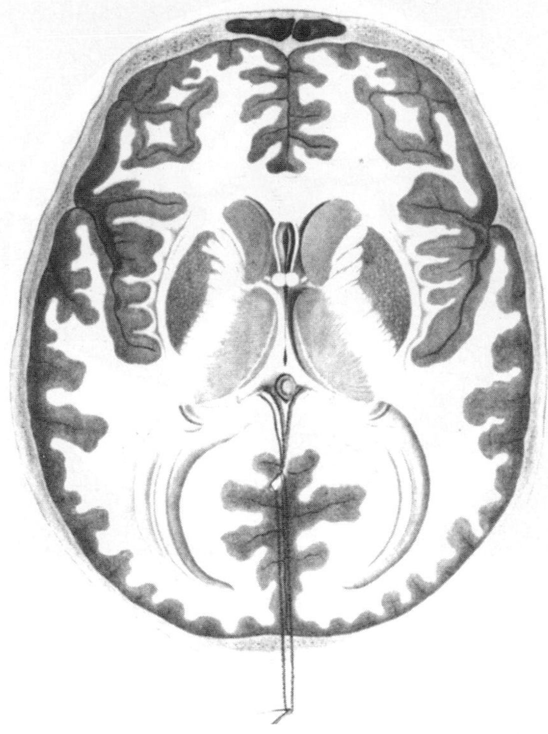

Fig. 1.18. Horizontal cut of the brain passing through the basal ganglia and the internal capsules (Felix Vicq d'Azyr 1786; Bibl. Museum National d'Histoire Naturelle, Paris)

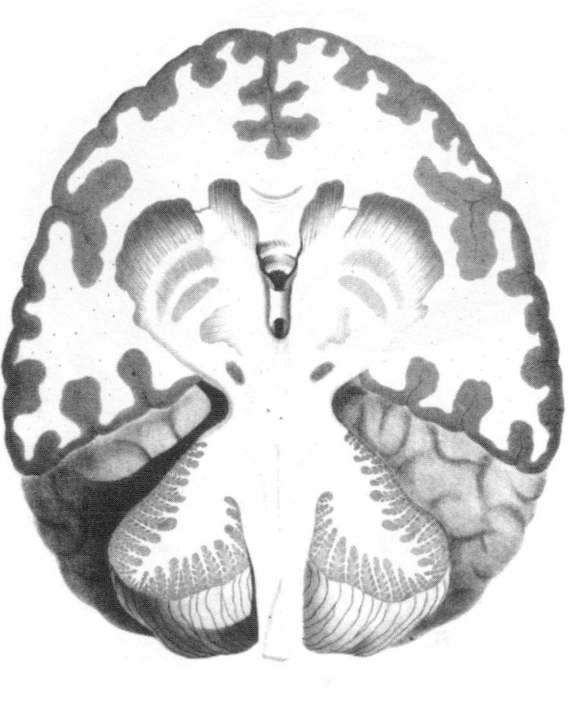

Fig. 1.19. Coronal cut of the brain through the basal ganglia and the brainstem (Felix Vicq d'Azyr 1786; Bibl. Museum National d'Histoire Naturelle, Paris)

The venous system of the brain was described by Stenon (1669), who used a sagittal brain section to demonstrate the importance of this system (Fig. 1.11). Highmorous used "cuts in profile" to show the superior sagittal sinus (Fig. 1.12) in his "Corporis Humani Disquisitio Anatomica"(1651).

Raymond Vieussens (1644–1716) from Montpellier described, in "Neurographia Universalis", the center semiovale in his studies of brain convolutions (Fig. 1.13).

The most true to life representation of the cerebral convolutions (Fig. 1.14) was presented by Godefroid Bidloo (1685) who, in his textbook comprising more than 500 figures, clearly displayed the central sulcus located between the frontal and the parietal lobes. The latter were named by Rolando 150 years later.

In a 50-page publication entitled " Adversaria Anatomica", Pierre Tarin in 1750 showed for the first time several sections of the brain in three planes: sagittal (Fig. 1.15), horizontal (Fig. 1.16) and frontal (Fig. 1.17). Sections through the lateral ventricle showed the hippocampus, the choroid plexus, optic tracts and the corpus callosum.

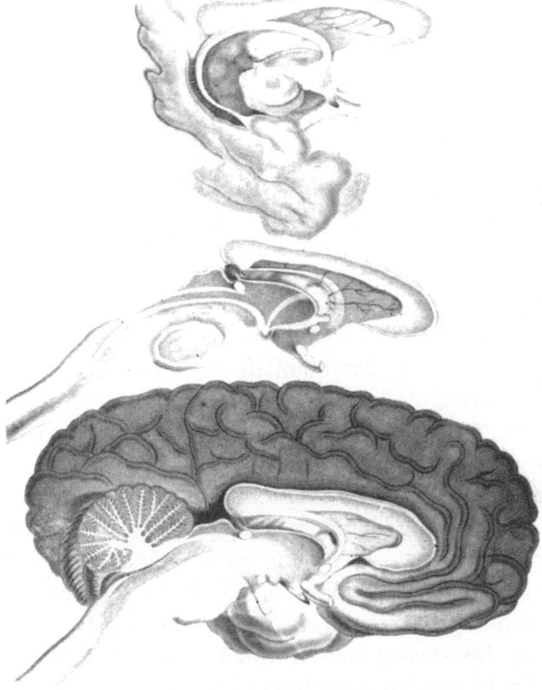

Fig. 1.20. Sagittal view of the brain and description of the uncus and the fornix (Felix Vicq d'Azyr 1786; Bibl. Museum National d'Histoire Naturelle, Paris)

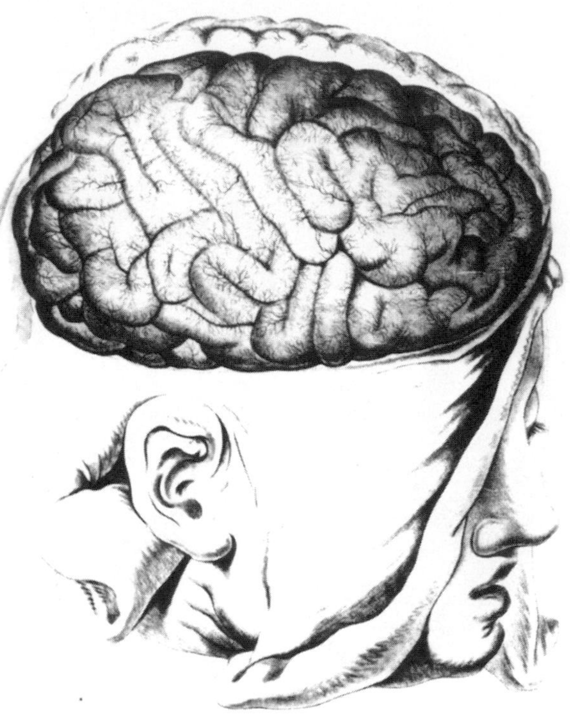

Fig. 1.21. Representation of brain convolutions and first attempt to provide a nomenclature preceding lobulation (Felix Vicq d'Azyr 1786; Bibl. Museum National d'Histoire Naturelle, Paris)

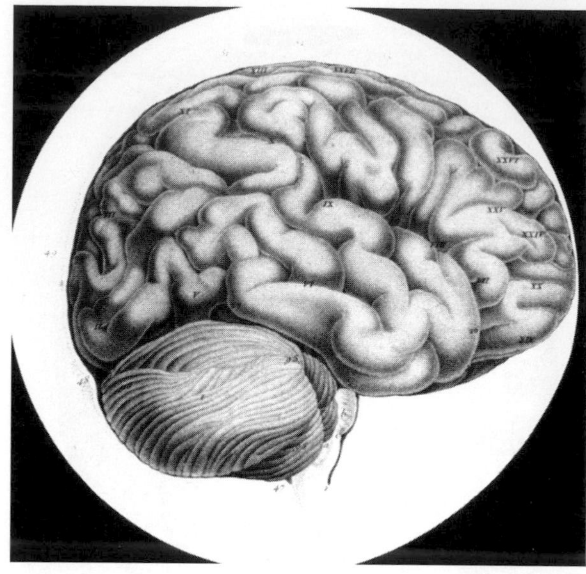

Fig. 1.22. Fairly good representation of brain anatomy and first attempt to ascribe neuropsychological functions to areas of the brain and skull (Francois-Joseph Gall 1810)

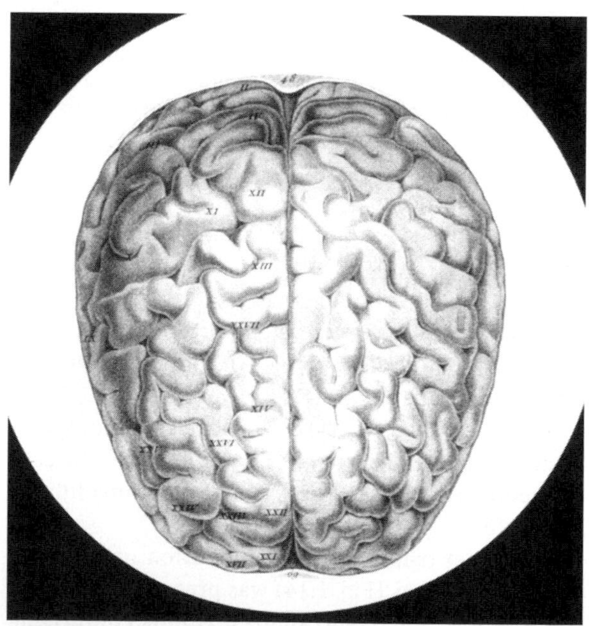

Fig. 1.23. First attempt at localization of brain functional areas based on phrenology (Francois-Joseph Gall 1810)

Towards the end of the eighteenth century, Felix Vicq d'Azyr (1748–1794), famous for the description of the "mamillothalamic" tract, in a treatise of anatomy and physiology published in 1786, showed well displayed anatomical brain cuts in different planes (Figs. 1.18, 1.19, 1.20). His works marked the earliest contribution to gyral anatomy, and described the pre- and postcentral convolutions and coined the term "uncus" (Figs. 1.20, 1.21).

In 1809 Johann Christian Reil (1759–1813) comprehensively described the insula, which was previously noted by Bartholin in 1641. Between 1810–1820, Francois-Joseph Gall published a 5-volume book, "Anatomie et Physiologie du Systeme nerveux en general et du Cerveau en particulier", dedicated to the anatomy and physiology of the brain. Morphology was adequately detailed (Figs. 1.22, 1.23). However, the correlations with mental functions were arbitrarily attributed, marking the prelude to phrenology. Although lacking any scientific foundation, this theory was accepted in Europe and the United States for more than 50 years.

With the discovery of lithography in the nineteenth century, Jean Marc Bourgery, a surgeon of Napoleon's army, published an extensive treatise in 14 volumes. This included color illustrations and is considered one of the most comprehensive works of anatomy to date (Fig. 1.24).

The first photograph of a preparation of a human brain was attempted by Emile Huschke (1797–1858) of Jena (Fig. 1.25). Photographs quickly replaced drawn illustrations.

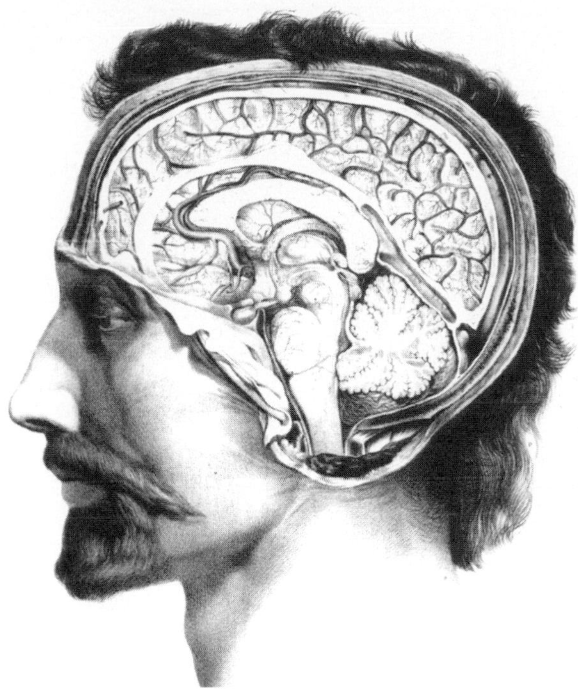

Fig. 1.24. Sagittal cut of the head and brain (Jean-Marc Bourgery 1844; A. Gordon)

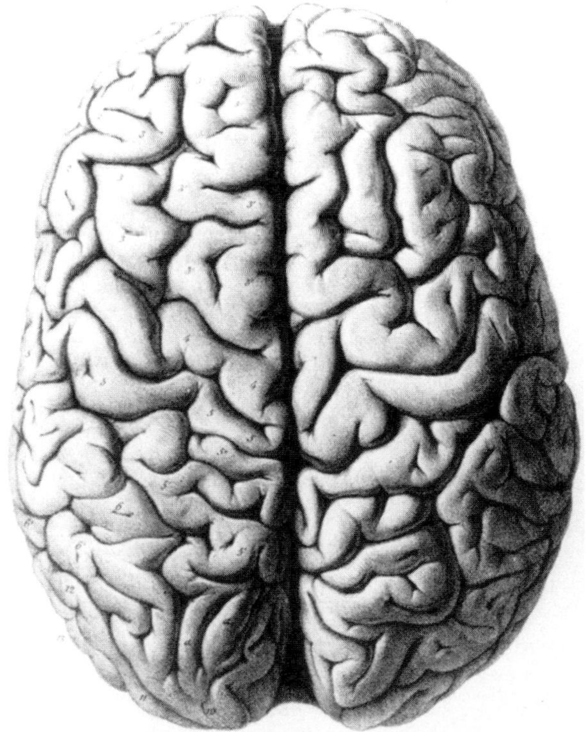

Fig. 1.25. Photograph of the superior aspect of an isolated brain (Emile Huschke 1854; Bibl. Med. Paris)

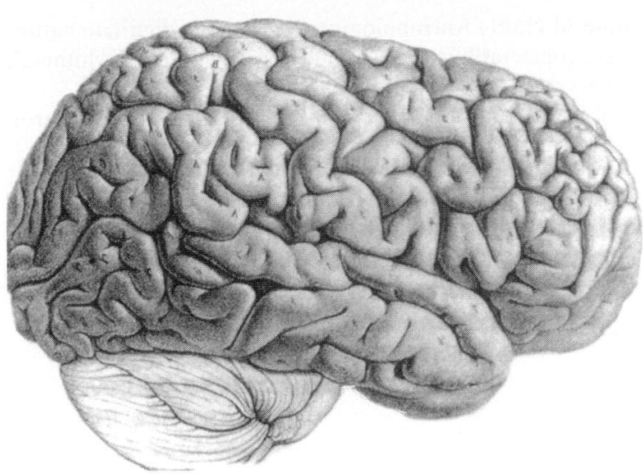

Fig. 1.26. First attempt to classify lobes and fissures of the brain, in "les circonvolutions restituées" (Louis-Pierre Gratiolet 1854; A. Gordon)

In the same year (1854), Louis Pierre Gratiolet, one of the most famous French anatomists, defined the lobes and fissures of the brain (Fig. 1.26). The nomenclature he devised is still in use today. He distinguished primary and secondary gyri based on their respective appearance phylogenetically. His interest was concentrated on the primate brain, and he introduced the study of comparative anatomy. His large collection of isolated brains is conserved in the French National Museum of Natural History, in Paris.

Other notable workers in the field included William Turner (1832–1916) of Edinburgh, who redefined the limits of the brain and its fissures, establishing the Rolandic fissure as the posterior limit of the frontal lobe, and Alexander Ecker from Freiburg who described in 1869 in great detail the sulci and gyri of the brain. This contribution is still valuable today.

References

Berengario di Carpi G (1523) Isagoge breves per lucidae anatomiam humani corporis. Mectoris Bibliopolam, Bolognae

Dagoty JG (1775) Exposition anatomique des organes des sens jointe à la névrologie entière du corps humain et conjectures sur l'électricité animale et le siège de l'âme. Demonville, Paris

Dryander J (1536) Anatomia capitis humani in Marpurgensis academia superiori anno pullice. Egenolphi, Marpurg

Ecker A (1869) Die hirnwindun gen des menschen, 2nd edn (1883). Vieweg, Braunschweig, p 56

Gratiolet LP (1854) Mémoire sur les plis cérébraux de l'homme et des primates. Bertrand, Paris

Hundt M (1501) Antropologium de hominis dignitate natura et proprietatibus. De elementis partibus corporis humani. Baccalorium Wolfgangi, Lipsae

Vesalius A (1543) De humanis corporis fabrica. Bernardi, Venetiis

Vicq d'Azyr F (1813) Traité de l'anatomie du cerveau, tome I et planches tome II, nouvelle édition. Duprat-Duverger, Paris

2 Cephalic Reference Lines Suitable for Neuroimaging

Both morphometric and topographic approaches to analyze brain structures require a careful choice of reliable anatomic landmarks in order to achieve appropriate imaging and clinical correlations. Therefore, a precise topographic analysis of brain structures ought to be performed using definite brain reference lines, which are based most efficiently on commissural landmarks. Whenever possible, correlations with cutaneous and cranial anthropologic points are necessary for multimodal imaging purposes (Broca 1873; Ariens Kappers 1947; Talairach et al. 1952; Guiot and Brion 1958; Delmas and Pertuiset 1959; Cabanis et al. 1978; Olivier et al. 1985, 1987; Baulac et al. 1990; Tamraz et al. 1990).

The ability of MRI to visualize tissues in any direction, due to its multiplanar and computerized capabilities, permits the evaluation of specific anatomic structures from the most suitable orientation by direct scanning either parallel or orthogonal to the long axis of the anatomic structure studied.

In this chapter, the various cranial reference lines will first be reviewed. Subsequently, the anatomic and physiologic cephalic orientations widely used in anatomic imaging will be covered.

Particular attention will be devoted to a new sylvian approach to brain anatomy based on recent ontogenetic, phylogenetic and anatomic data obtained using the reference system based on two specific reference lines, namely the "chiasmatico-commissural line" (CH-PC line), which is oriented parallel to the "sylvian fissure" and defines the "chiasmato-mamillo postcommissural plane"; and the "commissural-obex line" (PC-OB line), which is perpendicular to the latter and corresponds to the vertical long axis of the brainstem (Tamraz et al. 1989, 1990, 1991).

These orthogonal reference planes, suitable for multimodal imaging, can be used routinely in brain imaging with highly reproducible results. The anatomic landmarks defining these reference lines are easily seen on a midsagittal MR view, and are present in all vertebrates. From an anatomic point of view, both ontogenetically and phylogenetically, the accuracy of these midline structures located at the mid-brain-diencephalic junction need not be demonstrated.. Constant and statistically proven angular variations demonstrate the validity of these cephalic orientations both in vivo and in the cadaver: (1) the angular relationship between the CH-PC line and the bicommissural line (AC-PC), called the commissural angle (CH-PC-AC) is 24±2.3; (2) the angular relationship between the CH-PC line and the PC-OB brainstem vertical axis joining the posterior commissure to the obex, named the CH-PC-OB truncal angle, is 93±3.4.

It is worth noting that the bicommissural line (Talairach et al. 1952), which is very close to the orbitomeatal or canthomeatal lines used in conventional radiology, has great validity and continues to be used in brain imaging fields, despite its great deviations, due to its neurosurgical stereotactic validation (Talairach et al. 1957, 1967; Schaltenbrand and Bailey 1959; Schaltenbrand and Wahren 1977) and its neuroradiological evaluation (Salamon and Huang 1976; Szikla et al. 1977; Salamon and Lecaque 1978; Vanier et al. 1985; Talairach and Tournoux 1988; Bergvall et al. 1988). Its usefulness is obvious when interest is in the study of the central region of the brain. This is also true for the more recently described callosal reference plane demonstrated and validated for routine use by Olivier et al. (1985, 1987) and Lehman et al. (1992).

I Cranial Reference Lines and Planes

A Historical Background and Overview

More than 80 cephalic reference lines based on cranial and anthropological landmarks have been defined and reported. These reference systems were developed mainly by anatomists and anthropologists at the end of the eighteenth century.

Within the field of comparative craniology, a search for a horizontal plane for the skull was performed by Daubenton (Daubenton and Daele 1764), by Cuvier (1835) and later by Lucae (1872), along with many others. In his communication to the French Academy of Science in 1764, Daubenton described the importance of the plane of the foramen magnum as the horizontal plane tangent at the middle of its posterior border to the condylar processes of the skull. He pointed out that this plane is differently oriented in humans as compared with animals, passing through the inferior aspect of the orbits in man and considered by him as horizontal and perpendicular to the vertical axis of the body and neck when an erect position is assumed. This differs in monkeys, in which the plane passes beneath the mandible, becoming even more obliquely tilted downward in lower species such as the dog. Daubenton was convinced that horizontality is closely related to the orientation and position of the foramen magnum located in a central position at the base of the skull, stating "plus le grand trou occipital est éloigné du fond de l'occiput plus le plan de cette ouverture approche de la direction horizontale" (Daubenton and Daele 1950, p 570). His contribution to craniology and anatomy differs from previous contributions in this field, which lacked precision in the choice of anatomic landmarks.

These attempts were used a few decades later for works on racial morphologic differences which were extensively pursued at the end of the eighteenth century, and are well represented by the important contributions of Camper (1791), Blumenbach (1795), Doornik (1808) and many others. In 1791, Camper defined an interesting cephalic plane of orientation joining the spina nasalis inferior to both external auditory meati. About 20 years earlier, he had reported many lines and angles in order to show the differences which may be depicted on a face, reporting his results at the Academy of Painting in Amsterdam (1770). Camper's horizontal plane was slightly modified by Cuvier (1795)for use in his works on comparative anatomy. At the same time, Blumenbach defined the norma verticalis of the cranium when lying horizontally, as observed from above.

Cranial reference systems underwent a major additional development in the nineteenth century with the development of phrenologic craniometry as defined in Edinburgh by the Scotsman Combe (1839). From his research on brain proportions, Combe proposed a frontoparietal line, which was to be defined later by one of his pupils, Morton (1839), in the United States, as the line joining the frontal to the parietal ossification centers of the skull.

B The Need for a Consensus

Given the presence of several reference lines, an attempt to find a consensus became obvious and necessary. Following a meeting in Göttingen, German anthropologists adopted the line advocated by Von Baer, which corresponds to the superior border of the zygomatic arch, and named it the horizontal line of Göttingen (1860). This line modifies to some extent the line of Lucae (1872) who defined as the horizontal, the line passing through the axis of the zygomatic arches.

At the same time in France, Broca (1862), in one of his major contributions on the natural position of the head, observed that the horizontal plane corresponds to the alveolar-condylar plane, defined as the reference plane passing through the inferior aspect of the occipital condyles and joining the middle of the alveolar ridge. Broca considered and defended this plane as the horizontal plane of the cranium (1873). An alternative was proposed by Hamy, namely, the glabella-lambda plane, which was roughly parallel to the latter. From 1862 to 1877, Broca evaluated this plane with respect to many others, such as the masticatory plane, the glabellar-occipital, the nasion-opisthion, and the nasion-inion, pointing to their variability as compared to the alveolar-condylar plane (1862), which he considered as the skull reference baseline (1873), or the plane of the "vision horizontale" (1862), also called the "visual plane" (1873) and later the "bi-orbital" plane (1877) (Fig. 2.1). A century later, this plane was described, using computerized assisted tomography (CT), as the neuro-ocular plane (Cabanis et al. 1978).

According to Topinard (1882), the English anthropologists accepted Broca's choice of the visual plane as the reference plane, while the Germans remained attached to Merckel's "orbito-auditory" plane (1882), also named "auriculo-suborbital" plane by Ihering (1872), and modified by Virchow and Hoelder to become the "supra-auricular-infra-orbital" plane. The latter plane was retained during the Munich Con-

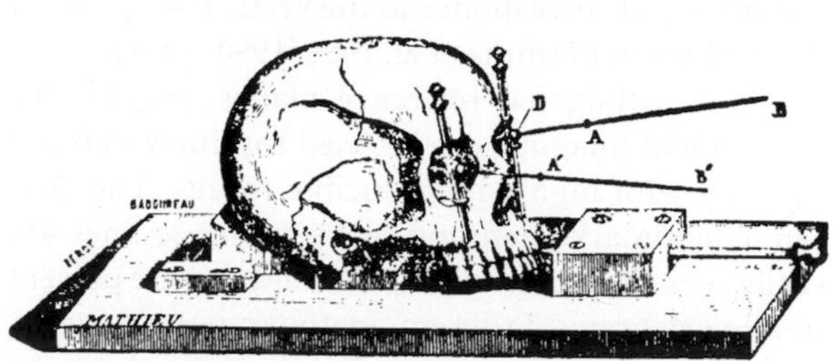

Fig. 2.1. The "bi-orbital" plane of Broca (1877)

gress (1877) and adopted in Frankfurt as the "infra-orbital-meatal" plane, widely known as the Frankfurt-Virchow plane, which received the general acceptance of most of the anthropologists of the time.

C Classification of the Cephalic Reference Planes

A great number of cranial and cephalic reference planes and lines have been described, which are of variable importance based on an anatomic, phylogenetic or anthropologic point of view. Saban (1980), in an attempt to codify the available data in this field, proposed a classification of these reference lines and planes based on anatomic grounds. The craniofacial references reported in his exhaustive review of the literature are grouped as follows: craniofacial planes based on external landmarks, including superior horizontal planes (Table 2.1), inferior horizontal planes (Table 2.2), base of the skull planes (Table 2.3) and vertical planes (Table 2.4); and craniofacial planes based on endocranial landmarks (Table 2.5).

Some of these are of great interest as they are used in anthropology as well as in radiology and are widely applied. This includes the Frankfurt-Virchow plane, the nasion-opisthion, the nasion-basion, and others. Olivier (1978) pointed out, in view of comparative studies on craniofacial planes, that the nasion-opisthion and the Frankfurt-Virchow planes are remarkably constant. Other reference planes have been rediscovered and reevaluated with respect to their potential accuracy in regional anatomy and imaging studies.

D The Choice of a Nomenclature

The development and diversification of increasingly complex radiology procedures made a unified and pragmatic approach to cephalic orientation a necessity. The need for a universal consensus was obvious. In a study meeting of the World Federation of Neurology, held in Milan in 1961 and oriented toward problems of projections and nomenclature, the commission of nomenclature retained as basal reference lines two so-called horizontal baselines of radiological importance: (1) the anthropological basal line, and (2) the orbitomeatal (or canthomeatal) basal line (WFN 1962). These lines meet at an angle of 10° (Fig. 2.2).

II Brain Horizontal Reference Lines and Planes

A total of six cephalic reference lines and planes are currently used in neuroimaging fields, which are suitable for diagnostic, functional or interventional purposes (Fig. 2.3, Table 2.6). These are: the bicommissural plane (Talairach et al. 1952), and the intercommissural plane (Schaltenbrand and Bailey 1959), the cephalic reference plane of Delmas and Pertuiset (1959), the neuro-ocular plane (Cabanis et al. 1978), the callosal plane (Olivier et al. 1985), and the chiasmatico-commissural plane (Tamraz et al. 1989, 1990).

Table 2.1. Superior horizontal cranial reference lines (modified from Saban 1980)

Literature reference	Reference line	Description
Hamy 1873	Glabella-lambda line	Roughly parallel to the alveolar-condylar plane of Broca
Krogmann 1931	Horizontal line	Parallel to Frankfurt plane, proceeding from the nasion
Lucae 1872		Axis of the zygomatic arches
Merkel 1882	Horizontal orbital-auditory line	Center of the external auditory meatus; inferior rim of the orbit
Morton 1839; Combe 1839	Horizontal plane	Plane passing through the four prominent points of the frontal and parietal bones
Perez 1922	Vestibian axis	
Virchow-Hoelder 1875 (Topinard 1882)	Supra-auricular-suborbital plane Horizontal line of Munich (1877)	Superior border of the external auditory meatus; inferior border of the orbit
Von Baer 1860	Horizontal line of Göttingen	Superior border of the zygomatic arch

Table 2.2. Inferior horizontal cranial reference lines (modified from Saban 1980)

Literature reference	Reference line	Description
Barclay 1803	Inferior facial plane	Tangent to inferior border of the mandible
Blumenbach 1795	Cranium in norma verticalis	Lying on its base over a horizontal plane
Broca 1862	Plane of mastication	Inferior border of the teeth of the maxilla
Broca 1862	Horizontal plane of the head Alveolar-condylar plane Cardinal plane of the cranium (1873)	Alveolar point at the inferior border of the alveolar ridge – inferior aspect of both occipital condyles
Broca 1862	Plane of horizontal vision, or visual plane (1873) or bi-orbital plane (1877)	The natural attitude of the head is that which permits the eyes to reach the horizon without muscular contraction
Daubenton and Daele 1764	Plane of the foramen magnum	Center of the posterior edge of the occiput – condylar facet
Camper 1791	Horizontal plane	Spina nasalis anterior – center of the external auditory meati
Doornik 1808	Horizontal line	Incisors – most prominent point of the occiput
His 1860, 1876	Horizontal line	Spina nasalis anterior – opisthion (plane perpendicular to midsagittal)
Lucae 1872	Horizontal line	Spina nasalis anterior – basion
Martin 1928	Line of the alveolar ridge or horizontal alveolar line	Alveolar border between median incisors and the molars (study of the mandible)
Martin 1928	Line of the base of the skull	Nasion-basion (perpendicular to midsagittal plane)
Spix 1815	Alveolar-condylar plane	Tangent to the inferior aspect of the occipital condyles – median-most declivitous point of the superior alveolar ridge

Table 2.3. Reference lines from the base of the skull (modified from Saban 1980)

	Literature reference	Reference line Description
Aeby 1862	Nasion-basilar plane	Base of the nose – basion
Barclay 1803	Inion-glabellar line	Horizontal of Schwalbe (glabella-inion line)
Broca 1872	Nasion-opisthion line	Base of the nose (nasion) – opisthion
Broca 1872	Nasion-inion line	Base of the nose (nasion) – inion
Bell 1805	Basion-supraorbital line	Basion – superior orbital rim
Keith 1910	Subcerebral plane	Median frontomalar symphysis – median parietomastoid symphysis
Martin 1928	Glabella-opisthion line	Glabella – opisthion

A The Bicommissural Reference Plane

The bicommissural plane (AC-PC) of Talairach et al. (1952), is defined as the plane through the line joining the upper border of the anterior commissure (AC) to the lower border of the posterior commissure (PC) (Figs. 2.3, 2.4). It is widely accepted and used by numerous neurosurgeons and a large community of neuroradiologists, mainly since the advent of CT. The intercommissural plane joins the center of both the anterior and posterior commissures (Schaltenbrand and Bailey 1954, 1959).

Table 2.4. Vertical reference lines of the skull (modified from Saban 1980)

Literature reference	Reference line	Description
Busk 1861	Vertical plane	Auriculo-bregmatic line
Bell 1806	Vertical axis of the cranium	Cranium maintained in equilibrium over a stick held through the center of the foramen magnum
Clavelin 1932	Vertical plane of the mandible	Glenion – posterior border of the mandible
Klaatsch 1909	Vertical line	Bregma – basion
Maly 1924	Vertical plane of the orbital aperture	Superior border – inferior border of the orbital aperture

Table 2.5. Cranial reference lines based on endocranial landmarks (modified from Saban 1980)

Literature reference	Reference line	Description
Barclay 1803	Palatine plane	Passing through the palatine vault
Beauvieux 1934	Plane of the ampullas	Passing through the three ampullas of the semicircular canals
Bjork 1947	Horizontal plane	Nasion – center of the sella turcica
Girard 1911	Plane of the horizontal semicircular canal	
Huxley 1863	Basi-cranial axis or basi-occipital line	Middle of the anterior border of the foramen magnum – anterior extremity of the sphenoid
Villemin and Beauvieux 1937	Nasion-opisthion line	
Walther 1802	Horizontal line	Crista galli-inioning)

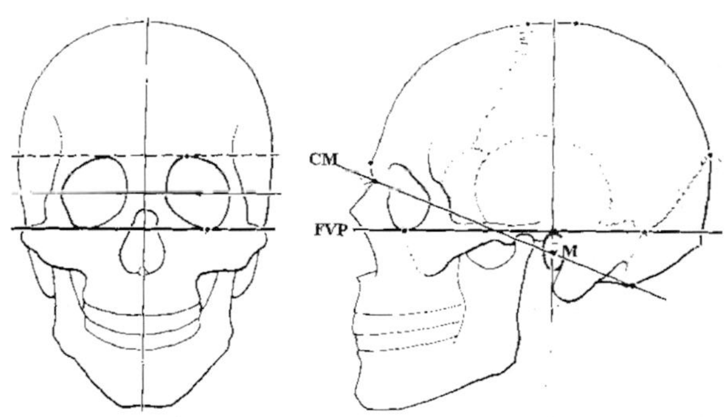

Fig. 2.2. Radiologic reference baselines, modified according to the WFN (1962). *CM*, canthomeatal baseline; *FVP*, anthropological baseline

Table 2.6. Major brain reference lines (suitable for neuroimag

Brain horizontal planes / lines:
1. Bicommissural plane (Talairach et al. 1952, 1957) and intercommissural plane (Schaltenbrand and Bailey 1954, 1959)
2. Cephalic plane (Delmas and Pertuiset 1959)
3. Neuro-ocular plane (Cabanis et al. 1978)
4. Callosal plane (Olivier et al. 1985)
5. Chiasmato-commissural plane (Tamraz et al. 1989, 1990)
Brain vertical planes / lines:
1. Commissuro-mamillary plane (Guiot and Brion 1958)
2. Commissural-obex plane (Tamraz et al. 1989, 1991)
3. Commissuro-mamillary plane (Baulac et al. 1990)

1 Biometric Data

The interest of a great number of anatomists, anthropologists and neurosurgeons in this reference line explains the importance of the data available in the scientific literature based on these bicommissural landmarks (Talairach et al. 1952, 1957, 1967; Schaltenbrand and Bailey 1959; Salamon and Huang 1976; Szikla et al. 1977; Talairach and Tournoux 1988).

Neuroradiology has provided stereotactic validation of this reference plane at least for the deep nuclear structures of the brain, explaining its frequent

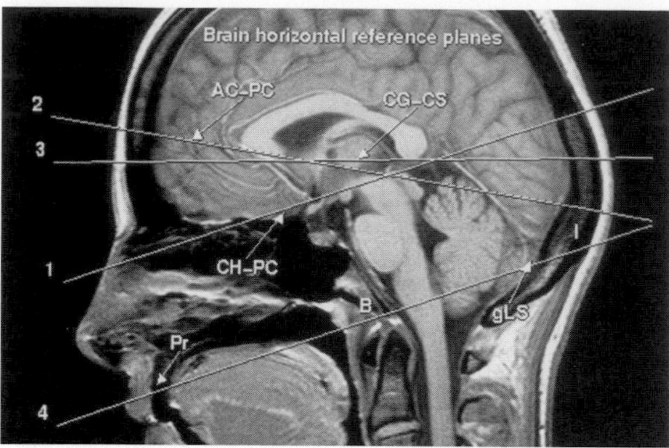

Fig. 2.3. Horizontal brain reference lines and planes. *AC-PC*, bicommissural plane; *CG-CS*, callosal plane; *CH-PC*, chiasmatico-commissural plane

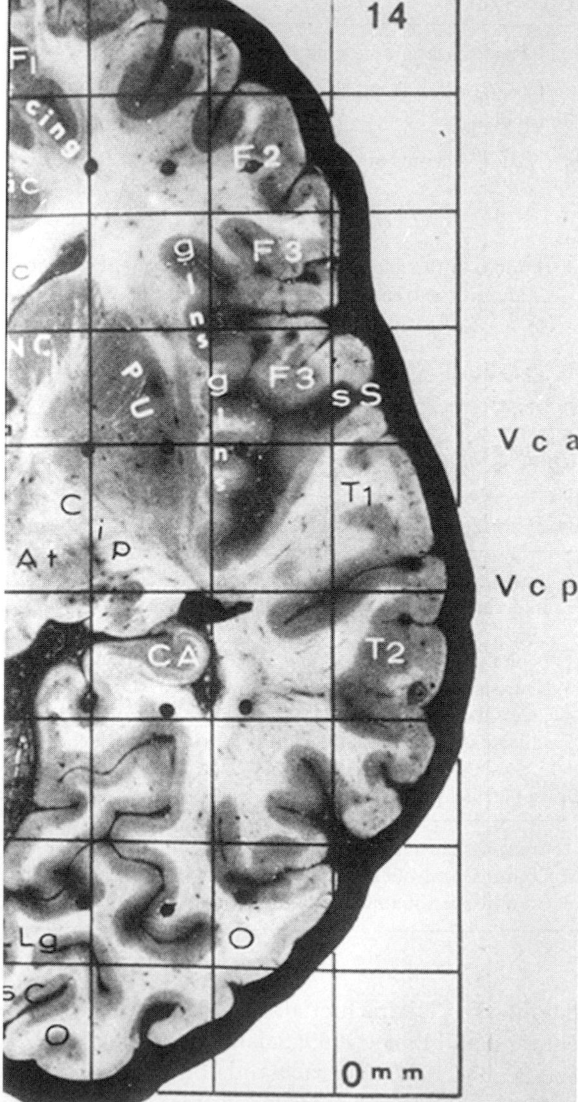

Fig. 2.4. The bicommissural plane of Talairach et al. (1952). (From Talairach et al. 1967)

use in brain imaging mainly since the advent of CT (Michotey et al. 1974; Salamon and Huang 1976; Szikla et al. 1977; Habib et al. 1984; Vanier et al. 1985; Gelbert et al. 1986; Bergvall et al. 1988; Rumeau et al. 1988).

According to Cabanis and Iba-Zizen the canthomeatal line (OM), retained as the radiological reference line (WFN 1962) which joins the outer canthus of the eye to the center of the auditory meatus, the latter corresponding cutaneously to the tragion, has been shown to be very close (1.4±2.7°) to the bicommissural line (Szikla et al. 1977) (Fig. 2.5). This observation has revived interest in external references. Other similar observations have been reported by Tokunaga et al. (1977) and Takase et al. (1977), who tried to demonstrate the approximate parallelism of the glabella-inion line (GIL), which joins the glabella to the inion, i.e., the external occipital protuberance and the fronto-occipital line (FOL) defined as the longest endocranial fronto-occipital diameter, with the bicommissural line (Fig. 2.6). Nevertheless, we agree with Bergvall et al. (1988) that these external landmarks, although suitable for different imaging modalities and helping patient positioning in the routine practice, are much too approximate and unreliable for precise anatomical and topometric studies. The opinion that the reference and the related target structure ought to pertain to the same ontogenetic system is still accepted.

Concerning the landmarks of the AC-PC line, i.e., the AC and the PC, significant variations responsible for potential errors may be observed with variations in AC diameter ranging from 2 to 5 mm, considering PC at a fixed position. Such variations may correspond to a difference of up to 7° in angle. To avoid such variations dependent on the diameter of the AC, Tokunaga et al. adopted a center-to-center positioning of the reference plane. On the other hand, a center-to-center orientation of the AC-PC line, called the intercommissural line (Amador et al. 1959), is used (Tokunaga et al. 1977) in order to minimize variation in the determination of the end points at the landmark levels since the center of AC is easier to define than its limiting border, which varies with the resolution of the MR system and slice thickness. From an imaging point of view such observations are obvious. Considering AC, we agree with Delmas and Pertuiset (1959) that the inferior border of AC is easier to delimit than its superior border, minimizing errors that could be introduced by the proximity of the anterior columns of the fornix (Tamraz et al. 1990). For accuracy and preciseness based on anatomic grounds, as presently obtained using midline

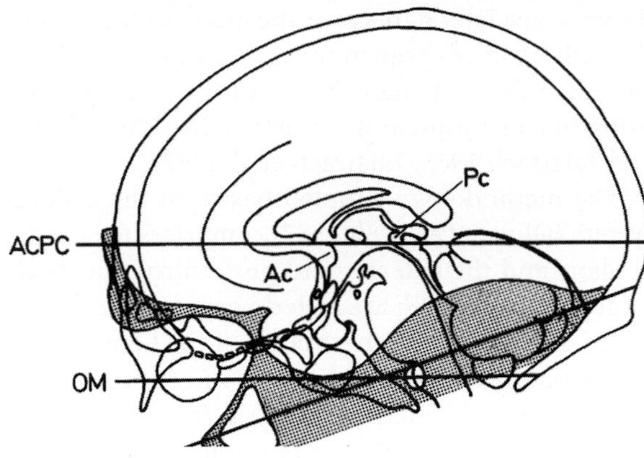

Fig. 2.5. Close parallelism between the canthomeatal line (*OM*) and the bicommissural line (*ACPC*). *AC*, anterior commissure; *PC*, posterior commissure. (According to Cabanis and Iba-Zizen; from Szikla et al. 1977)

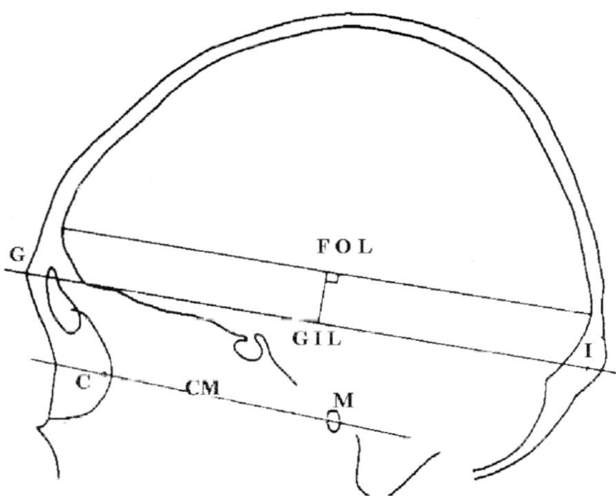

Fig. 2.6. Approximate parallelism of glabella-inion line (*GIL*) and fronto-occipital line (*FOL*), with the canthomeatal line (*CM*). (From Tokunaga et al. 1977, and Takase et al. 1977)

brain commissures, the choice of landmarks ought to be adapted to the imaging system being used.

Reference to stereotactic and topometric atlases is necessary in order to best achieve reliable clinical and anatomical correlations using MR imaging and accurate coordinates and landmarks (Talairach et al. 1957, 1967; Schaltenbrand and Bailey 1959; Delmas and Pertuiset 1959).

2 Anatomic and Imaging Correlations

This reference system provides a definite and accurate relationship to the central gray nuclei (Talairach et al. 1957; Schaltenbrand and Bailey 1959). Anatomically, this reference line roughly follows the direction of the hypothalamic sulcus, separating the thalamus and the hypothalamic region. Thus, it totally differs from the chiasmatico-commissural line on anatomic, ontogenetic and phylogenetic grounds, the latter being situated more caudally at the level of the diencephalon-mesencephalic junction.

The bicommissural line also maintains to some extent reliable relationships to telencephalic structures and helps in the localization of individual gyri on the brain cortex as demonstrated by numerous works carried out by Salamon and Talairach. The major brain sulci seem to maintain relatively constant relationships with respect to the bicommissural line (Szikla and Talairach 1965; Szikla 1967; Talairach et al. 1967). As pointed out by Rumeau et al. (1988), Talairach noted the increasing variations observed with respect to cortical topography. These may show differences in location up to 20 mm from central to peripheral regions. Moreover, in their neuroimaging and anatomic study of 30 brains oriented according to the bicommissural line, these authors reported difficulties in the identification of three major regions: the temporal parieto-occipital, the pars triangularis of the inferior frontal gyrus, and the paracentral lobule, due to important individual variations.

Localization of the central sulcus is one of the most important applications of the bicommissural line of Talairach, which is found between the anterior (VCA) and posterior (VCP) vertical lines perpendicular to the AC-PC. These are tangent to the posterior border of the AC and the anterior border of the PC, respectively. (Fig. 2.7). In axial cuts, as reported by Talairach et al. (1967), the central sulcus is found

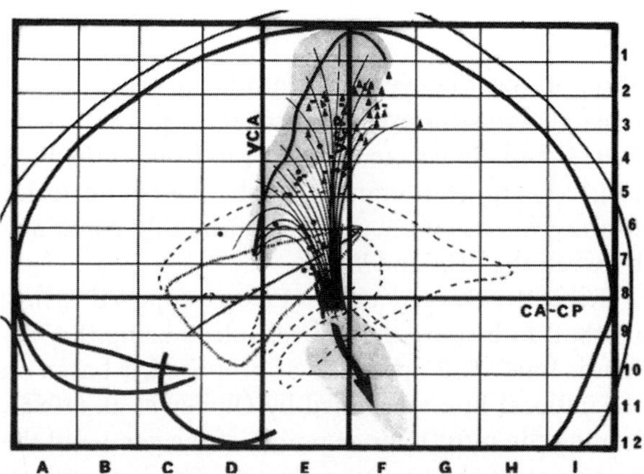

Fig. 2.7. The central sulcus: anatomic correlations using the bicommissural coordinates. (From Talairach et al. 1967)

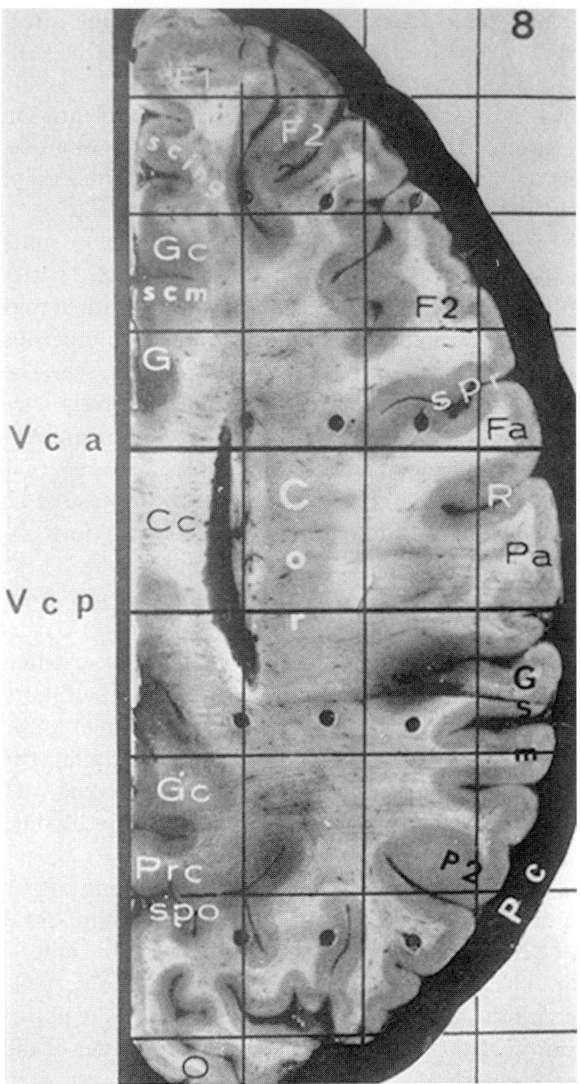

Fig. 2.8. The central sulcus: anatomic correlations using the bicommissural coordinates. (From Talairach et al. 1967)

about midway between the anterior to posterior extension of the supraventricular cuts (Fig. 2.8). It originates caudally, 0.5 cm behind or in front of the VCA (Fig. 2.9) and ends cranially at about 1 cm posterior to the VCP. Its sinuous course is roughly contained between the VCA and VCP.

Recently, Devaud et al. (1996), proposed a new method to localize the central sulcus using the "rolandic line". This approach, as proposed, is based on the callosal line as defined by Olivier et al. (1985), joining the most inferior points of the genu and the splenium of the corpus callosum. The long axis of the central sulcus follows the direction of the rolandic line which seems to be a reliable way to identify the axis on a lateral image of the brain. In the view of the authors this is even more accurate for central sulcus identification than the vertical planes defined using the bicommissural system of Talairach (Szikla and Talairach 1965; Talairach et al. 1967).

The methodology adopted based on the callosal system (Oliver et al. 1985, 1987) comprises the callosal plane and the anterior and posterior vertical callosal planes, to which are added a superior tangential plane, rising to the highest point of the hemisphere, and a parallel inferior plane, passing through the lowest point of the temporal fossa. The rolandic line is generated by joining the two intersection points between the callosal planes and the tangential hemispheric extending from the posterior superior to the anterior inferior points, parallel to the direction of the central sulcus (Fig. 2.10). According to the authors, the central sulcus can be identified on any sagittal cut using the rolandic line, which may also be displayed on the lateral angiograms. The inferior tangential line is traced from the lateral sagittal image at a distance of 30 mm from the midsagittal cut. The major anatomic correlations observed by the authors show that the rolandic line seems to follow the direction of the central sulcus, beginning at the sulcal fundus or at the depth of its midextension in nearly 90% of cases.

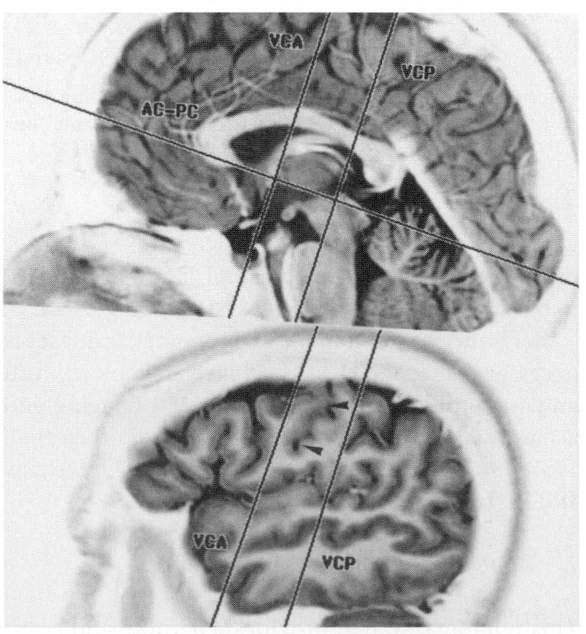

Fig. 2.9. MR correlations: lateral projections of VCA and VCP that could help to localize the central sulcus (*arrowheads*)

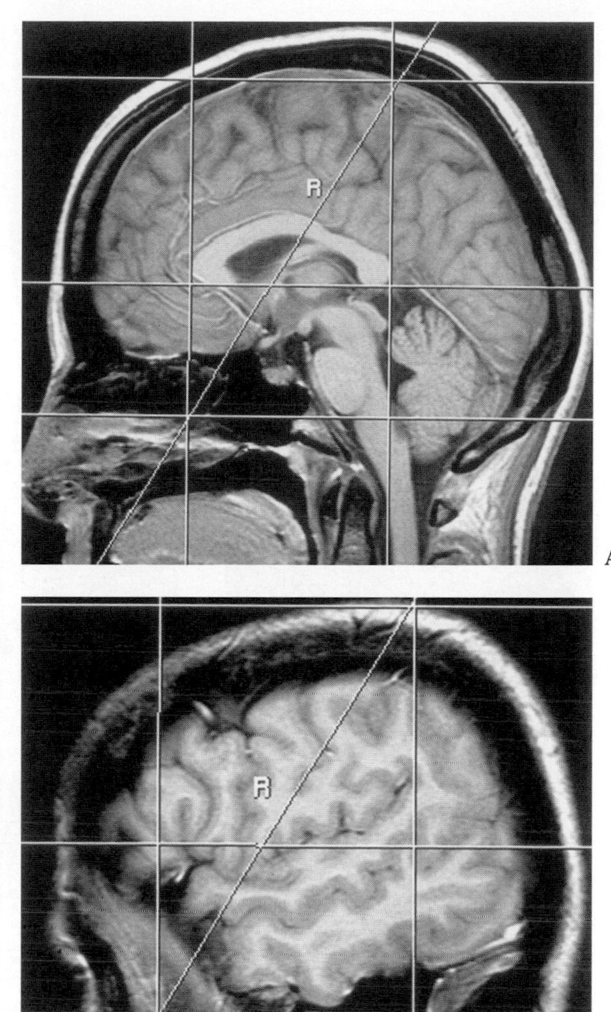

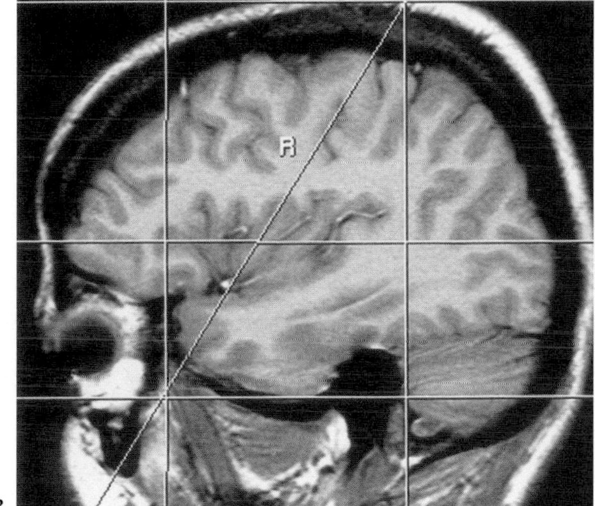

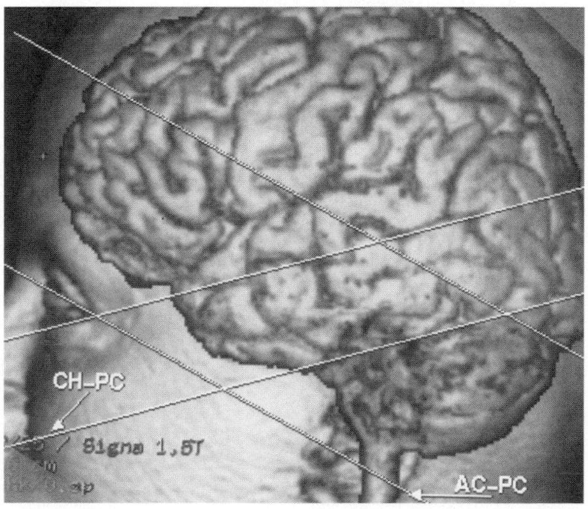

Fig. 2.10A–C. The rolandic line (*R*) based on the callosal orientation plane (Olivier et al. 1985). (According to Devaux et al. 1996)

C

To conclude, despite its deviations, the bicommissural brain reference line is most useful in the localization of the central gray nuclei and the identification of the central sulcus. The advent of MRI, with its direct multiplanar and three-dimensional capabilities, has modified our approach to brain anatomy and sectional imaging (Figs. 2.11–2.13).

Fig. 2.11. The bicommissural plane (*AC-PC*) most suitable for the study of the central region

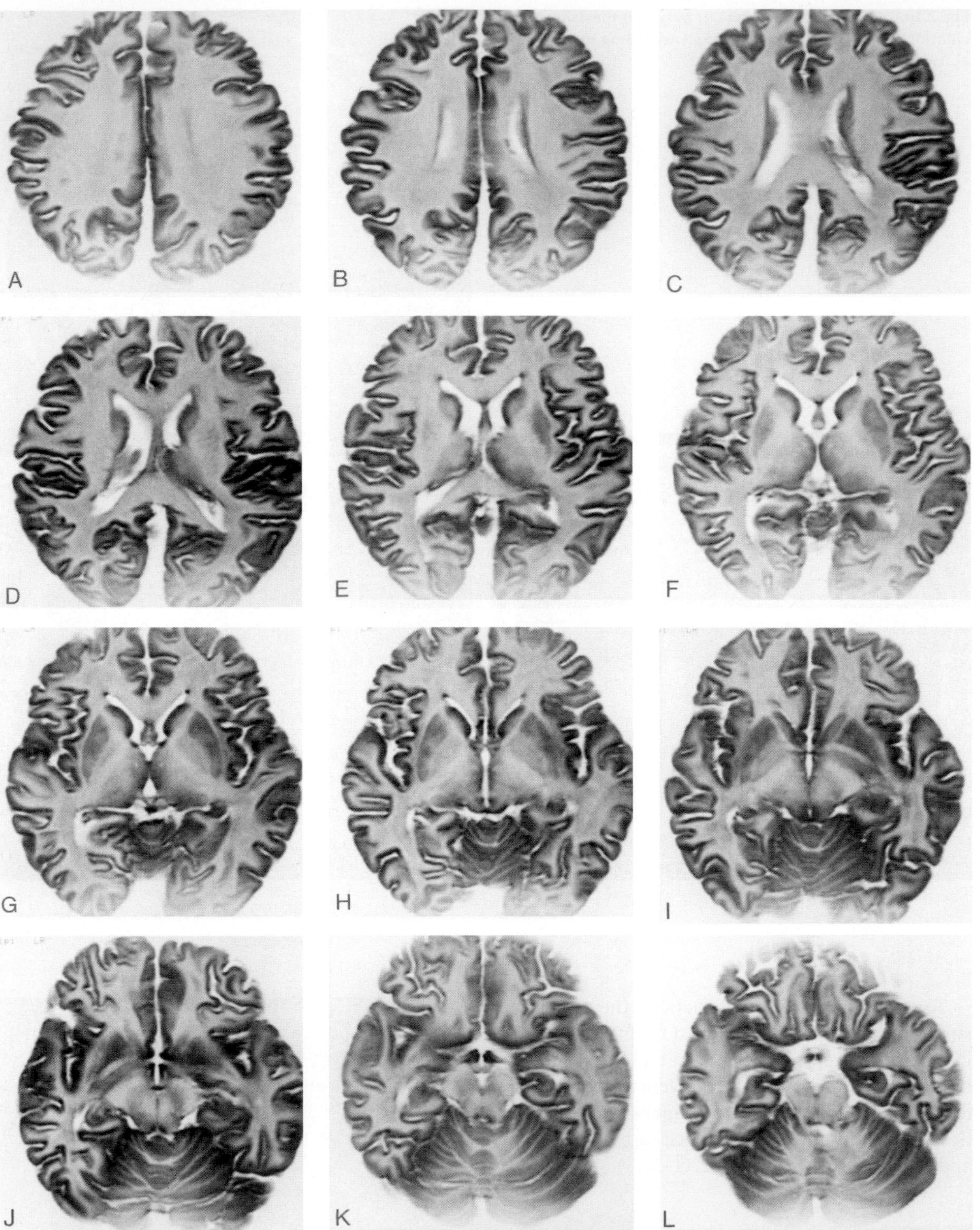

Fig. 2.12A–L. Successive 3 mm axial cuts of a formalin-fixed brain parallel to the AC-PC reference, as compared to the chiasmatico-commissural plane (*CH-PC*) most suitable for the study of the perisylvian region and the temporal lobes

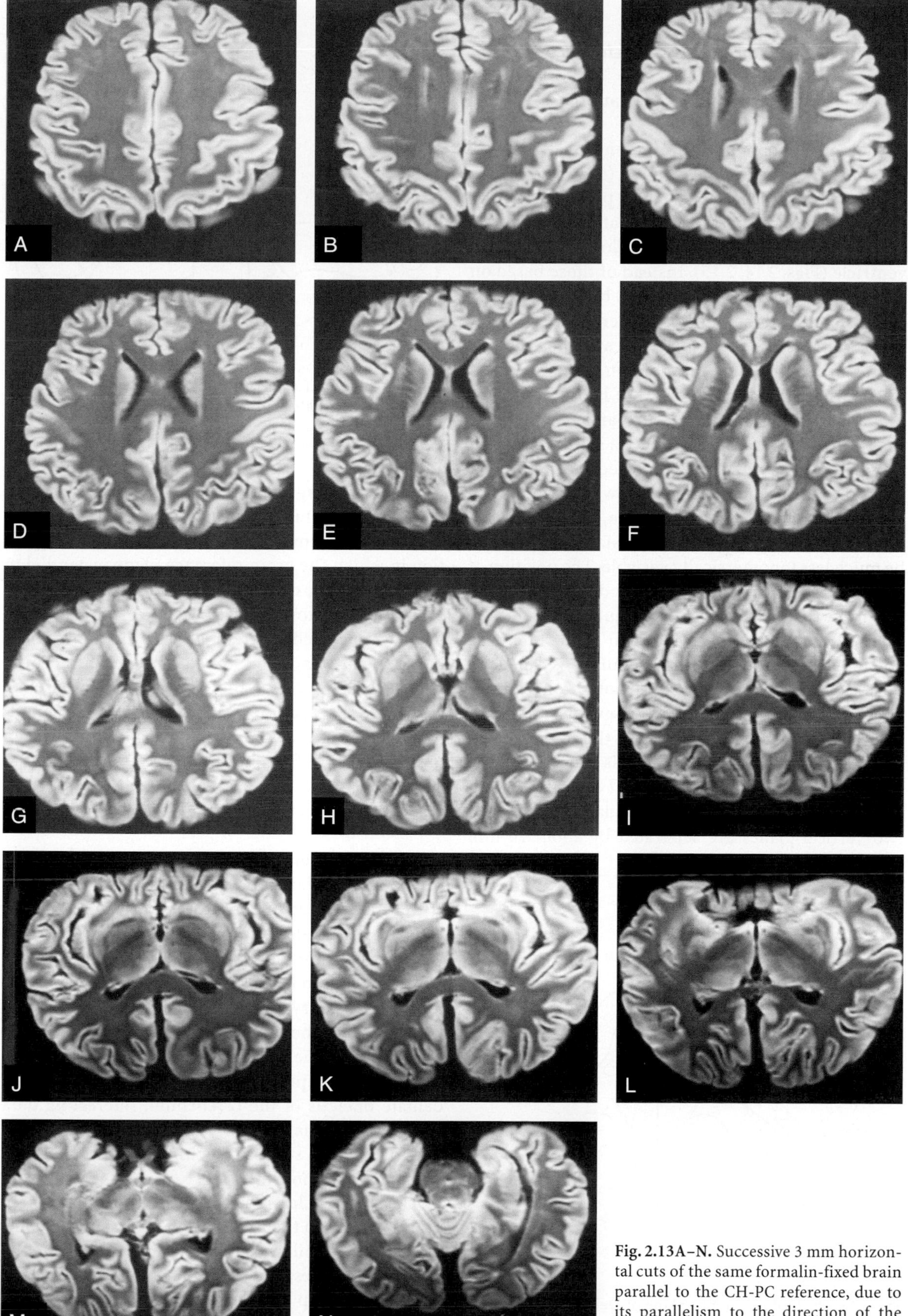

Fig. 2.13A–N. Successive 3 mm horizontal cuts of the same formalin-fixed brain parallel to the CH-PC reference, due to its parallelism to the direction of the parallel sulcus

B The Delmas and Pertuiset Reference Plane

1 Anatomic and Imaging Correlations

In their atlas "Topométrie crânio-encéphalique chez l'homme", Delmas and Pertuiset (1959) defined a horizontal brain reference plane passing rostrally through the lower part of the AC and caudally tangent to the highest part of the floor of the third ventricle (Figs. 2.14, 2.15). Instead of those based on the AC-PC plane, landmarks used by these authors better delineated the inferior border of the AC, freeing it from the close relation to the anterior columns of the fornix. This is, in our opinion, even more pertinent when a midsagittal MR cut is used to orient the slab. Partial volume effects, particularly in the case of thick slices, may introduce a significant positioning error, as previously reported for the AC-PC. The other posterior landmark shows a great advantage over PC, because this latter area, situated caudally to the posterior perforated substance, appears to be much less topometrically variable. The position of the PC varies with the degree of dilatation of the third ventricle and the cerebral aqueduct.

The frontal plane, perpendicular to the reference and tangent to the anterior border of PC, is called the posterior commissural plane. The other one, anteriorly located and parallel to the previous, as well as tangent to the posterior border of the AC, is named the anterior commissural plane. It is a more accurate reference for the study of adjacent structures, such as the pallidum, caudate, and amygdaloid nuclei. The two vertical planes are separated by about 20 mm according to the authors.

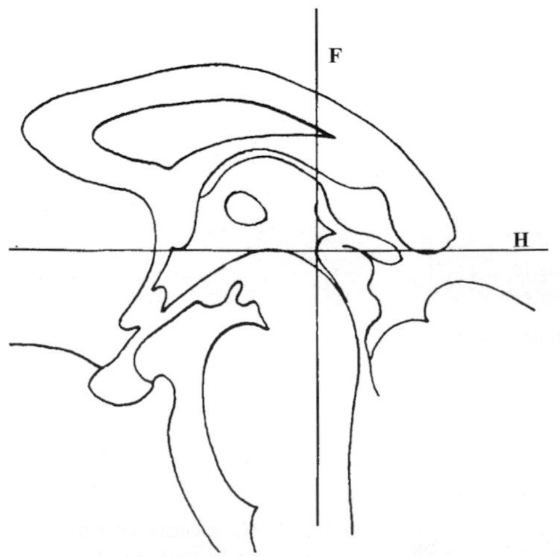

Fig. 2.14. The brain reference plane of Delmas and Pertuiset (1959)

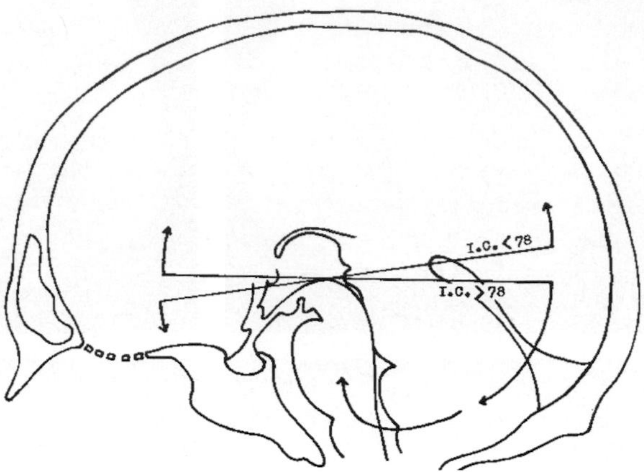

Fig. 2.15. Topometric variations of brain structures with respect to the cephalic index (*IC*) according to Delmas and Pertuiset (1959)

It is interesting to note, as reported by the authors, that the horizontal cuts included in the atlas of cross-sectional anatomy correspond to an anatomic position in which the brain reference plane is parallel to the cranial plane on which the head was oriented, the Frankfurt anthropological baseline. This atlas may be obviously used as a reference for anatomic imaging correlations when based on the infraorbital meatal baseline, i.e., the anthropologic baseline (WFN 1962), where the head is sectioned horizontally, as shown in the atlas, with a parallelism between the line of Frankfurt and the brain reference line.

2 Topometric Findings

This work, presented as a three-dimensional atlas, provides important topometric data for 21 anatomic structures studied by the authors which are: the anterior, centromedian, dorsomedian, ventral anterior, ventral posterior, lateral and medial pulvinar thalamic nuclei, the lateral and medial geniculate bodies, the mamillary body, the red nucleus, the subthalamic nucleus, the substantia nigra, the zona incerta, the amygdala, the pallidum, the caudate nucleus, the putamen, the superior and inferior colliculi, and the dentate nucleus of the cerebellum. Interesting data concerning variations in volume and position of such deep brain structures with respect to the cephalic index are shown.

The authors classified the 21 structures into three groups based on their volumes. The first group comprises the mamillary body, the lateral and medial geniculate bodies, and the superior and inferior colliculi. This group did not show any variations in volume or shape. The second group, represented by the nucleus subthalamicus, the putamen, the amygdala, and the dentate nucleus, showed symmetrical variations in volume. Of the remaining structures, some presented an asymmetric increase in volume, including the dorsomedian, centromedian, ventral posterior and the medial pulvinar thalamic nuclei, and the zona incerta, but most of the others failed to show statistically significant correlations.

Considering variations in position, the authors emphasized the close relation observed based on the cephalic index (Fig. 2.15) and separated the variations observed in individuals in which the cephalic indices were between 78 and 89 (Figs. 2.16, 2.17) from those in the 70 to 78 interval (Figs. 2.18, 2.19). The greatest statistical significance has been observed in the former category, i.e., in cases of mesocephaly rather than brachycephaly. On the other hand, these variations differ also with respect to the position of the anatomic structure as compared to the midsagittal plane. The medially located structures, including the red nucleus, substantia nigra, subthalamic nucleus, mamillary body, dentate nucleus, and the dorsomedian, centromedian and medial pulvinar thalamic nuclei, are displaced posteriorly and upward. The paramedial structures are displaced anteriorly in an upward or downward direction. This includes the thalamic anterior and ventral anterior nuclei, the medial geniculate body, and the amygdala. These two groups behave differently from the more laterally located structures, such as the lentiform and the caudate nuclei, which seem to vary in relation to the cortex.

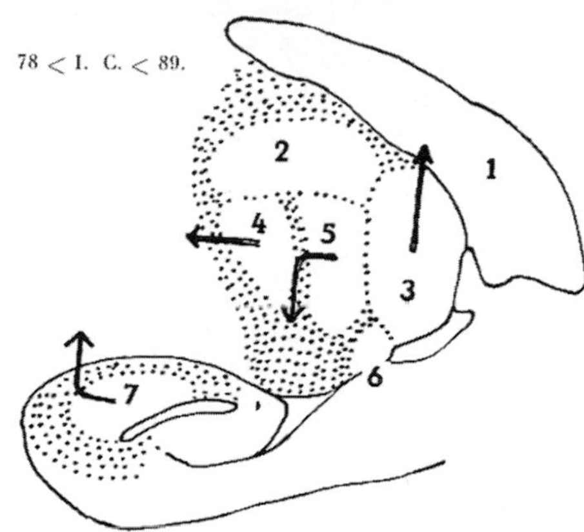

Fig. 2.17. Topometric variations observed in cephalic indices comprised between 78 and 89. *1*, lateral ventricle; *2*, ventral lateral thalamic nucleus; *3*, lateral pulvinar nucleus; *4*, ventral anterior thalamic nucleus; *5*, ventral posterior thalamic nucleus; *6*, lateral geniculate body; *7*, amygdala. (From Delmas and Pertuiset 1959)

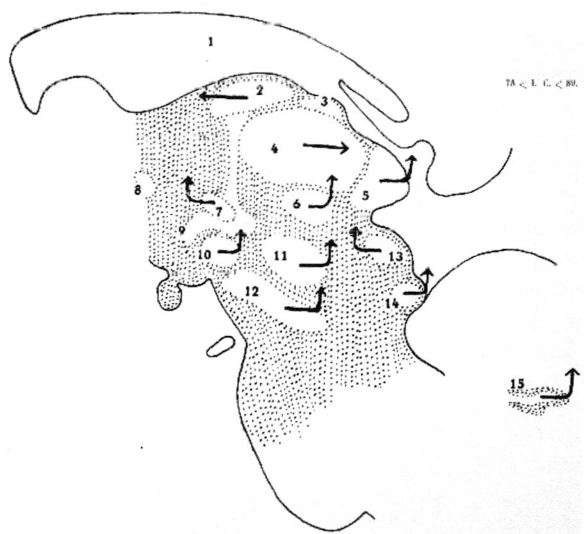

Fig. 2.16. Topometric variations observed in cephalic indices comprised between 78 and 89. *1*, lateral ventricle; *2*, anterior thalamic nucleus; *3*, lateral dorsal nucleus of thalamus; *4*, dorsomedial nucleus of thalamus; *5*, medial pulvinar nucleus; *6*, centromedian thalamic nucleus; *7*, zona incerta; *8*, anterior commissure; *9*, tegmental area; *10*, subthalamic nucleus; *11*, red nucleus; *12*, locus niger; *13*, superior colliculus; *14*, inferior colliculus; 15, dentate nucleus of cerebellum. (From Delmas and Pertuiset 1959)

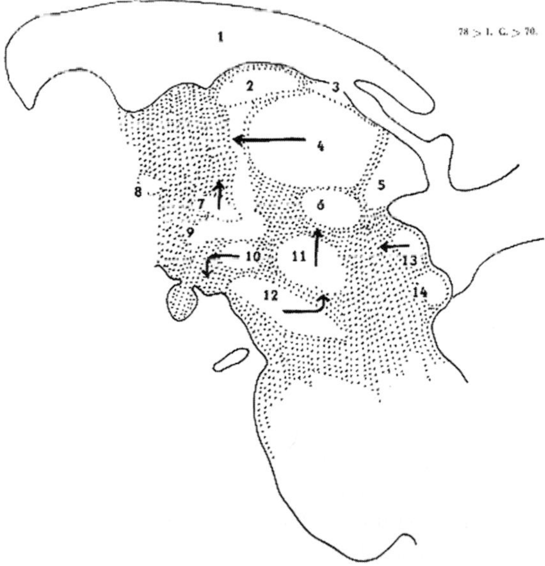

Fig. 2.18. Topometric variations observed in cephalic indices comprised between 70 and 78. *1*, lateral ventricle; *2*, anterior thalamic nucleus; *3*, lateral dorsal nucleus of thalamus; *4*, dorsomedial nucleus of thalamus; *5*, medial pulvinar nucleus; *6*, centromedian thalamic nucleus; *7*, zona incerta; *8*, anterior commissure; *9*, tegmental area; *10*, subthalamic nucleus; *11*, red nucleus; *12*, locus niger; *13*, superior colliculus; *14*, inferior colliculus; *15*, dentate nucleus of cerebellum. (From Delmas and Pertuiset 1959)

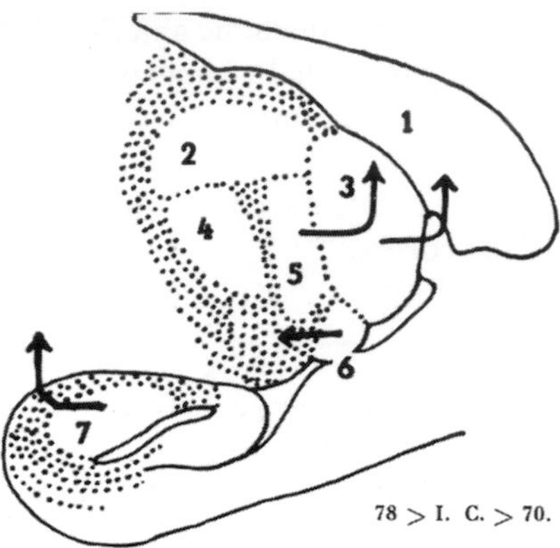

Fig. 2.19. Topometric variations observed in cephalic indices comprised between 70 and 78. *1*, lateral ventricle; *2*, ventral lateral thalamic nucleus; *3*, lateral pulvinar nucleus; *4*, ventral anterior thalamic nucleus; *5*, ventral posterior thalamic nucleus; *6*, lateral geniculate body; *7*, amygdala. (From Delmas and Pertuiset 1959)

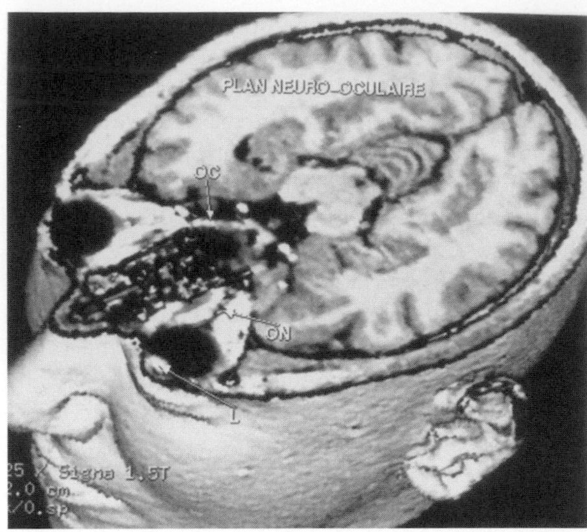

Fig. 2.20. The neuro-ocular plane (*NOP*) in a three-dimensional MR correlation, showing the cephalic landmarks in the axial plane: the lenses (*L*), the optic nerve heads (*ON*) and the optic canals (*OC*), as described by Cabanis et al. (1978)

C The Neuro-ocular Plane

The neuro-ocular plane (NOP), originally described in the CT study of the optic nerve in papilledema (Cabanis et al. 1978; Salvolini et al. 1978), best defines the cephalic orientation for scanning of patients with visual complaints. It is defined as the "plane passing through the lenses, the optic nerve heads and the optic canals, with the patient maintaining primary gaze" as shown on CT, and confirmed anatomically (Cabanis et al. 1978). It is now routinely used in CT and MR (Fig. 2.20), particularly in the exploration of patients presenting neuro-ophthalmological problems. The anatomic correlation obtained by Cabanis brought a definite confirmation to the clinical relevance of this cephalic orientation, which is most suitable for the exploration of the visual pathways (Fig. 2.21).

1 Anatomic and Imaging Correlations

NOP orientation provides the optimal conditions for CT or MR exploration of the intraorbital structures. The partial volume effect on the optic nerves is particularly reduced to a minimum (Cabanis et al. 1978; Brégeat et al. 1986). Anatomic, neuroradiologic, and clinical validations have been obtained (Tamraz 1983; Tamraz et al. 1984, 1985, 1988; Cabanis et al. 1981, 1982, 1988).

External cutaneous landmarks, experimentally determined and defined by the acanthion-tragion line (Fig. 2.22 A), are helpful to orient the patient's head in routine practice. Bony landmarks, defined by the prosthion-opisthion line, are also available and may be used on a sagittal localizer (Cabanis et al. 1982).

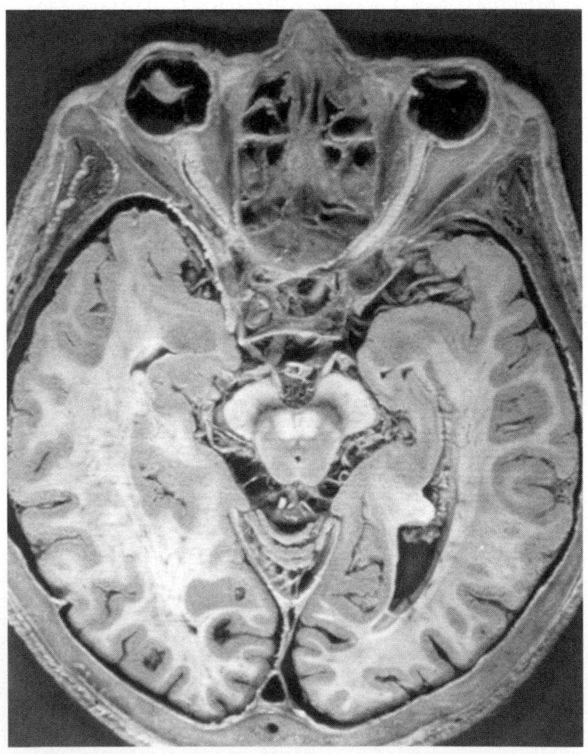

Fig. 2.21. The neuro-ocular plane (*NOP*), anatomic correlation. (Reprinted from Cabanis 1978)

The NOP is the most appropriate cephalic orientation for investigations in the axial and coronal

A
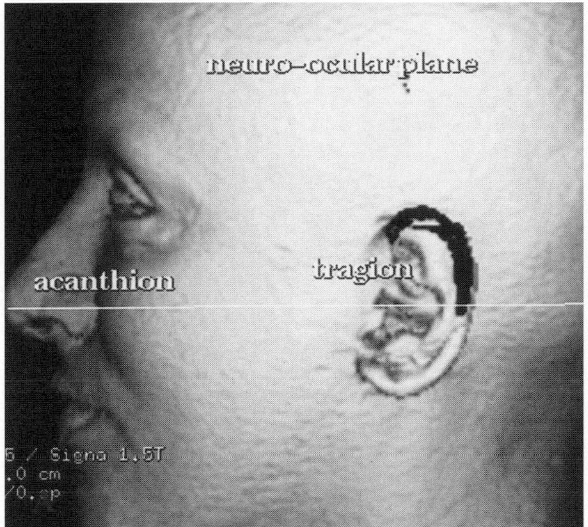

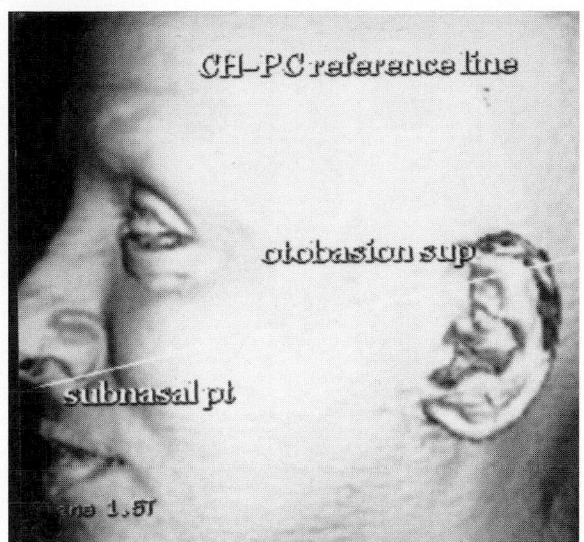

B

C
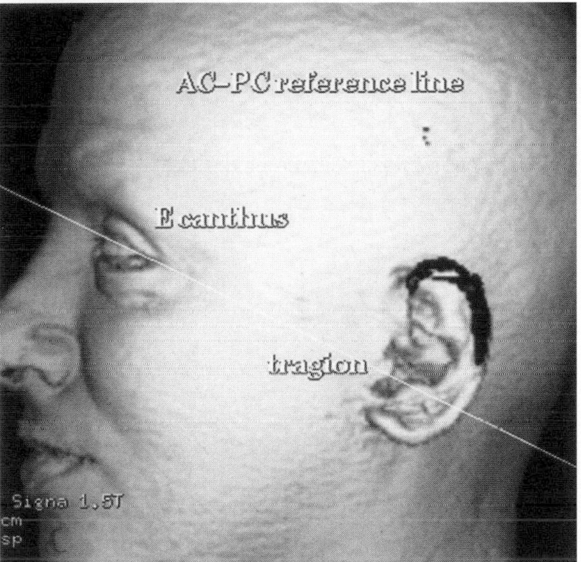

Fig. 2.22A–C. Cutaneous landmarks of the neuro-ocular plane (*NOP*) defined by the canthomeatal line (**A**) as compared to the CH-PC reference line (**B**) and the AC-PC reference line (**C**)

planes, for biometric studies, and for follow-up of eye diseases and examination of the intraorbital optic nerves. In fact, along its orbitocranial route, the visual pathway maintains a roughly horizontal orientation from the eyes to the calcarine fissure. For this reason, using the NOP as the cephalic reference plane appears to be the most accurate choice for the study of the brain and visual pathways, and the orbital optic nerves. This also applies to the screening and study of diseases involving the face and the skull base, due to a close parallelism with the Frankfurt-Virchow anthropologic reference baseline.

Such a reference atlas of cross-sectional anatomy of the head oriented in the NOP (Fig. 2.23), which includes the main anatomic correlations observed, may be used in routine practice for image interpretation (Tamraz 1983; Tamraz et al. 1984, 1985; Cabanis et al. 1988). The anatomic cuts in this work are detailed views based on these references. The coronal cuts used closely apply to the definition of the PC-OB line in the specimens reported. The perpendicular to the NOP is, in this case, presumably fortuitously parallel to PC-OB plane. It is not surprising that the respective MR correlations generally differ to some extent, as may also be observed in the published atlas (Fig. 2.37 p. 87). Actually, considering the axial landmarks, the perpendicular to the NOP is difficult to determine precisely and is angled about 10° as compared to the PC-OB plane. Similarly, the horizontal cuts reproduced in the atlas of Delmas and

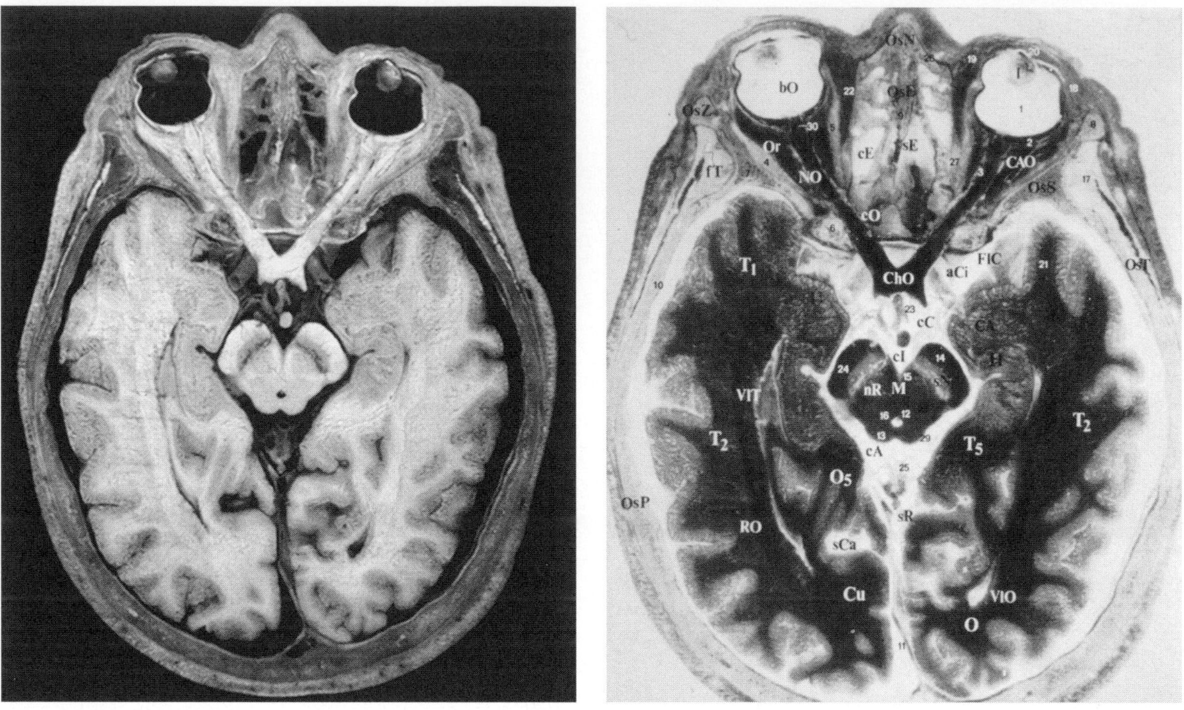

Fig. 2.23A,B. The neuro-ocular plane (*NOP*). Topometric findings. (From Tamraz 1983; Cabanis et al. 1988)

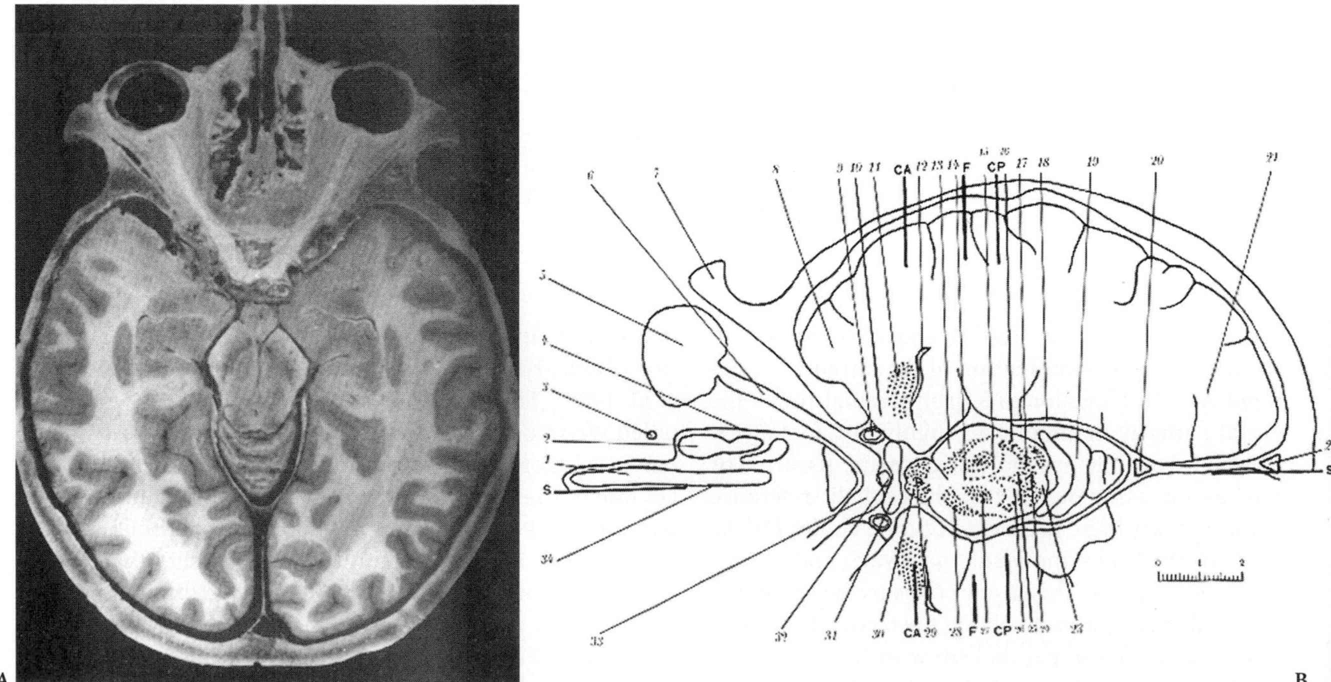

Fig. 2.24A,B. Axial anatomic cut (C27–HS, 19 mm) passing through the orbital and canalicular optic nerves, with the specimen oriented according to the Frankfurt-Virchow plane (anthropological baseline), and reported as fortuitously parallel, in the published case, to the defined brain reference. (From Delmas and Pertuiset 1959)

Pertuiset (1959) and oriented according to the Frankfurt-Virchow plane, as previously mentioned, show a close anatomic similarity as compared to the NOP (horizontal cut C27–HS 19 mm, Delmas and Pertuiset 1959 p. 267). In this particular specimen (Fig. 2.24), a NOP-like orientation cut is shown and may be considered as being roughly parallel to the anthropologic line. The topometric results derived from the work of Delmas may, therefore, be used in imaging interpretation of the slices oriented according to the NOP as defined by Cabanis et al. (1978).

2 Topometric and Biometric Findings

One of the great advantages of the NOP reference plane is the possibility to perform oculo-orbital topometry (Cabanis et al. 1980, 1982). Numerous distance measurements have been defined with respect to an external bicanthal line, joining the lateral orbital rims in the NOP, and these are used in routine practice. An overview of these biometric data is given in Chap. 9.

Many authors have proposed reference planes for visualizing the intraorbital optic nerves with the least partial volume effect phenomena and with reduction of the amount of radiation to the lens during slice acquisition. Different approaches have been proposed. Most of the procedures reported are based on simple calculations of the orbital references with respect to the reference cranial baselines previously defined, the OM (–20°) and the anthropologic line (Van Damme et al. 1977; Hilal and Trokel 1977; Vining 1977; Cabanis et al. 1978; Unsöld et al. 1980).

Actually, the mean angle between the NOP and the Frankfurt-Virchow plane (FVP) is about –7° (Fig. 2.25). As a reminder, the orbitomeatal plane, which is

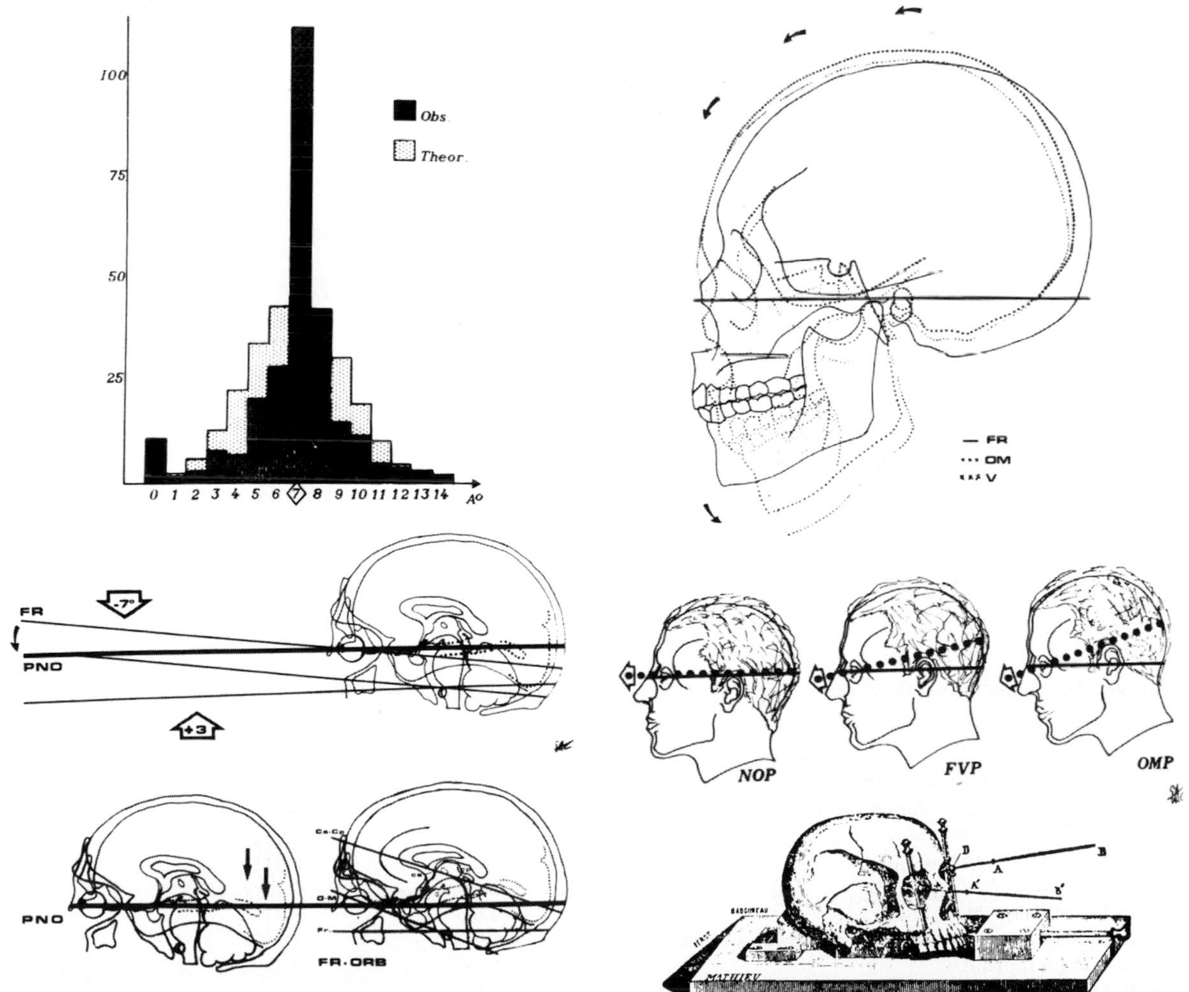

Fig. 2.25A,B. The neuro-ocular plane; biometric and topometric findings. (From Cabanis et al. 1982)

the classic radiologic reference plane (WFN 1962), is angled at approximately +10° relative to the FVP. Moreover, exhaustive work on the relation of the orbital axis plane to several craniofacial reference lines has been reported, including the important contribution from the comparative anatomy laboratory of Dr. Fenart in Lille (1982) to this field (Fig. 2.26, Table 2.7). Close parallelisms of the NOP with the alveolar-condylar plane, the hard palate plane and the prosthion-opisthion line (Saban 1980; Fenart et al. 1982), which may be used as external cranial landmarks to orient the slices on a lateral scout view of the skull by CT, may be retained and are actually helpful in routine practice.

In addition, such parallelisms explain the effectiveness of this cephalic orientation as a suitable reference for screening patients with diseases involving the orbitomaxillofacial region or the skull base.

The use of the NOP in comparative anatomic studies in vivo, reported in part in Chap. 9, and its angulation as compared to the FVP and the OM emphasizes its importance as a major anatomic and physiologic reference plane in hominids (Fig. 2.25). It is interesting to note also that the angle of the visual pathways with respect to the base of the skull changes with age due to the well-known occipital descent (Delattre and Fenart 1960). However, once maturation is complete, the angle between the visual pathways and the skull remains constant. Therefore, the angle between NOP and FVP becomes constant in the adult. As Delmas once stated: "...the vision of man rises to encounter the horizon".

D The Callosal Plane

The callosal plane was defined by Olivier et al. (1985, 1987) as the reference plane "passing by the lowest point of the genu and splenium of the corpus callosum and extending through the whole brain" (Fig. 2.3). The authors also defined orthogonal planes perpendicular to it. The planes tangent to the anterior border of the genu and to the posterior border of the splenium were named the anterior callosal and the

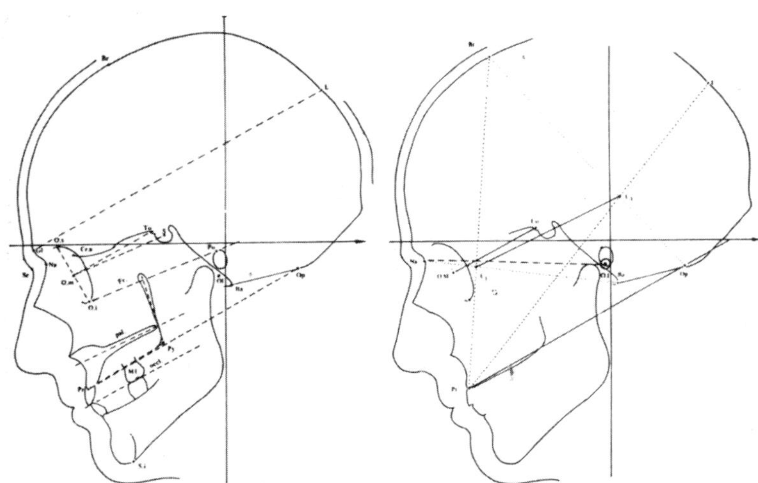

Fig. 2.26. The neuro-ocular plane, defined by the orbital axis (*OM-To*), as compared to various cranial reference lines. (According to Fenart et al. 1982; see Table 2.7 and Fig. 2.25). (In Cabanis et al. 1982)

Table 2.7. The orbital axis (*OM-To*) in relation to other cranial reference planes (from Fenart et al. 1982) (*n*=52)

Angle variations	Mean	Standard deviation
OM-To / midorbital axis – center of the sella turcica	6.27	1.47
OM-To / glabella-lambda plane	0.44	4.20
OM-To / prosthion-opisthion plane	–0.45	3.31
OM-To / Frankfurt-Virchow plane	7.08	4.12
OM-To / hard palate plane	4.63	3.91
OM-To / prosthion-pterygoalveolar (superior alveolar plane)	–2.19	4.23
OM-To / occlusal plane	2.05	4.15
OM-To / Cl-C3	3.32	4.70
OM-To / nasion-auricular plane	32.75	4.68

posterior callosal planes, respectively. A third perpendicular plane is drawn midway between the two and is called the midcommissural plane. The midcallosal plane, as defined, helps to localize the inferior part of the central sulcus (Fig. 2.27).

These landmarks are seen on midsagittal MR images and indirectly by digital subtraction angiography (DSA). The corpus callosum may be precisely localized on lateral projections showing both the arterial and venous phases. This permits the integration of MRI with angiographic data as well as data provided by positron emission tomography (PET), demonstrating that this reference is obviously suitable for multimodal imaging (Olivier et al. 1987).

The corpus callosum is the major telencephalic commissure influencing the shape of the adjacent cortical sulci, as may be demonstrated ontogenetically, emphasizing the suitability of this reference system for imaging within the telencephalon. It has been used for the preoperative identification of the central sulcus (Lehman et al. 1992). Integration of functional information with MR gyral data and stereotaxic implantation of depth electrodes for investigation of epilepsy have also been achieved using such coordinates.

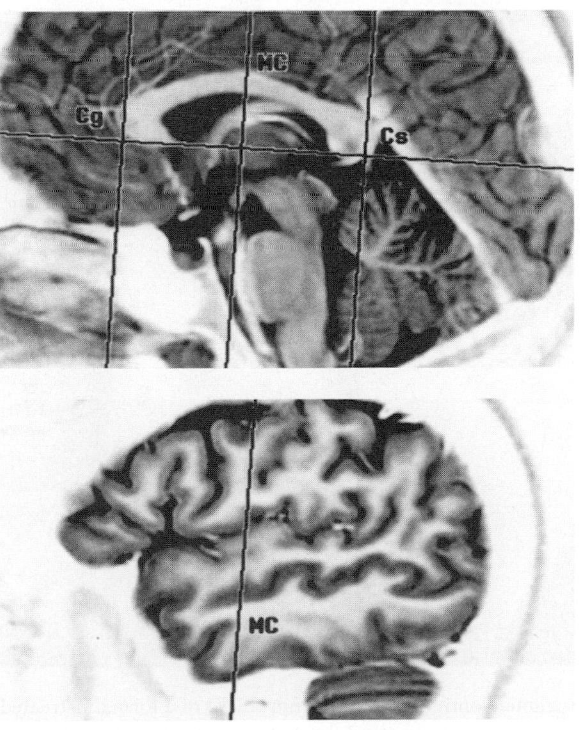

Fig. 2.27. The callosal reference plane. (After Olivier et al. 1985, 1987)

On the other hand, the relationship of this plane with the basal ganglia seems more tentative, as they are best analyzed using the AC-PC plane of Talairach.

E The Chiasmatico-Commissural Plane

This horizontal reference line, the CH-PC, runs tangential to the superior border of the CH anteriorly, and to the inferior border of the PC posteriorly (Figs. 2.3, 2.28). These landmarks, based on brain commissures, are well depicted and easily recognized on an in vivo midsagittal cut of human, as well as all vertebrate, brains (Tamraz et al. 1989, 1990, 1991). The horizontal plane through this line can also be used in the comparative anatomy of vertebrates if needed.

The consistency of the angle between this line and the AC-PC, as demonstrated, serves to validate the choice of this pivotal line, situated as it is at the midbrain-diencephalic junction corresponding to the related flexure during ontogenesis. The plane has been shown to be truly horizontal in that it is perpendicular to the main axis of the brainstem, defined as the line tangential to the anterior border of the PC and joining the lowest extremity of the calamus in the floor of the fourth ventricle behind the obex (Fig. 2.29).

If the NOP is accepted as the anatomic and physiologic plane permitting erect posture in humans, the CH-PC, which is roughly parallel to it as compared to the direction of the temporal horn of the lateral ventricle, may be considered as the anatomic plane defining the temporalization of the brain. It is parallel to the direction of the parallel sulcus and, thus, to the lateral fissure, and orthogonal to the long axis of the brainstem. It is possible to consider that the CH-PC is for the brain what the NOP is for the position of the head, the former being perpendicular to the brainstem long axis and the latter being anatomically and physiologically related to the vertical axis of the body and cervical spine. Both reference planes present progressive variations throughout phylogenesis, as demonstrated by the progressive closure of the truncal angle.

1 Biometric Findings

To study the anatomic and anthropometric usefulness of the CH-PC, in vivo MRI findings in 100 patients were analyzed, using high field MRI (1.5 T). The statistical analysis of the in vivo measurements confirmed the consistency of the angle between the reference lines CH-PC and AC-PC.

A

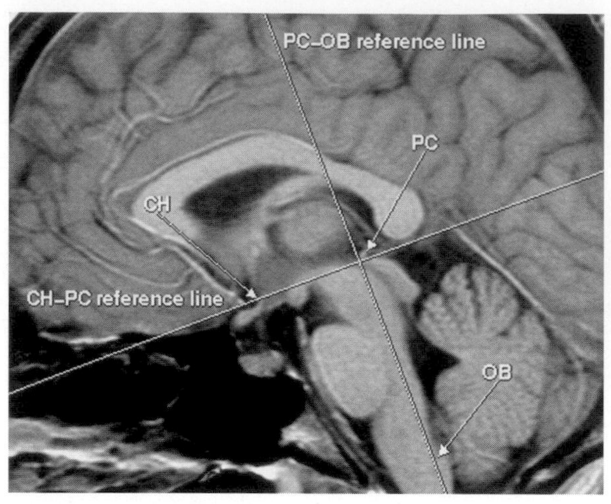

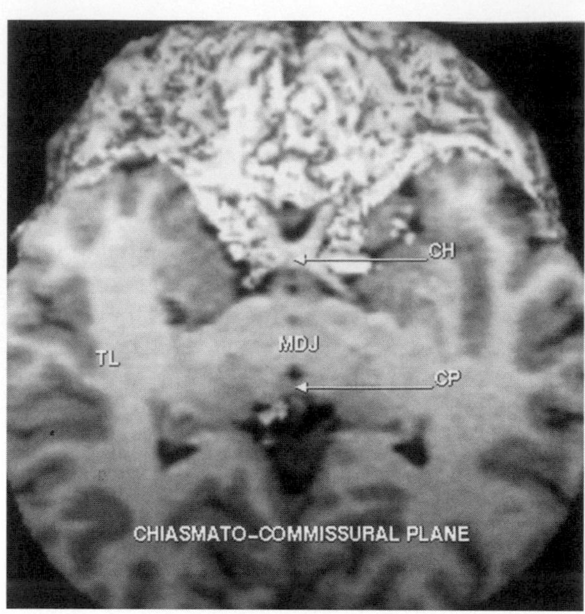

B

Fig. 2.28A,B. The chiasmatico-commissural (*CH-PC*) reference plane, defined as the plane tangent superiorly to the chiasmal point (*CH*) anteriorly, to the inferior border of the posterior commissure (*PC*) posteriorly, passing through the midbrain-diencephalic junction (*MDJ*) and showing the temporal lobes according to their long axis (*TL*). *PC-OB*, commissural-obex reference line. (Tamraz et al. 1990)

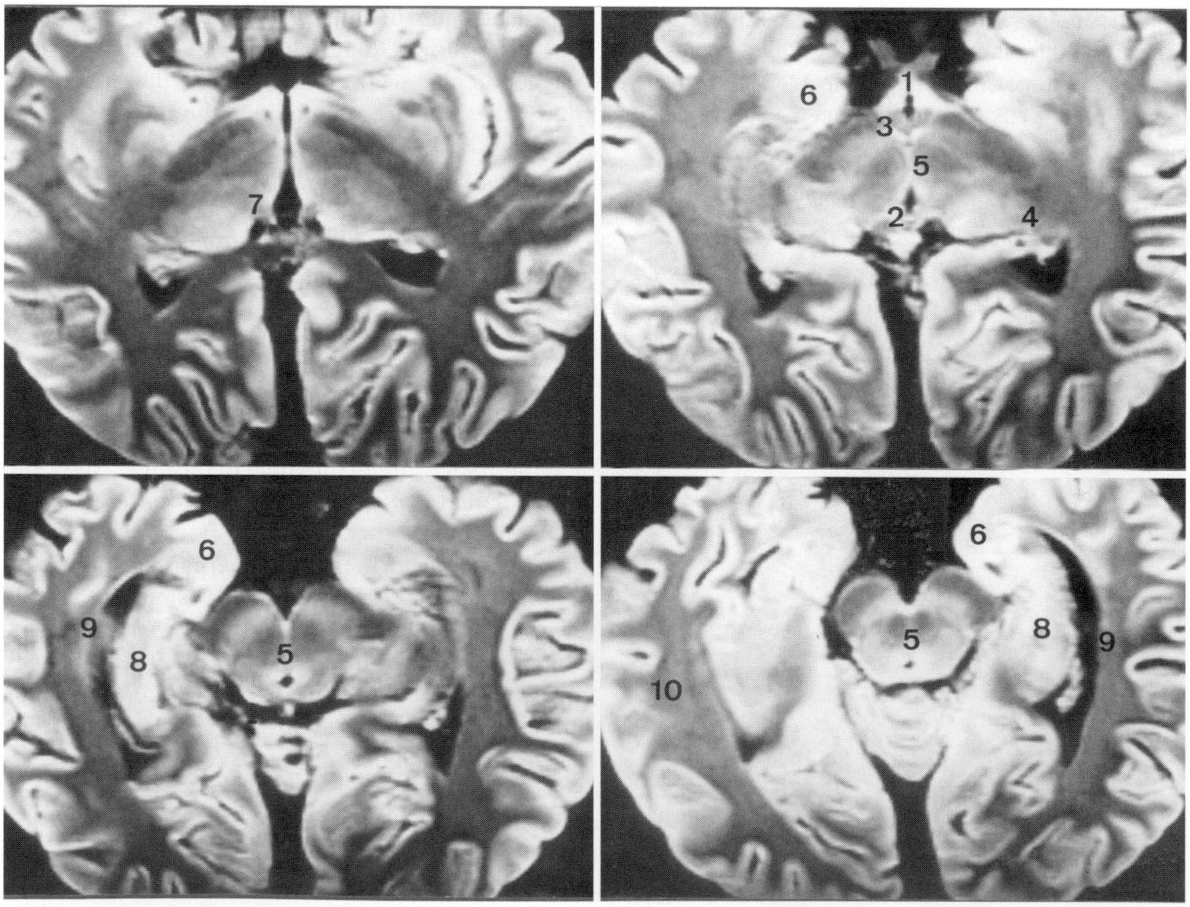

Fig. 2.29A–D. The chiasmatico-commissural reference plane. Horizontal contiguous cuts (3 mm thick) of a formalin-treated specimen showing the anatomic landmarks of the CH-PC reference plane (**B**), passing through the chiasmal point (*1*), the mamillary bodies (*3*) and the posterior commissure (*2*), on the midline, and involving laterally the lateral geniculate bodies (*4*) at the midbrain-diencephalic junction (*5*). The upper contiguous cut (**A**) passes through the habenula (*7*) and the lower part of the thalamus; the lower cuts (**C, D**) are oriented along the long axis of the temporal lobes (*10*) and temporal horns (*9*) and show the amygdala (*6*) – hippocampus (*8*) complex

The results obtained were the following (Fig. 2.30):

a) The mean value of the angle formed by the lines CH-PC and AC-PC, called the commissural angle or CH-PC-AC (Fig. 2.31), averaged 24.26° (range 19–30°, SD 2.3282) in the first group of 50 patients. This fell to 18.16° (range 13–25°, SD 2.4020) in the second group of 50 patients, in whom the tangent to the inferior border of the AC, as advocated by Delmas and Pertuiset (1959), was used.
b) The angle formed by the CH-PC line and the brainstem long axis is named the truncal angle (Fig. 2.32). Two angles are measured according to the definition of the brainstem axis. The first joins the anterior border of the AC to the inferior extremity of the floor of the fourth ventricle behind the obex, the CH-PC-OB, and appears to be at right angles to the main axis of the brainstem, measuring about 93° (range 83–102°, SD 3.4). The second joins the superior insertion of the superior medullary velum to the obex (CH-VI-OB) with CH-PC and is more variable, averaging 85° (range 71–101°, SD 4.4).

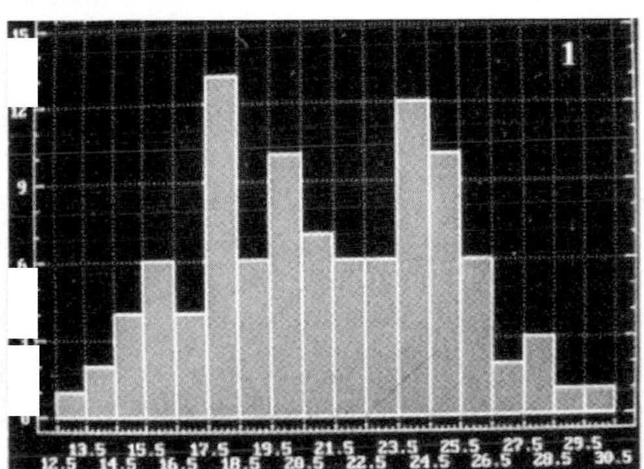

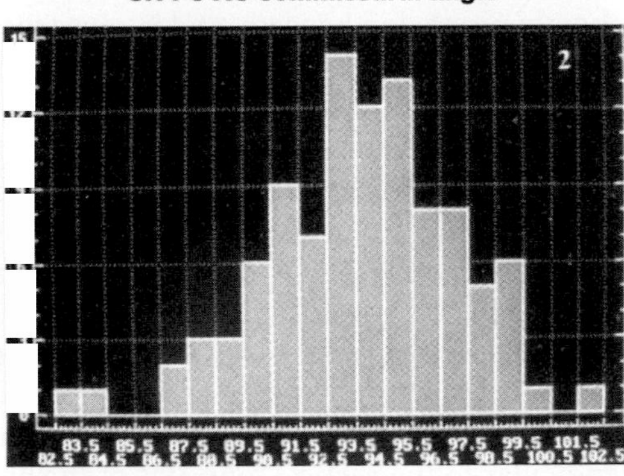

Fig. 2.30. The chiasmatico-commissural (*CH-PC*) reference plane: biometric findings. (From Tamraz et al. 1990)

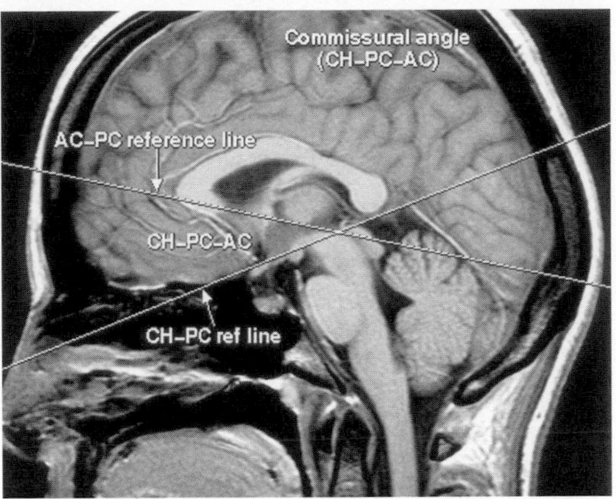

Fig. 2.31. The commissural angle (*CH-PC-AC*); biometric findings: average (24.26), median (24), standard deviation (2.32), minimum (19), maximum (30)

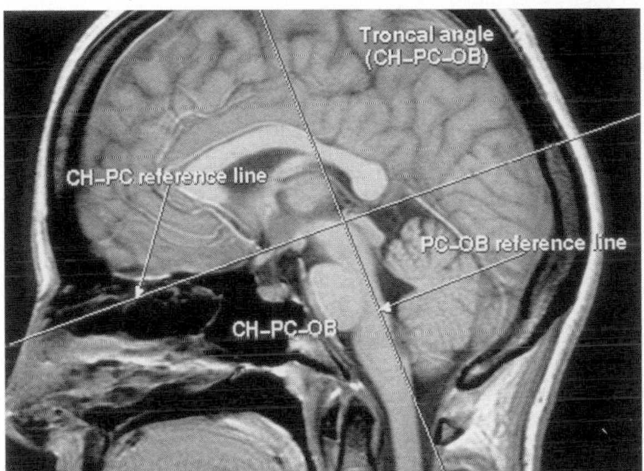

Fig. 2.32. The truncal angle (*CH-PC-OB*); biometric findings: average (93.7), median (94), standard deviation (3.42), minimum (83), maximum (102)

A measure of the distance between the chiasmal notch and the PC was quite uniform and averaged 26.23 mm (SD 1.58). This measure corresponds to the data reported by Lang (1987).

2 Anatomic and Imaging Correlations

The major anatomic correlations derived from the comparative analysis of the anatomy in the successive MR sagittal cuts were the following. First was the close parallelism of the CH-PC plane and the plane defined by the posterior branch of the lateral sulcus excluding its ascending terminal segment. In fact, the lateral projection of the plane on successive cuts, oriented parallel to CH-PC, shows close parallelism with the superior temporal sulcus (Fig. 2.33). Moreover, the projection onto the insular triangle of the parallel to the CH-PC line proves to be the same as the projection of the lateral fissure. The "lateral fissure plane" can thus be projected onto the median plane (Fig. 2.33).

This parallelism is demonstrated by the observed correspondence between the value of the angle CH-PC-AC (24°) and that of the angle formed by AC-PC and the lateral fissure, which averages 23–25° according to Szikla et al. (1977). The inclination of the central sulcus to the "sylvian plane" averages 58° according to these authors. Note that in the CH-PC orientation, the terminal portion of the central sulcus is approximately found at the junction of the anterior two-thirds and the posterior third, in the upper horizontal supraventricular cuts, contrary to what is observed in a bicommissural orientation of the axial cuts (Fig. 2.34).

It is, therefore, possible that this brain reference line is naturally the orientation of choice for horizontal cuts, particularly in the investigation of the temporal lobes, the superior temporal sulcus receiving the lateral projection of the CH-PC line and being recognized at the level of the carotid bifurcations on MR angiograms. The lateral temporal sulci are therefore displayed along their anterior-posterior long axis (Figs. 2.33, 2.35). The exploration of the perisylvian areas benefit even more significantly from such an orientation. Comparative evaluation of the planum temporale and studies of brain dominance are, therefore, best achieved with respect to this reference (Fig. 2.36). Moreover, angiographically, the arterial limits of the planum are depicted more precisely in the chiasmatico-commissural orientation than in the bicommissural plane (Szikla et al. 1977). MR angiography confirms such anatomical variations (Fig. 2.37).

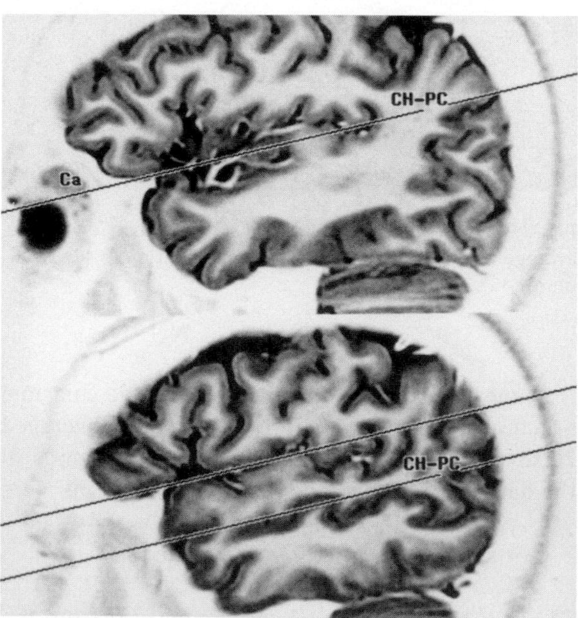

Fig. 2.33. The CH-PC plane: anatomic and imaging correlations, showing the close parallelism of the *CH-PC*, as projected on the parasagittal cuts, to the parallel sulcus (corresponding to the lateral projection of CH-PC), and to the sylvian fissure (*Ca*) with its correlated projection deeply onto the insular triangle. The CH-PC plane is therefore the ideal anatomic and angiographic reference for use when imaging the temporal lobes and the perisylvian regions

As a corollary, a close parallelism of CH-PC to the plane of the temporal horns of the lateral ventricles, and roughly to the choroidal fissure, seems obvious. It is, therefore, suitable for studying the hippocampus along its long axis (Fig. 2.38). Another interesting parallelism concerns the anterior portion of the body of the corpus callosum and its adjacent cingulate gyrus (Fig. 2.39).

The constant topography of the posterior prolongation of the CH-PC line passing through the ambient cistern between the inferior border of the splenium and the upper limit of the culmen and paralleling or intersecting the common stem of the parieto-occipital with the calcarine sulci also should be noted (Fig. 2.39). Thus, most of the calcarine fissure may reliably be found on the lower infra-CH-PC axial cuts in most circumstances. This plane therefore separates the cerebellum and the brainstem from the main mass of the cerebrum, except for the occipital lobes whose topography is a function of the cranial index and typology, as shown on this three-dimensional MR (Fig. 2.40). The CH-PC plane obviously separates the proencephalon (telencephalon and diencephalon) above, from the mesencephalon and rhombencephalon beneath, and is consequently of real embryologic, as well as phylogenetic, significance.

The coronal projection of the CH-PC plane to the commissural-obex vertical reference plane is constantly tangent to the superior border of the lateral geniculate bodies (Fig. 2.41), showing a constant topography at the diencephalon-mesencephalic junctional region, which is well displayed in the horizontal reference plane.

The last finding is that the CH-PC plane is almost perpendicular to the vertical long axis of the brainstem (Fig. 2.42). Thus, anatomic and clinical correlations, in the coronal and the axial cuts, of fine structures in the brainstem are possible and facilitated

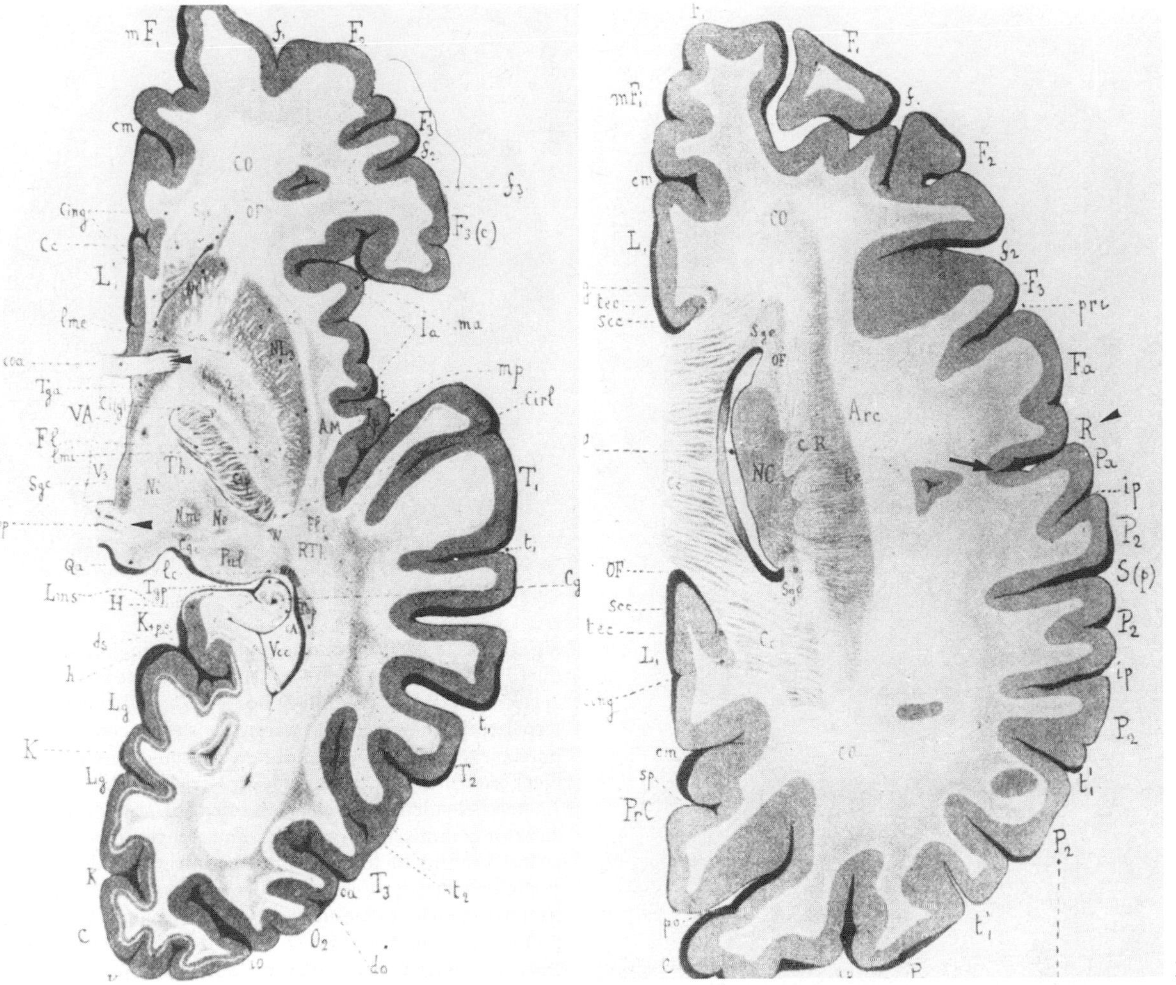

A B

Fig. 2.34A,B. Topography of the central sulcus: anterior-posterior variations with respect to the axial reference plane used and considering the supraventricular cuts. A Axial cuts through the anterior and posterior commissures and transcallosal (B). (From Déjerine 1895)

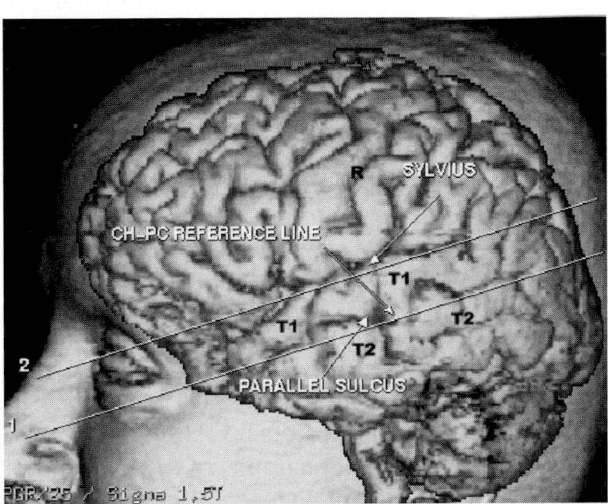

Fig. 2.35. The CH-PC reference plane as a "sylvian" orientation plane, most suitable for the study of the perisylvian region and the temporal lobes

(see Chap. 8). There is, as well, an easier and more definite reference to the tegmental areas beneath the floor of the fourth ventricle and, therefore, to the underlying nuclei and related fiber bundles.

On the other hand, in order to develop an in vivo morphometric approach to the brain, numbers of parallelisms to the CH-PC and PC-OB lines have been evaluated in a preliminary study in an attempt to determine the morphometric peculiarities and the eventual proportional variations that may help to differentiate individual brains (Fig. 2.43). All the parallel lines defining reference planes are chosen according to major anatomic landmarks found on the midsagittal MR cut and are considered as roughly parallel to the horizontal CH-PC reference plane. Three planes are defined dorsoventrally on each side of the CH-PC line, perpendicular to the PC-OB reference line.

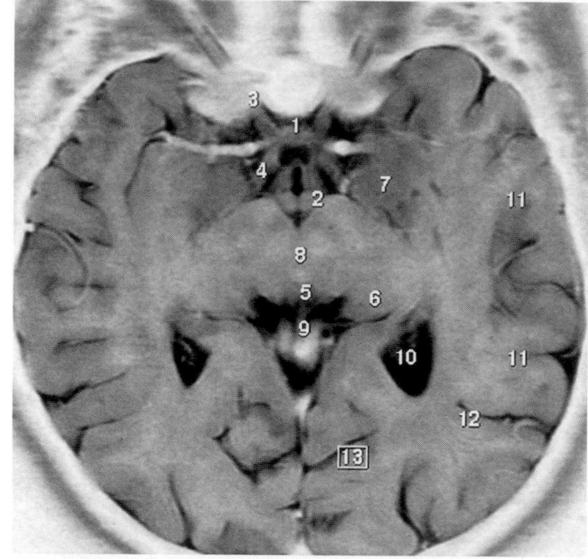

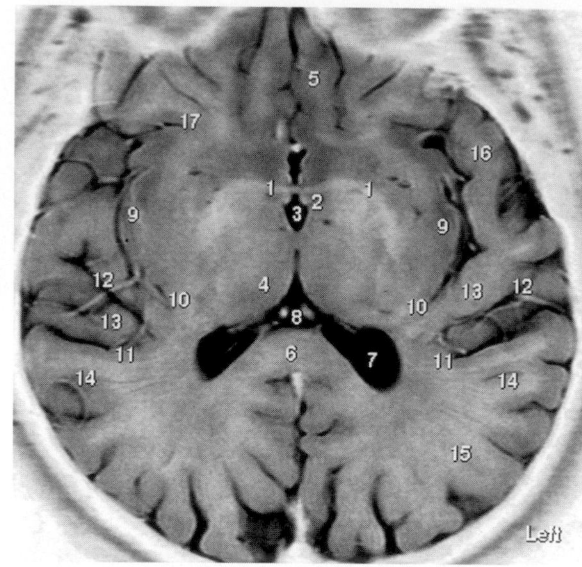

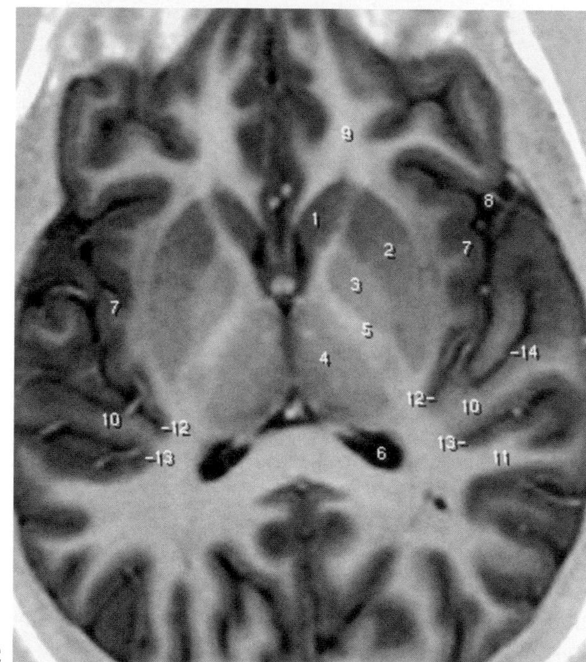

Fig. 2.36A–C. The planum temporale, imaging according to the CH-PC reference. **A** At the CH-PC reference level (case 1): *1*, Optic chiasm; *2*, mamillary bodies; *3*, canalicular and cisternal optic nerve; *4*, optic tract; *5*, posterior commissure; *6*, pulvinar; *7*, amygdala; 8, midbrain-thalamic junction; *9*, ambient cistern; *10*, atrium of lateral ventricle; *11*, lateral fissure; *12*, parallel sulcus; *13*, calcarine sulcus. **B** At the level of the anterior commissure (case 1): *1*, anterior commissure; *2*, anterior columns of fornix; *3*, third ventricle; *4*, thalamus; *5*, gyrus rectus; *6*, splenium of corpus callosum; *7*, atrium of lateral ventricle; *8*, ambient cistern; *9*, insula; *10*, posterior border of circular sulcus; *11*, transverse supratemporal sulcus; *12*, intermediate transverse supratemporal sulcus; *13*, Heschl gyrus (transverse supratemporal gyrus); *14*, planum temporale; *15*, supramarginal gyrus; *16*, temporal operculum; *17*, anterior border of circular sulcus. **C** At the midthalamus and basal ganglia level (case 2): *1*, caudate nucleus; *2*, putamen; *3*, pallidum, lateral part; *4*, thalamus; *5*, internal capsule, posterior limb; *6*, atrium of lateral ventricle; *7*, insula; *8*, lateral fissure; *9*, frontal lobe; *10*, superior temporal gyri of Heschl; *11*, planum temporale; *12*, circular sulcus, posterior border; *13*, transverse supratemporal sulcus; *14*, intermediate sulcus

Among the angles evaluated, one merits particular attention. It is defined as the basal callosal angle formed between the CH-PC plane and the tangent to the base of the corpus callosum. The importance of the latter in encephalometric studies has been stressed by Ariens Kappers in his work on racial differences in the brain (1947). The in vivo MR value of this CH-PC-CC angle, as determined statistically on a series of 86 normal exams (Tamraz 1991), averages 16.2209° (range 8–22°, SD 3.3690). The interesting anatomic correlation observed concerns its relation with the major telencephalic reference, defined by the callosal plane as described by Olivier et al. (1985). Actually, the mid-callosal plane of Olivier also shows some relation to the mamillary bodies, which are known to be very constant topometrically and are contained in the CH-PC plane (Fig. 2.44). Note the other interesting anatomic correlations, as projected on parasagittal cuts involving the hippocampal formation: the topography of the midcallosal plane, as pointed out by Olivier between the amygdala and the hippocampus; and the projection of the CH-PC plane approximately tangential superiorly to the amygdala and the tail of the hippocampus pass-

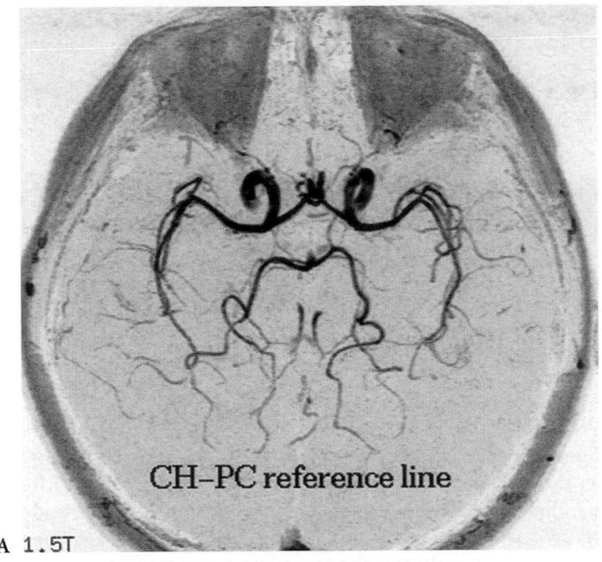

A

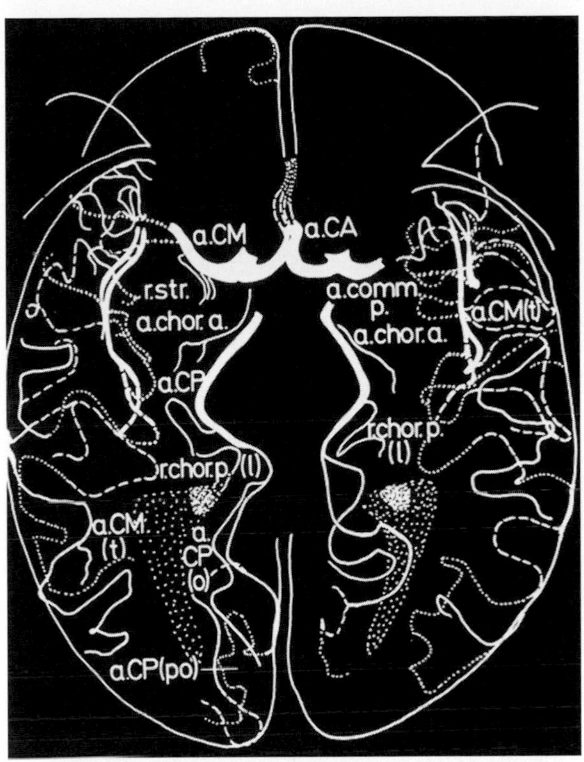

B

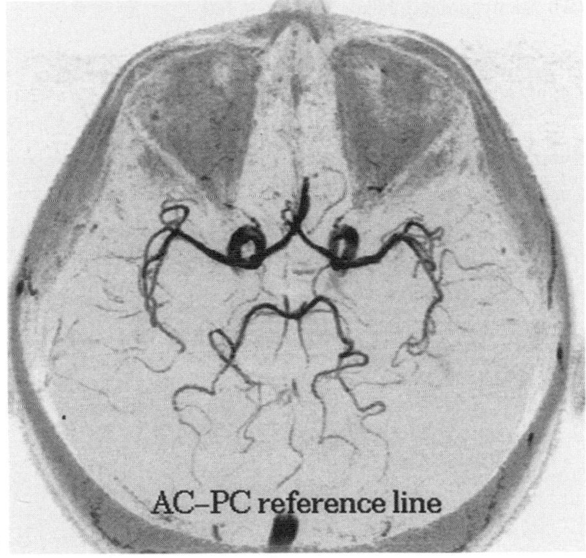

C

Fig. 2.37A–C. MR angiography according to the chiasmatico-commissural reference plane (*CH-PC*), suitable for multimodal imaging and for the investigation of the perisylvian region and the supratemporal plane (**A**) as compared to the bicommissural (*AC-PC*) orientation (**C**). The MR result is close to the angiogram obtained in the "sylvian" orientation (**B**) and shown by Cabanis and Iba-Zizen (in Szikla et al. 1977)

ing through the limen insulae. Such interrelations between the callosal reference and the CH-PC reference plane seem promising but need further anatomic and functional evaluations.

Finally, it appears that the CH-PC corresponds well with the anatomic facts, both anthropologically and phylogenetically. The consistent angulation with the AC-PC of neurosurgical stereotaxy, the close parallelism with the parallel sulcus and the lateral fissure, and the perpendicular relationship with the vertical long axis of the brainstem will facilitate both comparative biometric analysis of the living and the fixed brain, as well as the study of ontogenesis and phylogenesis of the brain based on a sylvian orientation.

F Anatomic and Physiologic Reference Planes

Anatomic and physiologic planes are mainly represented by the "horizontal vestibular plane", which is the plane of equilibration defined by Girard, Perez, Delattre and Fenart, and the "plane of the orbital axis", described by Broca, which corresponds to the "plane of the horizontal vision".

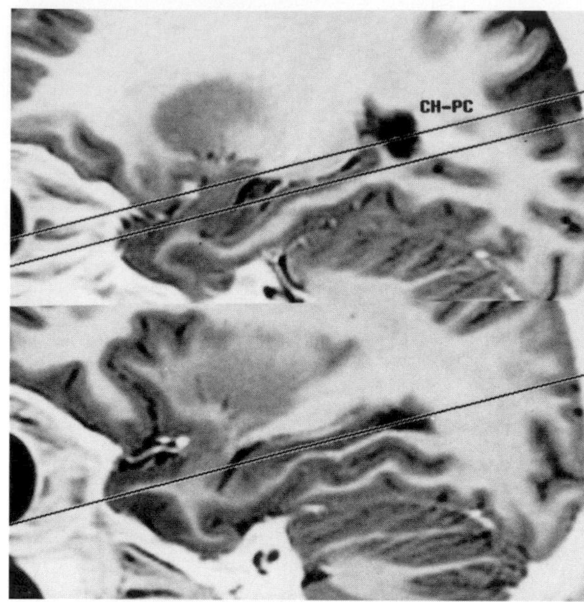

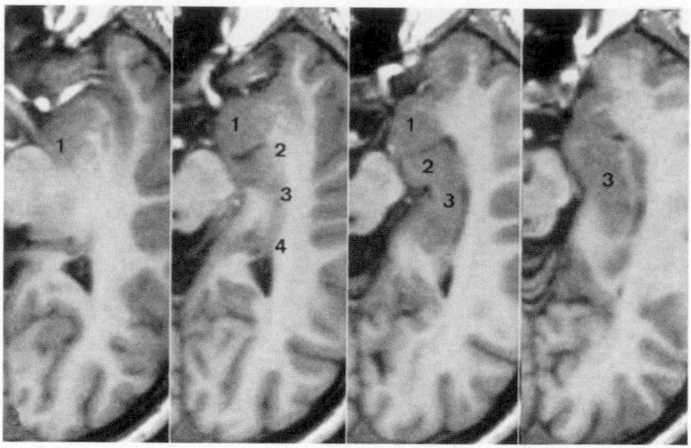

Fig. 2.38A,B. Close parallelism of CH-PC plane to the inferior horn of the lateral ventricle and to the hippocampal long axis, as shown on the lateral projections of the reference and its parallel through the hippocampal formation (**A**). The contiguous 2 mm axial cuts proceeding downward from the upper CH-PC level display the amygdala-hippocampal complex (**B**). *1*, amygdala; *2*, head; *3*, body; *4*, tail

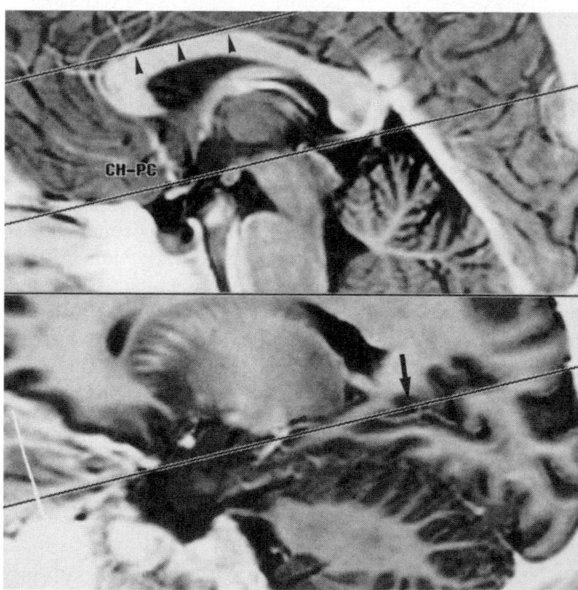

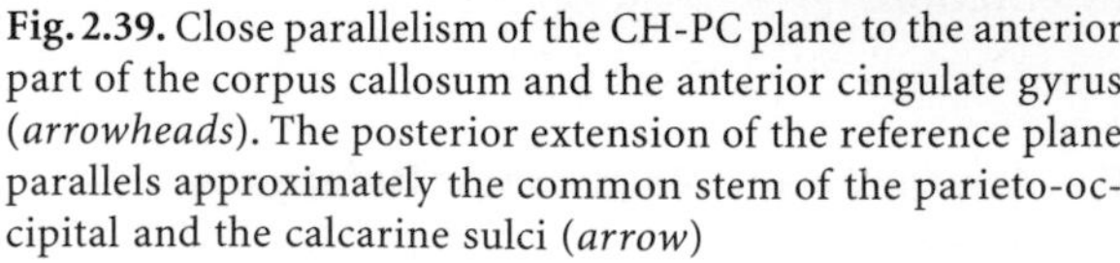

Fig. 2.39. Close parallelism of the CH-PC plane to the anterior part of the corpus callosum and the anterior cingulate gyrus (*arrowheads*). The posterior extension of the reference plane parallels approximately the common stem of the parieto-occipital and the calcarine sulci (*arrow*)

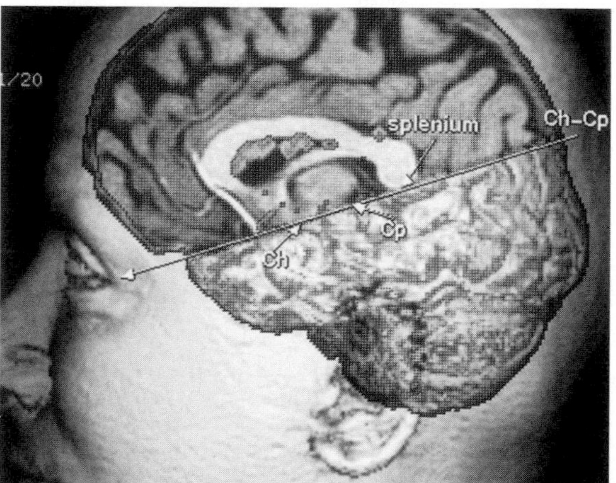

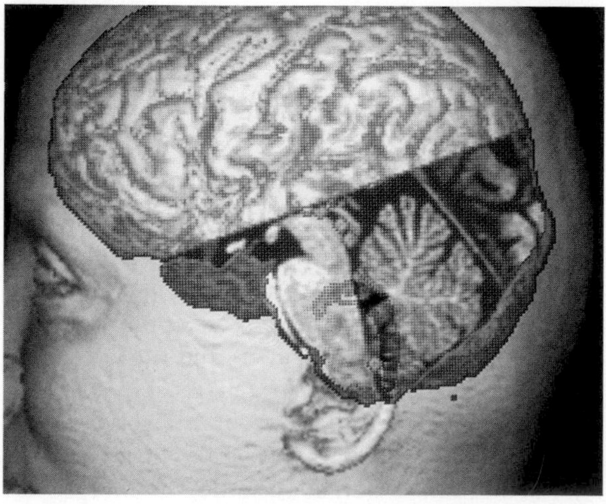

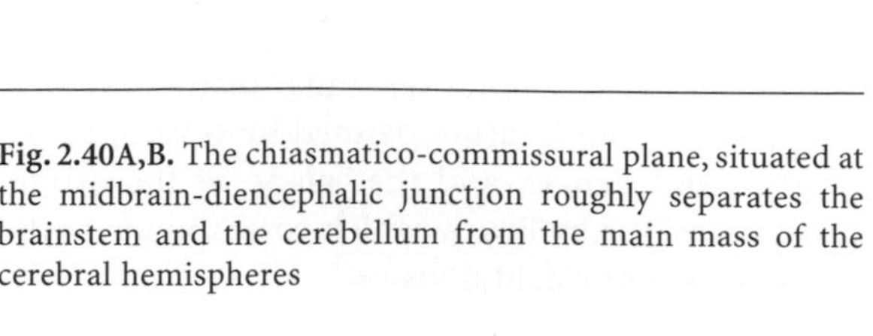

Fig. 2.40A,B. The chiasmatico-commissural plane, situated at the midbrain-diencephalic junction roughly separates the brainstem and the cerebellum from the main mass of the cerebral hemispheres

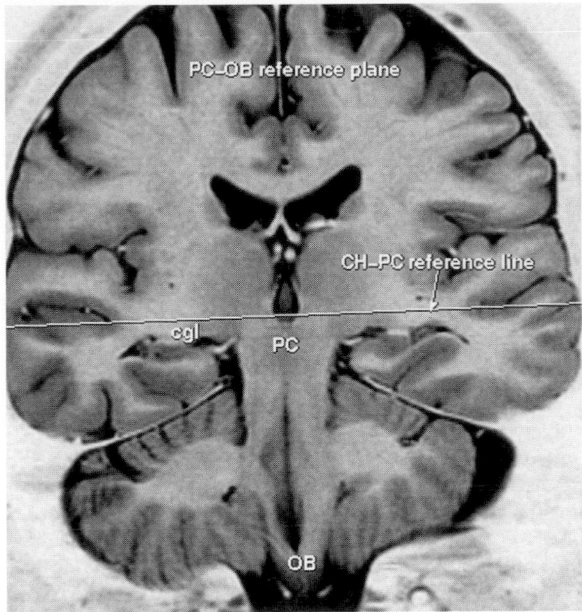

Fig. 2.41. The CH-PC reference plane is a pivotal plane at the midbrain-diencephalic junction; its projection onto the coronal commissural-obex (*PC-OB*) reference plane is constantly found tangent to the topometrically stable lateral geniculate bodies (*cgl*)

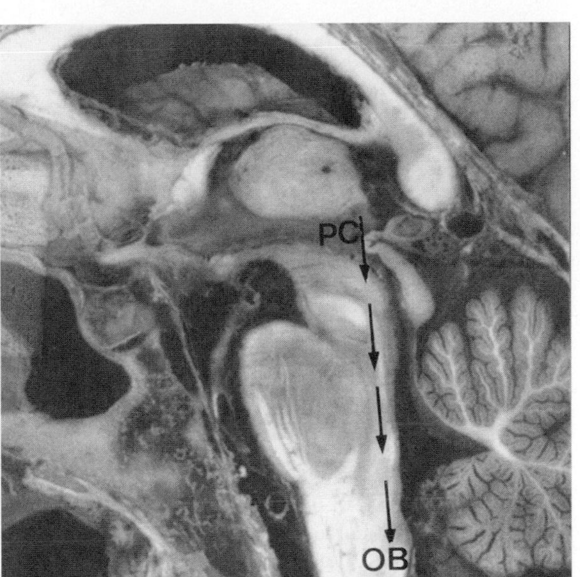

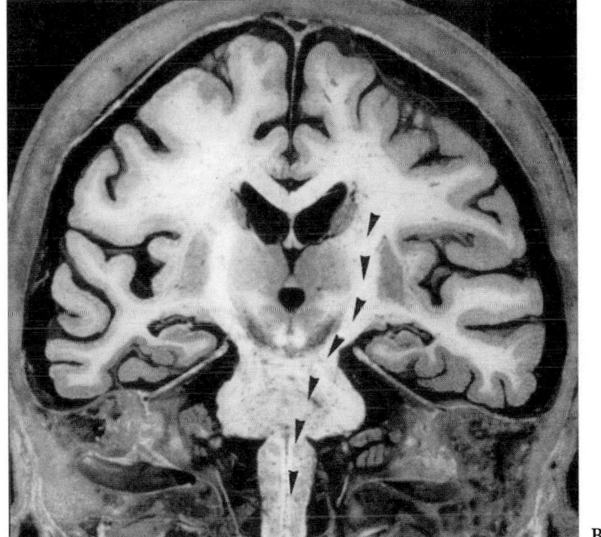

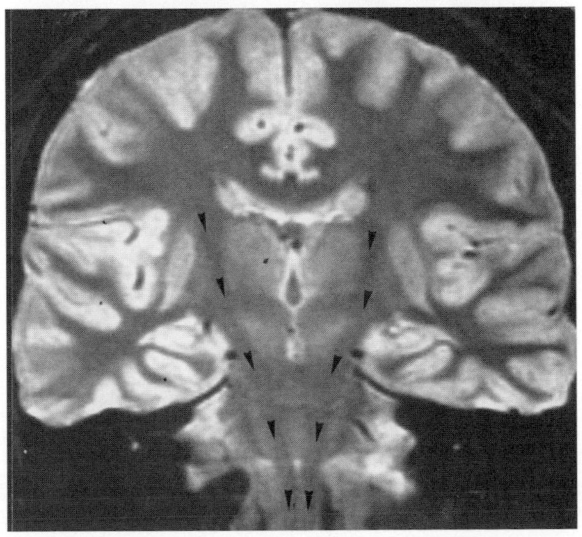

Fig. 2.42A–C. The CH-PC plane is almost perpendicular to the brainstem vertical long axis as defined by the parallel anterior to the PC-OB reference line (*arrows*) showing the whole brainstem-diencephalic continuum. The corticospinal tracts are nicely displayed in this orientation of the coronal cuts, as demonstrated routinely with MR (*arrowheads*)

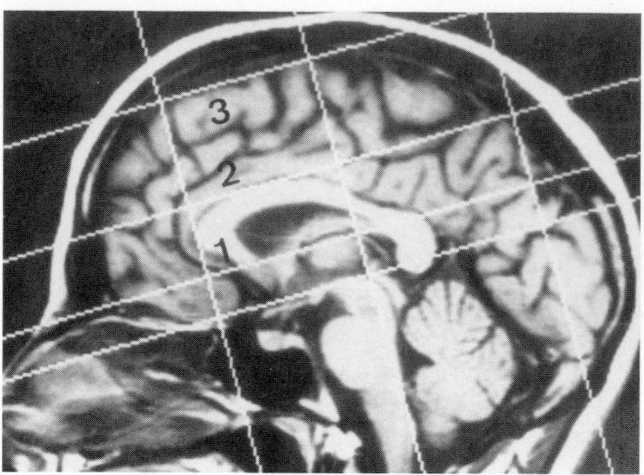

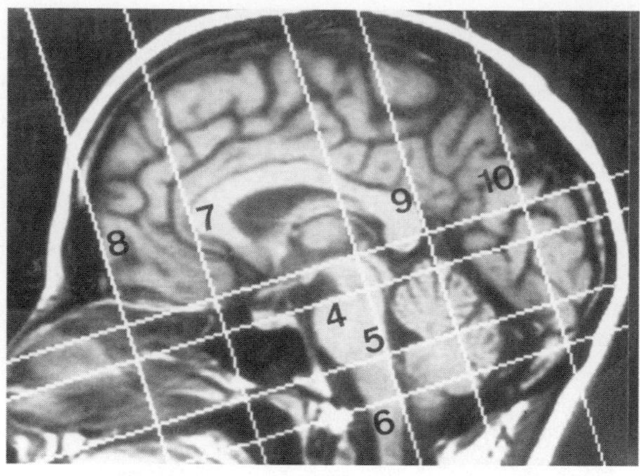

Fig. 2.43A,B. Brain morphometry based on the orthogonal references: CH-PC and PC-OB planes, as defined in the encephalometric study of patients presenting with genetic diseases due to chromosomal aberrations (Tamraz 1991). Parallel planes are traced: the horizontal supra-CH-PC planes, tangent to the inferior border of the rostrum (*1*), to the superior border of the callosal body (*2*), and to the vertex (*3*); the horizontal infra-CH-PC planes, passing through the tip of the interpeduncular space and the lower aspect of the tectal plate (*4*), at the pontomedullary junction (*5*), and at the obex level (*6*); the vertical planes, anterior to PC-OB, tangent to the genu of the corpus callosum (*7*) and to the frontal pole (*8*), and posterior to PC-OB, tangent to the splenium (*9*) and passing through the inferior tip of the occipital lobe (*10*)

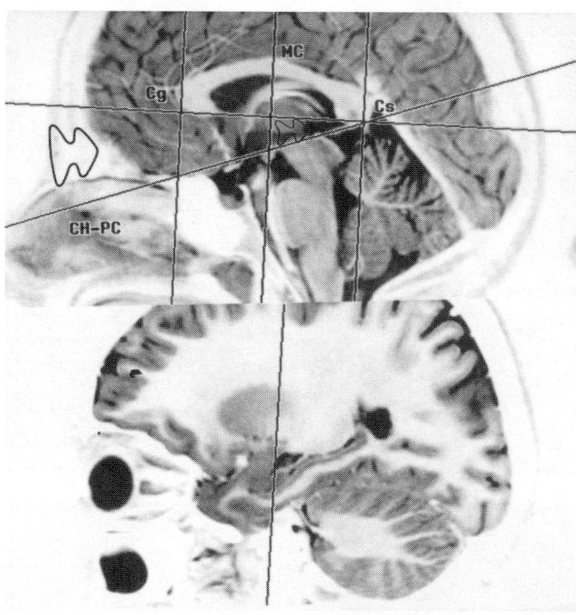

Fig. 2.44. The callosal angle (16∞), as defined between the chiasmatico-commissural plane (*CH-PC*) and the callosal plane (*Cg-Cs*)

1 The "Plan Vestibulaire Horizontal"

Following the works of Girard (1911) and Perez (1922) on the relations existing in man between the labyrinth and erect posture, Girard defined, in 1923, the "plan vestibulaire horizontal" as the line joining the centers of both foramina of the lateral semi-circular canal from one side. In 1952, Saban provided another definition of this plane as that passing through the ampullary portion of the lateral semicircular canal. Methods based on the vestibian axis were consequently developed and applied more precisely in the field of comparative craniology (Delattre and Daele 1950; Delattre and Fenart 1960; Fenart et al. 1966). Numerous applications have been reported using this methodological approach, in comparative anatomy, orthodontics ontogenesis and human paleontology. The localization of this reference system in vivo is, unfortunately, sometimes very difficult.

On the other hand, Caix and Beauvieux (1962) proposed a vestibulo-visual plane based on the superior oblique muscle of the eye and the semicircular canals. In man, this musculoskeletal plane is defined by the fact that the superior oblique muscle is oriented in the same plane as the lateral semicircular canal, its reflected tendon being parallel to the posterior canal.

2 The "Plan des Axes Orbitaires"

In his writings on the projections of the head, Broca stated: "the direction of gaze is the only characteristic of the living by which it may be determined that the head is horizontal. When man is standing and his visual axis is horizontal he is in his natural attitude" (Broca 1862, 1873 p. 578). He went on, in 1873, to describe two orbital axes, determined by two needles fixed in the optic canals and considered by him as passing through the pupils (Fig. 2.45). This was considered by him as a "sufficient approximation of the horizontal direction of gaze" (Broca 1873). Extending his research to animals, Broca defined, in 1877, the horizontal plane as "the plane determined in mammals by the two visual axes in an animal looking in the horizon direction", corresponding to the bi-orbital plane as defined for the cranium in animals, including man. He also demonstrated that this cephalic orientation lies close to the alveolar-condylar plane.

One century after his death, Broca's ideas regarding horizontality of the visual pathways were validated by CT. The NOP defines this cephalic orientation and orients the anatomic cuts (Cabanis et al. 1978).

III Brain Vertical Reference Lines and Planes

Three reference lines based on brain anatomic and midsagittal landmarks are retained (Fig. 2.46) and include the PC-OB used as a standard reference for the coronal investigation of the entire brain, and two other vertical lines described and proposed for more restricted anatomic areas, which are based on the AC and the mamillary bodies (MB).

A The Anterior Commissure-Mamillary Planes

The anterior commissure-mamillary vertical reference planes are based on the AC and the MB as the midsagittal landmarks. The first reference line, named the commissuro-mamillary (CA-CM) baseline, was defined by Guiot and Brion (1958), in an attempt to localize exactly the medial border of the globus pallidus, as well as its anterior aspect, in order to complete a stereotaxic pallidotomy for parkinsonian syndrome. The other plane, close to the former, has been described more recently by Baulac et al. (1990), based on the same anatomic landmarks used for imaging of the basal forebrain.

These vertical reference lines and planes differ to some extent (Fig. 2.37) if compared and applied to imaging. The plane used by Guiot and Brion in their stereotaxic approach to medial pallidum is defined as the line tangent to the posterior border of the AC passing through the premamillary notch (Fig. 2.47). This plane, close to the PC-OB plane, differs significantly from the CA-CM line which is defined as joining the center of the AC to the center of the MB (Fig. 2.48).

1 The Commissuro-Mamillary Reference Line

In this brain orientation, and according to the important work of the authors, which we have routinely verified using the coronal approach according to the PC-OB line by MRI, the anterior columns of the fornix are vertical from the level of the AC to the level of the premamillary notch, about 1.5 mm behind the CA-CM line.

According to Guiot and Brion (1958), this reference line gives the anterior topographic limit of the medial pallidum and, more precisely, its medial tip. The distance between the two landmarks averages 9.6 mm (8.5–11.5 mm) measured in 25 cases. This length appears very constant. The other interesting anatomic finding concerns the topography of the optic tract, which seems to follow a roughly parallel route, as compared to the base of the globus pallidus, and extends from its origin at the optic chiasm to the level of the MB. The optic tracts are separated from

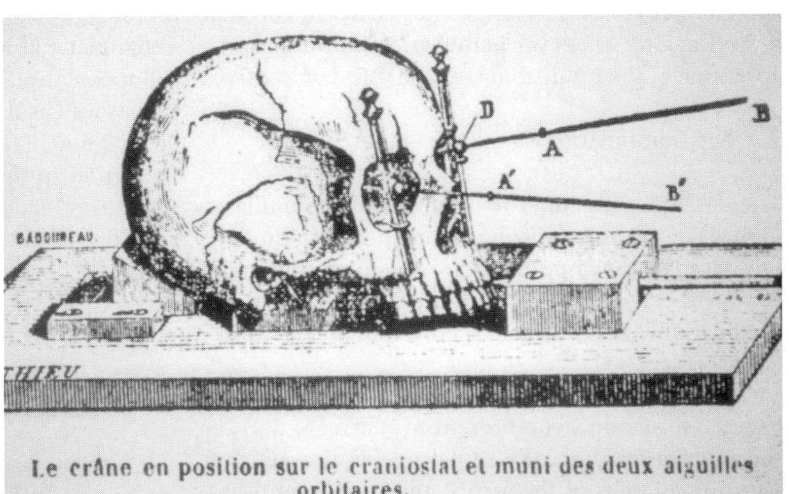
D
B
A
A'
B'
Le crâne en position sur le craniostat et muni des deux aiguilles orbitaires.

Fig. 2.45. The "bi-orbital" plane or the "plane of vision" of Broca (1873)

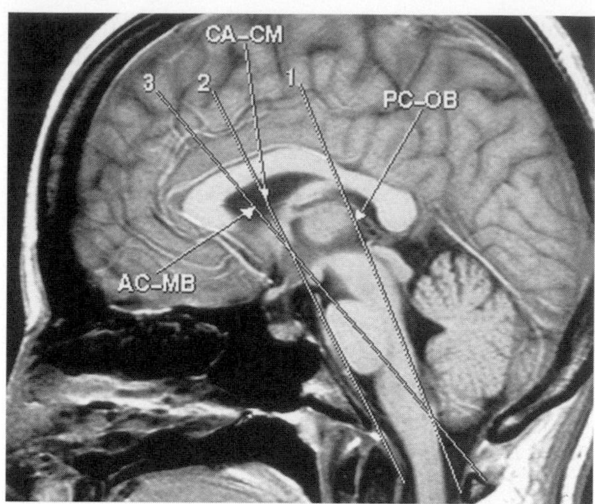

Fig. 2.46. Brain vertical reference lines and planes: *1*, PC-OB: commissural-obex plane (Tamraz et al. 1990, 1991); *2*, CA-CM: commissuro-mamillary plane (Guiot and Brion 1958); *3*, AC-MB: commissuro-mamillary plane (Baulac et al. 1990)

the basal aspect of the pallidum by 2 mm. This relationship explains, to some extent, the usual "X-shape" of the chiasm and tracts which are observed in the CH-PC line close to the perpendicular of the CA-CM line.

The CA-CM line shows constant topometric relation to the medial tip of the pallidum, which is difficult to localize anatomically due to its intrinsic relation with the pallidofugal bundles and the lenticular fasciculus. This is also true on MRI when contrast resolution is poor.

Considering the main anatomic correlations observed using this reference line, as it could be applied to brain imaging mainly for the basal ganglia, these results are close to the anatomic findings observed using the PC-OB reference line (see Sect. 10.IV) and, therefore, could be used as an alternative for coronal brain imaging whenever pathological conditions involve one of the brainstem (PC and OB) landmarks.

2 The Commissuro-Mamillary Plane

The obliqueness of the commissuro-mamillary plane is quite different from the former, even though it is based on the same anatomic structures, but joins center-to-center the AC and the MB, as is evident on the anatomic and MR cuts reported by Baulac et al. (1990) (Fig. 2.48).

This plane is utilized for the display of the anterior basal forebrain structures, from ventral to dorsal: the septum lucidum, the septal nuclei, the AC, the anterior columns of the fornix, and the MB projecting into the interpeduncular fossa. Note that this oblique plane is tilted more anteriorly as compared to the CA-CM line and, obviously, much more with respect to the parallel of the PC-OB plane, tangent to the posterior border of the AC (Fig. 2.49). It is interesting to note the similarity of these results with those obtained by Naidich et al. (1986) in their anatomic approach to the AC, which was considered a major landmark, at least in sagittal sections. According to these authors, the latter structure is nicely displayed in an axial oblique cut inclined 20–25° to the OM line.

Both orientations nicely display, from medial to lateral, the substantia innominata and the anterior perforated substance, easily seen beneath the AC. Note that the lateral temporal limbs of the AC are displayed in one single cut using the commissuro-mamillary orientation, its lateral extent being limited to the lateral aspect of the external pallidum, using the PC-OB orientation of the coronal cuts.

The anterior commissural plane, parallel to the PC-OB reference plane, may be considered as vertically limiting the anterior aspect of the ventral striatum and the CA-CM plane, defining more obliquely its rostrocaudal limit. Volumetric studies oriented to the study of the innominate substance of Reichert and, particularly, the basal nucleus of Meynert, in Alzheimer's disease or the various dementia syndromes of the Alzheimer type, may benefit from these landmarks.

A more extensive regional approach to cognitive and amnestic syndromes that may accompany the so-called extrapyramidal diseases would be more efficiently and globally evaluated on contiguous parallel slices oriented according to the vertical PC-OB reference line. This would cover an anterior-posterior region extending from the AC to the MB, involving the amygdala, or more largely from the chiasmal notch plane at least to the PC level (or the posterior callosal plane), to include the hippocampal formation as well as the septal-accumbens complex anterior to the AC (see the regional imaging approach to the septal-innominate and amygdalo-hippocampal structures, Chap. 6, and the synoptical atlas in the PC-OB orientation, chapt. 10.III).

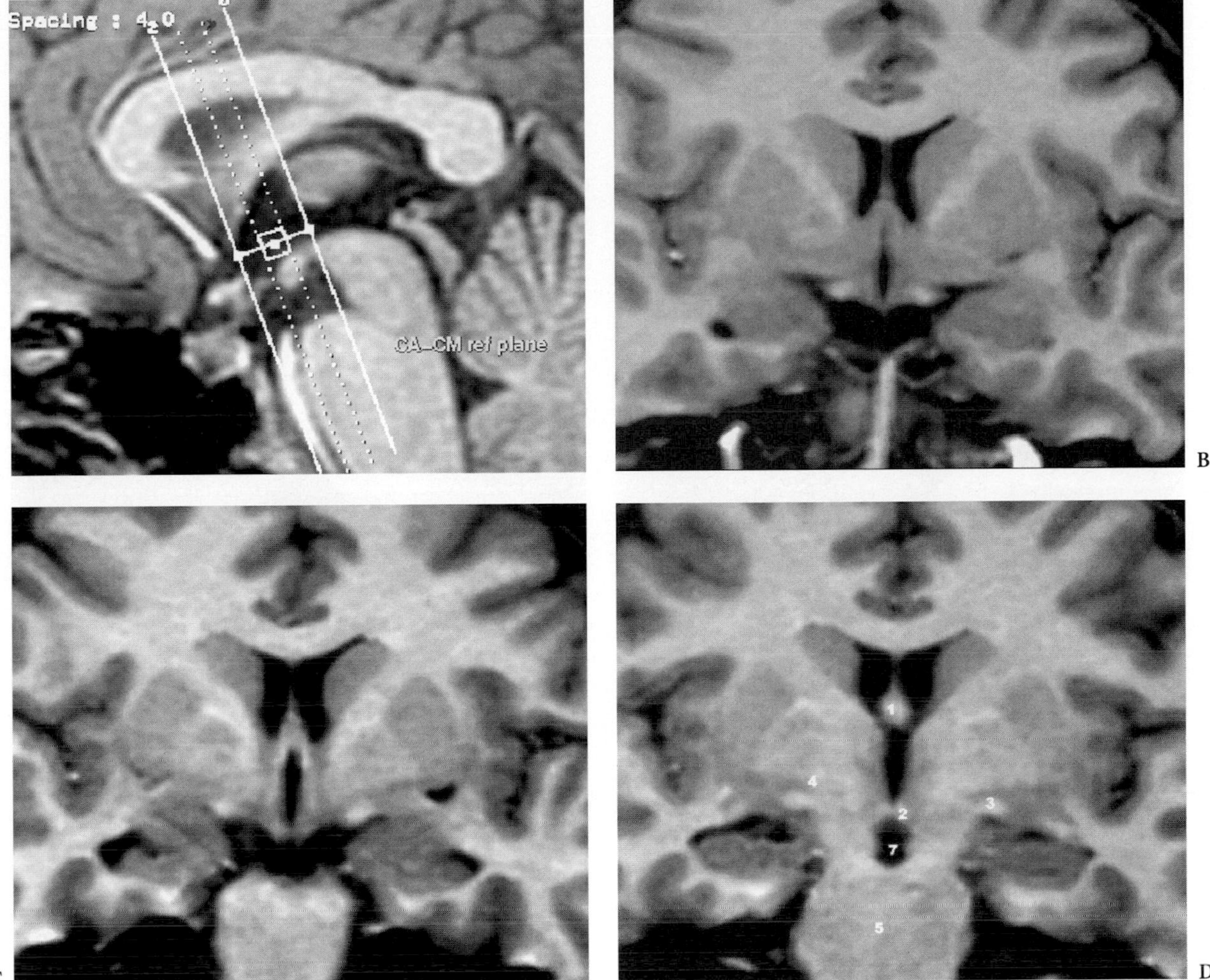

Fig. 2.47A–D. The CA-CM plane of Guiot and Brion (1958), defined as the line tangent to the posterior border of the anterior commissure and passing through the premamillary notch. This reference, defined to localize the medial tip of the medial pallidum, appears to be roughly parallel to the PC-OB reference plane and may therefore be used in regional imaging of the basal ganglia or the optic tracts and even the hippocampus. *1*, Anterior columns of fornix; *2*, mamillary bodies; *3*, pericrural optic tracts; *4*, tip of the medial globus pallidus; *5*, pons; *6*, medulla oblongata; *7*, interpeduncular cistern

B The Commissural-Obex Reference Plane

The commissural-obex reference line is defined as the line tangent to the anterior border of the PC, extending to the lower extremity of the calamus in the floor of the fourth ventricle behind the OB. This cephalic orientation describes, in our opinion, the main vertical axis of the brainstem and appears perpendicular to the CH-PC horizontal line, as previously demonstrated (Tamraz et al. 1990, 1991). With the sagittal plane, this line forms a coronal plane involving the brainstem cut along its long vertical axis (Fig. 2.46).

1 Biometric Findings

Two vertical reference lines are defined which could represent the vertical axis of the brainstem based on anatomic structures found in the midsagittal plane. They are reliable enough to permit reproducible alignment on follow-up exams if needed. The first line, called the PC-OB line, is tangent to the anterior border of the AC, superiorly, and extends to the inferior extremity of the floor of the fourth ventricle behind the OB, to which it is tangent anteriorly. The second line, called the VI-OB line, joins the superior insertion of the superior medullary velum at the

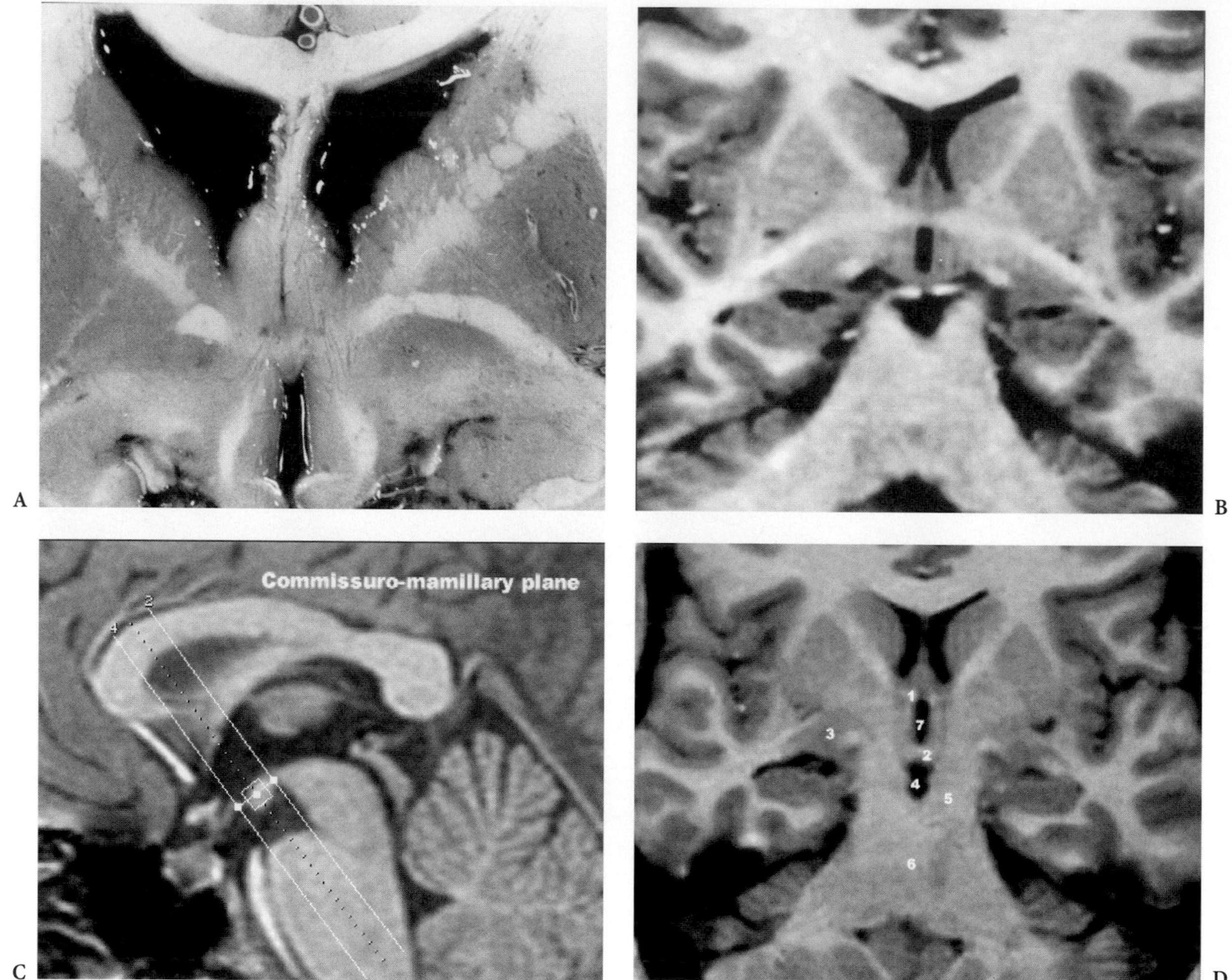

Fig. 2.48A–D. The commissuro-mamillary plane (Baulac et al. 1990), defined as joining the centers of the anterior commissure and the mamillary body, is proposed as the reference suitable for imaging of the anterior basal forebrain. The MR slice is 2 mm thick, T1 weighted, three-dimensional reformation. *1*, Anterior commissure; *2*, mamillary bodies; *3*, anterior basal forebrain; *4*, interpeduncular cistern; *5*, crus cerebri *6*, pons; *7*, third ventricle. (The anatomic cross-section provided by Baulac et al. 1990)

frenulum veli to the OB, to which it is tangent posteriorly. These lines intercept the horizontal CH-PC line with which they form two angles, CH-PC-OB and CH-VI-OB, respectively.

These two truncal angles were statistically evaluated and measured on a series of 100 in vivo MR exams. The CH-PC-OB angle appears to be at right angles to the main axis of the brainstem, measuring 93.7° (range 83–102°, SD 3.421). The CH-VI-OB proved to be more variable, averaging 85.54° (range 71–101°, SD 4.411). These two lines form an angle of about 8°. The former is retained as the brainstem vertical axis, approximately perpendicular to the CH-PC plane and considered as the reference for the coronal cuts of the brain.

2 Anatomic and Imaging Correlations

The PC-OB reference line intercepts, with the midsagittal plane, a PC-OB reference plane which laterally comprises the lateral geniculate bodies (Fig. 2.50). The lateral geniculate bodies, like the medial, are topometrically and volumetrically constant and do not show statistically significant variations between individuals, according to Delmas and Pertuiset (1959). They constitute lateral landmarks to this vertical reference, the horizontal CH-PC line projecting tangentially to their superior aspect.

Interestingly, the orientation of this plane is roughly parallel to the direction of the phylogenetically preserved, medial longitudinal fasciculi, easily

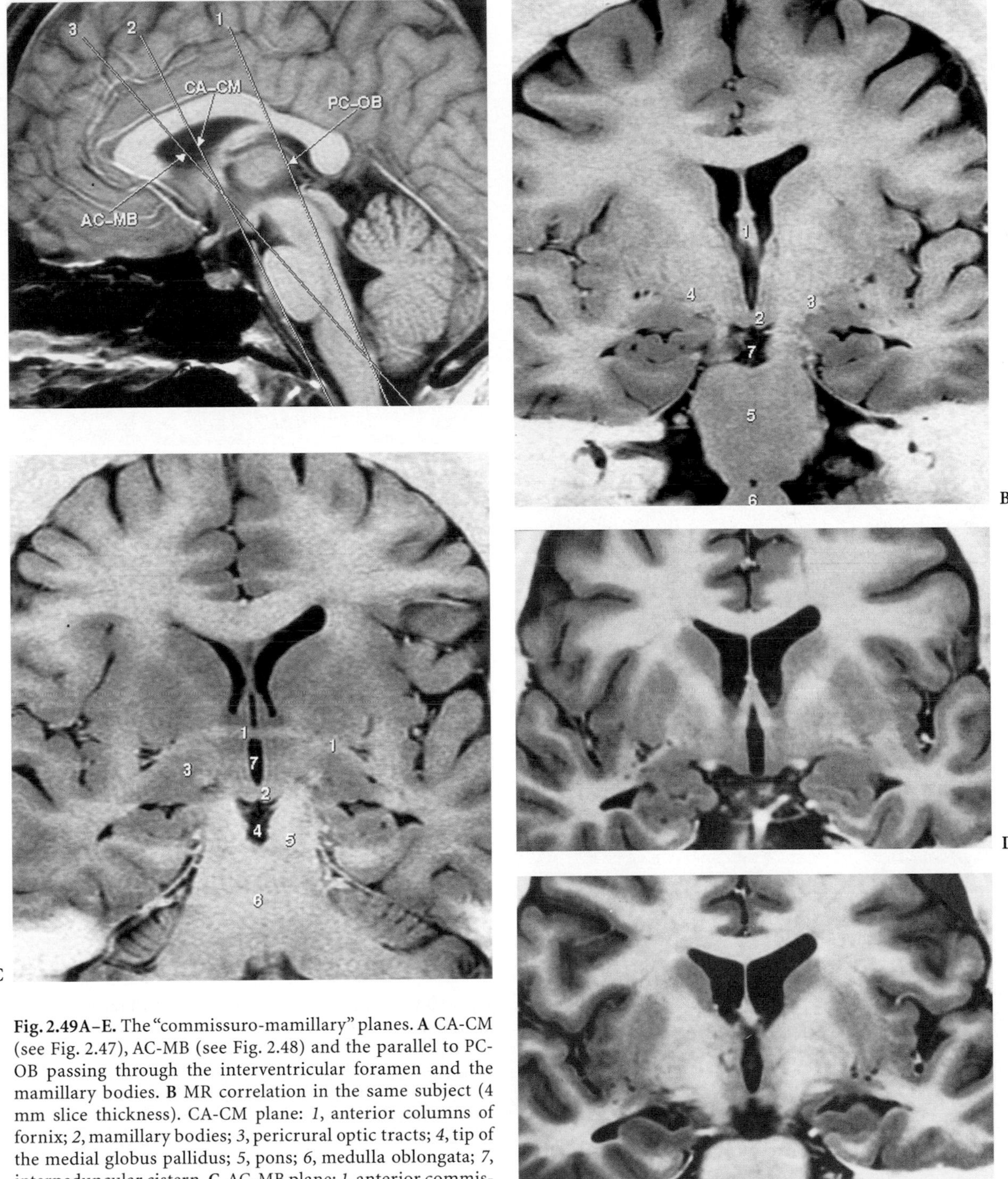

Fig. 2.49A–E. The "commissuro-mamillary" planes. **A** CA-CM (see Fig. 2.47), AC-MB (see Fig. 2.48) and the parallel to PC-OB passing through the interventricular foramen and the mamillary bodies. **B** MR correlation in the same subject (4 mm slice thickness). CA-CM plane: *1*, anterior columns of fornix; *2*, mamillary bodies; *3*, pericrural optic tracts; *4*, tip of the medial globus pallidus; *5*, pons; *6*, medulla oblongata; *7*, interpeduncular cistern. **C** AC-MB plane: *1*, anterior commissure; *2*, mamillary bodies; *3*, anterior basal forebrain; *4*, interpeduncular cistern; *5*, crus cerebri; *6*, pons; *7*, third ventricle. **D,E** Parallels to the PC-OB reference plane, passing through the anterior commissure and anterior columns of the fornix (**D**) and through the interventricular foramen and the mamillary bodies at their posterior notch (**E**)

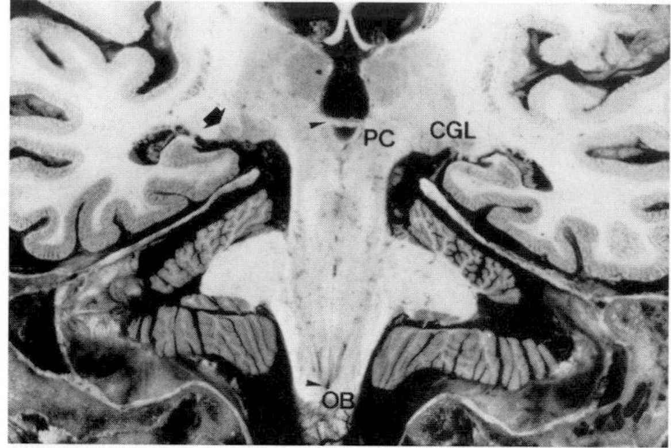

A

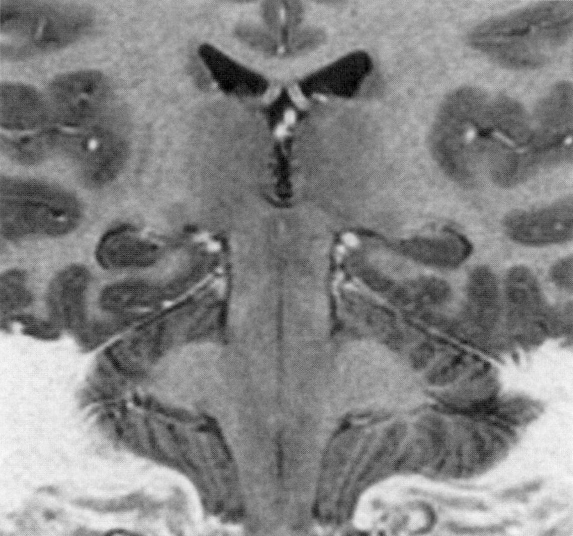
B

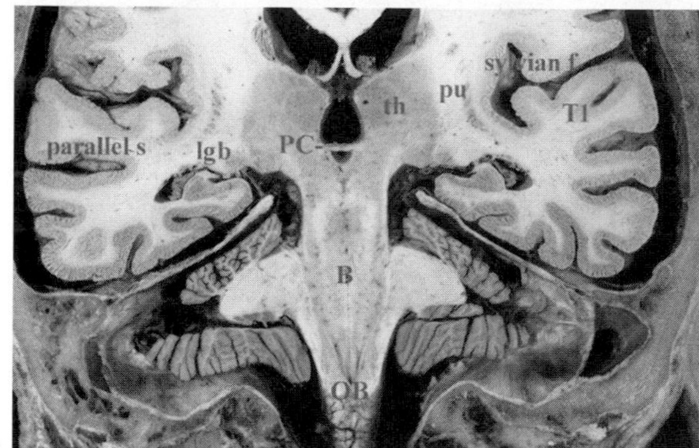

C

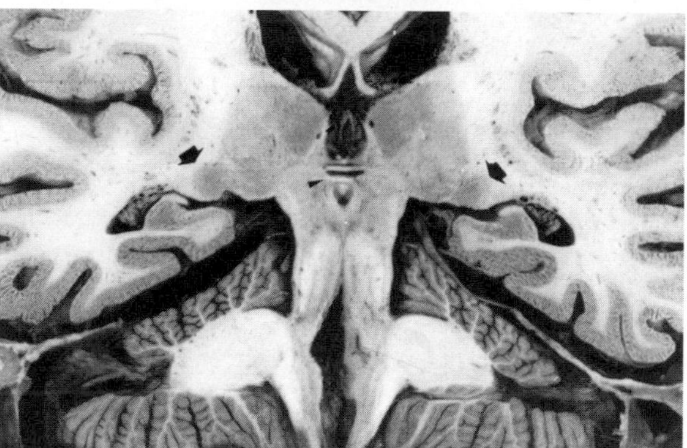
D

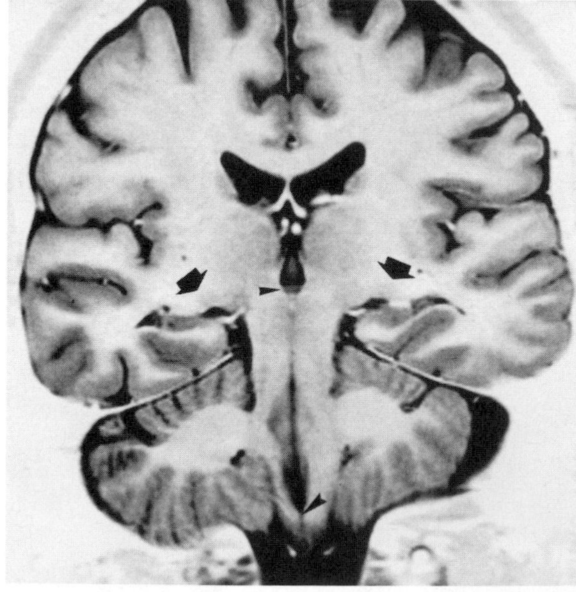
E

Fig. 2.50A–E. The commissural-obex (*PC-OB*) reference line: anatomic and MR correlations. The anatomic coronal cuts are separated by about 1 mm, showing the anatomic landmarks (*arrowheads*): the posterior commissure (*PC*) and the inferior extremity of the calamus behind the obex (*OB*). The lateral geniculate bodies (*CGL*) are contained in the cut, visualized laterally (*arrows*). Note that this reference cut limits the posterior boundary of the putamen and the insula

seen on the midsagittal cut (Fig. 2.51). Note that these tracts are found under the floor of the fourth ventricle, extending throughout the entire brainstem, and undergo a partial decussation in the PC, the upper landmark of the reference plane.

Such an orientation of the slices permits the study of the brainstem according to its vertical long axis, displaying both corticospinal tracts from the mid-brain-diencephalic junction to the inferior medulla at the level of their decussation. This is well shown on T2 weighted MRI in normal sections, as well as in degenerative or demyelinating diseased states (Fig. 2.52). Such an orientation differs from the perpendicular to both the AC-PC plane and the callosal plane, and is closely oriented to the intracerebral route of the cortico-spinal traets.

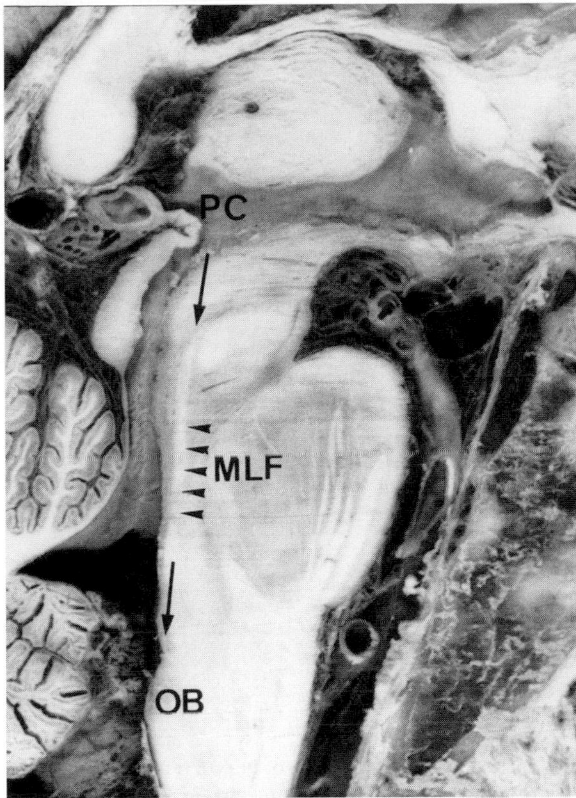

Fig. 2.51. The PC-OB plane follows roughly the direction of the sagittally oriented medial longitudinal fasciculi (*MLF*) (*arrowheads*)

Another significant parallelism is represented by the Monro-mamillary plane or cut, parallel to the PC-OB and comprising the interventricular foramina and the MB, both corresponding to highly constant anatomic structures that could be retained for imaging purposes as anterior alternative landmarks (Fig. 2.53). The topometric constancy of the MB is actually associated with the ontogeny of the interventricular foramina, as demonstrated by Delmas and Pertuiset (1959). This plane constitutes the anterior limit of the brainstem slices as well as the transthalamic limit (see Chap. 10).

The perpendicular relation of this reference to the CH-PC plane, as shown, explains its high accuracy for the study of the temporal lobes. The temporal pole is, in fact, usually included between the plane tangent to the genu of the corpus callosum (anterior callosal plane, CCg) or the "genu" of the cingulate sulcus (anterior cingulate plane, CSa) to include the tip of the temporal pole. The posterior extension, the posterior callosal plane (CCs), is arbitrarily provided by the plane tangent to the splenium of the corpus callosum. Both limiting planes are traced parallel to the PC-OB reference line.

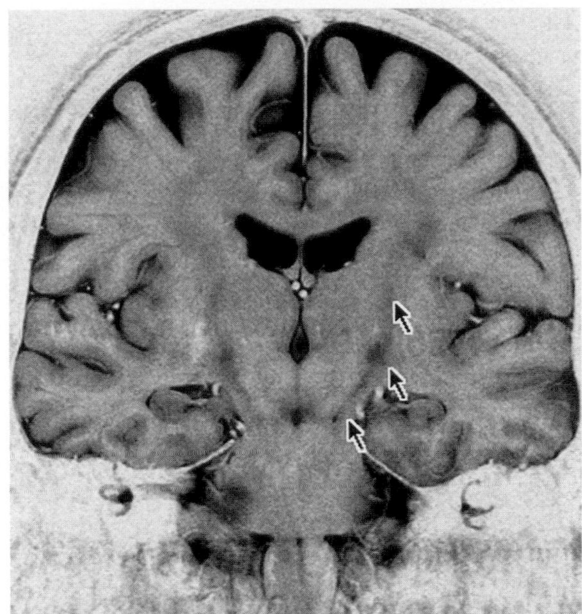

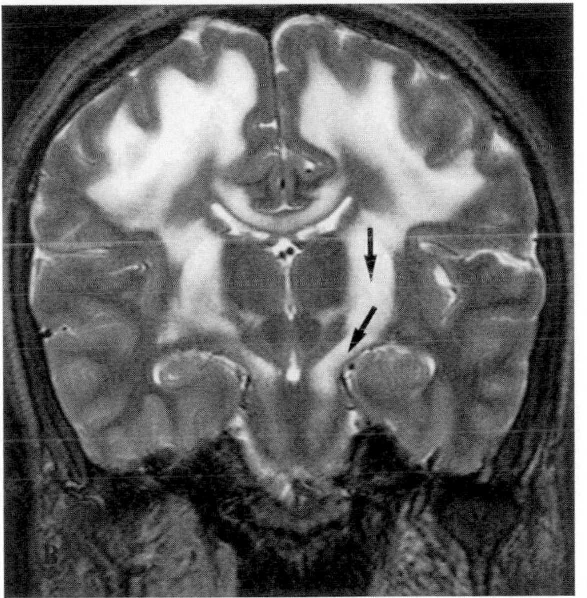

Fig. 2.52A,B. The PC-OB plane oriented roughly parallel to the corticospinal pathways displayed from the midbrain-diencephalic junction to the level of the medullary decussation, as shown on the MR coronal cut parallel to PC-OB (**A**) obtained from a patient presenting a toxic degeneration of these pathways, as compared to the perpendicular to the bicommissural plane (**B**)

This posterior plane passes through the superior inflection of the cingulate sulcus-marginal ramus on the mesial aspect of the hemisphere and at approximately the region of origin of the ascending rami of the lateral fissure on the lateral aspect of the hemisphere. This latter plane may be considered the pos-

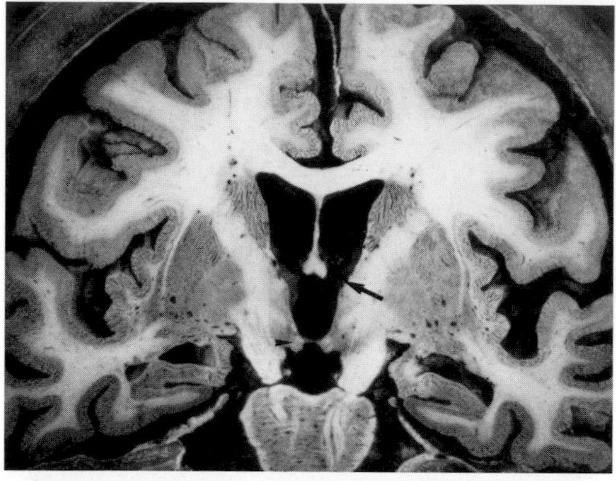
A

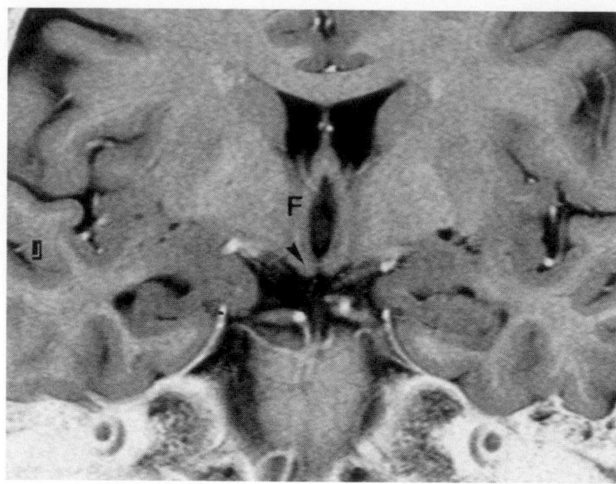

B

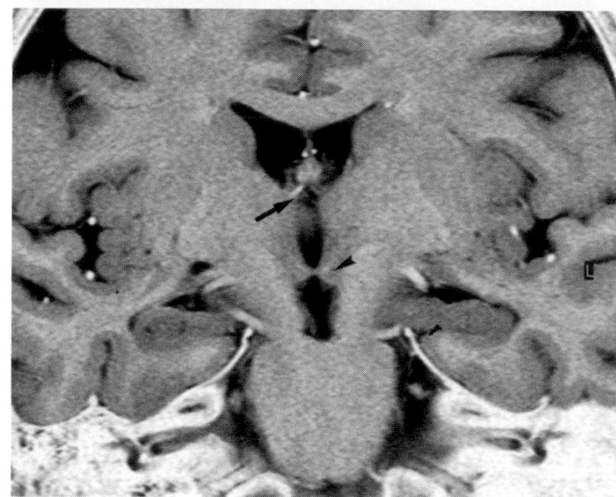
C

Fig. 2.53A–C. Close parallelism of PC-OB reference line to the Monro-mamillary plane: anatomic imaging correlation. Anatomic cut (6 mm thick) as compared to contiguous MR slices (3 mm thick) through the mamillary bodies, successively involving the anterior columns of the fornix (*F*) and, posteriorly, the interventricular foramen (*arrow*). Interventricular foramen of Monro (*arrow*); mamillary bodies (*arrowhead*)

terior boundary of the temporal lobe with the parieto-occipital inferior to the sylvian fissure.

The temporal pole may be arbitrarily limited posteriorly by the plane tangent to the genu of corpus callosum, passing anteriorly approximately through the anterior limit of the parallel sulcus.

The coronal slices from the CCg or the CSa anterior limiting plane to the CCs (Fig. 2.54) best evaluate the temporal gyri and sulci due to their approximate anterior-posterior parallelism and to the direction of the lateral fissure, surrounding the temporal horns of the lateral ventricles, at the lateral and inferomesial aspects of the cerebral hemispheres. The optic radiations coursing laterally along the external aspect of the temporal occipital horn are, consequently, well displayed in the white matter core, mainly on proton density or STIR sequences. Their relationship, with respect to the anterior temporal pole or to a temporal mass, may be evaluated as well in preoperative planning. The suprasylvian gyri may also benefit from such an orientation of the slices

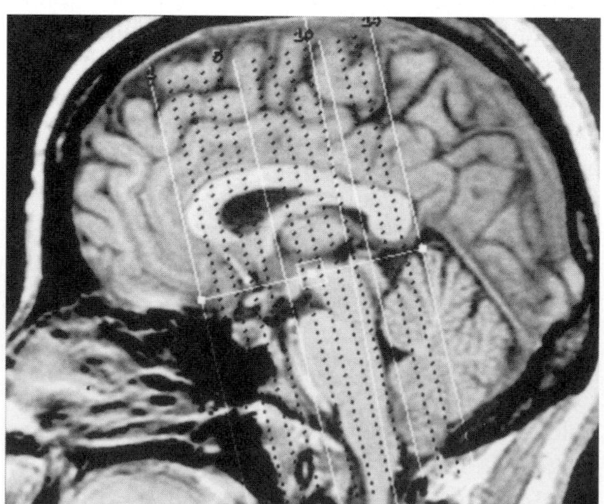

Fig. 2.54. Coronal imaging protocol for exploration of the temporal lobes according to the commissural-obex (*PC-OB*) brainstem reference plane

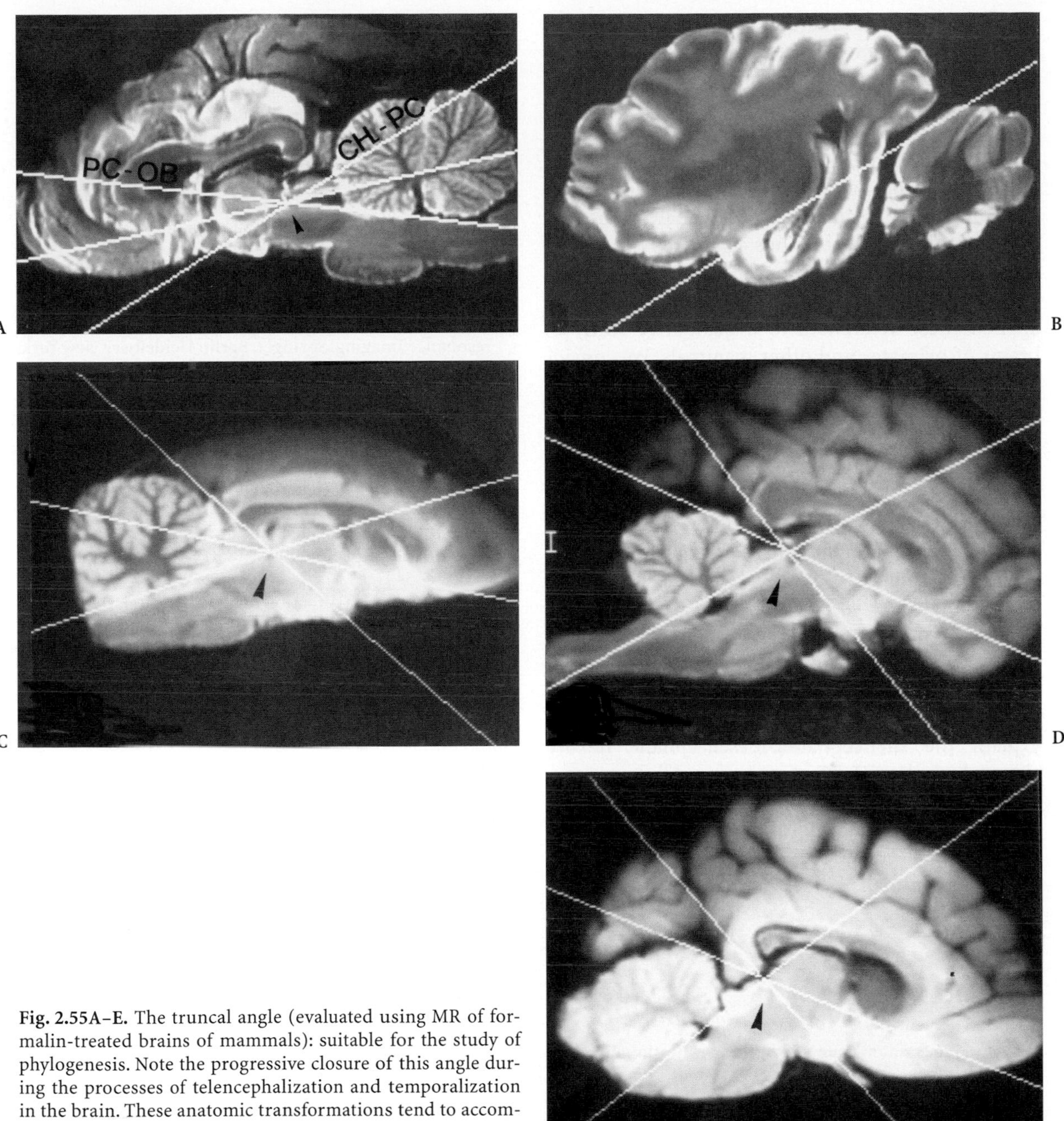

Fig. 2.55A–E. The truncal angle (evaluated using MR of formalin-treated brains of mammals): suitable for the study of phylogenesis. Note the progressive closure of this angle during the processes of telencephalization and temporalization in the brain. These anatomic transformations tend to accompany the evolutionary process toward erect posture. **A,B** ursus; **C** lemur; **D** orangutan; **E** chimpanzee

due to the parallelism of some of the adjacent sulci, such as the inferior frontal sulcus.

On clinical and pathological grounds, such a reference allows the evaluation of degenerative atrophic processes, such as those associated with dementia syndromes or mental retardation (Tamraz et al. 1987, 1991, 1993). The accuracy of this plane for the investigation of temporal lobe epilepsy is obvious, as it permits the direct evaluation of the mesial temporal region, as well as the temporal cortex and lobe, cut perpendicularly to their anterior-posterior axis. This has been well demonstrated in the successive cuts presented in the synoptical atlas by Tamraz et al. (1990, 1991, 1988; Tamraz 1994; Chap. 10). The hippocampal formations are sectioned perpendicular to their global long axis. To some extent, the results are close to the anatomic cuts presented by Duvernoy (1995) in his coronal approach to the hippocampus.

On comparative anatomic grounds, the PC-OB and CH-PC references, which are based on commissural landmarks found in all vertebrates, may be easily used in phylogenetic studies using MR imaging for primates or other lower mammalian species (Fig. 2.55). Comparative anatomy studies in vivo and in vitro may be performed as well, using these reference lines. For example, in order to analyze, the major anatomic transformations completed during the phylogenetic process of telencephalization which accompanied evolution toward the erect position, we applied these references to a qualitative study of brains of primates and other mammals. We considered the well known modifications of the "truncal angle", as named by Ariens Kappers (1947; Ariens Kappers et al. 1936, 1967), and replaced it by the previously defined CH-PC-OB angle (Tamraz 1991). This angle, which in lower mammals is open superiorly, tends to progressively open inferiorly in the primates to reach 90° in humans. Such transformations, which correspond to a progressive closure of the truncal angle, are associated with a rotation of the cerebral hemispheres, causing a posterior to anterior displacement of the temporal lobes, rotating around a transverse axis and a verticalization of the brainstem (Delattre and Fenart 1960). This process may explain the diencephalon-mesencephalic flexure along which the CH-PC plane passes. All these ontogenetic and phylogenetic modifications accompanying the temporalization of the cerebral hemispheres might to be correlated with the erect posture achieved in humans.

References

Aeby C (1862) Eine neue Methode zur Bestimmung der Schädelform von Menschen und Saugetieren. Westermann, Braunschweig

Amador LV, Blundell JE, Wahren W (1959) Description of coordinates of the deep structures. In: Schaltenbrand G, Bailey P (eds) Introduction to stereotaxis with an atlas of the human brain, vol 1. Thieme, Stuttgart pp 16–28

Ariens Kappers CU (1947)Anatomie comparée du système nerveux. Masson, Paris (with the collaboration of E.H. Strasburger)

Ariens Kappers CU, Huber GC, Crosby EC (1936) Comparative anatomy of the central nervous system of vertebrates, including man, vol 1 and 2. Macmillan, New York

Ariens Kappers CU, Huber GC, Grosby EC (1967) The comparative anatomy of the nervous system of vertebrates, including man, vol III. Hafner, New York

Baulac M, Iba Zizen MT, Granat O, Lehericy S, Vitte E, Signoret JL, Cabanis EA (1990) The commissuro-mamillary plane in MRI of the brain. Surg Radiol Anat 12:299–301

Barclay J (1803) A new anatomical nomenclature relating to the terms which are expressive of position and aspect in the animal system. Ross and Blackwood, Edinburgh

Beauvieux J (1934) Recherces anatomiques sur les canaux semi-circulaires des vertébrés. Thèse médecine, Bordeaux

Bell C (1805) Essay on the anatomy of expression in painting. London

Bell C (1806) The anatomy and philosophy of expression as connected with the fine arts. London

Bergvall U, Rumeau C, Van Bunnen Y, Corbaz JM, Morel M (1988) External references of the bicommissural plane. In: Gouaze A, Salamon G (eds) Brain anatomy and magnetic resonance imaging. Springer, Berlin Heidelberg New York, pp 2–11

Bjork A (1947) The face and profile. Svensk Tandl Tidskr 40:5

Blumenbach JF (1795) De generis humani varietate natura, 3rd edn. Thesis, Göttingen

Brégeat P, Cabanis EA, Iba-Zizen MT, Tamraz J, Stoffels C, Alfonso JM, Lopez A, Le Bihan D (1986) Nerf optique et Résonance magnétique. Bull Soc Ophthalmol France 5:86

Broca P (1862) Sur les projections de la tête, et sur le nouveau procédé de céphalométrie. Bull Soc Anthropol Paris 3(1):514–544

Broca P (1872) Sur la direction du trou occipital. Description du niveau occipital et du goniomètre occipital. Bull Soc Anthropol Paris 7(2):649–668

Broca P (1873) Nouvelles recherches sur le plan horizontal de la tête et sur le degré d'inclinaison des divers plans crâniens. Bull Soc Anthropol Paris 8(2):542–563

Broca P (1877) Sur l'angle orbito-occipital. Bull Soc Anthropol Paris 12(2):325–333

Busk G (1861) Observations on a systematic mode of craniometry. Trans Ethnol Soc London 1:341–348

Cabanis EA, Salvolini U, Radallec A, Menichelli F, Pasquini U, Bonnin P (1978) Computed tomography of the optic nerve, part II. Size and shape modifications in papilledema. J Comput Assist Tomogr 2:150–155

Cabanis EA, Haut J, Iba-Zizen MT (1980) Exopthtalmométrie tomodensitométrique et biométrie TDM oculo-orbitaire. Bull Soc Ophthalmol 80:63–66

Cabanis EA, Pineau H, Iba-Zizen MT, Coin JL, Newman N, Salvolini U (1981) CT scanning in the 'neuro-ocular plane': the optic pathways as a 'new' cephalic plane. Neuro-ophthalmology, vol 1(4). Aeolus, Amsterdam, pp 237–252

Cabanis EA, Iba-Zizen MT, Pineau H, Tamraz J et al (1982) Le plan neuro-oculaire (PNO) en tomodensitométrie (TDM ou scanner RX), détermination d'un "nouveau" plan horizontal de référence céphalique orienté selon les voies visuelles, the neuro-ocular plane (NOP) A new horizontal cephalic reference determined with CT by the optic pathways. Biometr Hum Paris 17:21–48

Cabanis EA, Tamraz J, Iba-Zizen MT (1988) Corrélations anatomiques normales dans 3 dimensions selon l'orientation du plan neuro-oculaire à 0,5 Tesla. In: Cabanis EA, Doyon D, Tamraz J et al (eds) Atlas d'IRM de l'encéphale et de la moëlle. Masson, Paris, pp 11–120

Caix M, Beauvieux J (1962) Note préliminaire sur le plan vestibulo-visuel. CR As Anat 48:396–407

Camper P (1791) Dissertation sur les variétés naturelles qui caractérisent la physionomie des Hommes des divers climats et les différents âges. Jansen, Paris

Clavelin P (1932) Sur le plan d'orientation du maxillaire inférieur. Rev Stomatol 34:705–708

Combe G (1839) Constitution of man considered in relation to external object. Maclach and Stewart, Edinburgh

Cuvier G (1835) Leçons d'anatomie comparée de Georges cuvier recueillies et publiées par M. Duméril. Paris, Crochard et Cie, 1, p 588

Daubenton A, Daele JM (1764) Sur les différences de la situation du grand trou occipital dans l'homme et dans les animaux. Mem Acad Sci Paris pp 568–575

Déjerine J (1895) Anatomie des centres nerveux. Rueff, Paris

Delattre A, Daele JM (1950) La méthode vestibulaire en craniologie. CR Acad Sci 230:1981–1982

Delattre A, Fenart R (1960) L'hominisation du crâne étudiée par la méthode vestibulaire. CNRS, Paris

Delmas A, Pertuiset B (1959) Topométrie crânio-encéphalique chez l'homme. Masson, Paris

Devaux B, Meder JF, Missir O, Turak B, Dilouya A, Merienne L, Chodkiewicz JP, Fredy D (1996) La ligne rolandique: une ligne de base simple pour le repérage de la région centrale. Masson, Paris, pp 6–18 (Journal of neuroradiology, vol 23)

Doornik JE (1808) Wysgeerig natuurkundig onderzoek aangaande den oorspronkelyken mensch en de oorspkerronglyke stammen van deszelfs gesachts (sur l'homme primitif et ses races), Amsterdam

Duvernoy H (1995) Brain anatomy. In: Kuzniecky R, Jackson G (eds) Magnetic resonance in epilepsy. Raven, New York

Fenart R, Empereur-Buissin R, Becart P (1966) Première application au vivant de l'orientation vestibulaire du crâne. J Sci Med Lille 84:189–195

Fenart R, Vincent H, Cabanis EA (1982) Le plan orbitaire chez l'adulte jeune, sa position relative à d'autres éléments architecturaux de la tête. Etude vestibulaire. Bull Mem Soc Anthropol Paris 9(XIII):29–40

Gelbert F, Bergvall U, Salamon G, Sobel D, Jiddane M, Corbaz JM, Morel M (1986) CT identification of cortical speech areas in the human brain. J Comput Assist Tomogr 9:140–153

Girard L (1911) Atlas d'anatomie chirurgicale du labyrinthe. Maloine, Paris

Girard L (1923) Le plan des canaux semiè-circulaires horizontaux considéré comme plan horizontal de la tête. Bull Mem Soc Anthropol Paris 4(7):14–33

Guiot G, Brion S (1958) La destruction stéréotaxique du pallidum interne dans les syndromes parkinsonniens. Ann Chir 17:1–20

Habib M, Rennuci RL, Vanier M, Corbaz JM, Salamon G (1984) CT assessment of right left asymmetries in the human cerebral cortex. J Comput Assist Tomogr 8:922–927

Hamy D (1873) Discussion sur le plan horizontal de la tête par P. Broca. Bull Soc Anthropol Paris 8(2):93

Hilal SK, Trokel SL (1977) Computerized tomography of the orbit using thin sections. Semin Roentgenol 12:137–147

His W (1876) Über die Horizontalebene des menschlichen Schädels. Arch Anthropol 9:271

Huxley TH (1863) Evidence as to man's place in nature. William B (ed), Norgate, London, p 159

Ihering HV (1872) Ueber das Wesen der Prognathie und ihr Verhaltnisse zur Schädelbasis. Arch Anthropol 5:359–407

International Anatomical Nomenclature Committee (1989) Nomina Anatomica, 6th edn. Livingstone, Edinburgh

Klaatsch H (1909) Kraniomorphologie und Kraniotrigonometrie. Arch Anthropol 8:101–123

Krogman WM (1931) Studies in growth changes in the skull and face of Anthropoids. Am J Anat 47:89–115; 325–365

Lang J (1987) Clinical anatomy of the head: neurocranium, orbit, cranio-cervical region. Springer, Berlin Heidelberg New York

Lehman RM, Olivier A, Moreau JJ, Tampieri D, Henri C (1992) Use of the callosal grid system for the preoperative identification of the central sulcus. Stereotact Funct Neurosurg 58:179–188

Lucae JCG (1872) Zur Morphologie des Saugethier-Schädels. Winter, Frankfurt

Maly J (1924) Sklon vchodu ocnice jako pomocne rovina orientacni. (L'inclinaison de l'ouverture orbitaire comme plan d'orientation du crâne). Anthropologie 2:224–230

Martin R (1928) Lehrbuch der Anthropologie in systematischer Darstellung, vol II. Kraniologie, osteologie, 2nd edn. Fischer, Jena, pp 582–591

Merckel F (1882) Zur Kenntniss der postembryonalen Entwicklung des menschlichen Schädel. Festschrift. Henle, Bonn

Michotey P, Grisoli F, Raybaud C, Salamon G (1974) Etude anatomique et radiologique de l'artère cérébrale moyenne. Procédé de repérage Ann Radiol 17:721–741

Morton SG (1839) Cranio americana. A comparative view of the skulls of various aboriginal nations of North and South America to which is prefixed an essay on the varieties of the human species. Dobson, Philadelphia, p 226

Naidich TP, Daniels DL, Pech P, Haughton VM, Williams A, Pojunas K (1986) Anterior commissure: anatomic-MR correlation and use as a landmark in three orthogonal planes. Radiology 158:421–429

Olivier A, Marchand E, Ethier R, Melanson D, Peters T (1985) A proposed anatomical methodology for MR scanning based on the corpus callosum. Proceedings, 4th Annual Meeting of Society of Magnetic Resonance in Medicine, 19–22 August, London

Olivier A, Peters TM, Clark JA, Marchand E, Mawko G, Bertrand G, Vanier M, Ethier R, Tyler J, de Lotbinière A (1987) Intégration de l'angiographie numérique, de la résonance magnétique, de la tomodensitométrie et de la tomotroencephalogr. Neurophysiol Clin 17:25–43

Olivier F (1978) Note sur la variabilité des axes basicrâniens. Bull Ass Anat 62:325–331

Ono M, Kubik S, Abernathey Chad D (1990) Atlas of the cerebral sulci. Thieme, Stuttgart

Perez F (1922) Craniologie vestibienne, ethnique et zoologique. Bull Mem Soc Anthropol Paris 3(7):16–32

Rumeau C, Gouaze A, Salamon G, Laffont J, Gelbert F, Einseidel H, Jiddane M, Farnarier P, Habib M, Perot S (1988) Identification of cortical sulci and gyri using magnetic resonance imaging: A preliminary study. In: Gouaze A, Salamon G (eds) Brain anatomy and magnetic resonance imaging. Springer, Berlin Heidelberg New York, pp 11–32

Saban R (1952) Fixité du canal semi-circulaire externe et variation de l'angle thyroidien. Mammalia 16:77–92

Saban R (1980) Les plans d'orientation de la tête. Cahiers Anthropol 3-4:285–313

Salamon G, Huang YP (1976) Radiologic anatomy of the brain. Springer, Berlin Heidelberg New York

Salamon G, Lecaque G (1978) Choice of the plane of incidence for computed tomography of the cerebral cortex. J Comput Assist Tomogr 2:937

Salvolini U, Cabanis EA, Rodallec A (1978) Computed tomography of the optic nerve, part I: normal results. J Comput Assist Tomogr 2:141–149

Schaltenbrand G, Bailey P (eds) (1959) Introduction to stereotaxis with an atlas of human brain. vol 2, Thieme, Stuttgart

Schaltenbrand G, Wahren W (1977) Atlas for stereotaxonomy of the human brain. 2nd edn. Thieme, Stuttgart

Spix (1815) Cephalogenesis sen capitis ossei structura formatio et signification per omnes animalium. Hubschmanni JS, Monachii, typis, p 72

Szikla G (1967) Topographie stéréotaxique de la scissure de Rolando et des réponse motrices évoquées au niveau du centre ovale par des stimulations liminaires de basse fréquence. Thesis, Paris

Szikla G, Talairach J (1965) Coordinates of the Rolandic sulcus and topography of cortical and subcortical motor responses to low frequency stimulation in a proportional stereotactic system. Confin Neurol (Basel) 26:474–475

Szikla G, Bouvier G, Hori T, Petrov V (1977) Angiography of the human brain cortex. Springer, Berlin Heidelberg New York

Takase M, Tokunaga A, Otani K, Horie T (1977) Atlas of the human brain for computed tomography based on the glabella-inion line. Neuroradiology 14:73–79

Talairach J, Tournoux P (1988) Co-planar stereotaxic atlas of the human brain. Three-dimensional proportional system: an approach to cerebral imaging. Thieme, Stuttgart

Talairach J, De Ajuriaguerra J, David M (1952) Etudes stéréotaxiques des structures encéphaliques chez l'homme. Presse Med 28:605–609

Talairach J, David M, Tournoux P, Corredor H, Kvasina T (1957) Atlas d'anatomie stéréotaxique des noyaux gris centraux. Masson, Paris

Talairach J, Szikla G, Tournoux P, Prossalentis A, Bordas-Ferrer M, Covello L, Iacob M, Mempel E (1967) Atlas d'anatomie stéréotaxique du télencéphale. Masson, Paris

Tamraz J (1983) Atlas d'anatomie céphalique dans le plan neuro-oculaire (PNO). MD thesis. Schering, Paris (1986)

Tamraz J (1991) Morphometrie de l'encephale par resonance magnetique: application à la pathologie chromosomique humaine, à l'anatomie comparée et à la teratologie. Thesis Doct Sci Paris V

Tamraz J (1994) Neuroradiologic investigation of the visual system using magnetic resonance imaging. J Clin Neurophysiol 11:500–518

Tamraz J, Iba-Zizen MT, Cabanis EA (1984) Atlas d'anatomie céphalique dans le plan neuro-oculaire (PNO). J Fr Ophtalmol 7(5):371–379

Tamraz J, Iba-Zizen MT, Atiyeh M, Cabanis EA (1985) Atlas d'anatomie céphalique dans le plan neuro-oculaire (PNO). Bull Soc Fr Ophtalmol 8-9(85):853–857

Tamraz J, Rethore MO, Iba-Zizen MT, Lejeune J, Cabanis EA (1987) Contribution of magnetic resonance imaging knowledge of CNS malformations related to chromosomal aberrations. Hum Genet 76:265–273

Tamraz J, Iba-Zizen MT, Cabanis EA (1988) Magnetic resonance imaging of the eyes and the optic pathways. In: Gouaze A, Salamon G (eds) Brain anatomy and magnetic resonance imaging. Springer, Berlin Heidelberg New York, pp 71–83

Tamraz J, Saban R, Reperant J (1989) The chiasmato-commissural plane. Scientific session (poster). Joint meeting of the European Society of Neuroradiology and the International Congress of Radiology, 6 July, Paris

Tamraz J, Saban R, Reperant J, Cabanis EA (1990) Définition d'un plan de référence céphalique en imagerie par résonance magnétique: le plan chiasmato-commissural. CR Acad Sci Paris 311(III):115–121

Tamraz J, Saban R, Reperant J, Cabanis EA (1991) A new cephalic reference plane for use with magnetic resonance imaging: the chiasmato-commissural plane. Surg Radiol Anat 13:197–201

Tamraz J, Rethore MO, Lejeune J, Outin C, Goepel R, Stievenart JL, Iba-Zizen MT, Cabanis EA (1993) Morphometrie encephalique dans la maladie du cri du chat. Ann Genet 36(2):75–87

Tokunaga A, Takase M, Otani K (1977) The glabella-inion line as a baseline for CT scanning of the brain. Neuroradiology 14:67–71

Topinard P (1882) Crâniomètre de Hoelder et méthode géométrique. Bull Mem Soc Anthropol Paris 5(3):402–414

Unsöld R, Newton TH, Hoyt WF (1980) CT examination technique of the optic nerve. J Comput Assist Tomogr 4:560–563

Van Damme W, Kosman P, Wackenheim C (1977) A standard method for computed tomography of orbits. Neuroradiology 13:139–140

Vanier M, Lecours AR, Ethier R, Habib M, Poncet M, Milette PC, Salamon G (1985) Proportional localization system for anatomical interpretation of cerebral computed tomogragrams. J Comput Assist 9(4):715–724

Villemin F, Beauvieux J (1937) Les relations des limites inféireures du crâne avec le plan horizontal de la tête chez les vertébrés. CR Soc Biol, Bordeaux

Vining DQ (1977) Computed tomography in ophthalmology. In: Smith L, (ed) Neuroophthalmology update. Masson, New York, pp 271–279

Von Baer (1860) Die Makrophalen in Boden der Kryn und Oesterreichs. Mem Acad St Petersburg 2:6

Walther FL (1802) Kritische Darstellung der Gallschen anatomisch-physiologischen Untersuchungen des Gehirns und Schädelbanes. Zurich

World Federation of Neurology (1962) Problem commission of neuroradiology: study meeting on projections and nomenclature. Br J Radiol 35:501–503

3 Brain Cortical Mantle and White Matter Core

I Historical Notes and Landmarks

In 1810, François-Joseph Gall initiated the study of the human cerebral cortex. In 1839, Leuret and his pupil, Gratiolet, attempted to classify the fissures of the human brain. However, the first to give a detailed account of the structure of the cerebral cortex was Baillarger (1840), who in addition described the gray and white matter. Meynert (1867, 1868) expanded on this finding and gave a detailed account of the regional variations existing in the cortical mantle and their structural and functional relationships. Following this major contribution, Betz (1874) described the motor area and its giant pyramidal cells which bear his name.

A large body of literature from the second part of the nineteenth and the early twentieth centuries reported on the frequency and variations of the sulcal pattern of the brain. These are found in the works of Zernov (1877), Cunningham and Horsley (1892), Retzius (1896), Kohlbrugge (1906), Landau (1910, 1911, 1914), Shellshear (1926), Van Bork-Feltkamp (1930), Slome (1932), Vint (1934), Chi and Chang (1941), Connolly (1950) and others.

Encephalometry, pioneered by Ariens Kappers (1847; Ariens Kappers et al. 1936), and later by von Economo (1929), was one of the most extensively used methods to study the brain. The brain index, also described by Ariens Kappers, was determined by measuring, on the lateral aspect of the brain, the length of the hemisphere and on the medial side, the occipital and temporal lobe length, (Fig. 3.1). He defined the callosal baseline connecting the basis of the genu to the basis of the splenium of the corpus callosum and measured accordingly the callosal length and height. Many brain indexes were subsequently reported, such as the callosal index, the central or the occipital index, as well as the temporal indexes of frontal height and frontal depth or length.

The relationship between the sulcation pattern of the cerebral hemispheres and genetics is still controversial despite the efforts of several authors (Karplus 1905, 1921; Sano 1916; Rossle 1937; Geyer 1940; Higeta 1940). We have recently reported using MR for in vivo brain morphology and morphometry on a series of patients with specific chromosomal aberrations (Tamraz et al. 1987,1990, 1991a,b, 1993). These preliminary qualitative morphometric results showed a clear cortical and brain phenotype accompanying the clinical syndromes.

The extensive work on racial differences in the early part of this century, aimed at disclosing brain morphological peculiarities, failed to a large extent. The anthropology of the human brain has not been adequately studied, as most series of brains analyzed from an encephalometric aspect are too small to yield significant results. If some racial differences do exist, it seems that they involve more particularly the lunate sulcus, the superior frontal sulcus and the temporal lobe and pole (Bailey and von Bonin 1951).

II Cytoarchitecture and Brain Mapping

Several methodologies were used in the assessment of the surface of the cerebral cortex, and the relative thickness of the cortical mantle in relation to particular anatomical regions, with slightly variable results, averaging 2000–2200 cm^2 (Wagner 1864; Calori 1870; Baillarger 1840; Jensen 1875; Giacomini 1878; Flechsig 1898; Campbell 1905; Benedikt 1906; Brodmann 1909; Henneberg 1910; Ramon y Cajal 1911; Jaeger 1914; Aresu 1914; von Economo and Koskinas 1925; Rose 1926; Kraus et al. 1928; Leboucq 1929; Lorente de No 1933; Filimonoff 1947).

Differences with respect to sex are emphasized by Aresu (1914) who reported values of 2300 cm^2 in males and 2000 cm^2 in females. A difference of about 136 cm^2 between brachicephalics and dolichocephalics in favor of the former was reported by Calori (1870). The ratio between external to buried surface has been reported by Henneberg (1910) and Jensen (1875). Both emphasized the larger development of the buried cortical surface averaging two thirds of the total cortical surface. This shows regional varia-

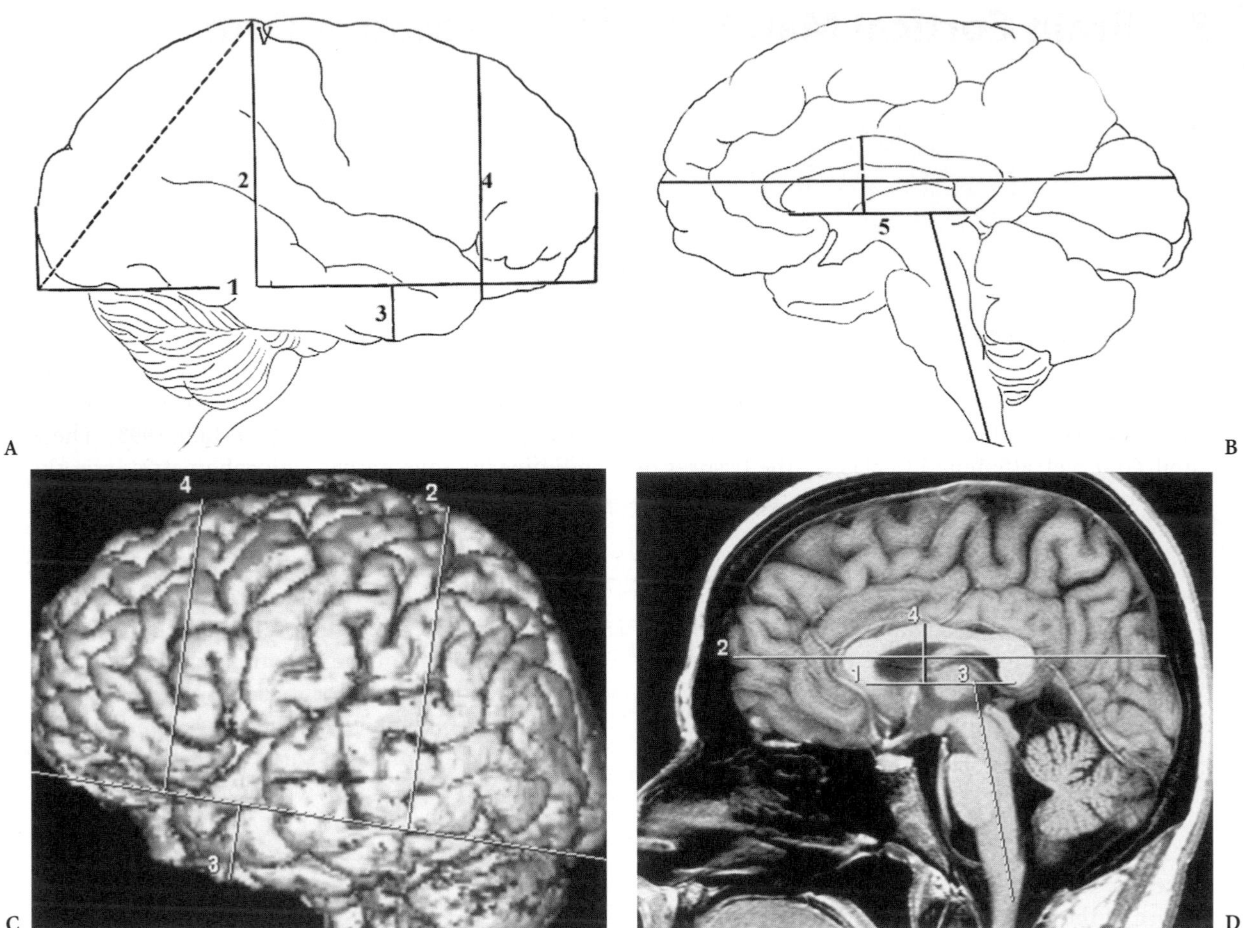

Fig. 3.1A–D. Encephalometry according to the methodology adopted by Ariens Kappers et al. (1936). **A** *1*, The horizontal lateral line, tangent to the ventral aspect of the occipital lobe and the fronto-orbital lobe; *2*, the parietal perpendicular line, from the highest parietal point; *3*, the temporal perpendicular line, from the lowest temporal point. **B** *4*, The callosal basal line tangent inferiorly to the genu and the splenium of the corpus callosum. **C,D** MR correlations

tions, ranging from as much as 4.5 mm in the precentral cortex to 1.5 mm in the depth of the calcarine sulcus. Actually, it increases from the frontal pole to the central cortex (2.2–3.3 mm), then decreases progressively in thickness from the postcentral gyrus toward the occipital pole (3.3–1.5 mm). The cortical thickness of the postcentral bank of the central sulcus is thinner than that of the precentral. The cortical ribbon of the central sulcus is thicker than the remaining part of the precentral gyrus. The cortical thickness decreases with age. The cortex is generally thicker on the apex of the convolution, decreasing in thickness in the depth of the sulci. In the future, high resolution MR, particularly with the use of small dedicated surface coils, will allow in vivo analysis of cortical thickness and will enhance the detection of focal abnormalities.

Jaeger (1914) measured the volume of the cortex at 540–580 cm^3 as compared to that of the white matter, about 400–490 cm^3. The number of cells in the cerebral cortex has been estimated by von Economo and Koskinas (1925) as averaging 15 billion neuronal cells.

The cytoarchitecture of the cortex is not uniform, showing wide variations in its intrinsic structural composition and thickness, as previously reported. Von Economo classifies the cerebral cortex into five fundamental types based on the partitioning of the pyramidal and granular cells. The homotypical type with the widest representation comprises the frontal (type II), the parietal (type III) and the polar (type IV). The heterotypical, limited to particular areas, comprises the agranular (type I) and the granular (type V) cortices. This classification differs from those previously proposed by Baillarger (1840) or Ramon y Cajal (1911).

Three different conceptual approaches were undertaken to map the human brain. The functional anatomical approach was inaugurated by Broca and followed by Jackson. The cytoarchitectural myelogenetic study was initiated by Baillarger, followed by Ramon y Cajal, and later popularized by Brodmann. The third approach was based on the study of the gyral and sulcal patterns. These three approaches converged as correlations between gross morphology, cytoarchitecture, myelogenesis and function progressively evolved.

Flechsig (1898) used the myelogenetic method based on the investigation of the spatiotemporal distribution of myelination in the immediate subcortical regions. He reported a myelogenetic map of the cerebral cortex with 40 cortical fields grouped into primordial (1–8), intermediate (9–32) and terminal (33–40) areas. The first eight are considered as sensory areas, the intermediate as associative, and the remaining terminal areas are specific to humans, as may be distinguished from the anthropoid brains (Fig. 3.2).

In 1905, Campbell presented his own map of the cerebral cortex based on cytoarchitectural patterns (Fig. 3.3). At the same time, Brodmann also proposed his widely used map of the human brain (Fig. 3.4) based on ontogenesis. Unfortunately, due to his premature death, it was without any accompanying description of the areas indicated on the drawings as he had provided for the cercopithecus.

Continuing in the same trend, Vogt and Vogt described more than 200 different cytoarchitectural ar-

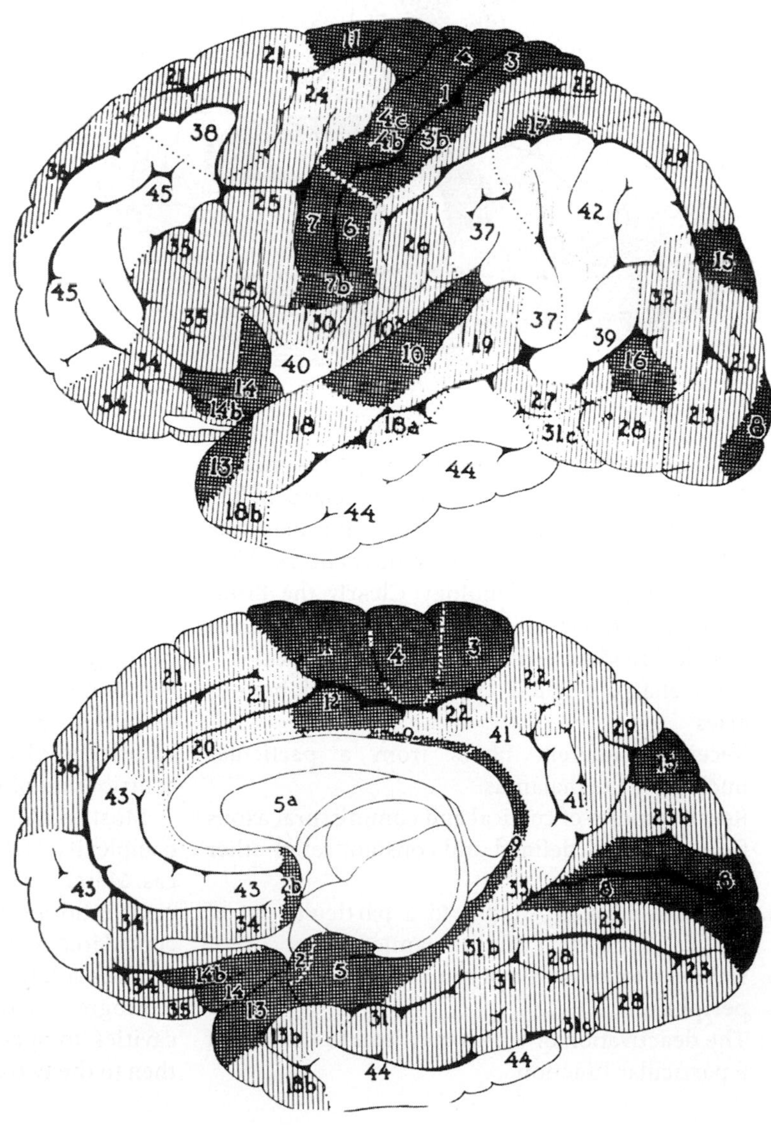

Fig. 3.2. Myelogenetic map of the cerebral cortex. Primordial areas numbered 1–8 (*cross-hatched areas*); terminal areas numbered 30–40 (*open areas*); intermediate areas numbered 9–32 (*lines*). (From Flechsig 1898)

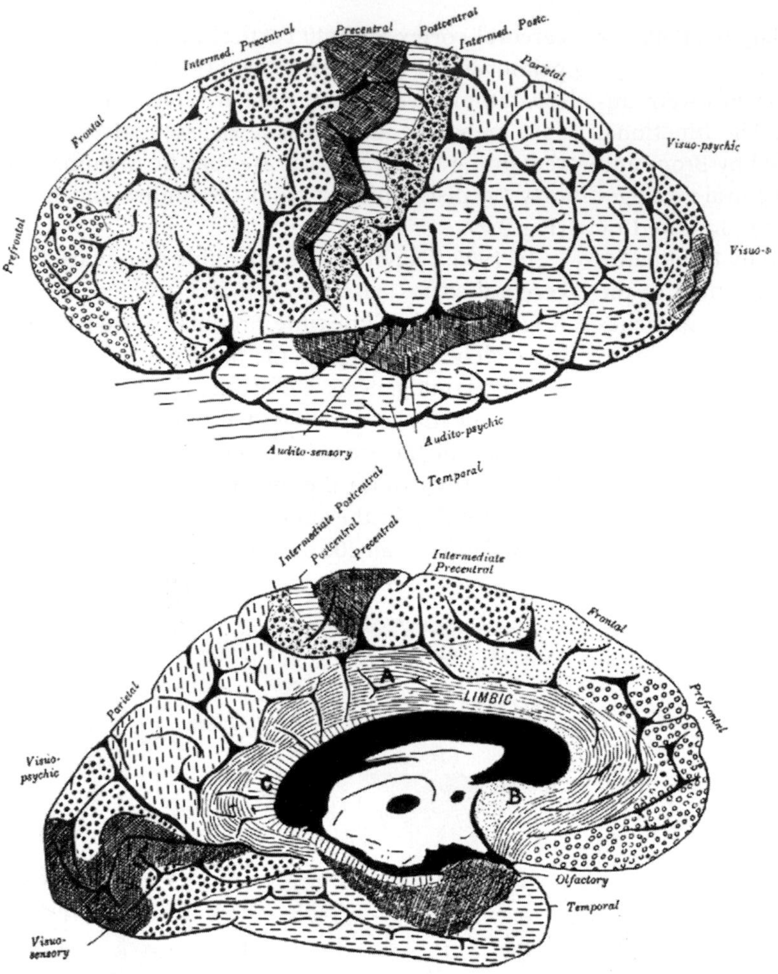

Fig. 3.3. Map of the cerebral cortex. (From Campbell 1905)

eas in the human brain cortex (Fig. 3.5). This attempt to "overparcelize" the cortex was criticized in the 1950s and 1960s. However, the Brodmann map survived these criticisms, and the numbers he used became the standard terminology. Clearly the Brodmann map is the closest to the modern definition of the cortical field, as defined by Jones as an area:

1. With sharp, singular cytoarchitectural boundaries
2. Receiving afferent fibers from a particular nucleus of the thalamus
3. Receiving a set of cortical and commissural axons from a limited, defined and constant set of other cortical areas
4. Giving a constant output to a particular set of cortical, subcortical, and thalamic targets
5. Having a topographic organization of a receptive periphery
6. The deactivation of which may lead to the loss of a particular function

A major contribution to cortical architecture and surface morphology was made by the work of von Economo and Koskinas (1925; von Economo 1927, 1929) (Fig. 3.6), who brought a highly detailed nomenclature of the cortical surface pattern accompanied by a description of cytoarchitectural peculiarities of each region (Fig. 3.7A–D). More recently, Bailey and von Bonin (1951) provided a new cytoarchitectural map (Fig. 3.8A–C). These authors increased our knowledge of cortical patterns following the initial contribution of Eberstaller (1884, 1890) (Fig. 3.9).

Most of the proposed maps, with their variable complexity, lack data concerning the transitional areas. Moreover, several authors have depicted significant inhomogeneities in cytoarchitectural areas considered distinctive.

The evolution of imaging followed a similar path. It progressed from investigation of the ventricular cavities, to opacification of the cerebral vasculature, then to the two dimensional sectional brain anatomy

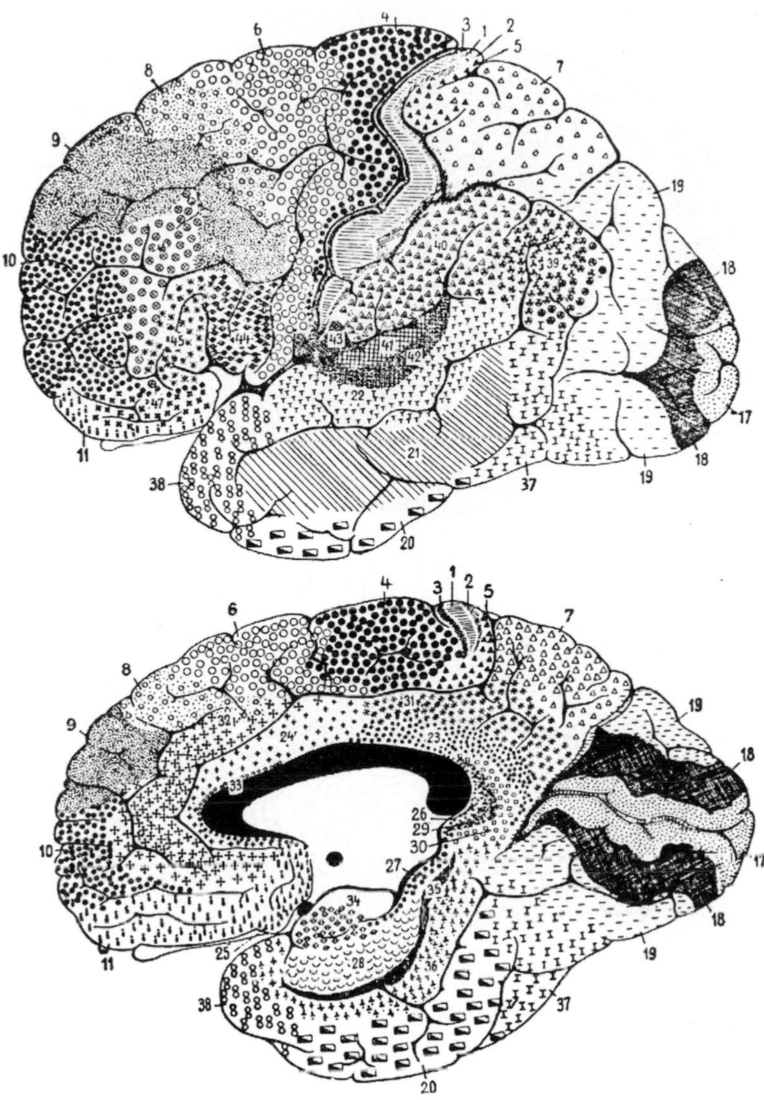

Fig. 3.4. Map of the cerebral cortex in man. Description of the cytoarchitectonic areas has been provided almost exclusively for the cercopithecus (1905), and only a few data concern areas 1, 3, 4, 6, 17, 18. (From Brodmann 1909)

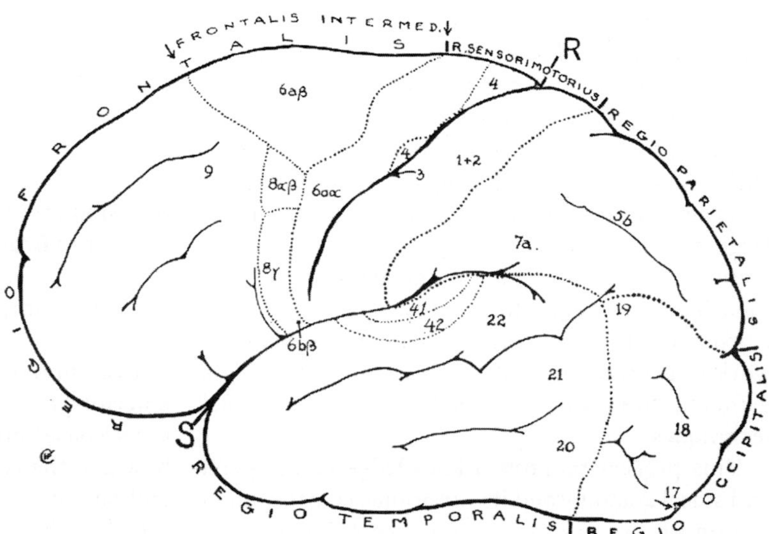

Fig. 3.5. Cytoarchitectonic map of the cortex. (Vogt and Vogt 1926)

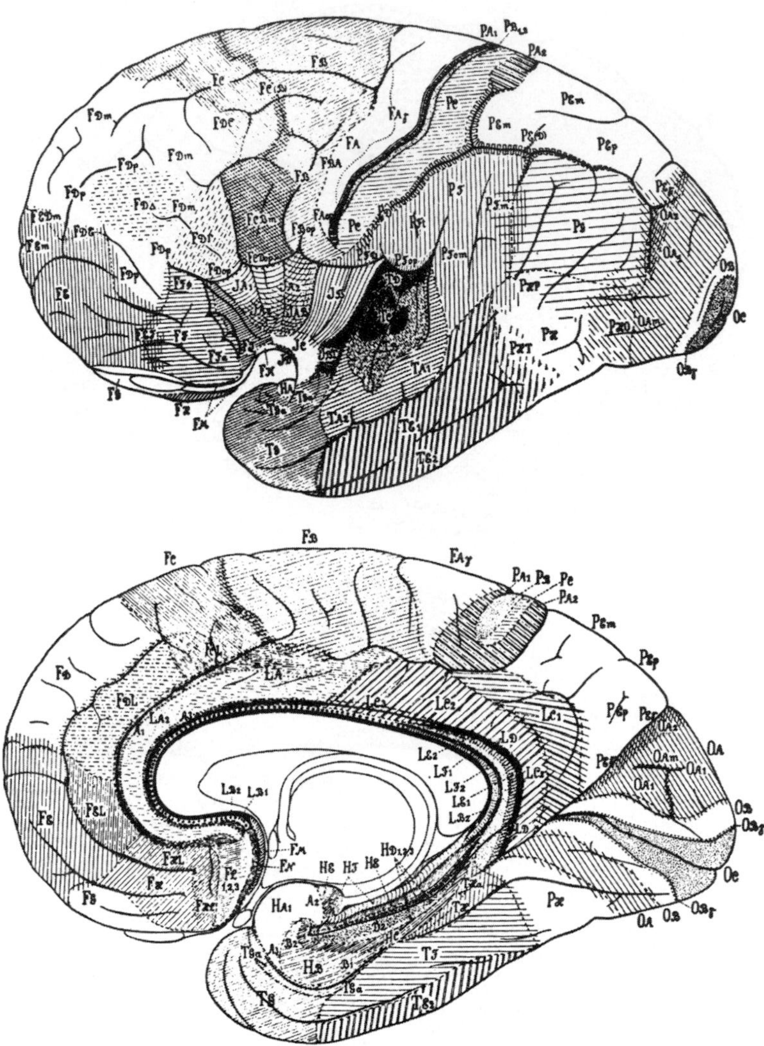

Fig. 3.6.. Cytoarchitectonic map of the cerebral cortex. (After von Economo 1925)

produced by CT scanning, and finally to the multiplanar method of MR, thus providing a sectional atlas of each imaged brain. Further advances in this technique rendered it possible, for the first time, to obtain a routine vision of an entire brain in three dimensions (3D). Furthermore, functional MR is presently available in vivo, allowing the establishment of links between morphology and function. This has in large part corroborated the precise work in brain mapping. The tedious work of the neuroscientists in their laboratories and the neurosurgeons in the operating rooms is progressively being replaced by the work of neuroradiologists, who are integrating data gathered from various metabolic and functional techniques.

This process requires a knowledge of the gyral and sulcal anatomy and its variations. Like the initial anatomists, we need to grasp the complexity of the cortical mantle as studied from various aspects: ontogenetic, phylogenetic, genetic and microscopic. Singly, these different approaches were limited and the results obtained suffered from lack of correlation between morphology and function.

A Gross Morphology and Fissural Patterns of the Brain

1 Gross Morphology

The cerebral hemispheres are ovoid in shape with an anterior-posterior long axis. Each hemisphere presents a base and a convexity. The base lies on the skull base and the convexity is related to the cranial vault and lateral aspects. The two hemispheres are separated by the interhemispheric fissure which penetrates deeply to the advent of the corpus callosum. The hemispheres are separated from the brainstem by the cerebral fissure of Bichat, which encircles the upper midbrain and extends posteriorly towards the ambient cistern, and merges anteriorly with the stem of the lateral fissures.

The cerebral hemisphere presents lateral, basal and medial aspects. The lateral and medial aspects are separated by the superior border of the hemisphere, while the lateral border separates the external from the basal aspects, and the medial border corresponds to the junction between the mesial and basal surfaces. Each hemisphere presents three poles: the frontal, occipital and temporal. The superior, mesial and lateral borders of each hemisphere converge towards the frontal and the occipital poles.

2 Brain Sulcation: Classifications

The distinction between fissures and sulci was made by Paul Broca who defined the fissures as folds of the wall pallium with an impression onto the ventricular walls and the sulci as indentations of the cortex. For the purpose of this work we will consider all furrows apart from the interhemispheric fissure as sulci. The classification of sulci into primary, secondary and tertiary has been adopted by most workers in this field.

Primary fissures were described using comparative and ontogenetic approaches The comparative approach was used and developed by Wernicke (1876, 1881–1883), Broca (1878), Turner (1891), Kükenthal and Ziehen (1895), von Bonin and Bailey (1947), and Bailey et al. (1950), among others. The ontogenetic approach was used by Cunningham and Horsley (1892), Retzius (1896) and His (1904).

The distinction made on the basis of comparative anatomy considered the sulci found in all gyrencephalic primates as primary (Fig. 3.10A,B). Embryologically, these fissures appear early in telencephalic development (Figs. 3.11A–C, 3.12). Upon reviewing previous works and the work of Larroche and Feess-Higgins (1987) we classified primary sulci as those appearing before the 30th week of gestation (Fig. 3.13A,B; Table 3.1). Secondary (Table 3.2) and tertiary sulci (Table 3.3) are those giving the brain its adult appearance. The classification of sulci remains controversial given the difficulties associated with the study of the human brain at birth and in infancy (Turner 1948, 1950; Bailey 1948; Bailey et al. 1950; Chi et al. 1977; Huang 1991) (Tables 3.4–3.8). MR data acquired in vivo from children will enable us to understand the progressive nature of sulcal development.

3 Sulcal and Gyral Anatomy

For a better understanding of the sulcal and gyral anatomy, we will first discuss the primary, followed by the secondary sulci. Tertiary sulci are difficult to identify on MRI since they are subject to marked individual variations; only those that are fairly constant will be discussed. In addition, this discussion is further complicated by the variable terminology used by different authors (Tables 3.9–3.11).

B The Lateral Surface of the Cerebral Hemisphere

The lateral aspect of the cerebral hemisphere is most efficiently investigated using 3D MRI surface renderings as reported in a previous work (Comair et al. 1996b). Anatomic correlations may be also achieved indirectly using multiplanar cross-sectional anatomic atlases based on definite reference markings (Déjerine 1895; Delmas and Pertuiset 1959; Talairach et al. 1967; Tamraz 1983; Cabanis et al. 1988; Salamon et al. 1990; Duvernoy et al. 1991) or by using two-dimensional (2D) contiguous MR slices (Naidich et al. 1995) extending from the lateral aspect of the hemisphere to reach the insular level.

1 Lateral Fissure of Sylvius

The lateral or Sylvian fissure, first described by Francois de Le Boë Sylvius (1652), is the major landmark on the lateral surface of the brain (Figs. 3.14–3.21). It is the most important and constant of the cerebral sulci. It is divided into three segments: the first extends from the lateral border of the anterior perforated substance and passes over the limen insulae in a posteriorly concave path that ends at the falciform sulcus, which separates the lateral orbital gyrus from the temporal pole. This part can be simply defined as the hidden or stem segment. The second, or horizontal segment, is the longest and deepest segment on the lateral surface of the hemisphere. We define the third segment as the segment limited anteriorly by the transverse supratemporal sulcus separating Heschl's gyri from the temporal planum and cutting into the superior temporal gyrus. This segment is complex, asymmetrical and correlates with hemispheric dominance. In right-handed individuals, it ascends at an acute angle on the right side and assumes an oblique course superiorly on the left.

Several branches are distinguished on the second or horizontal segment. Two sulci of almost similar

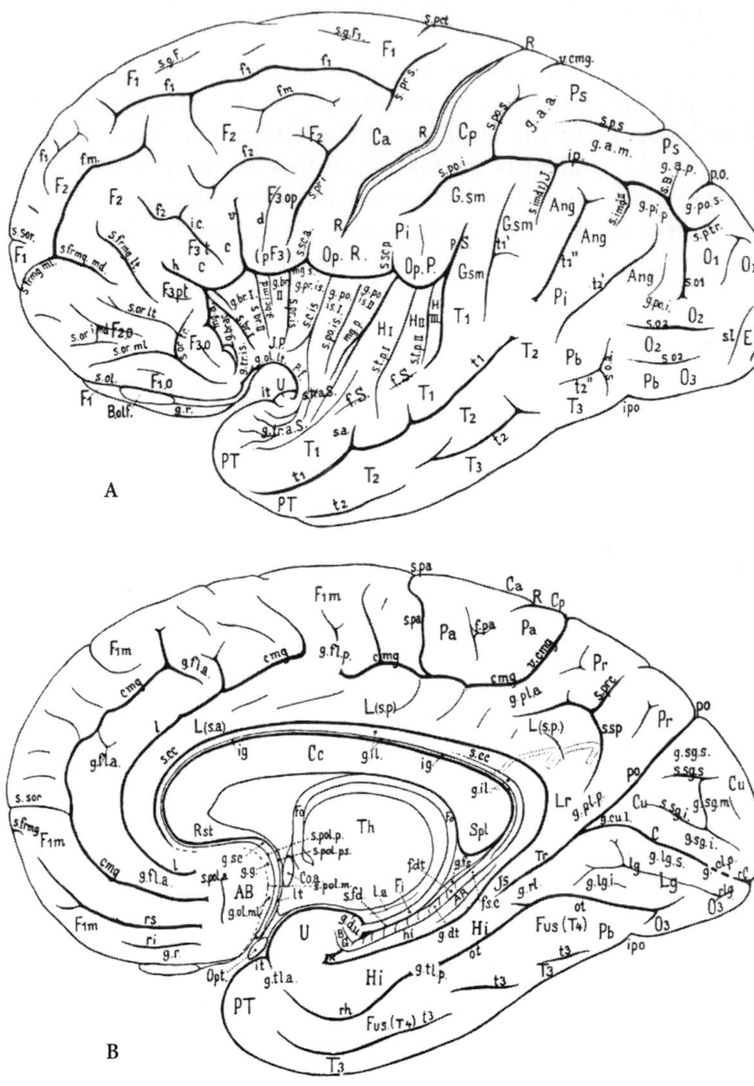

Fig. 3.7A–D. Fissural pattern of the human cerebral cortex. **A,B** Lateral and medial aspects; **C** inferior aspect; **D** superior aspect. (After von Economo and Koskinas 1925)

AB, Area parolfactoria of Broca (carrefour olfactif)
Ang, Lobulus angularis
Aq, Aqueduct
AR, Gyri Andreae Retzii
BB, Broca's band
BG, Bandelette of Giacomini
B.olf, Bulbus olfactorius
C, Fissura calcarina
Ca, Gyrus centralis anterior
Cc, Corpus callosum
Ch, Chiasma nervi optici
Coa, Commissura anterior
Cp, Gyrus centralis posterior
Cu, Cuneus
c, Cap
cmg, Sulcus callosomarginalis
d, Sulcus diagonalis (operculi)
E, Gyrus descendens of Ecker
F1, Gyrus frontalis primus
F2, Gyrus frontalis secundus
F3, Gyrus frontalis tertius
F3o, Pars orbitalis of F3 (F1o, F2o, F3o)
F3op, Pars opercularis of F3
F3pt, Pars praetriangularis of F3
F3t, Pars triangularis of F3 (Cap)
Fi, Fimbria
Fo, Fornix
Fus, Gyrus fusiformis
f1, Sulcus frontalis superior
f2, Sulcus frontalis inferior
f.dt, Fascia dentata
f.m, Sulcus frontalis medius
f.pa, Fossa paracentralis
fs.c, Fasciola cinerea
f.Sy, Fissura Sylvii
Gsm, Lobulus supramarginalis
g.a.a., Gyrus arcuatus anterior lobuli parietalis superioris
g.a.m., Gyrus arcuatus medius lobuli parietalis superioris
g.a.p., Gyrus arcuatus posterior lobuli parietalis superioris
g.amb, Gyrus ambiens
g.ant.o, Gyrus anticentralis operculi
g.ant.d, Gyrus antidiagonalis operculi
g.ant.pr.c, Gyrus antipraecentralis operculi
g.br.ac.(a), Gyrus brevis accessorius (anterior) insulae
<*ig.br.I,II,III*, Gyrus brevis primus, secundus, tertius, insulae
g.br.imd, Gyrus brevis intermedius insulae
g.cl.p., Gyrus cuneo-lingualis posterior
g.dt., Gyrus dentatus
g.d.u., Gyri digitati unci
g.fl.a, Gyrus frontolimbicus anterior
g.fl.p, Gyrus frontolimbicus posterior
g.fs, Gyrus fasciolaris
g.g, Gyrus geniculatus
g.il, Gyrus intralimbicus
g.imd, Gyrus brevis intermedius insulae
g.lg.s, Gyrus lingualis superior
g.lg.i, Gyrus lingualis inferior
g.ol.lt, Gyrus olfactorius lateralis
g.ol.ml, Gyrus olfactorius medialis
g.pip, Gyrus parietalis inferior posterior
g.pl.a, Gyrus parietolimbicus anterior
g.pl.p, Gyrus parietolimbicus posterior
g.po.i, Gyrus parieto-occipitalis inferior
g.po.s, Gyrus parieto-occipitalis superior
g.po.is.I, Gyrus postcentralis insulae primus
g.po.is.II, Gyrus postcentralis insulae secundus
g.pr.is, Gyrus praecentralis insulae
g.r, Gyrus rectus
g.rl, Gyrus retrolimbicus
g.sc, Gyrus subcallosus
g.sg.i, Gyrus sagittalis cunei inferior
g.sg.m, Gyrus sagittalis cunei medius
g.sg.s, Gyrus sagittalis cunei superior
g.sml, Gyrus semilunaris
g.str, Gyrus subtriangularis operculi
g.tl.a, Gyrus temporolimbicus anterior
g.tl.p, Gyrus temporolimbicus posterior
g.tr.a.S, Gyri temporales transversi anteriores of Schwalbe
g.tr.is, Gyrus transversus insulae
g.tr.op.I, Gyrus transversus operculi parietalis primus
g.tr.op.II, Gyrus transversus operculi parietalis secundus
g.tr.op.III, Gyrus transversus operculi parietalis tertius
H.I, Gyrus Heschl primus
H.II, Gyrus Heschl secundus
Hi, Gyrus hippocampi
h, Ramus horizontalis fissurae Sylvii
hi, Fissura hippocampi
Is, Isthmus
ic, Incisura capiti
ig, Indusium griseum
ip, Sulcus interparietalis
ipo, Incisura praeoccipitalis
it, Incisura temporalis
J, Incisura of Jensen or sulcus intermedius primus
Lg, Lingula
L.s.a, Gyrus limbicus superior pars anterior

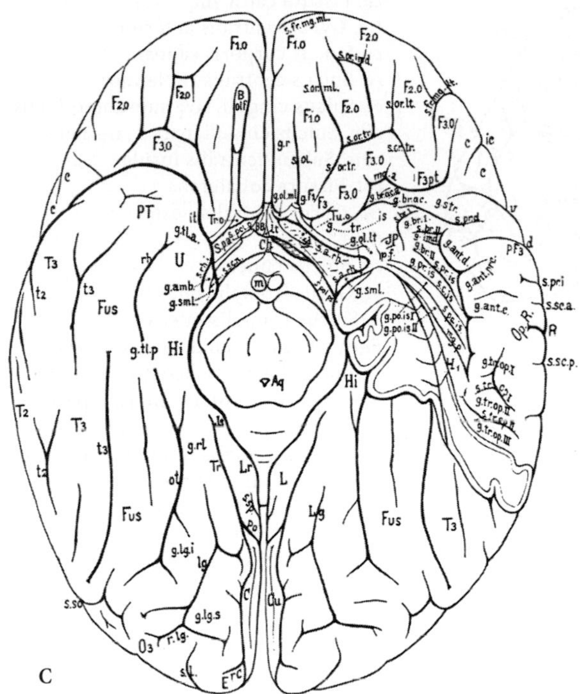

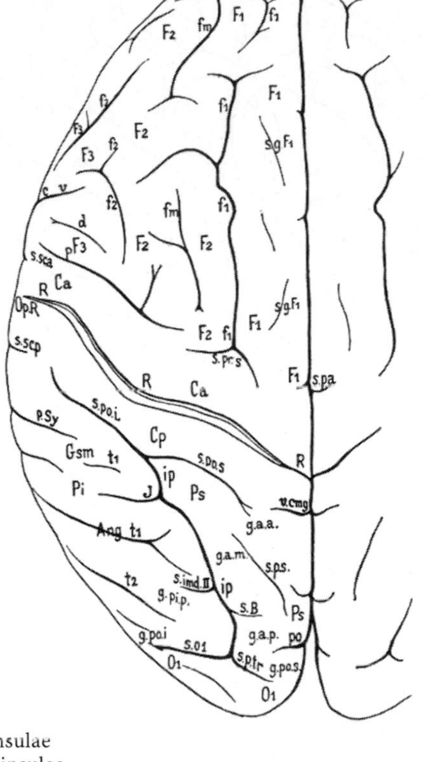

L.s.p, Gyrus limbicus superior pars posterior
Lr, Gyri limbici pars retrosplenialis
l, Sulcus intralimbicus
l.a, Lamina affixa
l.g, Sulcus lingualis
lt, Lamina terminalis
m, Corpus mamillare
mg.a, Margo anterior sulci circularis insulae
mg.p, Margo posterior sulci circularis insulae
O1, Gyrus occipitali primus
O2, Gyrus occipitali secundus
O3, Gyrus occipitali tertius
Op.P, Operculum parietale
Op.R, Operculum frontale of Rolando
Opt, Nervus opticus
ot, Fissura occipitotemporalis (collateralis)
Pa, Lobulus paracentralis
Pb, Regio parietalis basalis
Pi, Lobus parietalis inferior
Pr, Praecuneus
Ps, Lobus parietalis superior
PT, Gyrus temporopolaris
p.f, Incisura falciformis
po, Fissura parieto-occipitalis
p.Sy, Ramus posterior fissurae Sylvii
R, Sulcus of Rolando
Rst, Rostrum corporis callosi
rC, Fissura retrocalcarina
rh, Fissura rhinalis
ri, Sulcus rostralis inferior
rl, Sulcus retrolingualis
rs, Sulcus rostralis superior
S.p.a, Substantia perforata anterior
Spl, Splenium corporis callosis
s.a, Sulcus acusticus
s.a.rh, Sulcus arcuatus rhinencephali
s.B, Sulcus of Brissaud
s. br. I, Sulcus brevis primus insulae
s.b. II, Sulcus brevis secundus insulae
s.cc, Sulcus corporis callosi
s.c.is, Sulcus centralis insulae
s.d, Sulcus (parolfactorius) diagonalis
s.fd, Sulcus fimbriodentatus
s. frmg. ml, Sulcus frontomarginalis medialis
s.frmg.md, Sulcus frontomarginalis medius
s.frmg.lt, Sulcus frontomarginalis lateralis
s.g. F1, Sulcus gyri frontalis primi
s.imd.I, Sulcus intermedius primus of Jensen
s.imd.II, Sulcus intermedius secundus
s.l, Sulcus lunatus
so1, Sulcus occipitalis primus (praeoccipitalis, interoccipitalis)
so2, Sulcus occipitalis (secundus) lateralis
s.oa, Sulcus occipitalis (secundus) lateralis
s.ol, Sulcus olfactorius
s.or.lt, Sulcus orbitalis lateralis
s.or.ml, Sulcus orbitalis medialis
s.or.imd, Sulcus orbitalis intermedius
s.or.tr, Sulcus orbitalis transversus
s.pa, Sulcus paracentralis
s.po.i, Sulcus postcentralis inferior
s.po.s, Sulcus postcentralis superior
s.po.is, Sulcus postcentralis insulae
s.pol.a., Sulcus parolfactorius anterior
s.pol.m, Sulcus parolfactorius medius
s.pol.p, Sulcus parolfactorius posterior
s.pol.ps, Sulcus parolfactorius postremus
s.prc, Sulcus praecunei
s.prd, Sulcus praediagonalis
s.pr.i, Sulcus praecentralis inferior
s.pr.s, Sulcus praecentralis superior
s.pr.is, Sulcus praecentralis insulae
s.p.s, Sulcus parietalis superior
s.p.tr, Sulcus parietalis transversus
s.rh.i, Sulcus rhinencephali internus
s.san, Sulcus semiannularis
s.sc.a, Sulcus subcentralis anterior
s.sc.p, Sulcus subcentralis posterior
s.sg.s, Sulcus sagittalis cunei superior
s.sg.i, Sulcus sagittalis cunei inferior
s.so, Sulcus suboccipitalis
s.sor, Sulcus supraorbitalis
s.sp, Sulcus subparietalis
s.tp.I, Sulcus temporalis profundus primus
s.tp.II, Sulcus temporalis profundus secundus
s.tr.a.S, Sulci temporales transversi anteriores of Schwalbe
s.tr.op.I, Sulcus transversus operculi parietalis primus
s.tr.op.II, Sulcus transversus operculi parietalis secundus
T1, Gyrus temporalis primus
T2, Gyrus temporalis secundus
T3, Gyrus temporalis tertius
Th, Thalamus
Tr, Truncus fissurae parietooccipitalis et calcarinae
Tr.o, Trigonum (tuber) olfactorium
Tu.o, Tuberculum olfactorium or colliculus nuclei caudati
t1, Sulcus temporalis superior
t2, Sulcus temporalis medius
t3, Sulcus temporalis internus
U, Uncus
v, Ramus verticalis fissurae Sylvii
v.cmg, Ramus verticalis sulci callosomarginalis

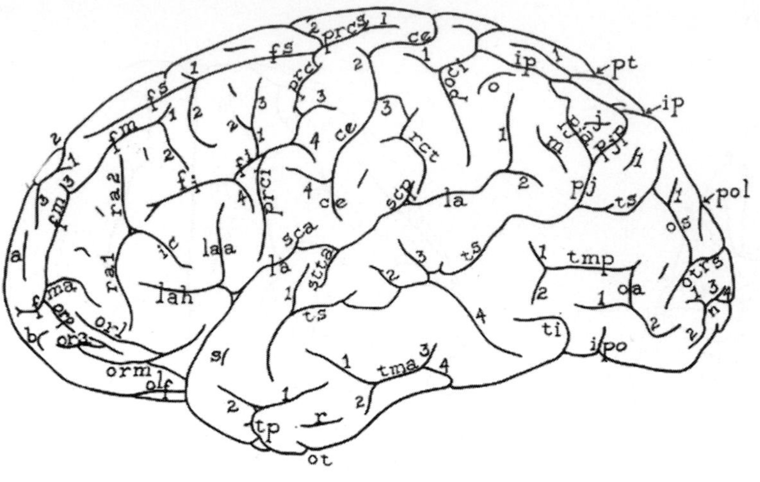

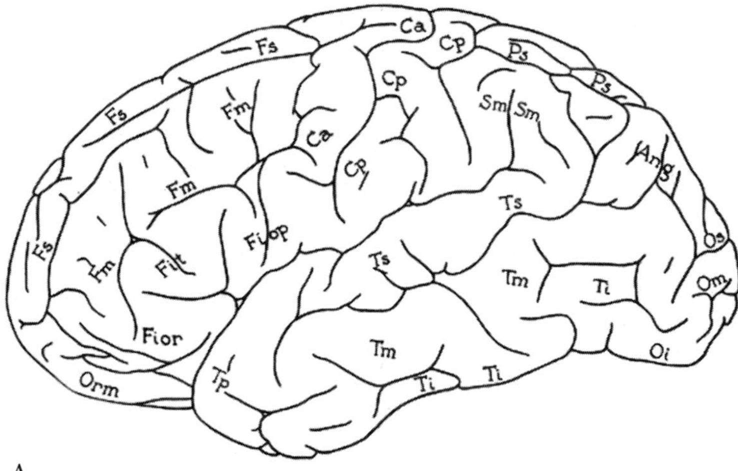

A

Fig. 3.8A–C. Fissural pattern of the human cerebral cortex. **A** Lateral aspect; **B** mesial aspect; **C** superior aspect. (After Bailey and von Bonin 1951)

aic, Sulcus arcus intercuneatus
Ang, Gyrus angularis (Huxley)
ca, Fissura calcarina
Ca, Gyrus centralis anterior
cc, Sulcus corporis callosi
ce, Sulcus centralis (Rolando)
ci, Sulcus cinguli, sive supramarginalis
cim, Sulcus cinguli, pars marginalis
cins, Sulcus centralis insulae
col, Fissura collateralis
Cp, Gyrus centralis posterior
Cu, Cuneus
cu, Sulcus cunei
Fi, Gyrus frontalis inferior
fi, Sulcus frontalis inferior
Fiop, Gyrus frontalis inferior, pars opercularis sive pedalis (Broca)
Fiorb, Gyrus frontalis inferior, pars orbitalis
Fit, Gyrus frontalis inferior, pars triangularis (cap de Broca)
Fm, Gyrus frontalis medius
fm, Sulcus frontalis medius
fma, Sulcus frontomarginalis (Wernicke)
Fs, Gyrus frontalis superior
fs, Sulcus frontalis superior
fsa, Sulcus frontalis superior anterior
ic, Incisura capitis
il, Sulcus intralimbicus
ip, Sulcus intraparietalis
ipo, Sulcus praeoccipitalis (Meynert)
L, Gyrus limbicus (sive cinguli)
La, Gyrus limbicus, pars anterior
Lp, Gyrus limbicus, pars posterior
la, Fissura lateralis (Sylvius)
laa, Fissura lateralis, ramus ascendens
lah, Fissura lateralis, ramus horizontalis
Lg, Gyrus lingualis
lo, Sulcus limitans operculi
mai, Sulcus marginalis anterior insulae
mii, Sulcus marginalis inferior insulae
msi, Sulcus marginalis superior insulae
oa, Sulcus occipitalis anterior (Wernicke)

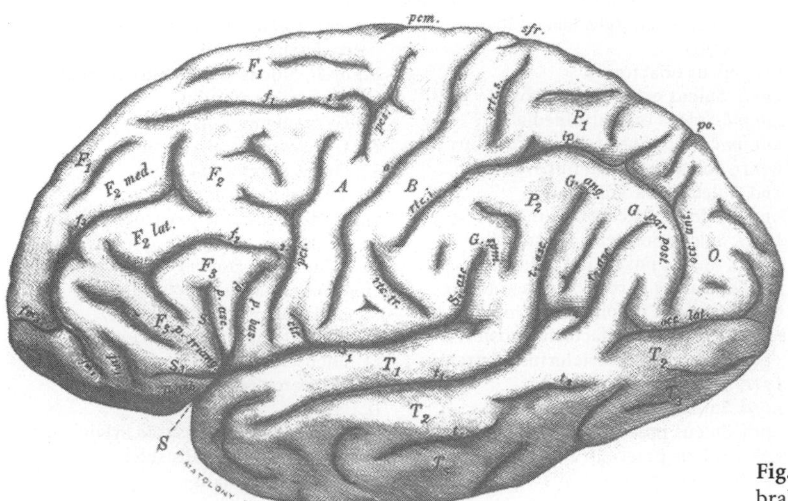

Fig. 3.9. Fissural pattern of the human cerebral cortex. (After Eberstaller 1890)

Oi, Gyrus occipitalis inferior
olf, Sulcus olfactorius
olri, Sulcus occipitalis transversus inferior
olrs, Sulcus occipitalis transversus superior
Om, Gyrus occipitalis medius
oper, Sulcus intraopercularis
ora, Sulcus orbitalis arcuatus
orl, Sulcus orbitalis lateralis
orm, Sulcus orbitalis medialis
orp, Sulcus orbitopolaris
Os, Gyrus occipitalis superior
os, Sulcus occipitalis superior (Ecker)
ot, Sulcus occipitotemporalis
ota, Sulcus occipitotemporalis accessorius
pa, Sulcus polaris anterior
pac, Sulcus paracentralis
Parc, Lobulus paracentralis
Pc, Praecuneus (Foville)
Pim, Gyrus parietalis inferior intermedius
pj, Sulcus parietalis intermedius (Jensen)
pja, Sulcus parietalis intermedius, ramus anterior
pjp, Sulcus parietalis intermedius, ramus posterior
po, Fissura parieto-occipitalis
poci, Sulcus postcentralis inferior
pocs, Sulcus postcentralis superior
pol, Sulcus parieto-occipitalis, pars lateralis
pom, Sulcus parieto-occipitalis, pars medialis
prc, Sulcus praecentralis
prci, Sulcus praecentralis inferior
prcs, Sulcus praecentralis superior
Ps, Lobulus parietalis superior
pt, Sulcus parietalis transversus (Brissaud)
ra, Sulcus radiatus
rct, Sulcus retrocentralis transversus
rh, Sulcus rhinalis
roi, Sulcus rostralis inferior
ros, Sulcus rostralis superior
sca, Sulcus subcentralis anterior
scp, Sulcus subcentralis posterior
Sm, Gyrus supramarginalis (Gratiolet)
sp, Sulcus subparietalis
sro, Sulcus suprarostralis
stta, Sulcus supratemporalis transversus anterior
sttm, Sulcus supratemporalis transversus medius
sttp, Sulcus supratemporalis transversus posterior
ti, Sulcus temporalis inferior
tma, Sulcus temporalis medius anterior
tmp, Sulcus temporalis medius posterior
tp, Sulcus temporopolaris
ts, Sulcus temporalis superior

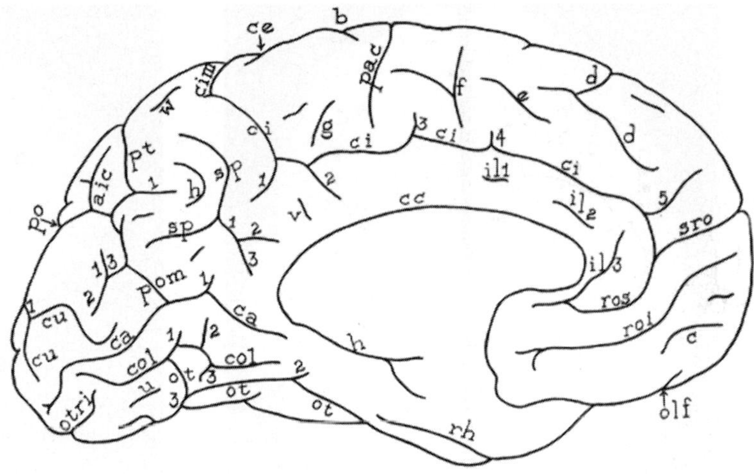

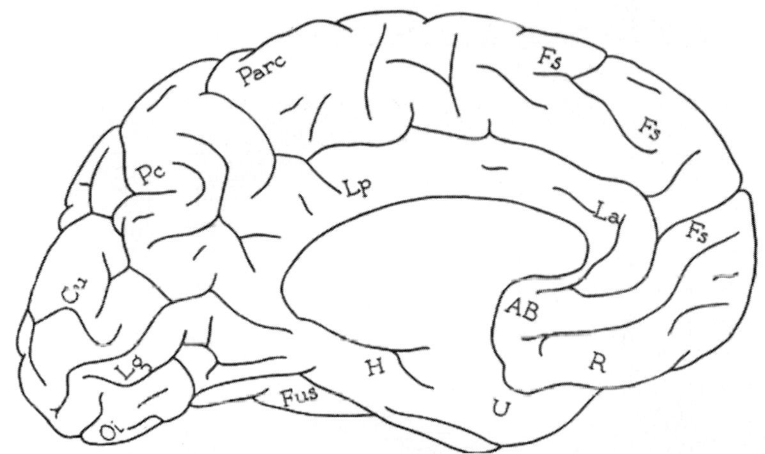

B

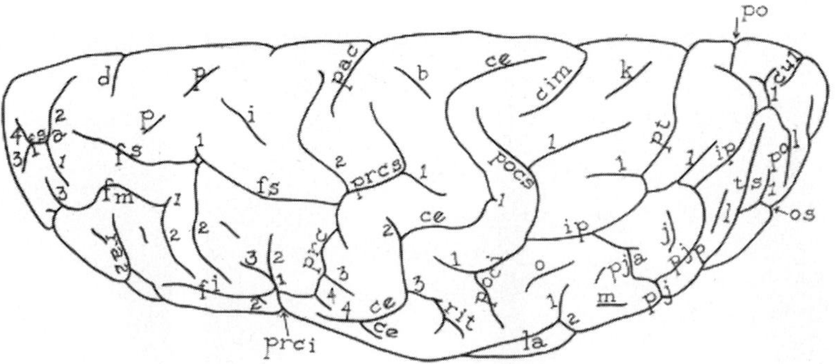

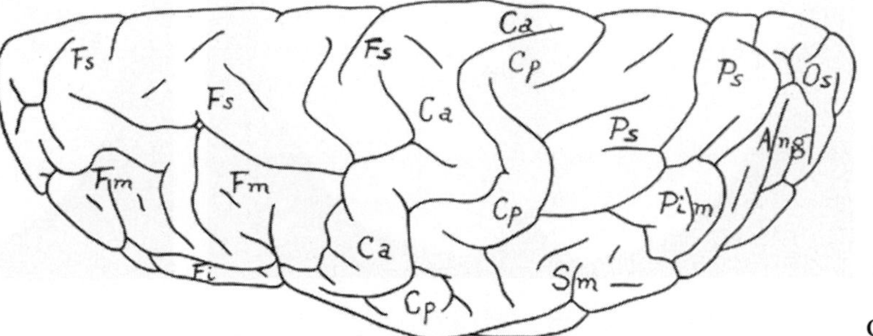

C

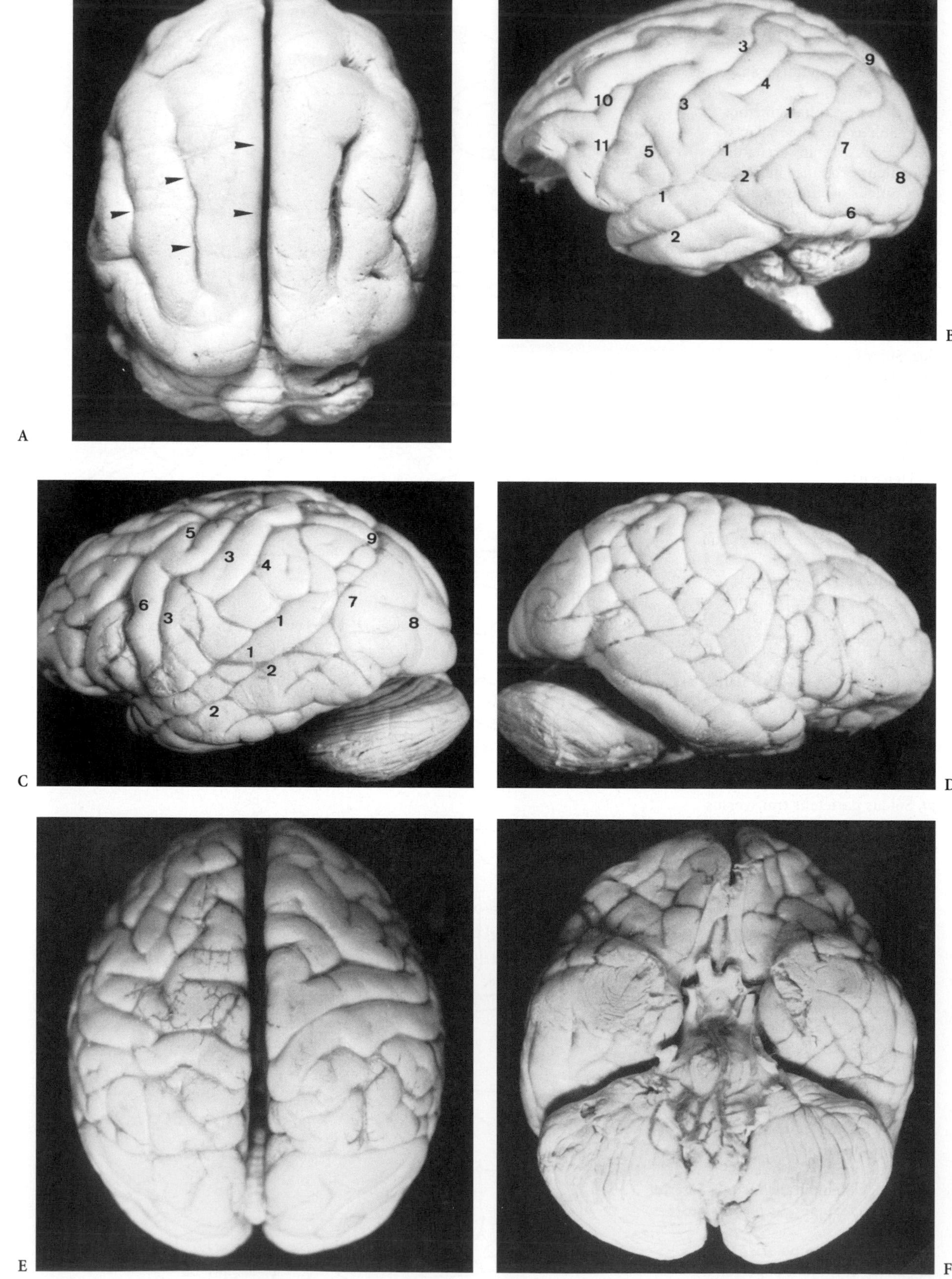
A
B
3
9
4
10
3
1
11
5
1
7
2
8
1
6
2
C
5
9
3
4
7
6
3
1
8
1
2
2
D
E
F

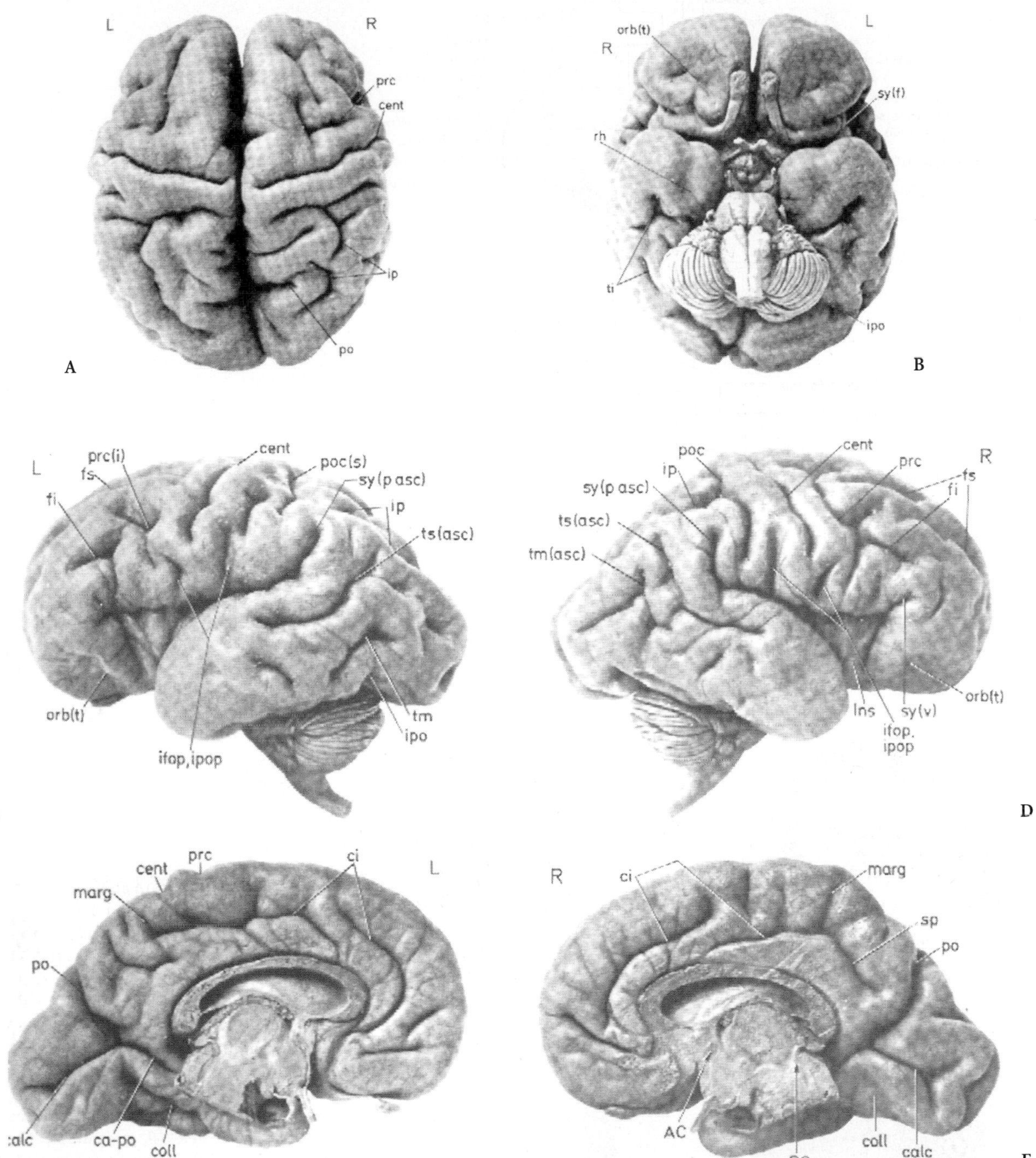

Fig. 3.11A–F. Fissural pattern of the fetal brain at 8 months. (After Retzius 1896)

◁ **Fig. 3.10A–F.** Brain sulcation of primates. **A** *Daubentonia* (lemurian, prosimian): most furrows show parallel orientation to the interhemispheric fissure as well to the sylvian fissure. **B** *Papio* (Cynomorpha): *1*, lateral fissure; *2*, superior temporal sulcus; *3*, central sulcus; 4, intraparietal sulcus; *5*, anterior subcentral sulcus; *6*, Inferior occipital sulcus; *7*, lunate sulcus; *8*, superior occipital sulcus; *9*, parieto-occipital sulcus; *10*, ramus superior of sulcus arcuatus; *11*, ramus infeior of sulcus arcuatus. **C–F** Chimpanzee (Anthropomorpha): *1*, superior temporal (parallel) sulcus; *2*, middle temporal sulcus; *3*, central sulcus; *4*, inferior postcentral and intraparital sulci; *5*, superior precentral sulcus; *6*, inferior precentral sulcus; *7*, sulcus lunatus; *8*, sulcus occipitalis diagonalis; *9*, lateral parieto-occipital incisure; *10*, fronto-orbital "H" (Museum National d'Histoire Naturelle, Paris; courtesy of R. Saban and J. Repérant)

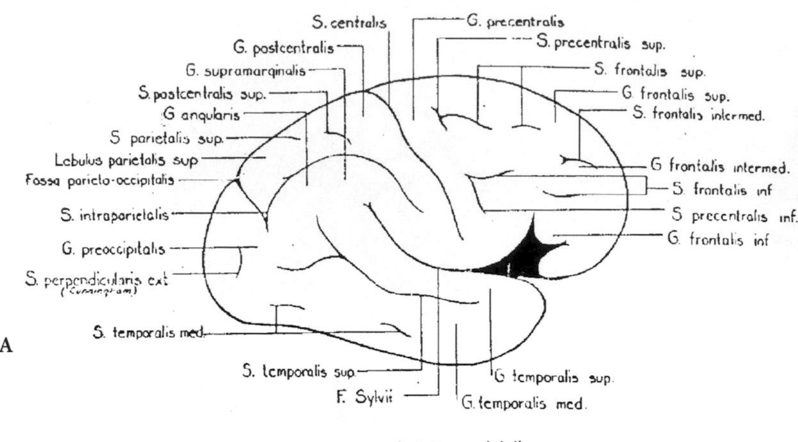

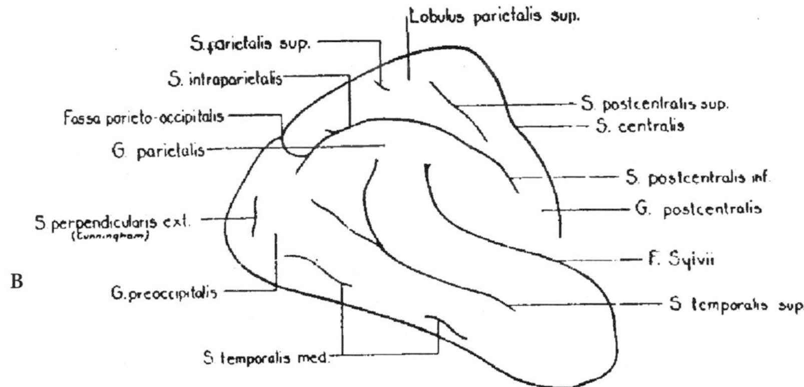

Fig. 3.12A,B. Fissural pattern of the fetal brain from the seventh month to birth. (According to Turner 1948)

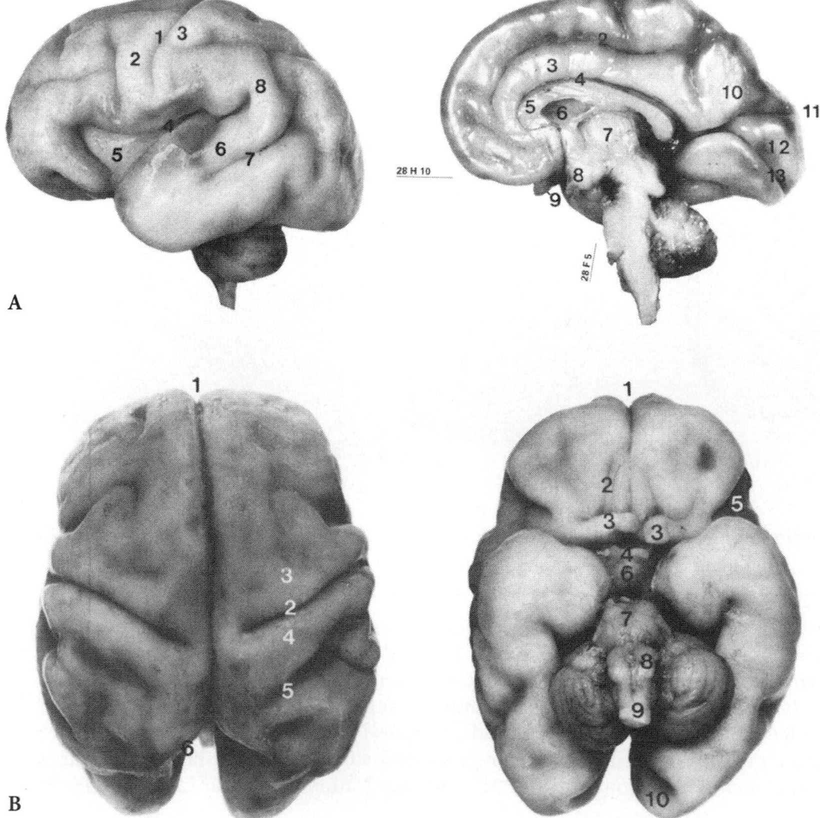

Fig. 3.13A,B. Fetal brain at 28–29 weeks of gestation. A Lateral ad mesial aspects. Lateral: *1*, central sulcus; *2*, precentral gyrus; *3*, postcentral gyrus; *4*, lateral sulcus; *5*, insula; *6*, superior temporal gyrus; *7*, superior temporal sulcus; *8*, supramarinal gyrus. Mesial: *1*, central sulcus; *2*, cingulate sulcus; *3*, cingulate gyrus; *4*, callosal sulcus; *5*, corpus callosum; *6*, cavum septi pellucidi; *7*, thalamus; *8*, infundibulum; *9*, olfactory tract; *10*, precuneus; *11*, parieto-occipital sulcus; *12*, cuneus; *13*, calcarine sulcus. B Superior and inferior aspects. Superior: *1*, interhemispheric fissure; *2*, central sulcus; *3*, precentral gyru; *4*, postcentral gyrus; *5*, postcentral gyrus; *6*, parieto-occipital sulcus. Inferior: *1*, interhemispheric fissure; *2*, olfactory sulcus; *3*, olfactory tract; *4*, optic chiasm; *5*, lateral fissure; *6*, infundibulum; *7*, pons; *8*, pyramid and uvula; *9*, spinal cod; *10*, calcarine sulcus. (According to Larroche and Feess-Higgins 1987)

Table 3.1. Classification of brain primary sulci

Weeks of gestation	Sulcal maturation
13–15	Early sylvian fissure
16–17	Cingulate sulcus
	Callosal sulcus
	Parieto-occipital sulcus
19–20	Calcarine
22–23	Circular sulcus (operculization)
25–26	Central sulcus
	Superior temporal (left) sulcus
	Superior part of precentral sulcus
	Olfactory sulcus
28–30	Intraparietal sulcus
	Inferior frontal sulcus
	Branching of lateral sulcus
	Paracentral sulcus
	Collateral sulcus
	Superior frontal sulcus

Table 3.2. Classification of brain secondary sulci

Lobe	Sulcus
Frontal lobe	Precentral
	Frontomarginal
	Orbitofrontal
	Rostral (superior, inferior)
Parietal lobe	Subparietal
Occipital lobe	Paracalcarine (ventral and dorsal)
	Lateral occipital
	Transverse occipital
	Lunate
Temporal lobe	Rhinal
	Transverse temporal
	Inferior temporal
Insular lobe	Sulcus centralis insulae

Table 3.3. Classification of fairly constant tertiary brain sulci

Lobe	Sulcus
Frontal Lobe	Intermediate frontal
	Diagonal
	Radiate
	Anterior subcentral
Parietal Lobe	Transverse parietal
	Intermediate (secondary, tertiary)
	Primary intermediate
Temporal lobe	Sulcus acousticus
Occipital lobe	Various individual variations and absence of consensus

Table 3.4. Chronology of sulcal maturation: lateral surface (From Chi et al. 1977)

Weeks of gestation	Sulcal maturation (lateral convexity)
10–15	Sylvian fissure
16–19	Circular sulcus
20–23	Central sulcus, superior temporal sulcus
24–27	Superior frontal sulcus, precentral sulcus, postcentral sulcus, intraparietal sulcus, lateral occipital sulcus, middle temporal sulcus
28–31	Inferior frontal sulcus, inferior temporal sulcus
32–35	Insular gyri, parietal sulci, secondary frontal sulci, secondary temporal sulci, secondary parietal sulci, superior and inferior occipital sulci
36–39	Secondary transverse temporal sulci, secondary inferior temporal sulci, tertiary frontal sulci, tertiary parietal sulci
40–44	Secondary insular sulci, tertiary inferior temporal sulci, tertiary superior and inferior occipital sulci

Table 3.5. Chronology of sulcal maturation: medial surface (From Chi et al. 1977)

Weeks of gestation	Sulcal maturation (medial surface)
10–15	Interhemispheric fissure
10–15	Hippocampal fissure
10–15	Callosal sulcus
16–19	Cingulate sulcus
16–19	Parieto-occipital sulcus
16–19	Calcarine sulcus
20–23	Collateral sulcus
32–35	Marginal sulcus
36–39	Secondary cingulate sulci
40–44	Secondary callosomarginal sulci

Table 3.6. Chronology of sulcal maturation: basal surface (From Chi et al. 1977)

Weeks of gestation	Sulcal maturation (inferior surface)
16–19	Olfactory sulcus, gyrus rectus
28–31	Medial and lateral orbital gyri
36–39	Anterior and posterior orbital gyri
40–44	Secondary orbital sulci

Table 3.7. Appearance of gyri during gestation (From Chi et al. 1977)

Weeks of gestation	Gyri
27	Middle frontal gyrus, cuneus, medial and lateral occipitotemporal gyri, superior and inferior occipital gyri
28	Callosomarginal gyrus, inferior frontal gyrus, supramarginal gyrus, angular gyrus, medial and lateral orbital gyri
30	Inferior temporal gyrus, external occipital temporal gyrus
31	Transverse temporal gyrus
35	Paracentral gyrus
36	Anterior and posterior orbital gyri

Table 3.9. Sulci of lateral surface. (Modified from Testut and Latarjet 1948, pp 783–785)

Sulci	Eponyms
Lateral fissure	Scissure de Sylvius, grande scissure interlobaire (Chaussier), fissura lateralis (Henle), fissura sive fossa Sylvii (Ecker)
Central sulcus	Scissure de Rolando, sulcus centralis (Ecker), fissura transversa anterior (Pansch), posteroparietal sulcus (Huxley)
Lateral parieto-occipital sulcus	Scissure perpendiculaire externe, sillon occipital transverse (Broca), occipitoparietal fissure (Huxley), parietooccipital fissure (Turner), pars superior sive lateralis fissure parieto-occipitalis (Ecker)
Superior frontal sulcus	Sillon frontal supérieur, scissure frontale supérieure (Pozzi), premier sillon frontal (Broca), superofrontal sulcus (Huxley)
Inferior frontal sulcus	Sillon frontal inférieur, scissure frontale inférieure ou sourcilière (Pozzi), deuxième sillon frontal (Broca), sillon inféro-frontal (Huxley), sillon frontal primaire (Pansch)
Precentral sulcus	Sillon prérolandique, scissure parallèle frontale (Pozzi), sillon antéro-pariétal (Huxley), sulcus precentralis (Ecker), descending ramus of middle frontal sulcus (Pansch)
Intraparietal sulcus	Sillon interpariétal, sillon pariétal (Broca, Pansch), intraparietal fissure (Turner), sulcus occipito-parietalis (Schwalbe), sulcus postcentralis (Ecker), ramus ascendens (Pansch)
Superior temporal sulcus	Sillon parallèle, premier sillon temporal, sillon temporal supérieur (Ecker), sulcus temporalis (Pansch), anterotemporal sulcus (Huxley)
Inferior temporal sulcus	Sillon temporal inférieur, deuxième sillon temporal, sulcus temporalis medius (Ecker), posterotemporal sulcus (Huxley)

Table 3.8. Ultrasound landmarks of cortical maturation at different stages of gestation (From Huang 1991)

Weeks of gestation	Landmarks
24–25	Prominent parieto-occipital sulcus, early branching calcarine sulcus
26–27	Matured calcarine sulcus, anterior cingulate sulcus
28–29	Whole cingulate sulcus, post central sulcus, insula partly covered
30–31	Insula covered completely, cingulate sulcus arcs, curves inferior temporal sulcus, with or without secondary cingulate sulci
32–33	Secondary cingulate sulci, partial insular sulci
34–35	Better insular sulci, more matured secondary sulci, with or without tertiary sulci
>36	Tertiary sulci, more matured insular sulci

Table 3.10. Sulci of medial surface. (Modified from Testut and Latarjet 1948, pp 783–785)

Sulci	Eponyms
Cingulate sulcus	Scissure calloso-marginale, Scissure festonnée (Pozzi), grand sillon du lobe fronto-pariétal (Gratiolet), sillon du corps calleux (Gromier), scissure sous-frontale (Broca)
Medial parieto-occipital sulcus	Scissure perpendiculaire interne, Occipitoparietal fissure (Huxley), pars medialis sive verticalis fissuræ occipitalis perpendicularis (Ecker), scissure occipitale (Broca), fissura occipitalis (Pansch), fissura posterior (Burdach), fissura occipitalis perpendicularis interna (Bischoff)
Calcarine sulcus	Scissure calcarine, scissure des hippocampes (Gromier), partie postérieure de la scissure des hippocampes (Gratiolet), fissura occipitalis horizontalis (Henle), fissura posterior (Huschke)

Table 3.11. Sulci of inferior surface. (Modified from Testut and Latarjet 1948, pp 783–785)

Sulci	Eponyms
Olfactory sulcus	Sillon olfactif, sulcus olfactorius (Ecker), scissure olfactive (Giacomini), sillon droit ou premier sillon orbitaire (Broca)
Orbital sulci	Sillon cruciforme, sulcus orbitalis (Ecker), scissure orbitaire (Giacomini), deuxième sillon orbitaire (Broca), triradialis sulcus (Turner); the two anteroposterior branches are termed, by Weisbach, l'interne sulcus longitudinalis medius and l'externe sulcus longitudinalis externus. The transversal branch is also called the transverse sulcus by the same author.
(Lateral) occipito-temporal sulcus	Sillon temporo-occipital externe, premier sillon temporo-occipital, sulcus temporo-occipitalis (Ecker)
(Medial) occipito-temporal sulcus (Collateral sulcus)	Sillon temporo-occipital interne, deuxième sillon temporo-occipital, sulcus longitudinalis inferior (Huschke), sulcus occipito-temporalis (Pansch), fissura collateralis (Huxley), fissura collateralis sive temporalis inferior (Bischoff), sulcus occipito-temporalis inferior (Ecker), sillon collatéral

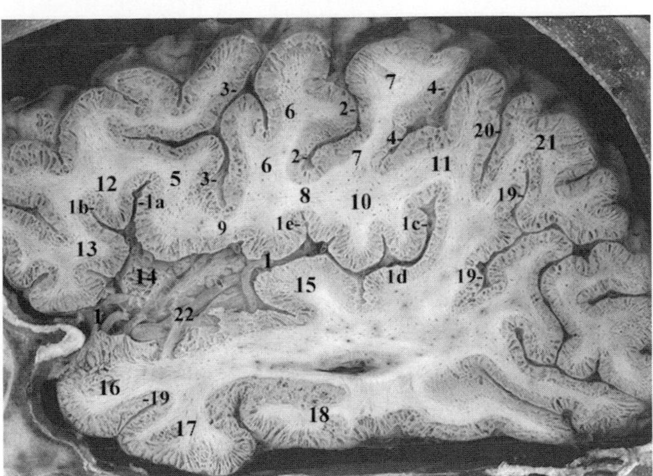

Fig. 3.16. Sagittal anatomical cut through the outer aspect of the insula showing the perisylvian region. *1*, Lateral fissure; *1a*, ascending ramus of lateral fissure; *1b*, horizontal ramus of lateral fissure; *1c*, terminal ascending tamus, *1d*, temporal planum *2*, central sulcus; *3*, inferior precentral sulcus; *4*, inferior postcentral sulcus (ascending segment of intraparietal); *5*, inferior frontal gyrus, pars opercularis; *6*, precentral gyrus; *7*, postcentral gyrus; *8*, central operculum; *9*, frontal operculum; *10*, parietal operculum; *11*, supramarginal gyrus; *12*, inferior frontal gyrus, pars triangularis; *13*, inferior frontal gyrus, pars orbitalis; *14*, insula; *15*, transverse temporal gyrus (Heschl); *16*, superior temporal gyrus; *17*, middle temporal gyrus; *18*, inferior temporal gyrus; *19*, superior temporal (parallel) sulcus; *20*, intermediate sulcus of Jensen; *21*, angular gyrus; *22*, insular branches of middle cerebral artery

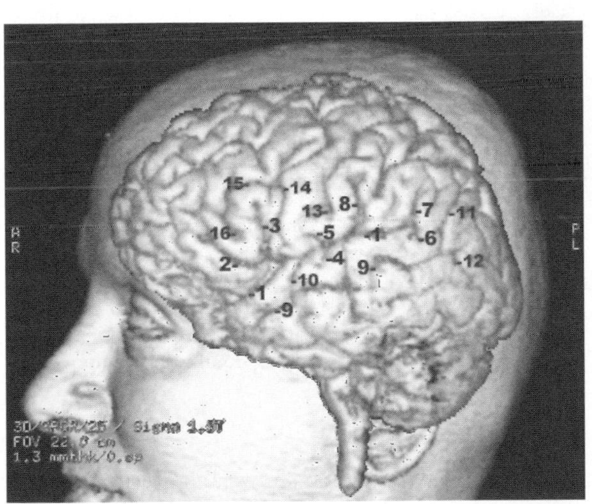

Fig. 3.14. 3D MR of the lateral aspect of the cerebral hemisphere showing the perisylvian sulci. *1*, Lateral fissure; *2*, horizontal ramus of lateral fissure; *3*, ascending ramus of lateral fissure; *4*, anterior transverse temporal sulcus; *5*, anterior subcentral sulcus; *6*, posterior transverse temporal sulcus; *7*, terminal ascending branch of lateral fissure; *8*, sulcus retrocentralis transversus (Eberstaller); *9*, superior temporal sulcus; *10*, sulcus acousticus; *11*, terminal ascending branch of temporal sulcus; *12*, descending branch of superior temporal sulcus; *13*, central sulcus; *14*, precentral sulcus; *15*, inferior central sulcus; *16*, radiate sulcus (incisura capitis)

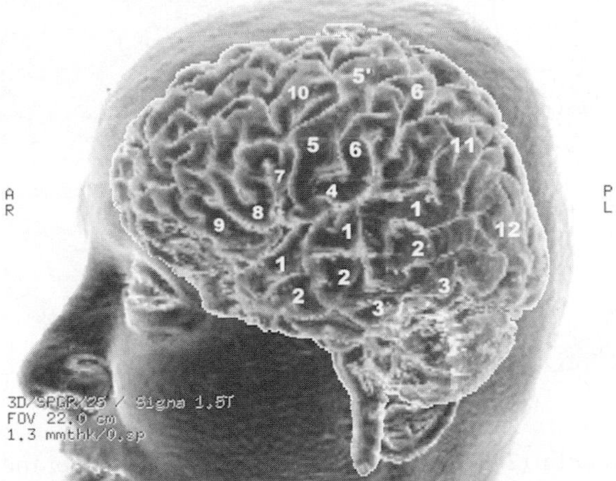

Fi. 3.15. 3D MR of the lateral aspect of the cerebral hemisphere showing the perisylvian gyri. *1*, Superior temporal gyrus; *2*, middle temporal gyrus; *3*, inferior temporal gyrus; *4*, fronto-parietal operculum; *5*, precentral gyrus (inferior enu); *5'*, precentral gyrus (superior genu); *6*, postcentral gyrus; *7*, inferior frontal gyrus, pars opercularis; *8*, inferior frontal gyrus, pars triangularis; *9*, inferior frontal gyrus, pars orbitalis; *10*, middle frontal gyrus; *11*, inferior parietal lobule; *12*, occipital lobe

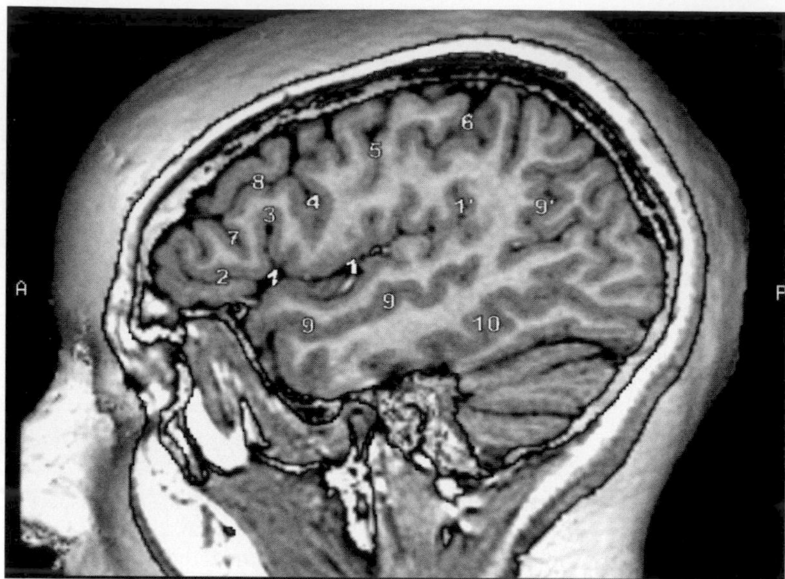

Fig. 3.17. Lateral 3D-MR view of the lateral fissure and its major rami. Sagittal cut into a 3D MR of the head showing the lateral surface of the brain. *1*, Lateral (sylvian) fissure; *1'*, ascending ramus of the lateral fissure; *2*, horizontal ramus of lateral fissure; *3*, ascending ramus of lateral fissure; *4*, inferior precentral sulcus; *5*, central (rolandic) sulcus; *6*, postcentral sulcus; *7*, radiate sulcus (incisura capitis); *8*, superior frontal sulcus; *9*, superior temporal (parallel) sulcus; *10*, inferior temporal sulcus

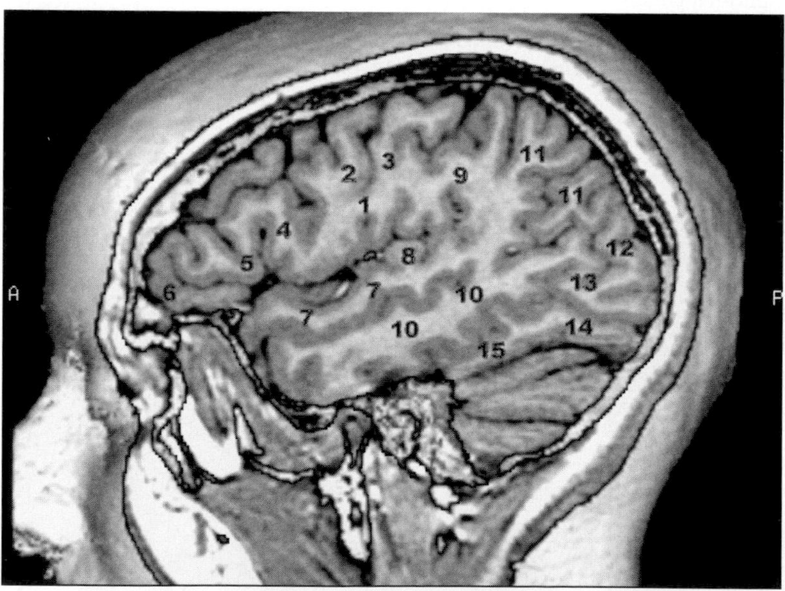

Fig. 3.18. Sagittal cut into a 3D MR of the head showing the lateral surface of the brain. *1*, Frontoparietal (central) operculum; *2*, precentral gyrus; *3*, postcentral gyrus; *4*, pars opercularis of inferior frontal gyrus; *5*, pars triangularis of inferior frontal gyrus; *6*, pars orbitalis of inferior frontal gyrus; *7*, superior temporal gyrus; *8*, transverse gyrus of Heschl; *9*, supramarginal gyrus; *10*, middle temporal gyrus; *11*, angular gyrus; *12*, superior occipital gyrus; *13*, middle occipital gyrus; *14*, inferior occipital gyrus; *15*, inferior temporal gyrus

length (2–3 cm) are noted in the frontal lobe: the horizontal ramus and the vertical ramus. These rami have a divergent course limiting a triangular space whose apex faces the sylvian fissure. These rami start from the sylvian fissure separately or from a common trunk (one third of cases). The terminal segment usually bifurcates at its end in about 70% of the cases forming long ascending and short descending parts. The latter is the posterior transverse temporal sulcus more frequently found on the right (70% of cases). This sulcus, which shows an anterior inferior oblique course, should not be confused with the transverse supratemporal sulcus, seen on the first temporal gyrus separating the posterior border of Heschl's gyri from the planum temporale. The cortical regions adjacent to the lateral sulcus are the frontal, parietal and temporal opercula, or lids, covering the insular lobe (Table 3.12).

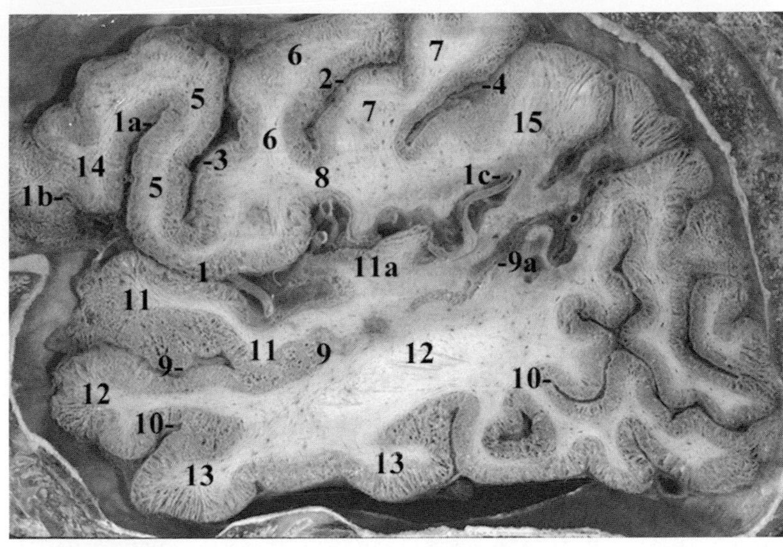

Fig. 3.19. Sagittal anatomical cut of the brain showing the lateral fissure and the perisylvian region. *1*, Lateral fissure; *1a*, ascending ramus of lateral fissure; *1b*, horizontal ramus of lateral fissure; *1c*, terminal ascending branch of lateral fissure; *2*, central sulcus; *3*, inferior precentral sulcus; *4*, inferior postcentral sulcus (ascending segment of intraparietal); *5*, inferior frontal gyrus, pars opercularis; *6*, precentral gyrus; *7*, postcentral gyrus; *8*, central operculum; *9*, superior temporal sulcus; *10*, inferior temporal sulcus; *11*, superior temporal gyrus; *11a*, transverse temporal gyri (Heschl); *12*, middle temporal gyrus; *13*, inferior temporal gyrus; *14*, inferior frontal gyrus, pars triangularis; *15*, supramarginal gyrus

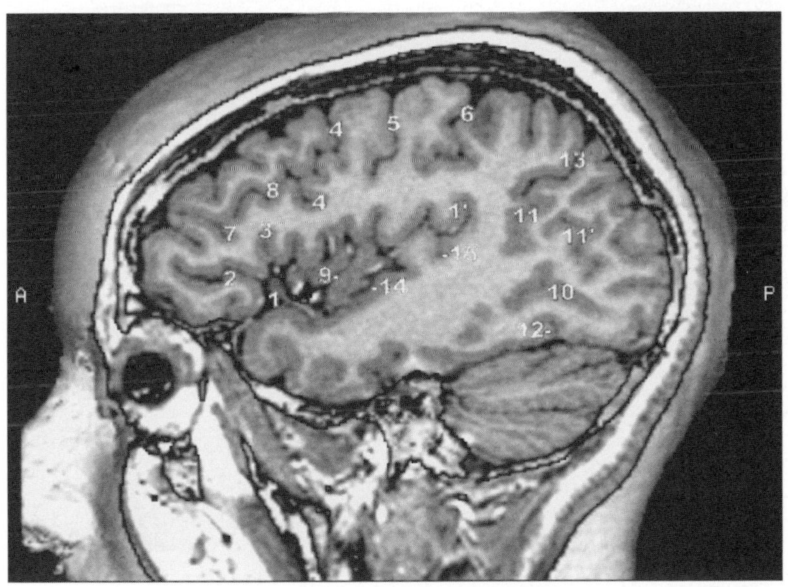

Fig. 3.20. Sagittal cut into a 3D MR of the head passing through the insular cortex and showing the main sulci. *1*, Lateral sylvian fissure; *1'*, ascending ramus of lateral fissure; *2*, horizontal ramus of lateral fissure; *3*, ascending ramus of lateral fissure; *4*, precentral sulcus; *5*, central sulcus; *6*, postcentral fissure; *7*, radiate sulcus (incisura capitis); *8*, inferior frontal sulcus; *9*, central sulcus of insula; *10*, inferior occipital sulcus; *11*, ascending ramus of parallel sulcus; *11'*, superior occipital sulcus; *12*, preoccipital incisure

2 Central Sulcus (Rolando)

Described by Rolando in 1829, the central sulcus separates the frontal from the parietal lobe (Figs. 3.22–3.31). Associated with it, Broca described three curves, a superior genu and an inferior genu. The cortex located between these genus represents the portion of the precentral gyrus innervating the arm. An increase in the depth of this sulcus is reported between the trunk and the arm motor field (Symington and Crymble 1913). The direction of this sulcus is anteriorly oblique from superior to inferior.

The rolandic sulcus is rarely interrupted and usually does not reach the sylvian fissure, resulting in most cases in a hook-like end. Anastomoses with the subcentral, precentral and postcentral sulci are fairly frequent, occurring in about 50% of cases. Extension into the sylvian fissure is found in about 20% of cases, generally as an anastomosis with the anterior or posterior subcentral sulci (Retzius 1896; Vint 1934).

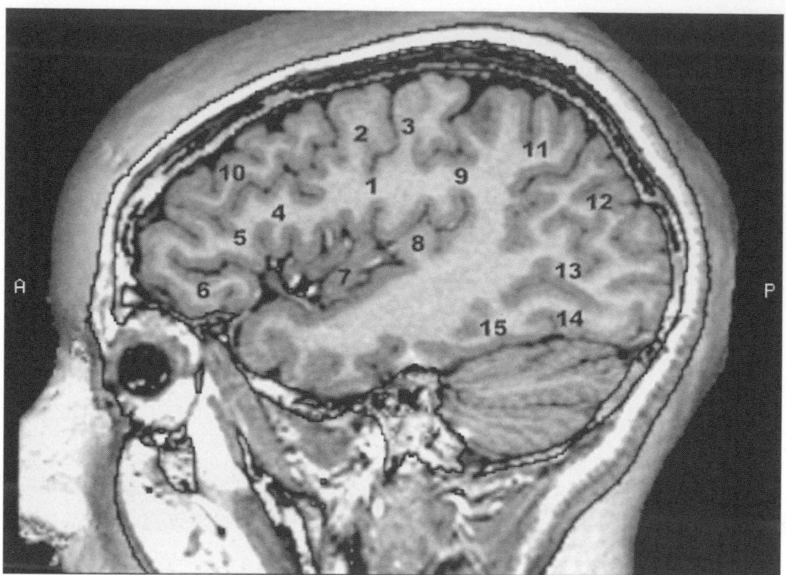

Fig. 3.21. Sagittal cut into a 3D MR of the head passing through the insular cortex and showing the main gyri. *1*, Frontoparietal operculum; *2*, precentral sulcus; *3*, postcentral sulcus; *4*, pars opercularis of inferior frontal gyrus; *5*, pars triangularis of inferior frontal gyrus; *6*, pars orbitalis of inferior frontal gyrus; *7*, insula; *8*, superior transverse gyrus of Heschl; *9*, supramarginal gyrus of inferior parietal lobule; *10*, middle frontal gyrus; *11*, angular gyrus of inferior parietal lobule; *12*, superior occipital gyrus; *13*, middle occipital gyrus; *14*, inferior occipital gyrus; *15*, inferior temporal gyrus

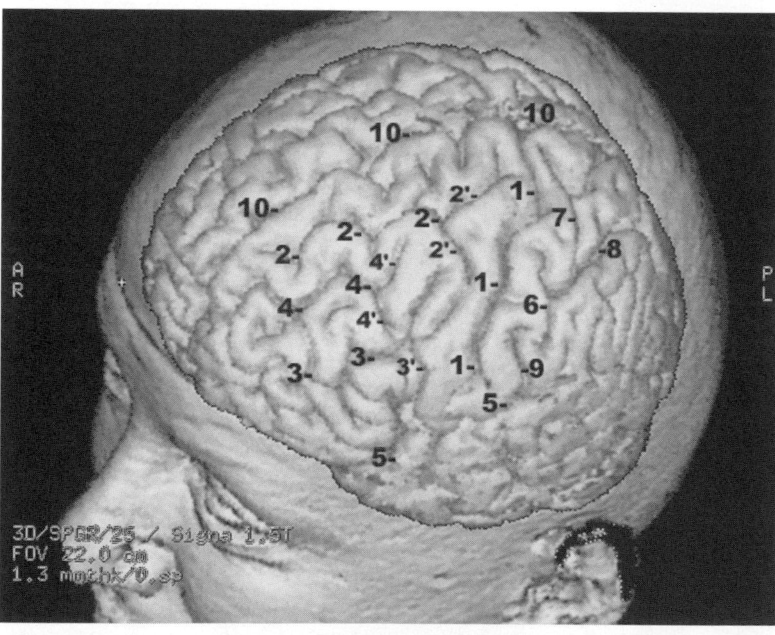

Fig. 3.22. 3D MR of the brain showing the frontal and central sulci. *1*, Central sulcus; *2*, superior frontal sulcus; *2'*, superior prefrontal sulcus; *3*, inferior frontal sulcus; *3'*, inferior precentral sulcus; *4*, intermediate frontal sulcus; *4'*, posterior Y-branching of intermediate frontal sulcus; *5*, lateral fissure; *6*, postcentral sulcus (ascending segment of intraparietal sulcus); *7*, superior postcentral sulcus; *8*, intraparietal sulcus; *9*, sulcus retrocentralis transversus; *10*, interhemispheric fissure

Table 3.12. Sylvian fissure opercula

After Ono et al. 1990	After Duvernoy et al. 1991
• Frontal operculum	• Frontal operculum
Pars orbitalis	Pars triangularis
Pars triangularis	Pars opercularis
• Frontoparietal operculum	• Central operculum
Pars opercularis	Precentral gyrus (inferior end)
Precentral gyrus	Subcentral gyrus
Postcentral gyrus	Postcentral gyrus (inferior end)
Inferior parietal lobule	• Parietal operculum: inferior parietal lobule
• Temporal operculum	• Temporal operculum
Superior temporal gyrus	Superior temporal gyrus

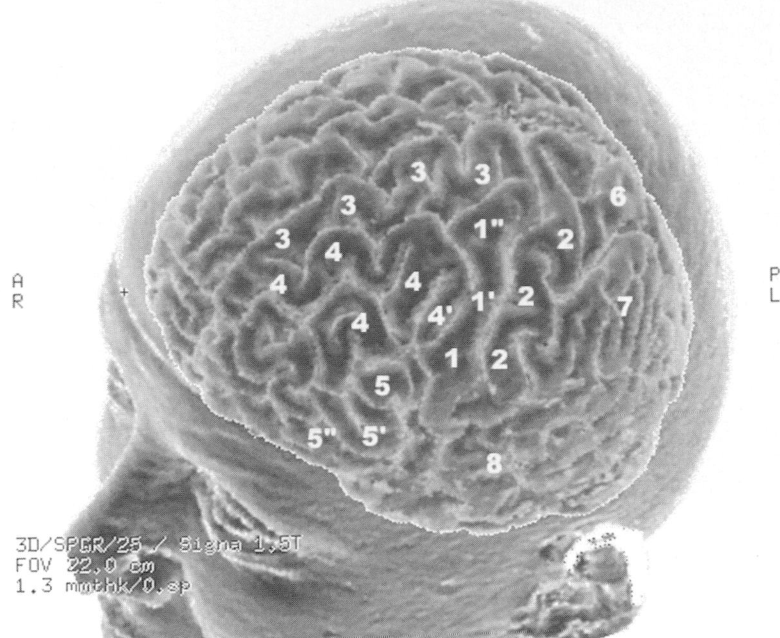

Fig. 3.23. 3D MR of the brain showing the frontal and central gyri. *1*, Central gyrus (inferior genu); *1'*, central sulcus (middle curve or genu); *1"*, central gyrus, superior genu; *2*, postcentral gyrus; *3*, superior frontal gyrus; *4*, middle frontal gyrus; *5*, inferior frontal gyrus; *5'*, inferior frontal gyrus, pars triangularis; *5"*, inferior frontal gyrus, pars opercularis; *6*, superior parietal gyrus; *7*, inferior parietal lobule; *8*, temporal lobe

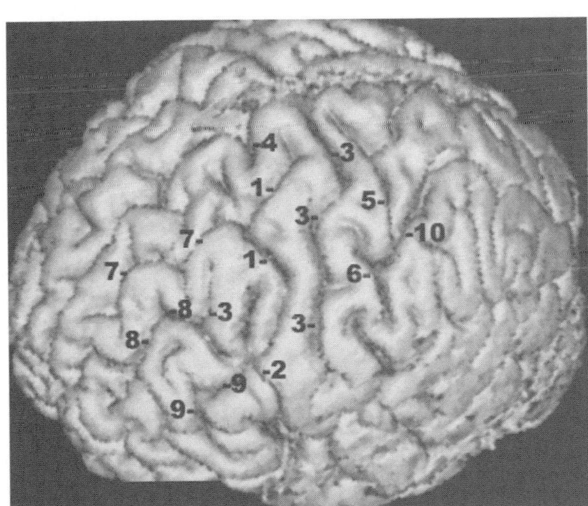

Fig. 3.24. 3D MR of the brain showing the pericentral sulci (lateral view). *1*, Precentral sulcus (superior segment); *2*, precentral sulcus (inferior segment); *3*, precentral gyrus (intermediate segment); *4*, medial precentral sulcus; *5*, postcentral sulcus, superior segment; *6*, postcentral sulcus, inferior segment; *7*, superior frontal sulcus; *8*, middle frontal sulcus; *9*, inferior frontal sulcus; *10*, intraparietal sulcus

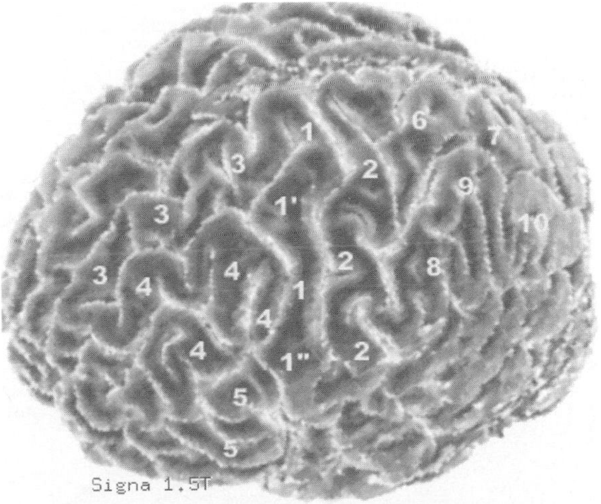

Fig. 3.25. 3D MR of the brain showing the pericentral gyri (lateral view). *1*, Precentral gyrus; *1'*, superior genu of precentral gyrus; *1"*, inferior genu of precentral gyrus; *2*, postcentral gyrus; *3*, superior frontal gyrus; *4*, middle frontal gyrus; *5*, inferior frontal gyrus; *6*, superior parietal lobule, anterior portion; *7*, superior parietal lobule, posterior portion; *8*, supramarginal gyrus; *9*, angular gyrus; *10*, posterior parietal gyrus

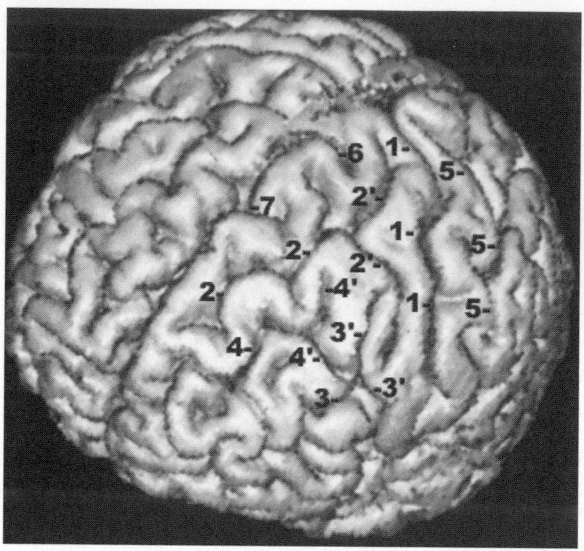

Fig. 3.26. 3D MR of the brain showing the central and frontal sulci (oblique anterior view). *1*, Precentral sulcus; *2*, superior frontal sulcus; *2'*, superior precentral sulcus; *3*, inferior frontal sulcus; *3'*, inferior precentral sulcus; *4*, intermediate frontal sulcus; *4'*, posterior branching of intermediate frontal sulcus; *5*, postcentral sulcus; *6*, medial precentral sulcus; *7*, paracentral sulcus

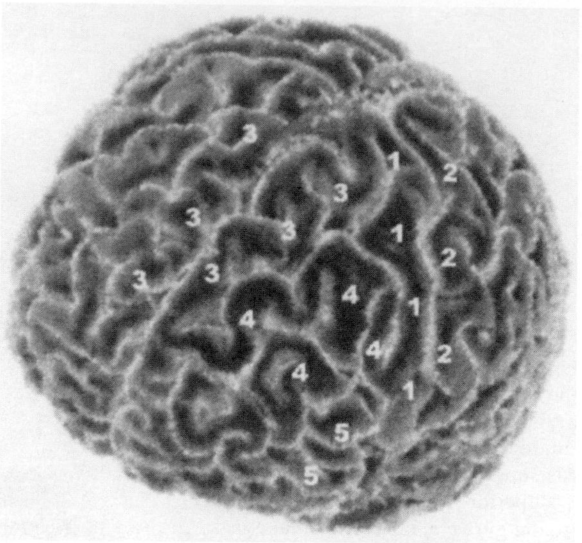

Fig. 3.27. 3D MR of the brain showing the central and frontal gyri (oblique anterior view). *1*, Precentral gyrus; *2*, postcentral gyrus; *3*, superior frontal gyrus; *4*, middle frontal gyrus; *5*, inferior frontal gyrus

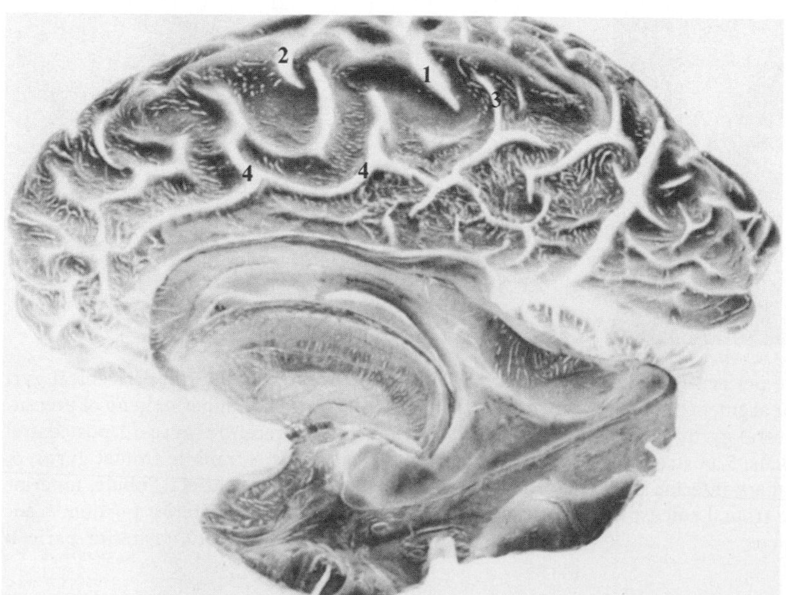

Fig. 3.28. The paracentral lobule: sulcal anatomy of the mesial aspect of the hemisphere. *1*, Central sulcus, medial extent; *2*, medial precentral sulcus; *3*, marginal ramus of cingulate; *4*, cingulate sulcus. (Brain specimen from Klingler; Ludwig and Klingler 1956)

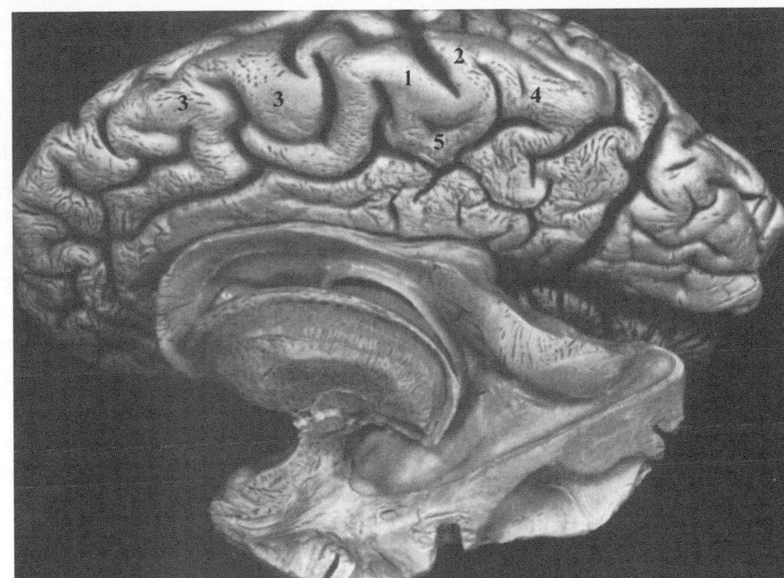

Fig. 3.29. The paracentral lobule: gyral anatomy of the mesial aspect of the hemisphere. *1*, Precentral gyrus, superior and medial extent; *2*, postcentral gyrus, superior and medial extent; *3*, medial frontal gyrus (superior frontal); *4*, precuneus; *5*, paracentral lobule. (Brain specimen from Klingler; Ludwig and Klingler 1956)

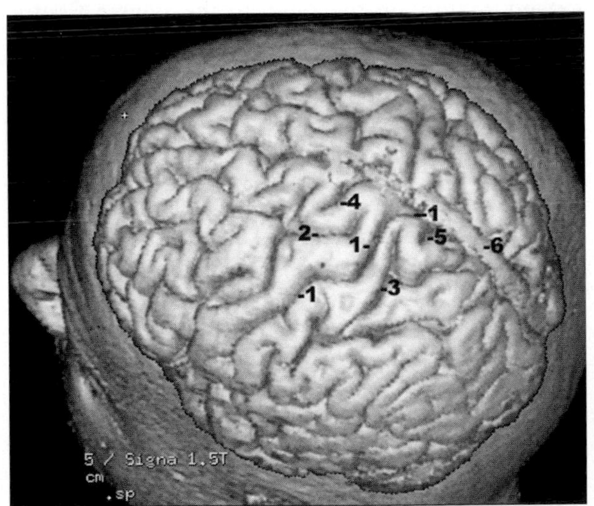

Fig. 3.30. 3D MR of the superior aspect of the brain showing the sulcation of the upper central region. *1*, Central sulcus; *2*, superior precentral sulcus; *3*, superior postcentral sulcus; *4*, medial precentral sulcus; *5*, marginal sulcus; *6*, superior sagittal sinus

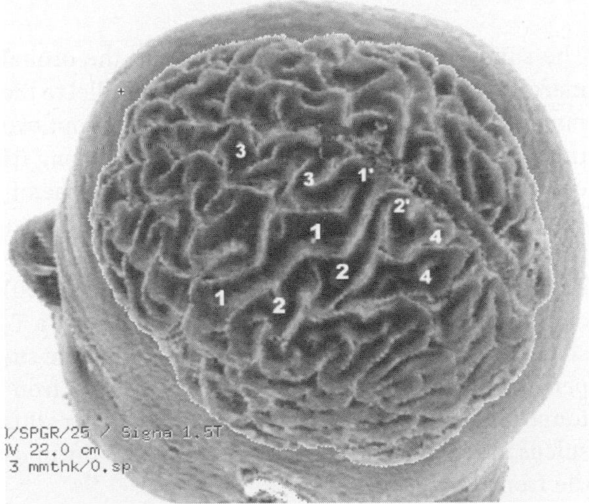

Fig. 3.31. 3D MR of the superior aspect of the brain showing the gyral pattern of the central region. *1*, Precentral gyrus; *1'*, superior extent of precentral gyrus; *2*, postcentral gyrus; *2'*, superior extent of postcentral gyrus; *3*, superior frontal gyrus; *4*, superior parietal gyrus

Superiorly, the rolandic sulcus reaches the superior border of the hemisphere and may extend over the mesial aspect of the hemisphere as a small sulcus, the "crochet Rolandique" (about 80% of cases). This mesial extension is considered as being constant according to Eberstaller. It was found in 88% of the hemispheres according to Lang but was observed in only 64% of the cases as reported by Retzius.

3 Inferior Frontal Sulcus

This sulcus arises anteriorly at the level of the lateral orbital gyrus presenting an Y-shape bifurcation, and courses roughly parallel to the lateral sulcus (Figs. 3.32, 3.33). Eberstaller places its anterior extent at about the middle of the pars triangularis (1890). The inferior frontal sulcus is a deep sulcus almost reaching the insular plane and ending at the inferior precentral sulcus, where a submerged gyrus is very frequently found according to Eberstaller (1890). This "pli de passage" may come to the surface separating the inferior frontal sulcus from the inferior precentral. More developed and constant than the superior frontal sulcus, it is interrupted in about 30% of cases, usually in the middle of this sulcus by two "plis de passage". The inferior frontal sulcus is continuous in approximately 50% of cases.

4 Superior Frontal Sulcus

The superior frontal sulcus arises from the orbital margin of the hemisphere and courses parallel to the interhemispheric fissure, extending along about two thirds of the frontal lobe (Figs. 3.34, 3.35). Along its course, it gradually separates from the interhemispheric fissure. It is frequently doubled and varies from race to race. Frequently this sulcus is interrupted (26–50% of cases, according to Ono et al. 1990) and ends posteriorly at the precentral sulcus in a T-shaped branching (50% of cases). Anteriorly, the superior frontal sulcus may anastomose with the frontomarginal sulcus. According to Eberstaller this sulcus may anastomose (45% of cases) with the middle frontal sulcus.

5 Precentral Sulcus

This sulcus is usually divided into a superior and an inferior precentral sulci (75%) separated by a connection between the precentral and the middle frontal gyrus (Figs. 3.34, 3.26). It may be composed of three segments (15%), the third constituting an intermediate precentral sulcus. The precentral sulcus courses parallel to the central sulcus and is formed by the posterior bifurcations of the inferior and the superior frontal sulci. The superior end of the inferior precentral sulcus is located anteriorly to the inferior end of the superior precentral sulcus. The inferior end of the inferior precentral sulcus may connect with the sylvian fissure either directly or through the anterior subcentral or the diagonal sulcus (Eberstaller 1890; Giacomini 1878). The superior precentral sulcus is usually smaller than the inferior precentral sulcus. It generally does not reach the superior border of the hemisphere and is separated from it by an inconstant horizontal marginal precentral sulcus (Cunningham and Horsley 1892), a small dimple medial to the superior precentral sulcus. Just anterior to the latter may be found a medial precentral sulcus (Eberstaller 1890) which cuts into the dorsal margin of the hemisphere.

6 The Intraparietal Sulcus

The intraparietal sulcus is divided into three parts(Figs. 3.36–3.41), the ascending postcentral, horizontal and descending or occipital segments (Wilder 1886). The ascending segment is a vertical segment which corresponds to the inferior portion of the postcentral sulcus (Turner 1948), and may extend, mainly on the right, to the sylvian fissure. According to Cunningham (1890; Cunningham and Horsley 1892), the horizontal or true intraparietal segment has variable relationships with the inferior and superior postcentral sulci (Jefferson 1913). The most frequent pattern is represented by the type IV in which the intraparietal is continuous with both the inferior and superior postcentral sulci (40% of cases). The inferior postcentral segment is continuous with that of the superior postcentral in more than 60% of the cases. The third descending or occipital segment almost always terminates in the occipital lobe and may even reach its pole. The intraparietal sulcus is a very deep sulcus almost reaching the roof of the lateral ventricles, as identified on coronal and parasagittal cuts.

The occipital segment of the intraparietal or superior occipital sulcus, shows a T-shaped ending in about 70% of cases (Ono et al. 1990), described as the transverse occipital sulcus. The superior end of the postcentral sulcus terminates most frequently on the lateral aspect of the hemisphere without extension to the medial aspect, in a Y-shaped configuration. At this Y-shaped end, it is joined by the marginal ramus

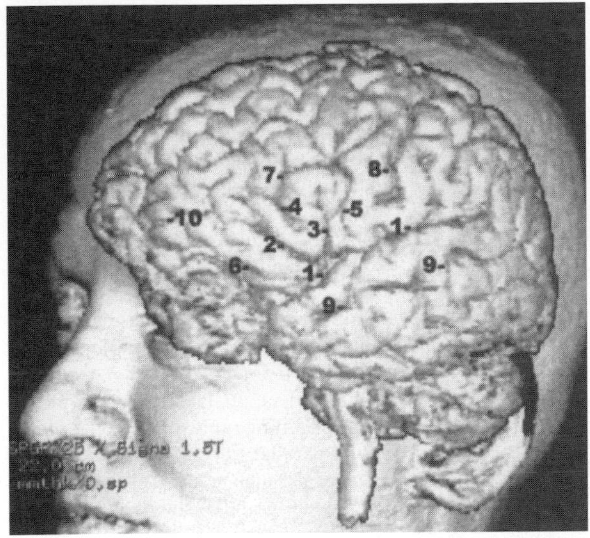

Fig. 3.32. 3D MR of the brain showing the sulcal pattern of the inferior frontal region. *1*, Lateral fissure; *2*, horizontal ramus of lateral fissure; *3*, ascending ramus of lateral fissure; *4*, radiate sulcus (incisura capitis); *5*, inferior precentral sulcus; *6*, lateral orbital sulcus; *7*, inferior frontal sulcus; *8*, central sulcus; *9*, superior temporal (parallel) sulcus; *10*, frontomarginal sulcus

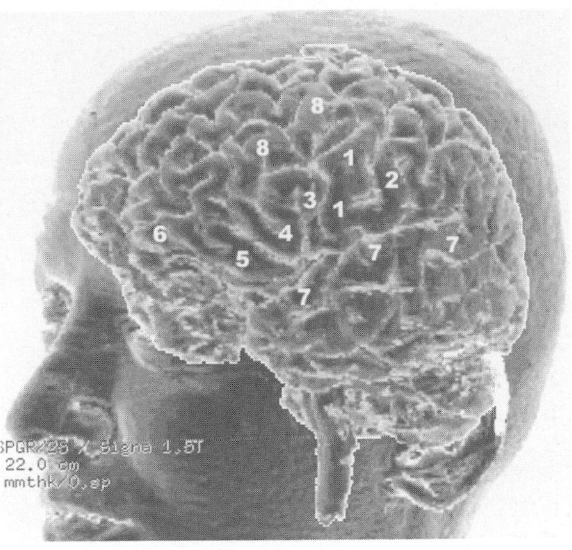

Fig. 3.33. 3D MR of the brain showing the gyral pattern of the inferior frontal region. *1*, Central gyrus; *2*, postcentral gyrus; *3*, pars opercularis of inferior frontal gyrus; *4*, pars triangularis of inferior frontal gyrus; *5*, pars orbitalis of inferior frontal gyrus; *6*, frontomarginal gyrus; *7*, superior temporal gyrus; *8*, middle frontal gyrus

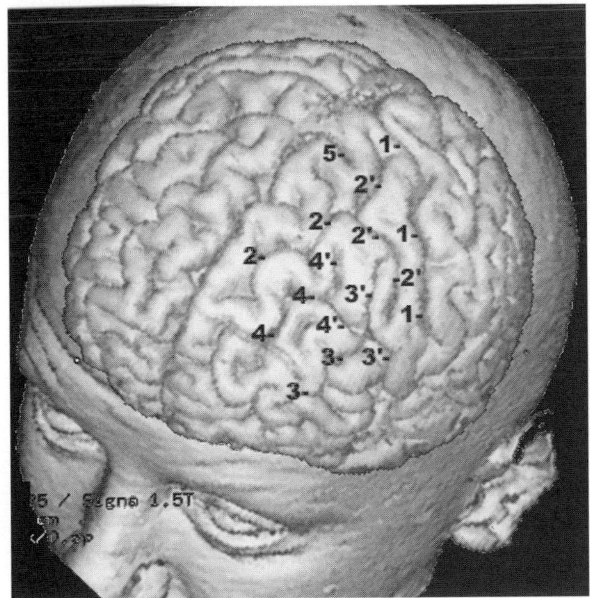

Fig. 3.34. Sulcal anatomy of the frontal lobe using 3D MR. *1*, Central sulcus; *2*, superior frontal sulcus; *2'*, superior precentral sulcus; *3*, inferior central sulcus; *3'*, inferior precentral sulcus; *4*, intermediate frontal sulcus; *4'*, posterior branching of intermediate frontal sulcus; *5*, medial precentral sulcus

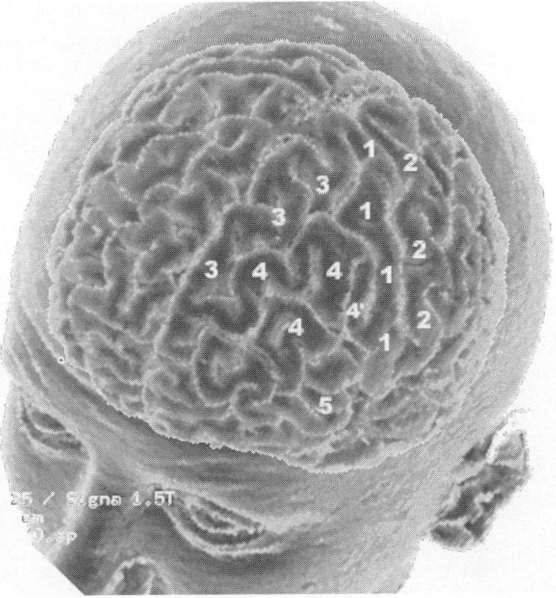

Fig. 3.35. Gyral anatomy of the frontal lobe using 3D MR. *1*, Central gyrus; *2*, postcentral gyrus; *3*, superior frontal gyrus; *4*, middle frontal gyrus; *4'*, pli de passage between middle frontal gyrus and precentral gyrus; *5*, inferior frontal gyrus

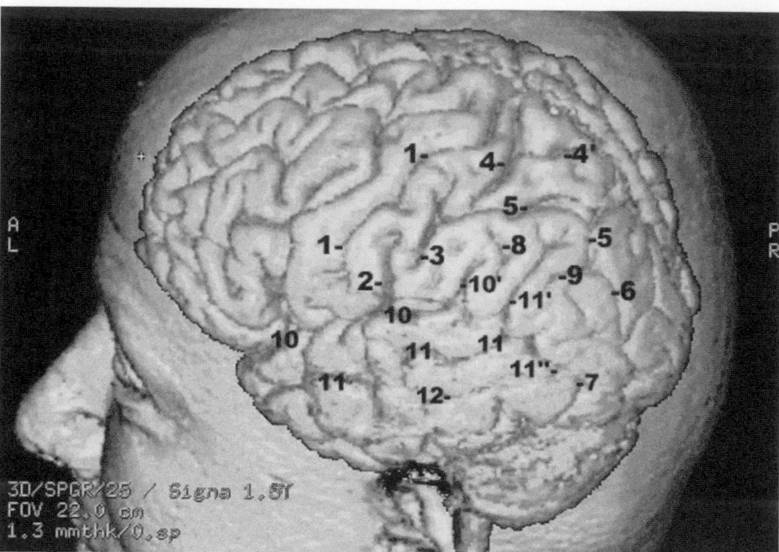

Fig. 3.36. 3D MR of the lateral aspect of the brain showing the sulcal anatomy of the temporal and parietal lobes. *1*, Central sulcus; *2*, sulcus retrocentralis transversus; *3*, inferior postcentral sulcus (ascending ramus of intraparietal sulcus); *4*, superior postcentral sulcus; *4'*, superior Y-branching of superior postcentral sulcus; *5*, intraparietal sulcus (horizontal segment); *6*, intraparietal sulcus (descending or occipital segment); *7*, preoccipital incisure; *8*, sulcus intermedius primus (Jensen); *9*, sulcus intermedius secundus (Eberstaller); *10*, lateral fissure, posterior ascending ramus; *11*, superior temporal parallel sulcus; *11'*, ascending ramus of parallel sulcus; *11''*, descending ramus of parallel sulcus; *12*, middle temporal sulcus

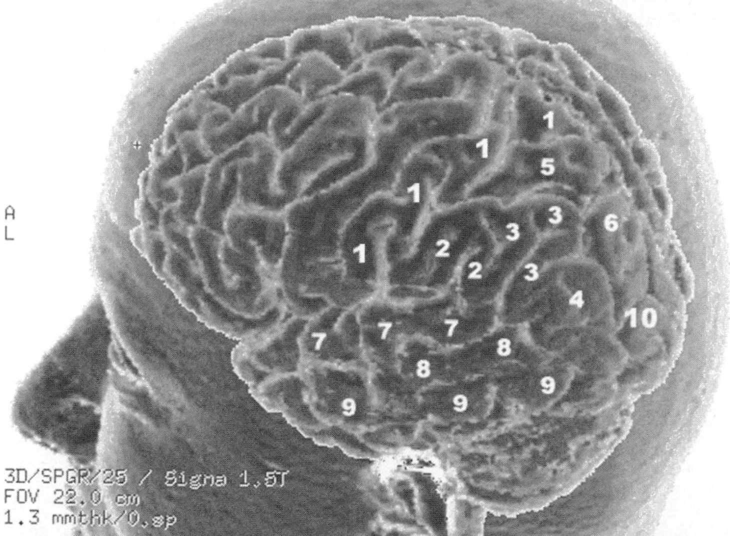

Fig. 3.37. 3D MR of the lateral aspect of the brain showing the gyral anatomy of the temporal and parietal lobes. *1*, Central gyrus; *2*, supramarginal gyrus (inferior parietal lobule); *3*, angular lobe (inferior parietal lobule); *4*, posterior parietal gyrus (inferior parietal lobule); *5*, superior parietal lobule (anterior portion); *6*, superior parietal lobule (posterior portion); *7*, superior temporal gyrus; *8*, middle temporal gyrus; *9*, inferior temporal gyrus; *10*, occipital lobe

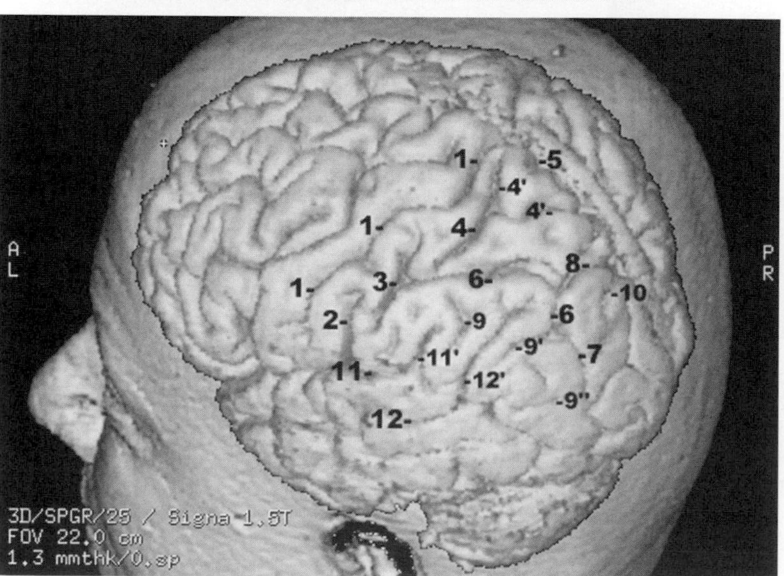

Fig. 3.38. 3D MR of the lateral aspect of the brain showing the sulcal anatomy of the inferior parietal region. *1*, Central sulcus; *2*, sulcus retrocentralis transversus (Eberstaller); *3*, inferior postcentral sulcus (ascending segment of intraparietal sulcus); *4*, superior postcentral sulcus; *4'*, end branches; *5*, marginal ramus of cingulate sulcus; *6*, intraparietal sulcus (horizontal segment); *7*, intraparietal sulcus (descending segment or superior occipital sulcus); *8*, sulcus parietalis transversus (Brissaud); *9*, sulcus intermedius primus (Jensen); *9'*, sulcus intermedius secundus (Eberstaller); *9''*, sulcus intermedius tertius (Eberstaller); *10*, lateral parieto-occipital sulcus; *11*, lateral fissure; *11'*, terminal ascending ramus of lateral fissure; *12*, superior temporal (parallel) sulcus; *12'*, ascending ramus of parallel sulcus

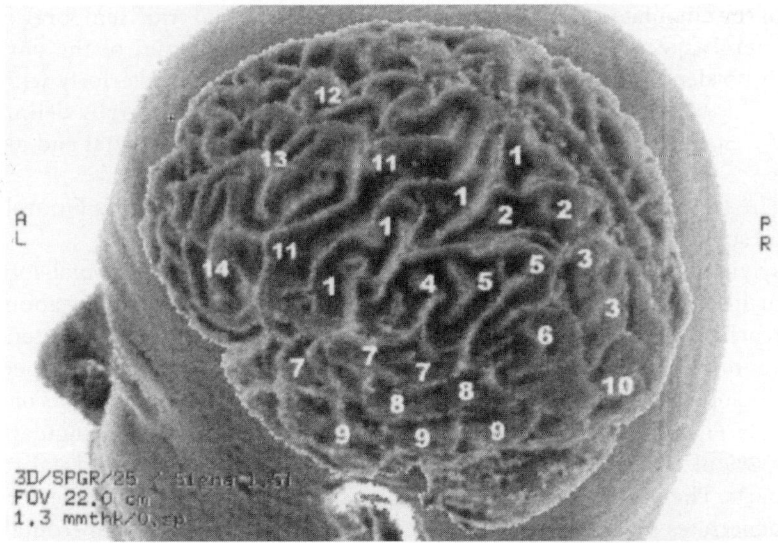

Fig. 3.39. 3D MR of the lateral aspect of the brain showing the gyral anatomy of the inferior parietal region. *1*, Postcentral gyrus; *2*, superior parietal gyrus (anterior portion); *3*, superior parietal gyrus (posterior portion); *4*, supramarginal gyrus (inferior parietal lobule); *5*, angular gyrus (inferior parietal lobule); *6*, posterior parietal gyrus; *7*, superior temporal gyrus; *8*, middle temporal gyrus; *9*, inferior temporal gyrus; *10*, occipital lobe; *11*, precentral gyrus; *12*, superior frontal gyrus; *13*, middle frontal gyrus; *14*, inferior frontal gyrus

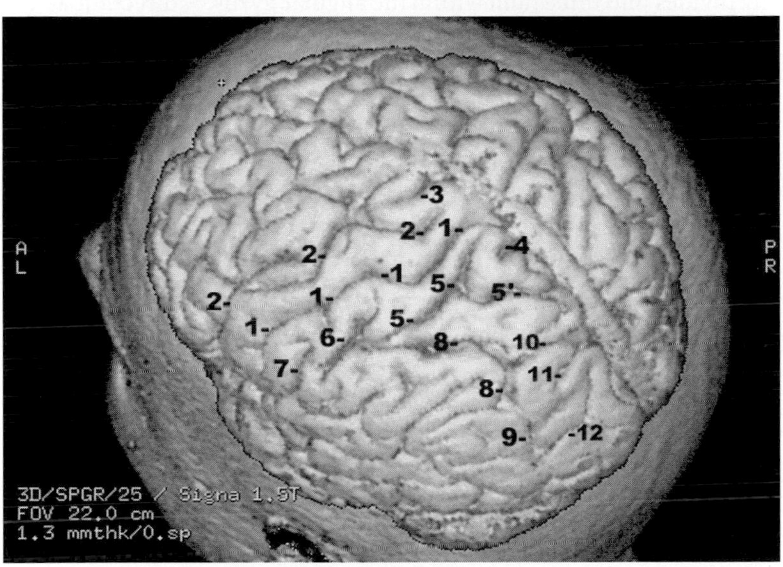

Fig. 3.40. 3D MR of the superior aspect of the brain showing the sulcal anatomy of the superior parietal region. *1*, Central sulcus; *2*, precentral sulcus; *3*, medial precentral sulcus; *4*, marginal sulcus (lateral extent); *5*, superior postcentral sulcus; *6*, inferior postcentral sulcus (ascending ramus of intraparietal sulcus); *7*, sulcus postcentralis transversus (Eberstaller); *8*, intraparietal sulcus (horizontal segment); *9*, intraparietal sulcus (descending or occipital segment); *10*, transverse parietal sulcus (Brissaud); *11*, parieto-occipital sulcus (lateral extent); *12*, transverse occipital sulcus

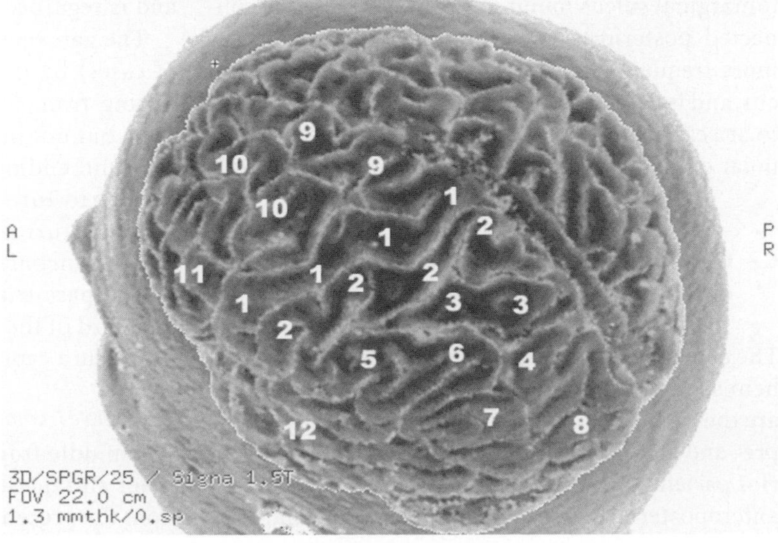

Fig. 3.41. 3D MR of the superior aspect of the brain showing the gyral anatomy of the superior parietal region. *1*, Precentral gyrus; *2*, postcentral gyrus; *3*, superior parietal gyrus; *4*, arcus parieto-occipitalis; *5*, supramarginal gyrus; *6*, angular gyrus; *7*, posterior parietal gyrus; *8*, occipital pole; *9*, superior frontal gyrus; *10*, middle frontal gyrus; *11*, inferior frontal gyrus; *12*, temporal lobe

of the cingulate sulcus terminates as it extends to the lateral aspect of the hemisphere indenting its superior border.

7 Superior Temporal Sulcus

The superior temporal sulcus is also called the parallel sulcus because it follows closely the course of the sylvian fissure. This sulcus is one of the oldest of the primate brain. It is a deep sulcus (2.5–3 cm) almost reaching the level of the inferior border of the insula, coursing roughly parallel to the opercular surface of the superior temporal gyrus as shown on the coronal cuts(Figs. 3.42–3.45). It is a rarely interrupted sulcus (32% of cases) divided into anterior and posterior parts. The posterior part is the angular sulcus which penetrates into the inferior parietal lobule and usually divides into three rami within the angular gyrus.

Its most consistent interruption point is below the inferior end of the central sulcus and its anterior extremity never extends into the temporal tip. This explains the apparent extension of the superior temporal gyrus to form the temporal pole. The superior temporal sulcus limits the superior temporal gyrus inferiorly. At the level of the central sulcus, this gyrus may show an inconstant sulcus acousticus which originates from the parallel sulcus and courses towards the lateral fissure, limiting the anterior extent of Heschl gyri.

8 Frontomarginal Sulcus

Described by Wernicke (1876), the frontomarginal sulcus is fairly constant and deep and is found at the frontal pole. It courses parallel to the orbital margin (Figs. 3.32, 3.33, 3.46). It corresponds to the frontomarginal sulcus found in the orangutan. It is connected posteriorly with the middle frontal sulcus more frequently than with the superior frontal sulcus, and is deeper than the latter, from which it seems to arise. This sulcus separates the transverse frontopolar gyri from the frontomarginal gyrus inferiorly.

C Gyri of the Lateral Surface of the Cerebral Hemisphere

The convolutions on the lateral aspect of the cerebral hemisphere determined by these primary fissures are the inferior, middle and superior frontal gyri, the pre- and postcentral gyri, and the inferior and superior parietal convolutions, in the suprasylvian region anteroposteriorly, and the superior, middle and inferior temporal gyri, in the infrasylvian region. The gyri of the parietal and the temporal lobes merge posteriorly with the variable occipital gyri, and are generally delimited by a superior occipital, a lateral occipital and an inferior occipital sulci.

1 The Frontal Lobe

The frontal lobe is the largest of the hemisphere, occupying about one third of its surface. It comprises four gyri extending from the lateral to the medial and basal aspects of the hemisphere. Medially, this lobe consists of a hook-like gyrus bounded inferiorly by the cingulate sulcus, and anteriorly corresponds to the orbital region. The gyri on the lateral aspect are the inferior frontal, the middle frontal and the superior frontal gyri. They follow a roughly parallel direction as compared to the lateral fissure and the superior border of the hemisphere. The fourth gyrus, the precentral gyrus, parallels the central sulcus and is almost perpendicular to the others.

a Inferior Frontal Gyrus

The inferior frontal gyrus is the smallest one and is situated between the lateral fissure and the inferior frontal sulcus, in relation with the horizontal and vertical rami of the lateral fissure (Figs. 3.15, 3.17, 3.19, 3.32, 3.33). These rami divide the gyrus into three parts: the pars orbitalis, the pars triangularis and the pars opercularis. The orbital part passes into the basal orbital aspect of the hemisphere and the opercular part continues with the lower extension of the precentral gyrus, constituting the frontal operculum. This gyrus is more developed on the left side in right-handed subjects, particularly in its triangular and opercular parts. It is called Broca's convolution and is regarded as the motor speech area.

The pars opercularis is frequently traversed (70% of cases) by the diagonal sulcus (Eberstaller 1890) arising from the precentral or the inferior frontal sulci, but not involving the circular sulcus of the insula, and ending at or about the sylvian fissure. According to Turner (1948) this sulcus would be a characteristic furrow of the human brain. Nevertheless, it remains inconstant.

The pars triangularis is traversed in more than one third of the cases by the radiate sulcus (Fig. 3.44) or incisura capitis (Eberstaller).

b Middle Frontal Gyrus

The middle frontal gyrus is located between the inferior and the superior frontal sulci and is separated from the precentral gyrus posteriorly by the branch-

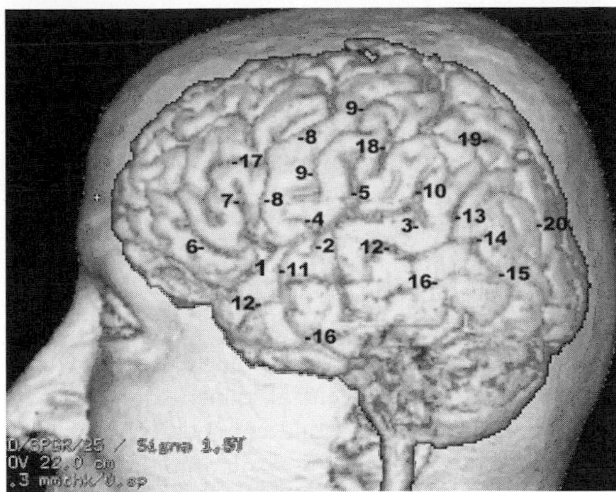

Fig. 3.42. Sulcal anatomy of the lateral surface of the cerebral hemisphere using 3D MR. *1*, Lateral fissure; *2*, transverse supratemporal sulcus; *3*, posterior transverse temporal sulcus; *4*, anterior subcentral sulcus; *5*, sulcus retrocentralis transversus; *6*, horizontal ramus of lateral fissure; *7*, ascending ramus of lateral fissure; *8*, precentral sulcus; *9*, central sulcus; *10*, ascending ramus of lateral fissure; *11*, sulcus acousticus; *12*, superior temporal (parallel) sulcus; *13*, ascending ramus of superior temporal sulcus; *14*, horizontal or descending ramus of parallel sulcus; *15*, lateral occipital sulcus; *16*, inferior temporal sulcus; *17*, inferior frontal sulcus; *18*, central sulcus (ascending ramus of intraparietal sulcus); *19*, intraparietal sulcus, horizontal segment; *20*, intraparietal sulcus (descending or occipital segment)

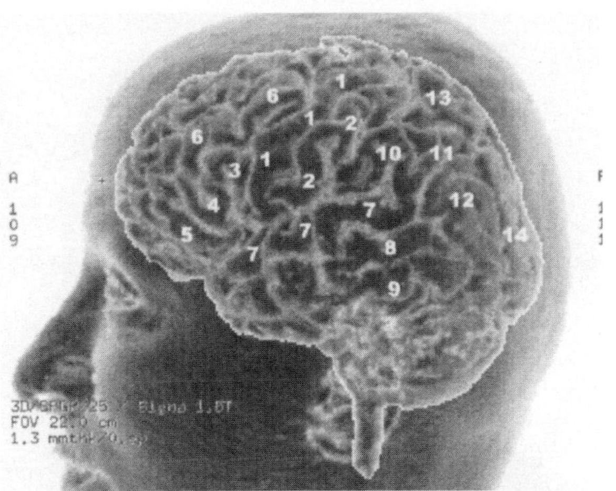

Fig. 3.43. Gyral anatomy of the lateral surface of the cerebral hemisphere using 3D MR. *1*, Central gyrus; *2*, postcentral gyrus; *3*, pars opercularis of inferior frontal gyrus; *4*, pars triangularis of inferior frontal gyrus; *5*, pars orbitalis of inferior frontal gyrus; *6*, middle frontal gyrus; *7*, superior temporal gyrus; *8*, middle temporal gyrus; *9*, inferior temporal gyrus; *10*, supramarginal gyrus; *11*, angular gyrus; *12*, posterior parietal gyrus; *13*, superior parietal gyrus; *14*, superior occipital gyrus

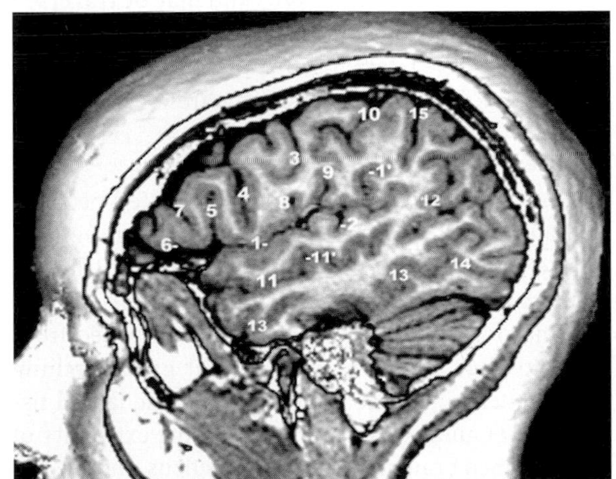

Fig. 3.44. Sulcal anatomy of the lateral surface of the cerebral hemisphere based on a sagittal lateral MR cut. *1*, Lateral sylvian fissure; *1'*, ascending ramus of lateral fissure; *2*, transverse temporal sulcus; *3*, central sulcus; *4*, inferior precentral sulcus; *5*, ascending ramus of lateral fissure; *6*, horizontal ramus of lateral fissure; *7*, radiate sulcus (incisura capitis); *8*, anterior subcentral sulcus; *9*, posterior subcentral sulcus; *10*, postcentral sulcus; *11*, superior temporal (parallel) sulcus; *11'*, sulcus acousticus; *12*, ascending ramus of parallel sulcus; *13*, middle temporal sulcus; *14*, inferior occipital sulcus; *15*, intraparietal sulcus

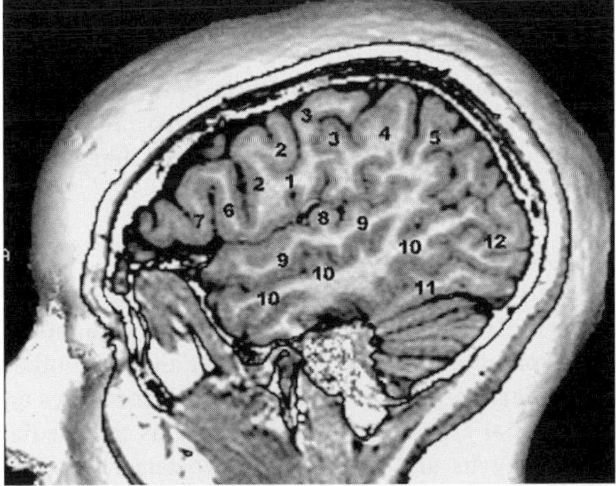

Fig. 3.45. Gyral anatomy of the lateral surface of the cerebral hemisphere based on a sagittal lateral MR cut. *1*, Frontoparietal operculum; *2*, precentral gyrus; *3*, postcentral gyrus; *4*, supramarginal gyrus; *5*, angular gyrus; *6*, pars opercularis of inferior frontal gyrus; *7*, pars triangularis of inferior frontal gyrus; *8*, superior transverse gyrus; *9*, superior temporal gyrus; *10*, middle temporal gyrus; *11*, inferior temporal gyrus; *12*, middle occipital gyrus

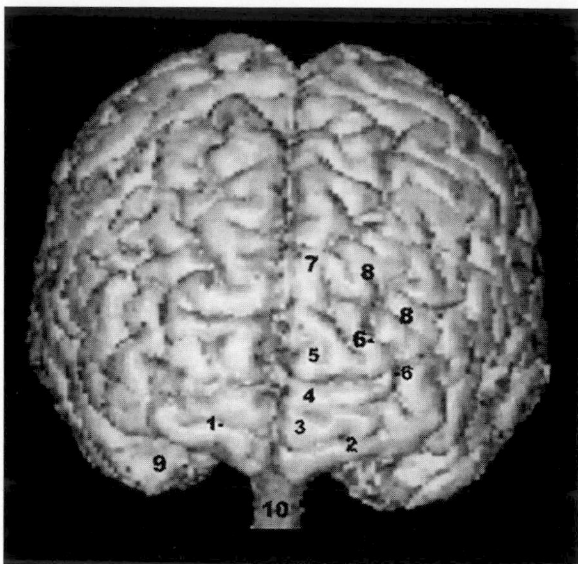

Fig. 3.46. 3D MR anatomy of the frontal pole (anterior view). *1*, Frontomarginal sulcus; *2*, frontomarginal gyrus; *3*, inferior transverse frontopolar gyrus; *4*, middle transverse frontopolar gyrus; *5*, superior transverse frontopolar gyrus; *6*, intermediate frontal sulcus; *7*, superior frontal gyrus; *8*, middle frontal gyrus; *9*, temporal pole; *10*, spinal cord

es of the precentral sulci (Figs. 3.22, 3.23, 3.26, 3.27). It is connected to the precentral gyrus by a deep annectent gyrus. The middle frontal gyrus is traversed by an inconstant intermediate or middle frontal sulcus which courses parallel to the inferior and superior frontal sulci, and shows a great variability in length. It originates about halfway between the precentral gyrus and the orbital margin, and usually ends in a bifurcation at the orbitodorsal margin as a part of the frontomarginal sulcus.

c Superior Frontal Gyrus

The superior frontal gyrus is situated between the superior frontal sulcus and the dorsal margin of the hemisphere and is therefore longer than the other frontal parallel gyri (Figs. 3.34, 3.35). It continues on the medial aspect of the hemisphere as the medial frontal gyrus and is connected posteriorly to the central gyrus.

d Precentral Gyrus

Also called the ascending frontal gyrus (circonvolution frontale ascendante), the precentral gyrus is located posteriorly between the central sulcus and between the inferior and superior frontal sulci anteriorly (Figs. 3.22–3.25, 3.30). Its is limited inferiorly by the lateral fissure and extends superiorly to reach the superior border of the hemisphere where it is continuous with the paracentral lobule on the medial aspect of the hemisphere. Its lower end may be traversed by the anterior subcentral sulcus, a sulcus of variable length arising from the upper bank of the lateral fissure and ending in the precentral gyrus behind the inferior precentral sulcus with which it may anastomose.

2 The Parietal Lobe

The parietal lobe is located superior to the lateral fissure and behind the central sulcus, extending posteriorly to an arbitrary line connecting the lateral extent of the parieto-occipital sulcus to the preoccipital notch. It extends to the medial aspect of the hemisphere as the precuneus gyrus and to the medial postcentral gyrus anteriorly. Its largest portion is on the lateral surface of the hemisphere where it is divided into three gyri by the intraparietal sulcus: the inferior parietal, the superior parietal and the postcentral gyri. The inferior parietal gyrus is usually further subdivided into three small gyri.

a Postcentral Gyrus

Also called the ascending postcentral gyrus, it is found posterior to the central sulcus, bounded caudally by the inferior and superior postcentral sulci (Figs. 3.24, 3.25, 3.40, 3.41). Its lower end is connected to the inferior precentral gyrus and may be traversed by a posterior subcentral sulcus (Marchand 1895) arising from the lateral fissure and ending as a small indentation in the parietal operculum.

b Inferior Parietal Gyri

The inferior parietal gyri lobule is situated between the lateral fissure inferiorly, the horizontal segment of the intraparietal sulcus superiorly, and the ascending postcentral segment of the intraparietal sulcus anteriorly (Figs. 3.36, 3.37). It is composed from front to back as the supramarginal gyrus arching over the terminal ascending ramus of the lateral fissure, the angular gyrus arching over the extremity of the upturned branch of the parallel sulcus, and the last corresponding to the posterior parietal gyrus which may cap the posterior end of the inferior temporal sulcus. The supramarginal and the angular arched convolutions are separated by a short sulcus, the primary intermediate sulcus of Jensen (1870) which is usually fused with the intraparietal but may anastomose with the lateral fissure. The angular gyrus may be separated from the posterior parietal gyrus by another secondary intermediate sulcus (Eberstaller 1884) which may anastomose with the parallel sulcus.

c Superior Parietal Gyrus

Located dorsal to the inferior parietal lobule, the superior parietal gyrus is limited inferiorly by the intraparietal sulcus, anteriorly by the superior postcentral sulcus, and extends posteriorly to the lateral extremity of the parieto-occipital sulcus, beyond which it passes into the occipital lobe forming the arcus parieto-occipitalis (Figs. 3.38, 3.39). The superior parietal gyrus may be divided into an anterior and a posterior portion by the transverse parietal sulcus (Brissaud 1893) originating on the medial side and extending to the lateral side of the superior aspect of the hemisphere where it is found between the postcentral sulcus and the parieto-occipital sulcus. The superior parietal gyrus extends posteriorly along the superior lateral aspect of the hemisphere to the lateral occipital lobe, arching over the lateral extent of the parieto-occipital sulcus to form the superior parieto-occipital "pli de passage" of Gratiolet (1854).

3 The Temporal Lobe

Somewhat pyramidal in shape, the temporal lobe has lateral, basal and dorsal aspects and an anterior apex or pole. The lateral aspect is bounded superiorly by the lateral fissure which separates it from the fronto-parietal lobes. Caudally, it is continuous with the inferior parietal lobule superiorly, and with the occipital lobe, inferiorly. Ventrally the temporal lobe extends to the collateral sulcus at the basal aspect of the hemisphere, which separates it from the limbic lobe. The lateral convolutions of the temporal lobe are three in number, oriented anteroposteriorly and roughly parallel to the lateral fissure. From superior to inferior these are: the superior, middle and inferior temporal gyri.

a Superior Temporal Gyrus

The superior temporal gyrus is located between the lateral fissure above and the parallel sulcus below (Figs. 3.15, 3.42, 3.43, 3.45). Its anterior extent participates in the formation of the temporal pole and its posterior extremity merges with the supramarginal gyrus. At its caudal extremity, this gyrus is continuous with the supramarginal gyrus. The dorsal surface of this gyrus which forms the lower boundary of the sylvian fissure, called the operculo-insular surface, extends over 9 cm from anterior to posterior. It is divided into an opercular and an insular segment. The former is located in relation to the frontal and parietal opercula and the latter is related to the insula. One or two transverse temporal gyri, the Heschl gyri (Heschl 1878), cross the dorsal aspect of the superior temporal gyrus, obliquely forward, at the depth of the lateral fissure. More frequently doubled on the right side (Pfeifer 1936), these gyri are separated at least partly by an intermediate transverse temporal sulcus. These gyri are posteriorly separated from the planum temporale, by the transverse supratemporal sulcus (Holl 1908) originating from the lateral fissure and are frequently noticed on the lateral aspect of the superior temporal gyrus. Even the intermediate temporal sulcus may cut into the lateral surface of the first temporal gyrus. The frontal boundary of the Heschl gyri is marked by the anterior limiting sulcus of Holl. The anterior extent of the of these gyri is demarcated by the sulcus acousticus, originating from the parallel sulcus and cutting into the lateral aspect of the first temporal gyrus.

b Middle Temporal Gyrus

The middle temporal gyrus is almost parallel to the superior gyrus and is separated from the superior temporal gyrus by the superior temporal or parallel sulcus and bounded inferiorly by the inferior temporal sulcus which is a regularly interrupted sulcus (Figs. 3.15, 3.17, 3.37, 3.45). This gyrus is continuous at its posterior extremity with the angular gyrus superiorly, and with the occipital lobe inferiorly, following the inferior branching of the inferior temporal sulcus, namely the anterior occipital sulcus. This gyrus is more flexuose and larger than the superior temporal gyrus.

c Inferior Temporal Gyrus

The inferior temporal gyrus is bounded superiorly by the inferior temporal sulcus and extends inferiorly over the basolateral border of the cerebral hemisphere, to the inferior surface, limited at this level by the occipitotemporal sulcus (Fig. 3.15). It is largely discontinuous (70% of cases), mainly posteriorly, extending like the occipitotemporal gyrus close to the preoccipital notch. At this level, it is continuous posteriorly and inferiorly with the inferior occipital gyrus.

4 The Occipital Lobe

The occipital lobe is the smallest of all hemispheric lobes occupying the posterior aspect of the hemisphere and lying on the tentorium cerebelli (Figs. 3.18, 3.47A–C). It is limited anteriorly in apes by the lateral parieto-occipital sulcus which in humans is reduced to a notch on the superior border of the hemisphere due to the characteristic presence of two

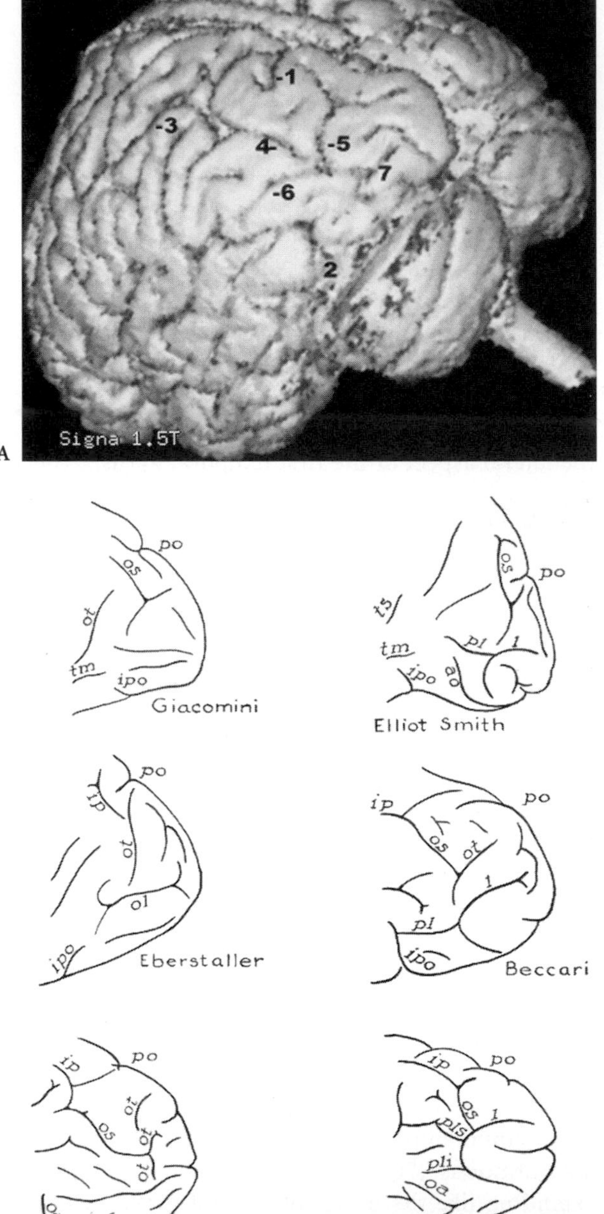

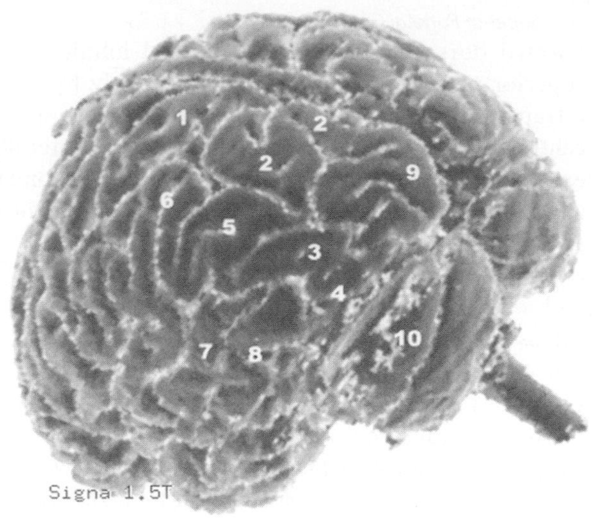

Fig. 3.47. A 3D MR sulcal anatomy of the occipital lobe (posterior lateral view). *1*, Lateral parieto-occipital sulcus; *2*, preoccipital incisure; *3*, intraparietal sulcus; *4*, superior occipital sulcus (occipital segment of intraparietal); *5*, transverse occipital sulcus; *6*, lateral occipital (middle) sulcus; *7*, lunate sulcus. **B** 3D MR gyral anatomy of the occipital lobe (posterior lateral view). *1*, Superior parietal gyrus; *2*, superior occipital gyrus (arcus parieto-occipitalis or 1st pli de passage parieto-occipital of Gratiolet); *3*, middle occipital gyrus (2nd pli de passage parieto-occipital of Gratiolet); *4*, inferior occipital gyrus; *5*, posterior parietal gyrus; *6*, angular gyrus; *7*, superior temporal gyrus; *8*, middle temporal gyrus. **C** Variations of the fissural pattern of the lateral aspect of the occipital lobe. *Left*, vertical type; *right*, horizontal type (from Bailey and von Bonin 1951)

longitudinal parieto-occipital "plis de passage" of Gratiolet. The first occupies the superior aspect of the hemisphere, paralleling the superior border of the hemisphere and joining the superior parietal gyrus to the superior, or first occipital, gyrus, limited laterally by the occipital segment of the intraparietal sulcus. This segment is therefore also called the superior occipital sulcus which may be crossed at its end by the transverse occipital sulcus. The latter shows variable length across the lateral aspect of the occipital lobe and may correspond to the end branching of the pars occipitalis of the intraparietal sulcus (Wilder's paroccipital sulcus). The other parieto-occipital "pli de passage" joins the angular gyrus to the middle or second occipital gyrus. This middle or lateral occipital gyrus is the largest of the lateral aspects of the occipital lobe and may be subdivided into superior and inferior portions by the middle occipital or lateral sulcus which may anastomose anteriorly with the parallel sulcus. Its posterior end joins the inconstant concave lunate sulcus posteriorly the existence of which, in humans, remains controversial. The middle occipital gyrus is bounded superiorly by the superior occipital sulcus and inferiorly by the inferior occipital sulcus. Two other temporal occipital "plis de passage", which are separated by an inconstant inferior occipital sulcus that may correspond to a side branch of the inferior temporal sulcus, occupy the inferior lateral aspect of the occipital lobe. These flexuose plis de passage are found in all primates. The inferior occipital sulcus medially limits the inferior occipital gyrus, or third occipital gyrus, extending posteriorly just anterior to the occipital pole. The anterior extent of the inferior occipital gyrus is ill-defined and found at the level of the preoccipital incisure (inferior preoccipital sulcus of Meynert, 1877), a sulcus indenting the inferior lateral border of the hemisphere. It is continuous anteriorly with the inferior temporal gyrus.

The sulcal and gyral configuration of the inferior temporal-occipital region shows wide unsettled morphological variations which explain the lack of consensus between authors. The sulci are shallow and may show numerous variable ramifications which has lead to the divergent descriptions (Testut and Latarjet 1948; Paturet 1964; Duvernoy et al. 1991).

5 The Insula of Reil

The insula of Reil is the smallest of the cerebral lobes found in the depth of the lateral fissure (Figs. 3.48, 3.49, 3.50, 3.51). It is best shown after excision of the lateral fissure opercula. It is triangular in shape with an apex directed anteriorly and inferiorly, called the monticulus. The latter is connected to the anterior perforated substance through the limen insulae. The insula is separated from the frontoparietal and the temporal opercula by the circular sulcus.

The insular cortex is constituted of convergent gyri presenting a fan-like arrangement, usually separated into three short and one or two long convolutions by the central sulcus of the insula, the deeper of all insular furrows always reaching the circular sulcus. The two insular lobules separated by the central sulcus, are connected with the third frontal gyrus and the superior temporal gyrus by two "plis de passages", fronto-insular and temporo-insular.

D The Mesial Surface of the Cerebral Hemisphere

The development of the specific gyral pattern characteristic of the interhemispheric area is influenced by the development of the callosal connections. Absence of the corpus callosum will lead to vertically oriented sulci and absence of the cingulate sulcus (Fig. 3.52). Sulci and gyri of the mesial aspect of the hemisphere are evident on the sagittal and parasagittal cuts of the brain (Fig. 3.53).

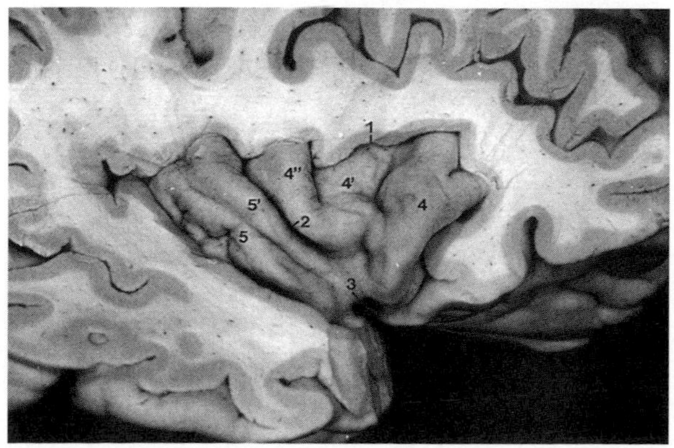

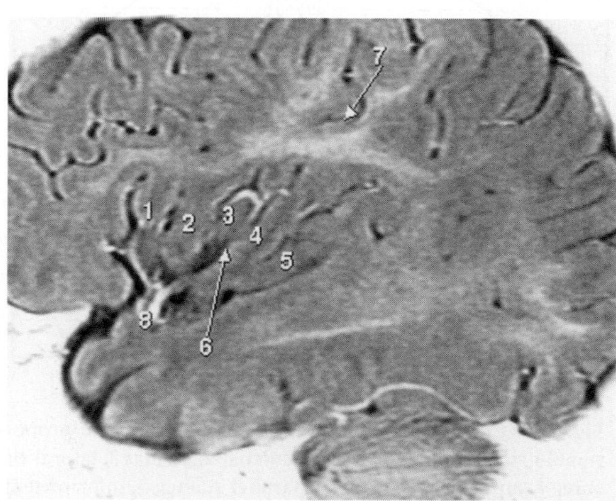

Fig. 3.48. A The insular cortex, anatomic dissection. *1*, Circular sulcus of insula; *2*, central sulcus of insula; *3*, falciform sulcus; *4*, *4'*, *4"*, short insular gyri; *5*, *5'*, long insular gyri. (from Duvernoy et al. 1991) **B** MR correlation in the sagittal plane, using STIR pulse sequence with inverse video display. *1*, *2*, *3*, Short insular gyri (anterior lobe of insula); *4*, *5*, long insular gyri; *6*, central sulcus of insula; *7*, central sulcus, inferior end; *8*, sylvian artery and its insular branches

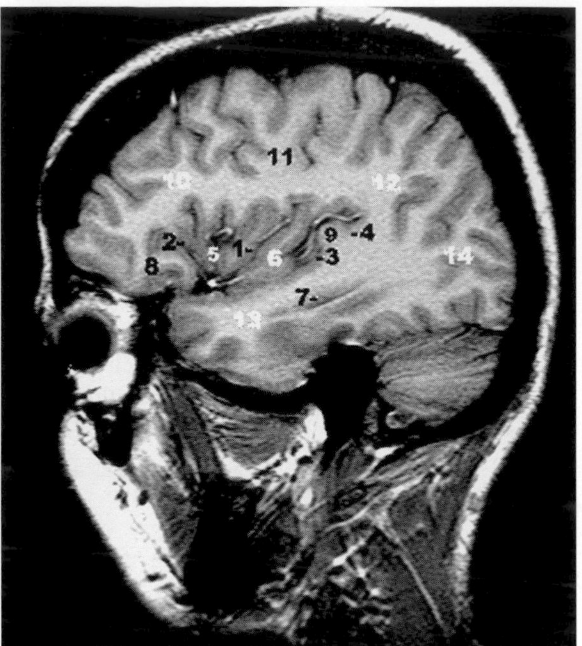

Fig. 3.49. Sagittal MR cut through the insula. *1*, Central insular sulcus; *2*, circular sulcus of insula; *3*, anterior transverse supratemporal sulcus (anterior limiting sulcus of Holl); *4*, posterior transverse supratemporal sulcus; *5*, short insular gyri; *6*, long insular gyri; *7*, inferior horn of lateral ventricle; *8*, lateral orbital gyrus; *9*, transverse temporal gyrus; *10*, inferior frontal gyrus; *11*, central operculum; *12*, inferior parietal lobule; *13*, temporal lobe; *14*, occipital lobe

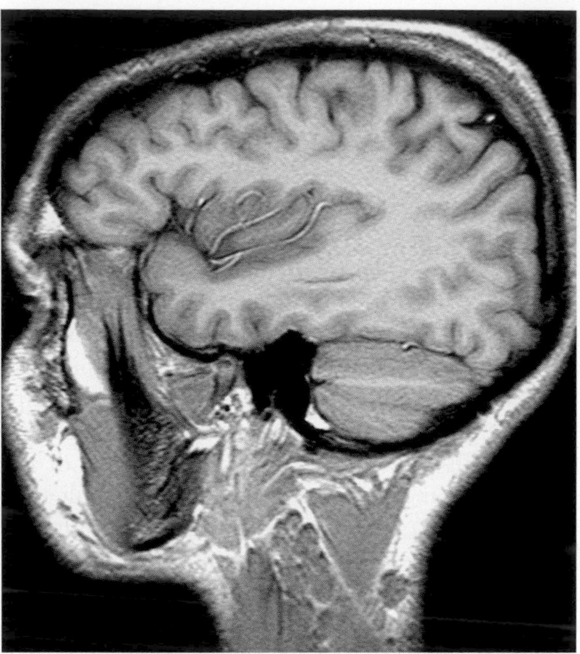

Fig. 3.51. Parasagittal MR cut showing the insular branches of the middle cerebral artery

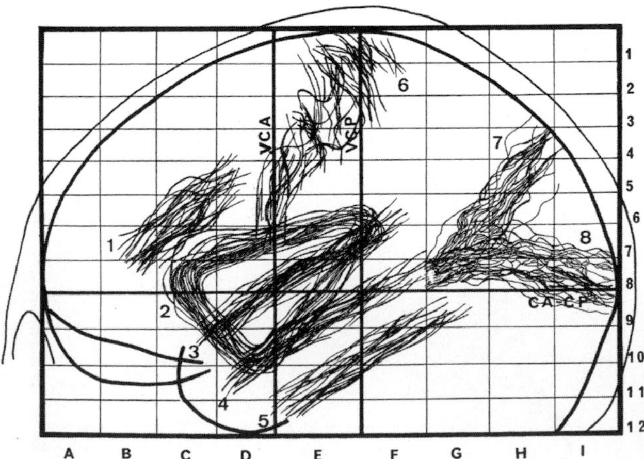

Fig. 3.50. Constant localization of the insula on the proportional grid. *1*, Superior frontal sulcus; *2*, insula; *3*, lateral fissure; *4*, superior temporal or parallel sulcus; *5*, inferior temporal sulcus; *6*, central sulcus; *7*, parieto-occipital sulcus; *8*, calcarine sulcus. Note the approximate parallelism of the frontal (excluding the central) and temporal sulci to the lateral fissure. (According to Szikla et al. 1977)

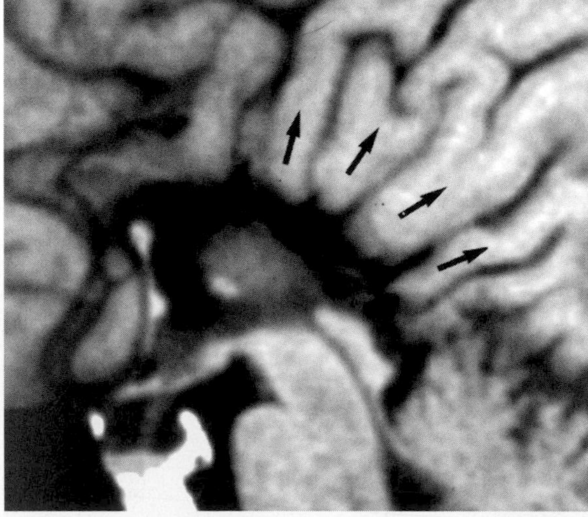

Fig. 3.52. Midsagittal MR cut showing the characteristic abnormal radiate pattern of the brain convolutions (*arrows*)

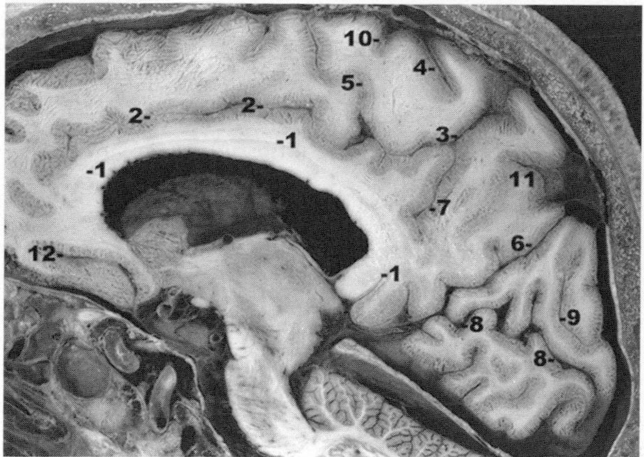

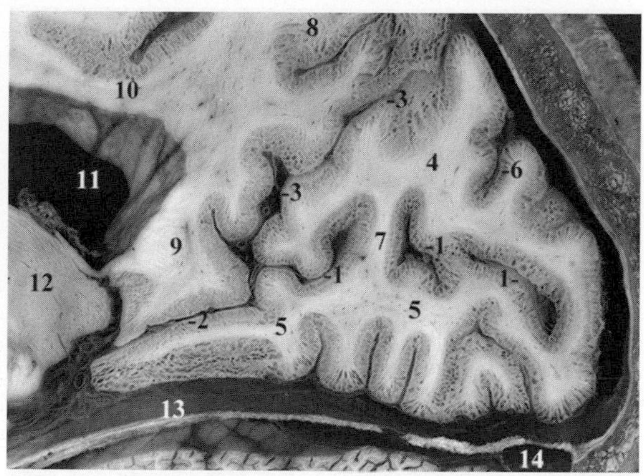

Fig. 3.53. A Anatomic parasagittal cut of the brain, showing the main sulci of the medial aspect of the hemisphere. *1*, Callosal sulcus; *2*, cingulate sulcus; *3*, marginal ramus of cingulate sulcus; *4*, central sulcus; *5*, paracentral sulcus; *6*, parieto-occipital sulcus; *7*, subparietal sulcus; *8*, calcarine sulcus; *9*, dorsal paracalcarine sulcus; *10*, medial precentral sulcus; *11*, transverse parietal sulcus; *12*, superior rostral sulcus. **B** The calcarine and parieto-occipital sulci: medial parasagittal anatomical cut. *1*, Calcarine sulcus, posterior segment; *2*, calcarine sulcus, anterior segment; *3*, parieto-occipital sulcus; *4*, cuneus; *5*, lingual gyrus; *6*, sulcus cunei; *7*, anterior cuneolingual gyrus; *8*, precuneus; *9*, isthmus; *10*, cingulate gyrus; *11*, lateral ventricle body; *12*, thalamus; *13*, tentorium cerebelli; *14*, transverse sinus

1 Cingulate Sulcus

Also called the callosomarginal sulcus (Huxley 1861) or scissure limbique (Broca 1878), the cingulate sulcus begins below the rostrum of the corpus callosum, in the subcallosal region before it sweeps around the genu paralleling the corpus callosum (Figs. 3.54, 3.55). This sulcus separates the medial frontal gyrus from the cingulate gyrus posteriorly, ending as a marginal ramus in the parietal lobe, and separating the precuneus from the paracentral lobule. The marginal ramus has a fairly constant relationship to the central sulcus, ending about 10 mm (range 8–12 mm) posterior to it in 96% of examined hemispheres. The cingulate sulcus is duplicated in 24% of examined hemispheres, mainly in its anterior segment, giving rise to an accessory intralimbic sulcus. Doubling of the anterior cingulate sulcus occurs twice as frequently in the left hemisphere according to Weinberg (1905). Up to three interruptions are frequently (40%) noted along its course. These interruptions lead to invaginations of the mesial frontal gyrus into the cingulate gyrus, corresponding to the "plis de passage fronto-limbiques" of Broca.

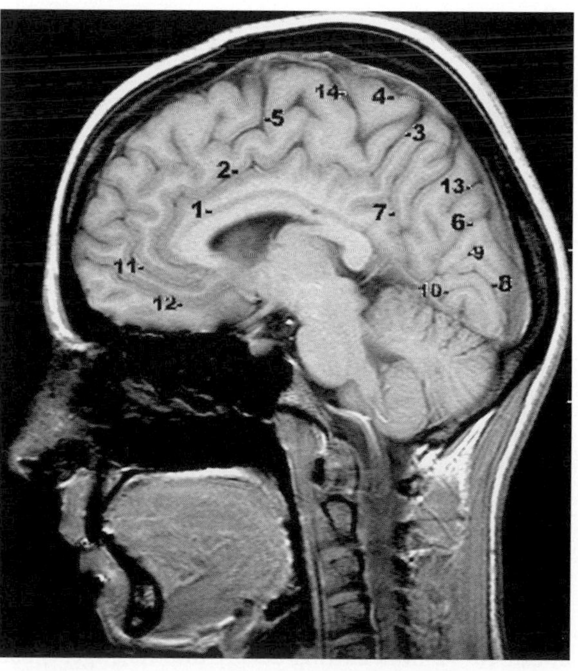

Fig. 3.54. : Parasagittal MR cut showing the sulcal anatomy of the mesial aspect of the cerebral hemisphere. *1*, Callosal sulcus; *2*, cingulate sulcus; *3*, marginal sulcus; *4*, central sulcus; *5*, paracentral sulcus; *6*, parieto-occipital sulcus; *7*, subparietal sulcus; *8*, calcarine sulcus; *9*, dorsal paracalcarine sulcus; *10*, ventral paracalcarine sulcus; *11*, superior rostral sulcus; *12*, inferior (accessory) rostral sulcus; *13*, transverse parietal sulcus; *14*, medial precentral sulcus

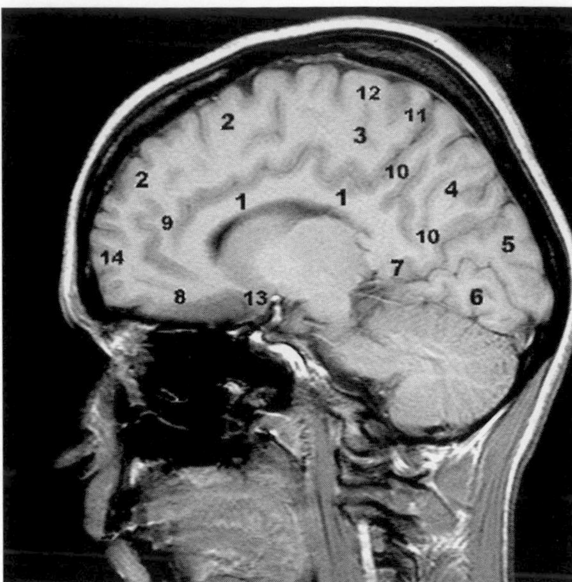

Fig. 3.55. Parasagittal MR cut showing the gyral anatomy of the mesial aspect of the cerebral hemisphere. *1*, Cingulate gyrus; *2*, medial frontal gyrus; *3*, paracentral lobule; *4*, precuneus; *5*, cuneus; *6*, lingual gyrus; *7*, isthmus; *8*, medial orbital gyrus; *9*, frontolimbic "pli de passage"; *10*, parietolimbic "pli de passage"; *11*, postcentral gyrus; *12*, precentral gyrus; *13*, subcallosal gyrus; *14*, fronto-orbital gyri

2 Parieto-occipital Sulcus

First analyzed by Gratiolet (1854), the parieto-occipital sulcus is deep (2–2.5 mm), constant and characteristic of the primate brain. Situated principally on the posterior mesial aspect of the hemisphere, it extends downward from the dorsal margin of the hemisphere forward to the caudal aspect of the splenium where it joins the stem of the calcarine fissure (Figs. 3.54, 3.55, 3.56). At this level it forms a Y-shaped sulcus. Actually, this sulcus is frequently separated from the calcarine by the cuneolimbic gyrus connecting the apex of the cuneus to the isthmus and shows a number of folds connecting the cuneus to the precuneus in its depths. The parieto-occipital sulcus continues as the external incisure on the lateral aspect of the hemisphere for a short distance of about 10–12 mm, cutting deeply into its edge. Close to the dorsal margin this sulcus may diverge into the sulcus limitans precunei which connects in 25% of the cases with the intraparietal sulcus. A line connecting the parieto-occipital incisure to the preoccipital notch draws the arbitrary boundary on the lateral surface separating the occipital lobe from the temporal and parietal lobes.

3 Calcarine Sulcus

The calcarine sulcus arises behind and just below the splenium of the corpus callosum and proceeds backward toward the occipital pole where it ends in a bifurcation, but it may encroach, most frequently by its superior ramus, on the lateral aspect of the hemisphere (Figs. 3.54, 3.55, 3.56). This deep sulcus (2.5–3 cm) is divided into two segments at the point of its junction with the parieto-occipital sulcus. The first, cephalad to this junction, having its counterpart in the calcar avis, is the anterior calcarine sulcus and the other caudal division is the posterior calcarine sulcus. The posterior calcarine sulcus ends posteriorly in a bifurcation found in half the cases on the medial aspect of the hemisphere. The superior branch extends more frequently to the lateral aspect of the occipital lobe (Zuckerkandl 1906). The course and bend of the posterior calcarine sulcus is variable. Its variations in relation with the cephalic index remain unclear.

One or two submerged gyri, the anterior and the posterior cuneolingual folds of Déjerine, may be found within the posterior calcarine segment. Exceptionally, one of these anastomotic folds may become superficial and interrupt the calcarine sulcus. The upper and the lower lips of the posterior calcarine sulcus and the lower lip only of the anterior calcarine correspond to the striate cortex (area 17).

4 Rostral Sulci

The superior rostral sulcus of Eberstaller (1884) or "incisure susorbitaire" of Broca courses anteroposteriorly around the rostrum of the corpus callosum, originating near the "carrefour olfactif " of Broca, and ends closely behind the frontal pole (Fig. 3.57). It is independent and roughly parallel to the anterior cingulate sulcus in two thirds of the cases according to Beccari (1911) and is very frequently doubled by the inferior shallower rostral sulcus, also named the accessory rostral sulcus.

5 Gyri of the Mesial Surface of the Cerebral Hemisphere

Seven gyri constitute the mesial hemisphere (Comair et al. 1996a). These are described as follows, from anterior to posterior.

a The Gyrus Rectus

The gyrus rectus is limited anteriorly by the floor of the anterior cranial fossa, laterally by the olfactory

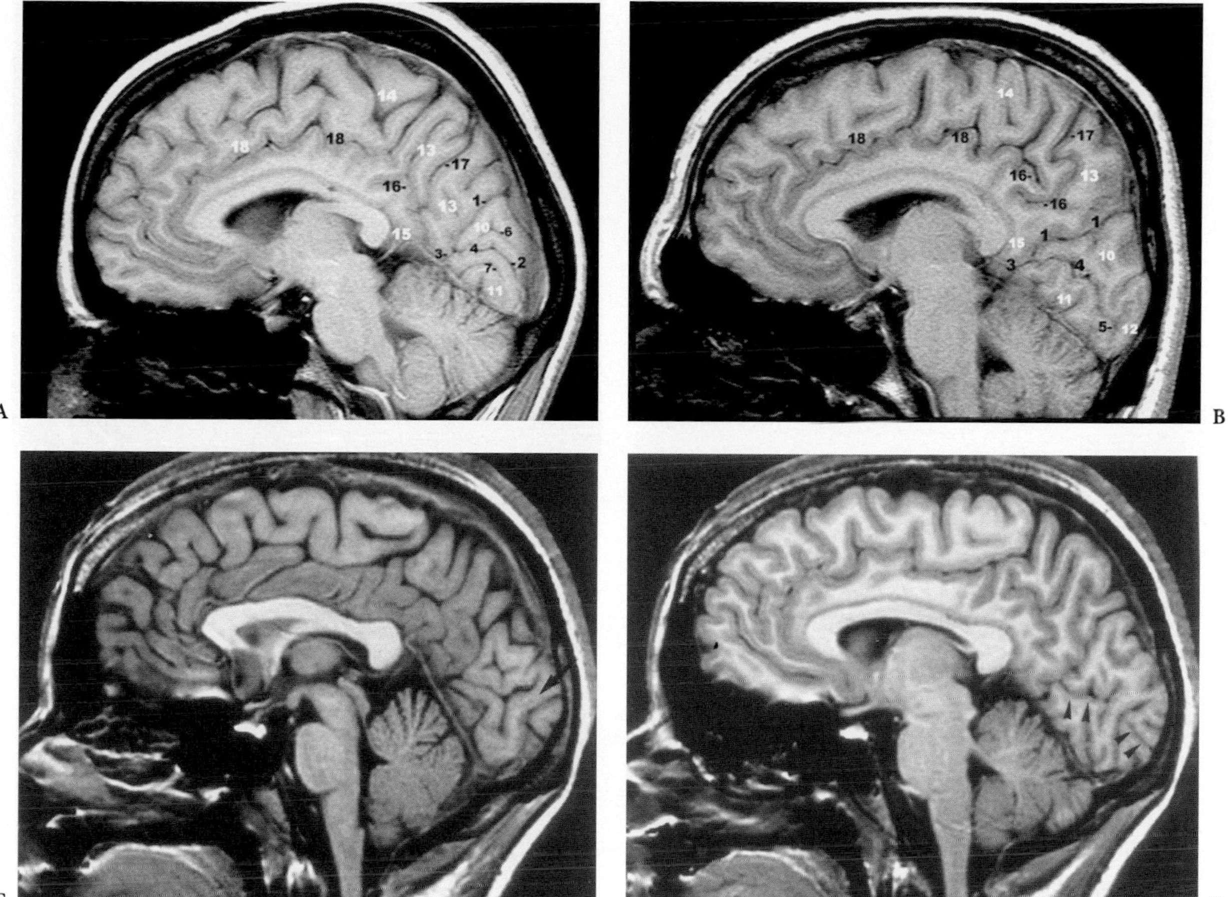

Fig. 3.56. A,B The mesial occipital lobe: MR correlations. *1*, Parieto-occipital sulcus; *2*, calcarine sulcus; *3*, anterior calcarine sulcus; *4*, posterior calcarine sulcus; *5*, retrocalcarine sulcus; *6*, paracalcarine sulcus (dorsal); *7*, paracalcarine sulcus (ventral); *8*, pli de passage, anterior cuneolimbic; *9*, pli de passage, posterior cuneolimbic; *10*, cuneus; *11*, lingual gyrus; *12*, gyrus descendens of Ecker; *13*, precuneus; *14*, paracentral lobule; *15*, isthmus cinguli; *16*, subparietal sulcus; *17*, transverse parietal sulcus; *18*, cingulate sulcus. **C,D** Cuneolingual gyrus (*arrow*) connecting the cuneus to the lingual gyrus through the calcarine sulcus (*arrowheads*) and showing a fairly unusual pattern

sulcus and superiorly by the superior rostral sulcus. A transverse rostral sulcus separates the gyrus rectus from the carrefour olfactif or subcallosal gyrus (Figs. 3.58–3.64). This latter was observed in about 60% of cases by Beccari.

b *The Cingulate Gyrus*

The cingulate gyrus is limited ventrally by the callosal sulcus, ventrally and anteriorly by the anterior paraolfactory sulcus, superiorly by the cingulate sulcus, superiorly and posteriorly by the subparietal sulcus, and posteriorly and inferiorly by the anterior calcarine sulcus (Figs. 3.53, 3.54, 3.55). It is continuous with the parahippocampal gyrus through the isthmus, a "pli de passage temporo-limbique". This arched convolution may be subdivided into three portions: the anterior located beneath the rostrum and in front of the genu of the corpus callosum, the intermediate middle portion roughly horizontal and parallel to the superior aspect of the body of the corpus callosum, and the last portion which is concave anteriorly, sweeps around the splenium and continues inferiorly and forward with the isthmus. The latter links the posterior cingulate gyrus with the parahippocampal gyrus. The anterior cingulate is followed in the subcallosal region, where it abuts the subcallosal gyrus, which is limited anteriorly by the anterior subcallosal sulcus (or transverse rostral sulcus of Beccari) and bounded posteriorly by the posterior subcallosal, the latter limiting anteriorly the paraterminal gyrus. The cingulate gyrus forms with the subcallosal, the isthmus hippocampi and the parahippocampal gyri, the limbic lobe.

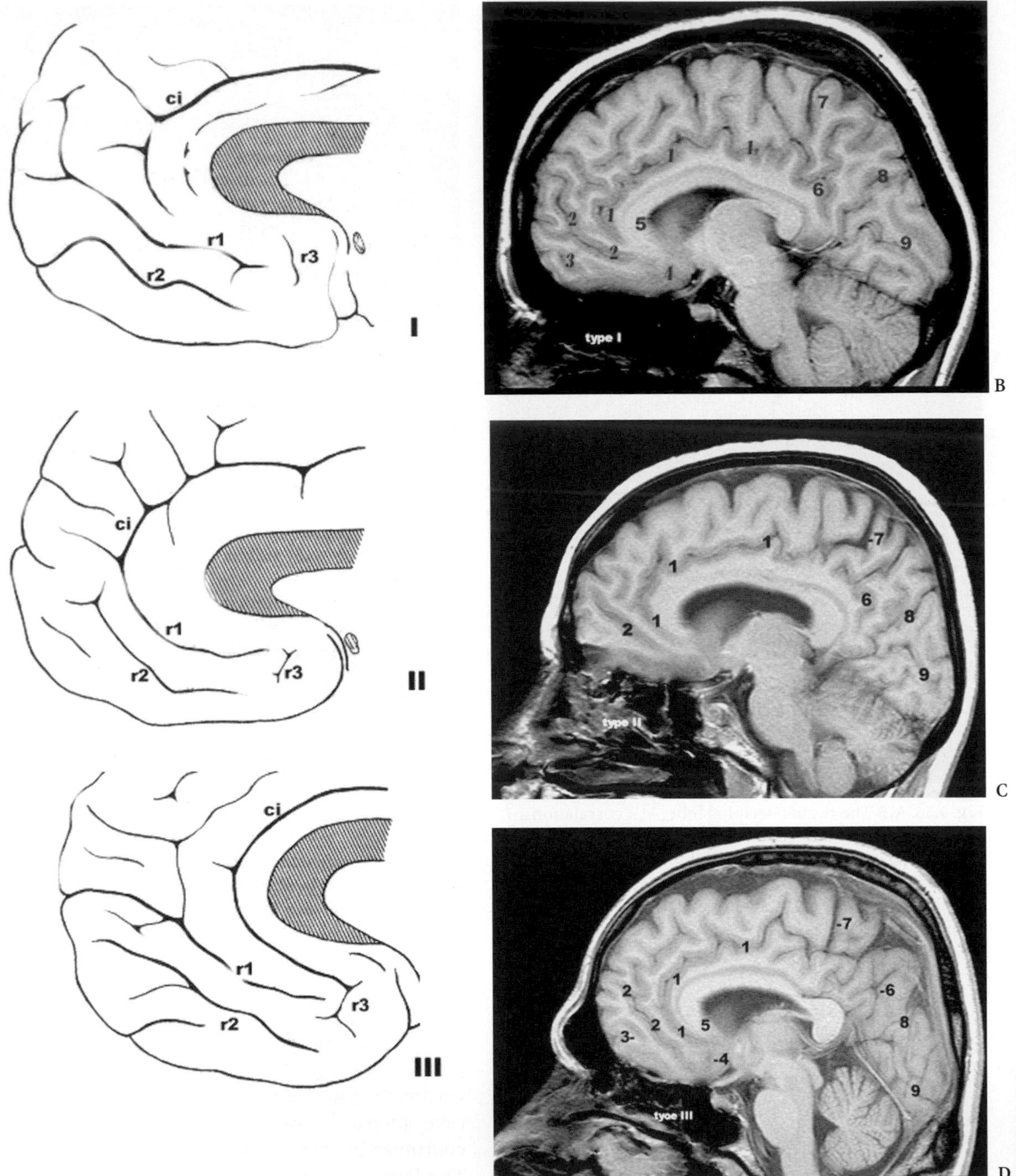

Fig. 3.57A–D. The rostral sulci with MR correlations. **A** Three major configurations are noted: type I (23%), type II (25%), type III (52%). *r1*, Superior rostral sulcus; *r2*, inferior rostral sulcus or accessory rostral sulcus; *r3*, transverse rostral sulcus; *ci*, cingulate sulcus. **B–D** *1*, Cingulate sulcus; *2*, superior rostral sulcus; *3*, inferior rostral sulcus; *4*, parolfactory sulcus; *5*, corpus callosum, genu and rostrum; *6*, subparietal sulcus; *7*, marginal ramus of cingulate sulcus; *8*, parieto-occipital sulcus; *9*, calcarine sulcus. (After Beccari 1911)

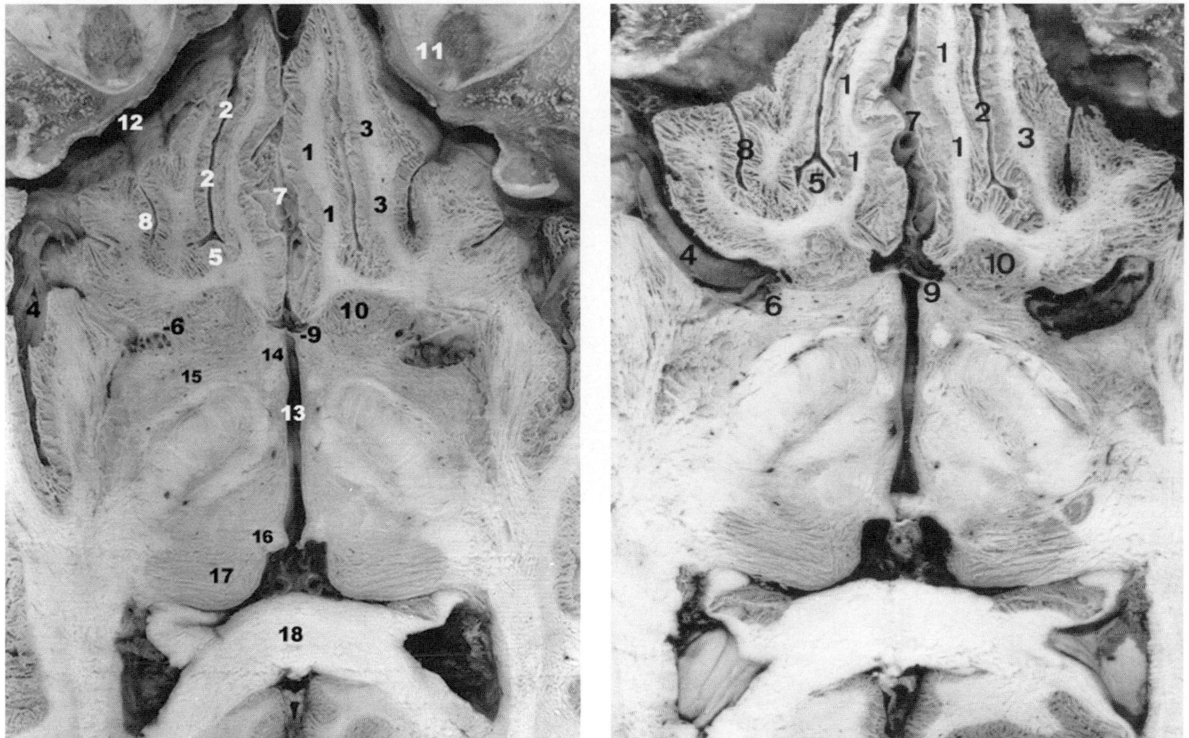

Fig. 3.58A,B. Horizontal cut of the brain showing the fronto-orbital sulci and gyri. *1*, Gyrus rectus; *2*, olfactory sulcus; *3*, medial orbital gyrus; *4*, lateral fissure; *5*, branching of olfactory sulcus; *6*, anterior perforated substance; *7*, interhemispheric fissure; *8*, medial fronto-orbital sulcus; *9*, lamina terminalis; *10*, ventral striatum; *11*, roof of the orbit; *12*, anterior cranial fossa; *13*, third ventricle; *14*, hypothalamus; *15*, innominate substance; *16*, habenula; *17*, pulvinar thalami; *18*, splenium of corpus callosum

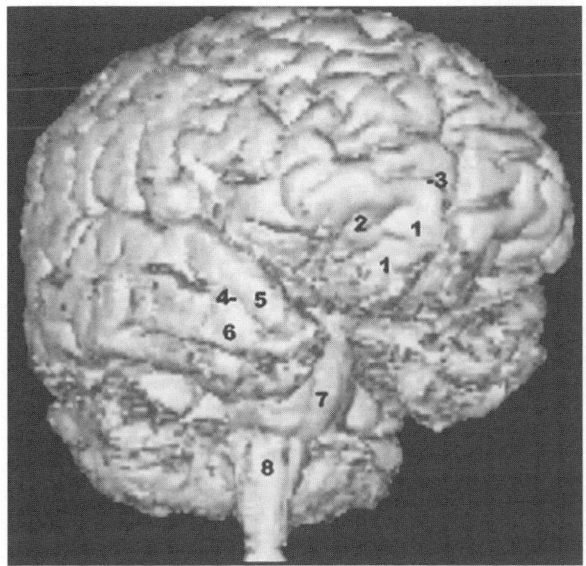

Fig. 3.59. 3D MR of the temporal pole and fronto-orbital region. *1*, Gyrus rectus; *2*, fronto-orbital gyri; *3*, supramarginal sulcus; *4*, superior temporal sulcus; *5*, superior temporal gyrus; *6*, middle temporal gyrus; *7*, pons; *8*, medulla oblongata

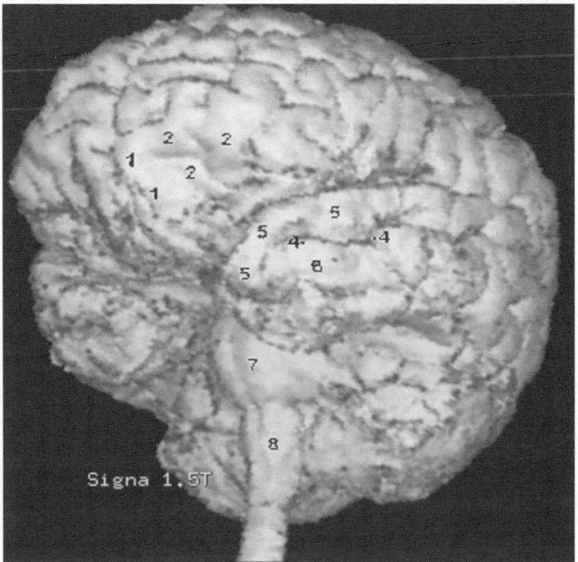

Fig. 3.60. 3D MR of the brain showing the frontal and temporal polar regions. *1*, Gyrus rectus; *2*, fronto-orbital gyri; *4*, superior temporal sulcus; *5*, superior temporal gyrus; *6*, middle temporal gyrus; *7*, pons; *8*, medulla oblongata

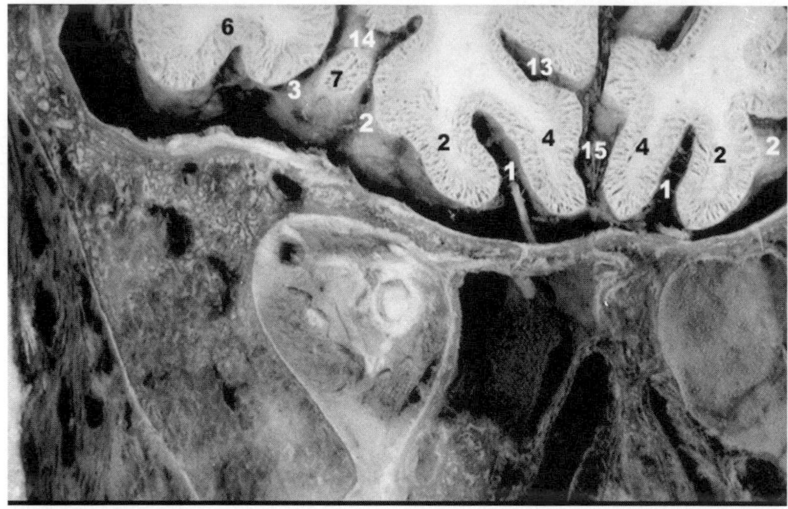

Fig. 3.61. Coronal anatomical cut showing the sulcal and gyral anatomy of the fronto-orbital lobe. *1*, Olfactory sulcus; *2*, medial orbital sulcus; *3*, lateral orbital sulcus; *4*, gyrus rectus; *5*, medial orbital gyrus; *6*, lateral orbital gyrus; *7*, anterior orbital gyrus; *8*, cingulate sulcus; *9*, cingulate gyrus; *10*, superior frontal sulcus; *11*, superior frontal gyrus; *12*, middle frontal gyrus; *13*, superior rostral sulcus; *14*, arcuate orbital sulcus; *15*, interhemispheric fissure

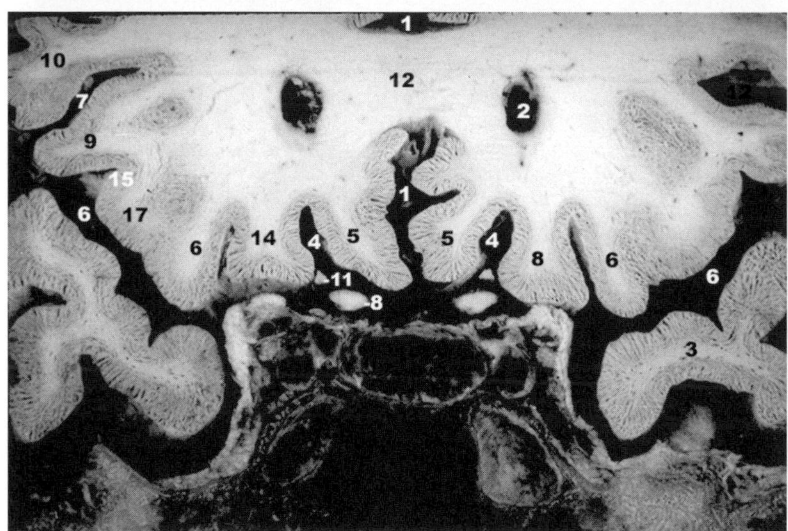

Fig. 3.62. Coronal anatomical cut of the fronto-orbital gyri. *1*, Interhemispheric fissure; *2*, tip of frontal horn; *3*, temporal pole; *4*, olfactory sulcus; *5*, gyrus rectus; *6*, posterior orbital gyrus; *7*, horizontal ramus of lateral fissure; *8*, cisternal optic nerve; *9*, inferior frontal gyrus, pars orbitalis; *10*, inferior frontal gyrus, pars triangularis; *11*, olfactory tract; *12*, corpus callosum, genu; *13*, inferior frontal sulcus; *14*, medial orbital gyrus; *15*, lateral orbital sulcus; *16*, cingulate sulcus; *17*, lateral orbital gyrus

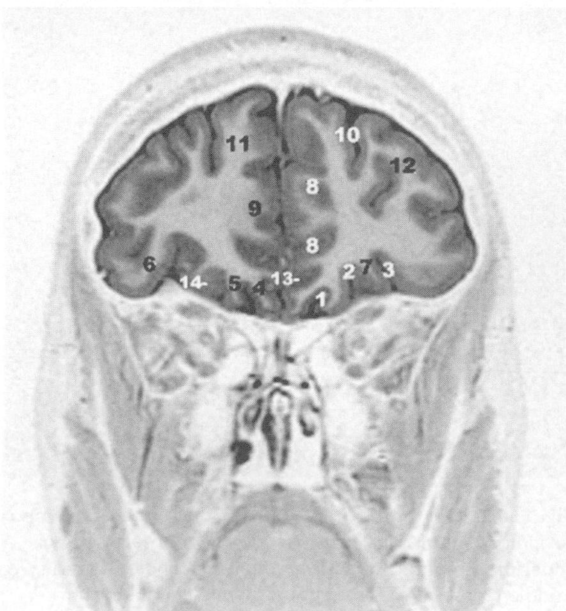

Fig. 3.63. MR coronal cut of the brain through the orbitofrontal lobes, parallel to PC-OB. *1*, Olfactory sulcus; *2*, medial orbital sulcus; *3*, lateral orbital sulcus; *4*, gyrus rectus; *5*, medial orbital gyrus; *6*, lateral orbital gyrus; *7*, anterior orbital gyrus; *8*, cingulate sulcus; *9*, cingulate gyrus; *10*, superior frontal sulcus; *11*, superior frontal gyrus; *12*, middle frontal gyrus; *13*, superior rostral sulcus; *14*, arcuate orbital sulcus

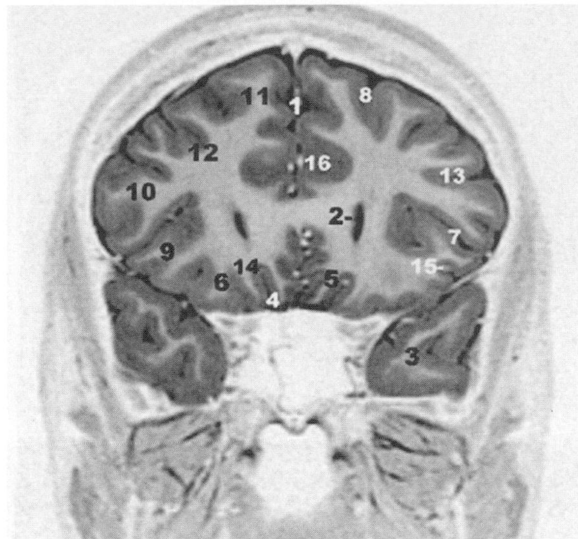

Fig. 3.64. Coronal anatomical cut of the brain passing through the genu of corpus callosum and the tip of the frontal ventricular horns. *1*, Interhemispheric fissure; *2*, tip of frontal horn; *3*, temporal pole; *4*, olfactory sulcus; *5*, gyrus rectus; *6*, posterior orbital gyrus; *7*, horizontal ramus of lateral fissure; *8*, superior frontal sulcus; *9*, inferior frontal gyrus, pars orbitalis; *10*, inferior frontal gyrus, pars triangularis; *11*, superior frontal gyrus; *12*, middle frontal gyrus; *13*, inferior frontal sulcus; *14*, medial orbital gyrus; *15*, lateral orbital sulcus; *16*, cingulate sulcus

c The Medial Frontal Gyrus

The medial frontal gyrus is limited ventrally and anteriorly by the gyrus rectus (Figs. 3.53, 3.62, 3.64). Superiorly it constitutes the superior border of the hemisphere and posteriorly it is limited by the paracentral sulcus, a well-demarcated sulcus that has its most constant portion in contact with the cingulate sulcus. This sulcus occasionally extends throughout the mesial surface and abuts the superior part of the hemisphere, being situated anterior to the medial precentral sulcus. Because of the interruptions of the cingulate sulcus, the medial frontal gyrus can invaginate into the cingulum.

d The Paracentral Lobule

The paracentral lobule is limited superiorly by the superior border of the hemisphere and anteriorly by the paracentral sulcus (Figs. 3.52, 3.53, 3.65). When the paracentral sulcus is only visible in contact with the cingulate sulcus its extension up to the medial border marks the anterior limit of the lobule. Posteriorly, the paracentral lobule is limited by the marginal ramus, an extension of the cingulate sulcus. The marginal ramus ends at the hemispheric border and in 80% of examined hemispheres it extends to the lateral surface. Two sulci are most frequently noted. The central sulcus extends into the paracentral lobule in 65% of examined hemispheres and assumes a characteristic shape, being oriented sharply posteriorly. More anteriorly, the medial precentral sulcus constitutes the most superior extent of the interrupted precentral sulcus, marking the anatomic limit of the primary motor area. The paracentral lobule proper usually extends anterior to the precentral sulcus.

Despite numerous reported stimulation studies, the relationship of the marginal ramus to the central area has not been adequately assessed. Anatomically, the marginal ramus has a relatively constant relationship with the central sulcus and ends posterior to the central sulcus in 97% of examined hemispheres. The precentral sulcus on the lateral border of the hemisphere has an extremely complex anatomy. It is frequently an interrupted sulcus, arising inferolaterally in contact with the sylvian fissure as the inferior precentral sulcus and delineating the anterior border of the ascending frontal gyrus (frontale ascendante). The posterior superior limit of the first frontal convolution is complex and is constituted by the marginal precentral and the medial precentral sulci, respectively. The latter extends over the mesial hemisphere. The paracentral sulcus is frequently anterior to the medial precentral sulcus. Since the medial precentral sulcus is usually shallow and does not extend down to the cingulate, the anterior limit of the primary motor area over the mesial hemisphere tends to be unclear. The postcentral sulcus extends to the mesial surface in 20% to 40% of examined hemispheres. Most commonly, it is posterior to the marginal ramus. Thus the primary sensory leg/foot area appears to extend anatomically beyond the limits of the paracentral lobule.

e The Precuneus

The precuneus is limited anteriorly by the marginal ramus, superiorly by the superior border of the hemisphere, posteriorly by the parieto-occipital sulcus and inferiorly by the subparietal sulcus (Figs. 3.53, 3.65). The superior parietal sulcus extends to the medial aspect and cuts into the precuneus. The parieto-occipital sulcus is a deep constant sulcus which demarcates the precuneus from the cuneus of the occipital lobe. The subparietal sulcus is a variable sulcus which may show various branching (H-shaped or "split H") or may appear as a posterior branching of the cingulate sulcus. It is frequently traversed by one or two "plis de passages" parietal limbic. Inferior to the subparietal sulcus, the cingulate gyrus becomes wide and then tapers sharply at the level of the splenium of the corpus callosum.

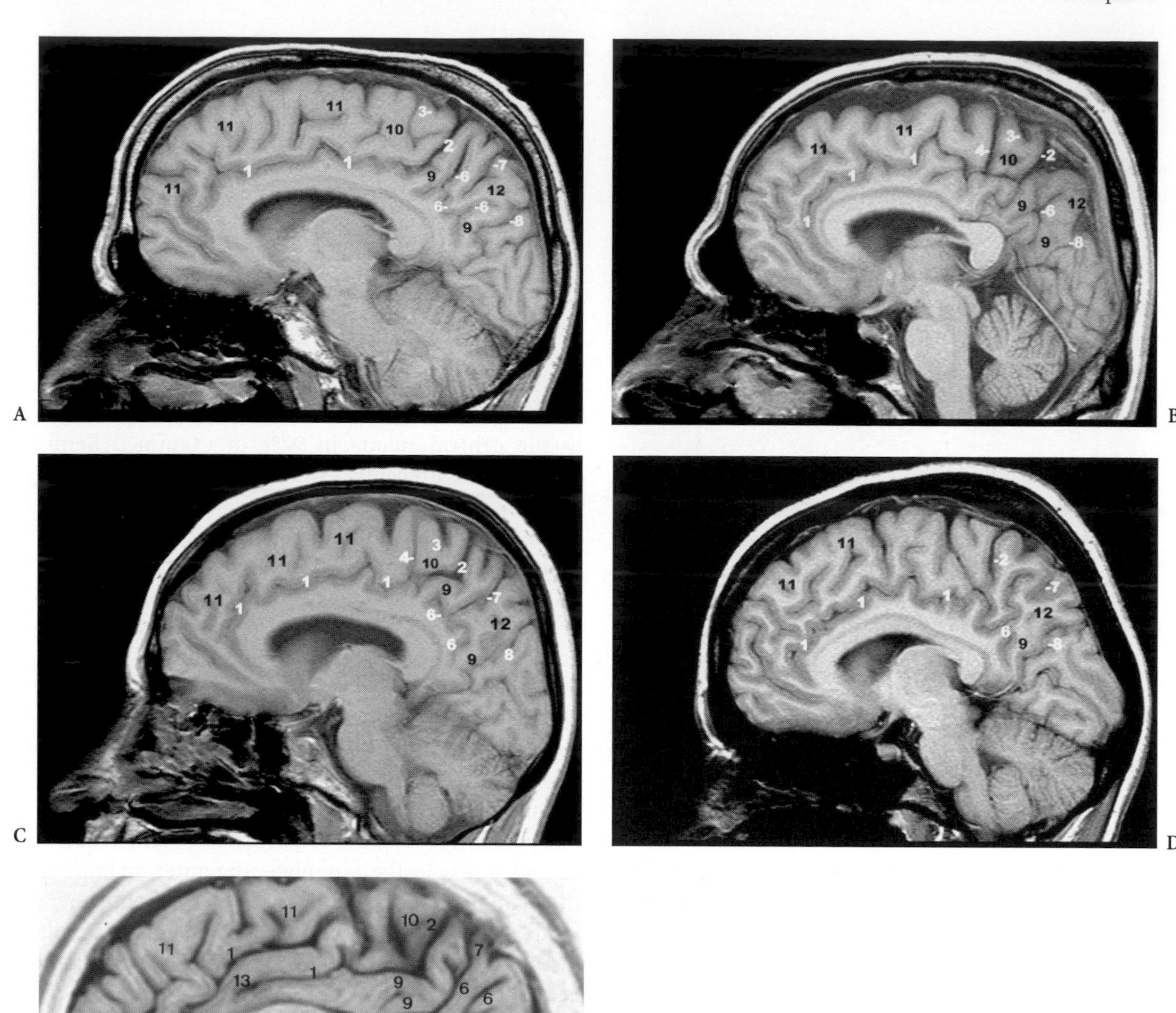

Fig. 3.65A–E. The precuneus and paracentral lobule, and medial frontal gyrus: MR correlations. *1*, Cingulate sulcus; *2*, marginal ramus of cingulate sulcus; *3*, central sulcus; *4*, paracentral sulcus; *5*, medial precentral sulcus; *6*, subparietal sulcus; *7*, superior parietal sulcus; *8*, parieto-occipital sulcus; *9*, pli de passage, parietolimbic; *10*, paracentral lobule; *11*, medial frontal gyrus; *12*, precuneus; *13*, pli de passage, frontolimbic

f The Cuneus

Triangular in shape, the cuneus is the only occipital gyrus to be well delimited. It is in fact bounded anteriorly by the parieto-occipital sulcus, superiorly by the superior and posterior borders of the hemisphere and inferiorly by the posterior calcarine sulcus (Figs. 3.55, 3.56). It is continuous with the lateral surface. The calcarine sulcus extends anteriorly and stops at the most posterior extent of the collateral sulcus, where the isthmus of the cingulate gyrus extends into the parahippocampal gyrus. The cuneus is connected to the posterior aspect of the adjacent cingulate gyrus by the deeply situated cuneolimbic pli de passage of Broca. In all primates except the gibbon, this gyrus is superficial and separates the parieto-occipital from the calcarine sulci. At the occipital pole, the calcarine sulcus terminates as the vertical retrocalcarine sulcus behind which is found the gyrus descendens of Ecker (1869). The latter may sometimes be located on the lateral aspect of the hemisphere, or bounded posteriorly by an occipital polar sulcus limiting the striate area.

g *The Lingual Gyrus*

The lingual gyrus constitutes the inferior and mesial aspect of the occipital lobe and is bordered superiorly by the calcarine sulcus (Figs. 3.55, 3.56). It is connected to the cuneus through the retrocalcarine sulcus by one or two cuneolingual gyri, "plis de passage cuneo-limbiques of Broca" (Déjerine 1895). It is continuous anteriorly with the parahippocampal gyrus. An inconstant lingual sulcus may further subdivide the lingual gyrus into superior and inferior parts, both connected anteriorly to the parahippocampal gyrus.

E The Basal Surface of the Cerebral Hemisphere

Sulci and gyri of the basal aspect of the frontotemporal lobes are best imaged and analyzed on coronal cuts as performed parallel to the commissural-obex brain reference line (Tamraz et al. 1990, 1991). Coronal anatomic correlations are available in previous works (Tamraz 1983; Cabanis et al. 1988). In the following sections we will separate the basal surface into the anterior basal orbitofrontal lobe and the posterior basal temporal lobe.

1 The Frontal Orbital Lobe

The orbital surface of the frontal lobe presents a primary sulcus, the olfactory sulcus and a secondary composite sulcus showing great individual variations and named the orbital sulci (Figs. 3.58–3.64, 3.66).

a *Olfactory Sulcus and Gyrus Rectus*

The olfactory sulcus originates at the anterior border of the anterior perforated substance in two rami, of which the longer lateral branch may anastomose with the lateral fissure or, less frequently, with the arcuate orbital sulcus. It courses from back to front roughly parallel to the anterior interhemispheric fissure, to end about 15 mm behind the frontal pole, relatively close to the interhemispheric fissure. It is related to the olfactory tract.

This sulcus separates the gyrus rectus medially from the orbital gyri laterally. The gyrus rectus is easily distinguished as the narrow strip of cortex of about 1 cm width, mesial to the olfactory sulcus and is a part of the longitudinal arciform region corresponding to the orbital portion of the superior frontal convolution.

b *Orbital or Orbitofrontal Sulci and Gyri*

The orbital or orbitofrontal sulci show numerous variations (Kanai 1938) consisting of two longitudinal sulci connected by a transverse furrow. These sulci are arranged in the shape of "H" (incisure en H of Broca), an "X" or a "K" (Figs. 3.66, 3.67). The longitudinal sulci are the medial and the lateral orbital sulci, which divide the orbital surface into medial and lateral orbital gyri and an intermediate orbital cortex. This is subdivided transversely into anterior and posterior middle orbital gyri by the arcuate orbital sulcus, which is situated near the frontal pole with a convex border directed toward the pole. Such subdivisions are not independent but are parts of the superior and inferior frontal gyri of the lateral aspect of the hemisphere. The lateral orbital sulcus limits the orbitofrontal lobe from the lateral aspect of the inferior frontal gyrus.

2 The Temporal Basal Lobe

The ventral surface of the temporal lobe extends laterally from the inferior and lateral border of the hemisphere to the mesial temporal border at the lateral wing of the transverse fissure (Figs. 3.68–3.71). It extends from the temporal pole to the inferior occipital lobe without definite anatomic demarcation other than the preoccipital notch. An arbitrary line joining this notch to the isthmus behind the splenium posteriorly limits the ventral temporal gyri. From mesial to lateral, two longitudinal sulci, the collateral sulcus and the occipitotemporal sulcus divide the inferior temporal lobe into three longitudinal gyri, the parahippocampal gyrus, the fusiform gyrus and the inferior temporal gyrus at the junction between the lateral and the inferior aspects of the hemisphere.

a *Collateral Sulcus and Parahippocampal Gyrus*

The collateral sulcus, a primary sulcus also called the medial occipitotemporal sulcus, is a constant, elongated S-shaped sulcus of the basal aspect of the temporal lobe. According to Landau (1911) it is interrupted in about half the cases but according to Ono

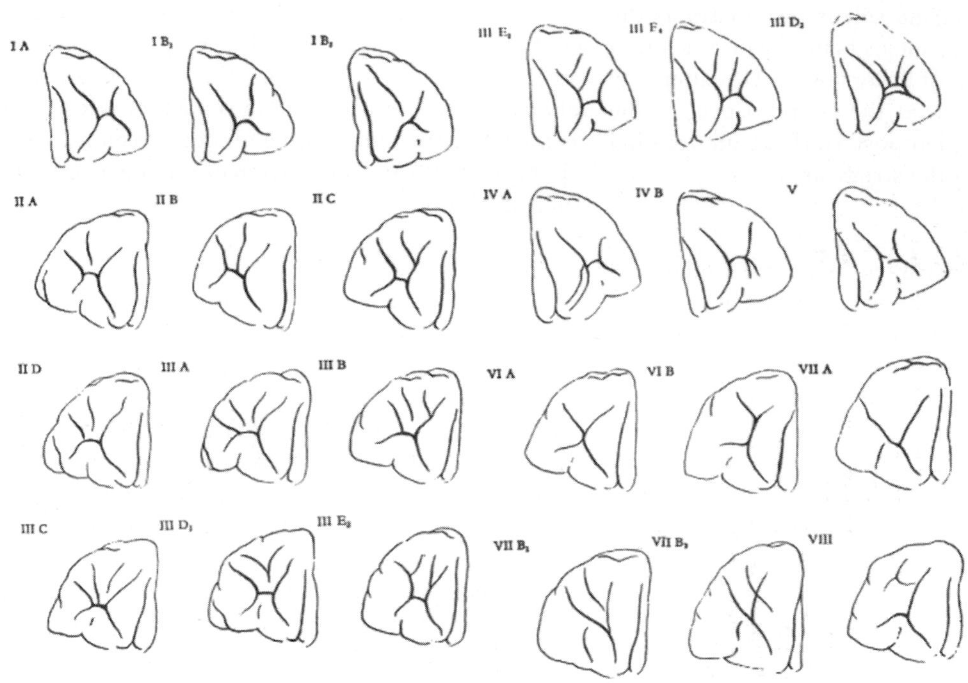

Fig. 3.66. Fissural patterns of the fronto-orbital region. (After Kanai 1938)

A

B

C

D

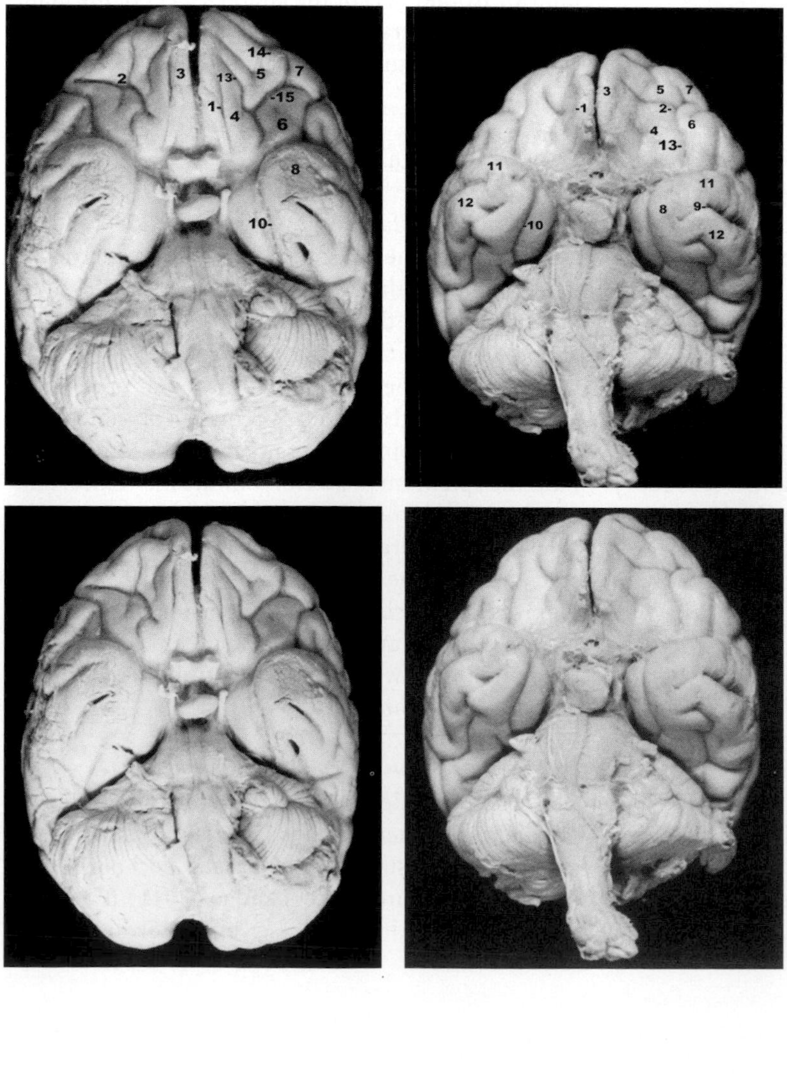

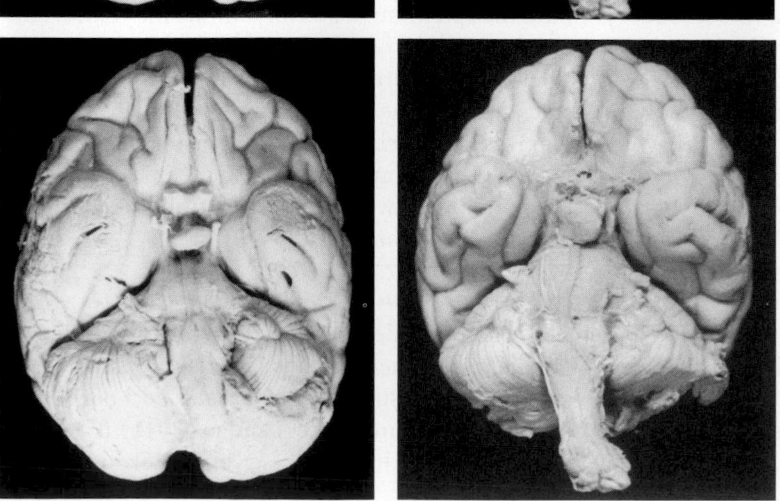

Fig. 3.67A–D. Inferior aspect of the brain showing the fissural pattern of the fronto-orbital lobe and the temporal poles, in anthropoids. A,C Gorilla, B,D orangutan. *1*, Olfactory sulcus; *2*, fronto-orbital "H-shape" sulci (cruciform); *3*, gyrus rectus; *4*, medial orbital gyrus; *5*, anterior orbital gyrus; *6*, posterior orbital gyrus; *7*, lateral orbital gyrus; *8*, temporal pole; *9*, parallel sulcus; *10*, rhinal sulcus; *11*, superior temporal gyrus; *12*, middle temporal gyrus; *13*, medial orbital sulcus; *14*, lateral orbital sulcus; *15*, arcuate sulcus

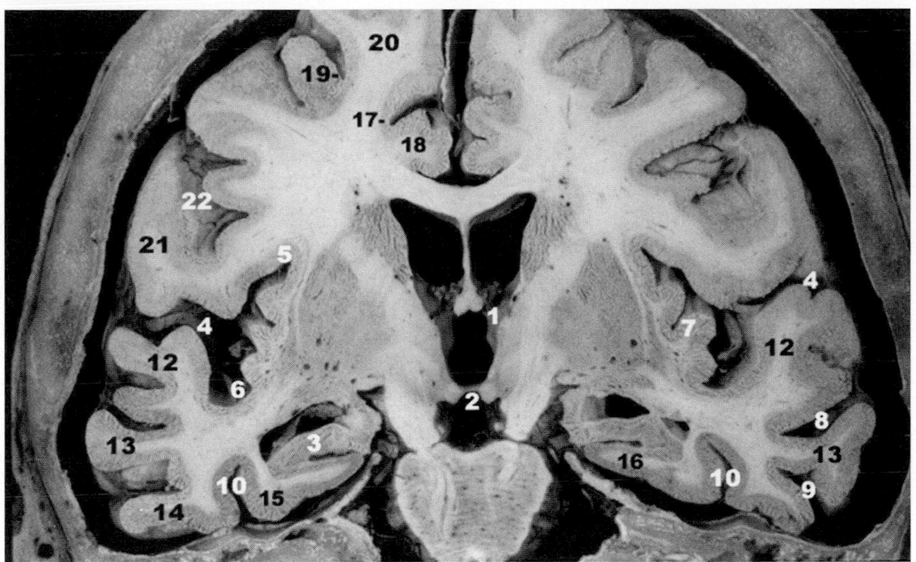

Fig. 3.68. Coronal anatomical cut of the brain through the interventricular foramina and the mamillary bodies. *1*, Interventricular foramen; *2*, mamillary body; *3*, hippocampal head; *4*, lateral fissure; *5*, superior circular sulcus; *6*, inferior circular sulcus; *7*, insula; *8*, superior temporal (parallel) sulcus; *9*, inferior temporal sulcus; *10*, occipitotemporal sulcus; *11*, collateral sulcus; *12*, superior temporal gyrus; *13*, middle temporal gyrus; *14*, inferior temporal gyrus; *15*, fusiform gyrus; *16*, parahippocampal gyrus; *17*, cingulate sulcus; *18*, cingulate gyrus; *19*, superior frontal sulcus; *20*, superior frontal gyrus; *21*, precentral gyrus; *22*, central sulcus.

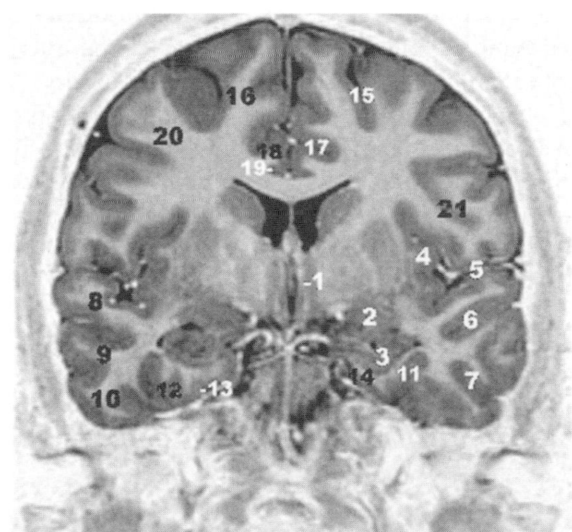

Fig. 3.69. MR coronal cut of the brain through the anterior columns of the fornix and the mamillary bodies, parallel to PC-OB.*1*, Anterior columns of fornix; *2*, amygdala; *3*, hippocampal head; *4*, insula; *5*, lateral fissure; *6*, superior temporal (parallel) sulcus; *7*, inferior temporal sulcus; *8*, superior temporal gyrus; *9*, middle temporal gyrus; *10*, inferior temporal gyrus; *11*, occipitotemporal sulcus; *12*, fusiform gyrus; *13*, collateral sulcus; *14*, parahypocampal gyrus; *15*, superior frontal sulcus; *16*, superior frontal gyrus; *17*, cingulate sulcus; *18*, cingulate gyrus; *19*, callosal sulcus; *20*, middle frontal gyrus; *21*, precentral gyrus

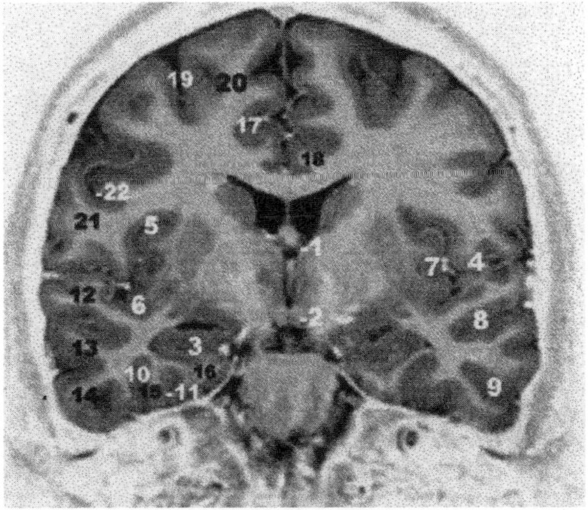

Fig. 3.70. MR coronal cut of the brain through the interventricular foramina and the mamillary bodies, parallel to PC-OB. *1*, Interventricular foramen; *2*, mamillary body; *3*, hippocampal head; *4*, lateral fissure; *5*, superior circular sulcus; *6*, inferior circular sulcus; *7*, insula; *8*, superior temporal (parallel) sulcus; *9*, inferior temporal sulcus; *10*, occipito-temporal sulcus; *11*, collateral sulcus; *12*, superior temporal gyrus; *13*, middle temporal gyrus; *14*, inferior temporal gyrus; *15*, fusiform gyrus; *16*, parahippocampal gyrus; *17*, cingulate sulcus; *18*, cingulate gyrus; *19*, superior frontal sulcus; *20*, superior frontal gyrus; *21*, precentral gyrus; *22*, central sulcus

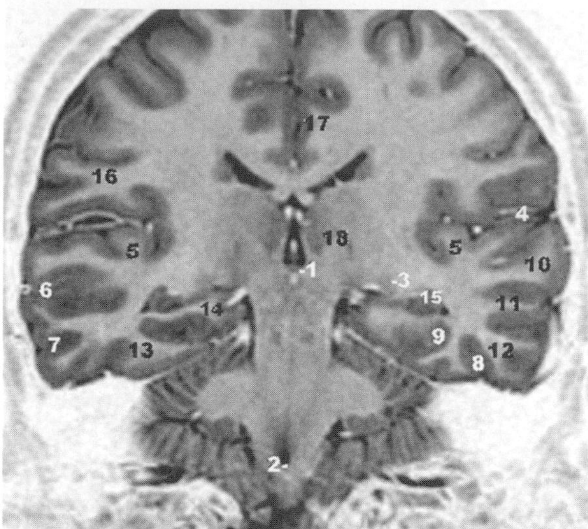

Fig. 3.71. MR coronal cut of the brain passing through the posterior commissure and the obex, according to the PC-OB orientation. *1*, Posterior commissure; *2*, obex; *3*, lateral geniculate body; *4*, lateral fissure; *5*, transverse gyrus of Heschl; *6*, superior temporal sulcus; *7*, inferior temporal sulcus; *8*, occipitotemporal sulcus; *9*, collateral sulcus; *10*, superior temporal gyrus; *11*, middle temporal gyrus; *12*, inferior temporal gyrus; *13*, fusiform gyrus; *14*, parahippocampal gyrus; *15*, hippocampus; *16*, supramarginal gyrus; *17*, cingulate gyrus; *18*, thalamus

et al. (1990), it is uninterrupted. It usually originates in a transverse collateral sulcus, near the temporal pole and ends in another transverse occipitotemporal sulcus which may show one (sulcus sagittalis gyri fusiformis of Retzius) or several small oblique connections with the inferior temporal sulcus. At this end, the collateral sulcus may fuse with the calcarine sulcus. The collateral sulcus laterally separates the parahippocampal gyrus and the lingual gyrus from the fusiform gyrus. Its depth impresses the inferior wall of the atrium and the temporal horn of the lateral ventricle, as observed on coronal cuts.

b Occipitotemporal Sulcus and Fusiform Gyrus

The lateral occipitotemporal sulcus is a secondary sulcus coursing lateral to the collateral sulcus, near the inferolateral margin of the hemisphere and ending close to the preoccipital notch in about two thirds of the cases. It shows frequent interruptions, being continuous in less than 40% of the cases according to Ono et al. (1990). It constitutes the outer boundary of the occipitotemporal or fusiform gyrus, and is limited medially by the collateral sulcus or medial occipitotemporal sulcus. This gyrus does not reach the temporal pole anteriorly. Its width increases from the pole to its posterior extremity before it decreases again to merge with the inferior occipital lobe.

F White Matter Core and Major Association Tracts

Raymond Vieussens, well known for his labeling of "centrum semi-ovale", first reported that the hemispheric white matter consists of fiber bundles. Baillarger (1840) emphasized that the gray and white matter are intimately linked. Meynert (1877) made a major contribution with a classification of the myelinated fibers into three major groups: (1) the association fibers, which interconnect different cortical regions and consist of most of the white matter substance; (2) the commissural fibers which link both hemispheres and cross through the corpus callosum, the anterior commissure and the fornix; (3) the projection fibers between the cortex and the subcortical centers, which contribute to the formation of the corona radiata (Fig. 3.72).

We will focus on the long association fibers which may be routinely clearly identified on MR (particularly in coronal cuts) using proton density, T2 or STIR pulse sequences (Fig. 3.73). Diffusion-weighted imaging sequences are more powerful for disclosing such bundles and will certainly modify the microsurgical approach to resections of brain tumors.

The medullary white matter with the very long association fibers bundles is found deep inside the white matter core on the medial or the lateral sides of the corona radiata. These fiber systems are at present

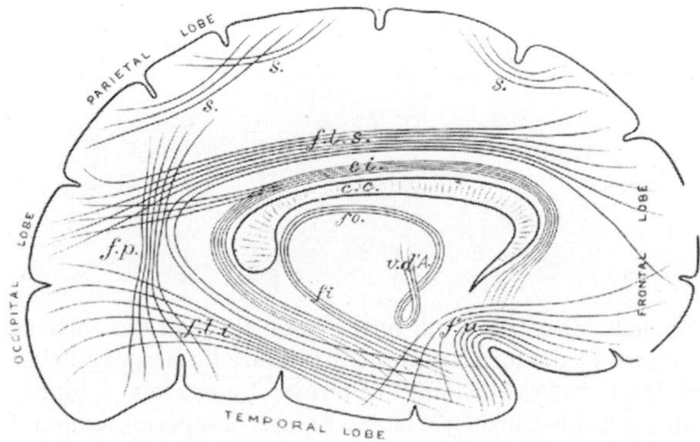

Fig. 3.72. The intrahemispheric association fibers. *s*, short association fibers between adjacent gyri; *f.l.s.*, superior longitudinal fasciculus; *ci.*, Cingulate fasciculus; *f.l.i.*, inferior longitudinal fasciculus; *f.u.*, uncinate fasciculus; *f.p.*, perpendicular fasciculus; *f.i.*, fimbria; *f.o.*, fornix; *v.d' A.*, thalamic fasciculus of Vicq d'Azyr; *c.c.*, corpus callosum. (After Meynert 1877)

best recognized from the macroscopic dissections as described in the major contributions of Meynert (1877), Déjerine (1895) and Klingler (1935) (Fig. 3.74). For MR correlations we will use the anatomical dissections as performed by Ludwig and Klingler (1956) at the Basel Institute of Anatomy.

Seven association fiber systems may be disclosed in the cerebral hemisphere: (1) the cingulum; (2) the superior fronto-occipital; (3) the superior longitudinal; (4) the arcuate; (5) the inferior fronto-occipital; (6) the uncinate; and (7) the inferior longitudinal fasciculus.

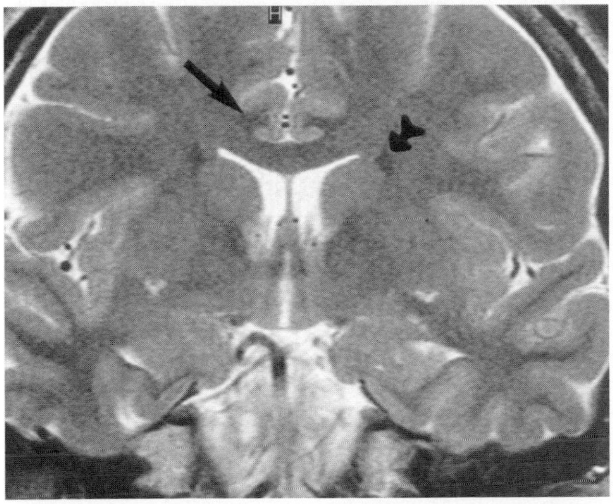

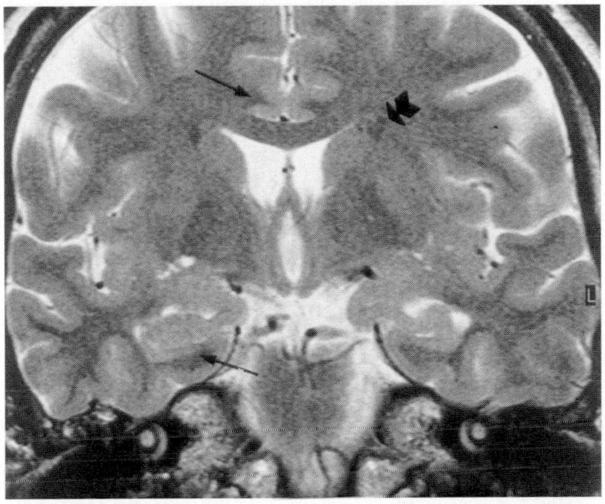

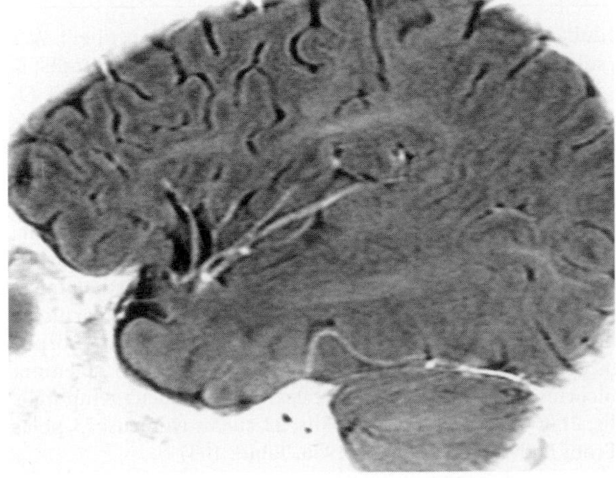

Fig. 3.73A–E. Brain long association fiber bundles as visualized by coronal FSE-T2 weighted MR. **A,B** Cut through the anterior columns of the fornix; **C,D** cut through the anterior brainstem at the fundus of the interpeduncular cistern. Both cuts are parallel to the PC-OB reference line. These cuts show the cingulum (*long arrow*) in the gyral white matter of the cingulate gyrus; the parahippocampal gyrus; the superior fronto-occipital fasciculus (*short arrow*) at the angle between the corpus callosum and the superolateral border of the lateral ventricle; the superior longitudinal fasciculus (*triple arrowheads*) dorsal to the upper border of the insula; and the inferior fronto-occipital fasciculus (*single arrowhead*) in the floor of the lateral fissure, beneath the claustrum and the external capsule. **E** Parasagittal MR cut in an infant showing the early myelinated arcuate fasciculus.

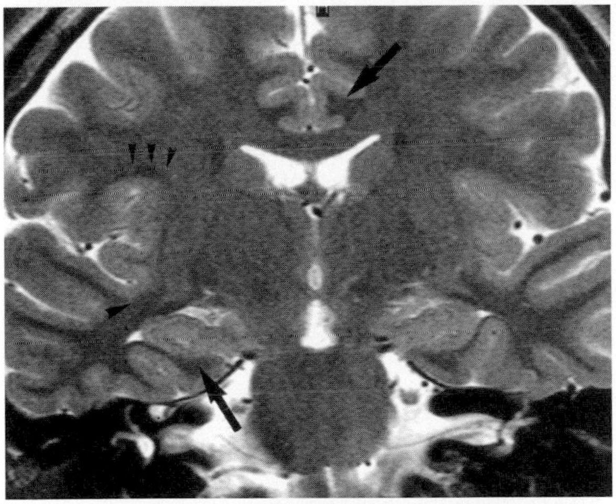

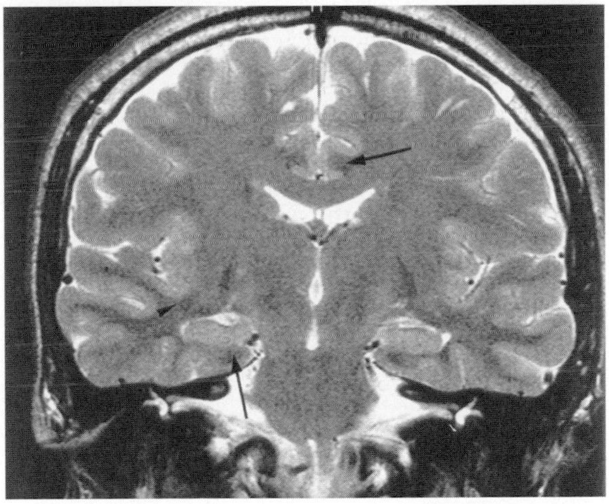

1. The cingulum is a bundle of long association fibers easily depicted on frontal MR cuts in the gyral white matter of the cingulate and the parahippocampal gyri. It is found above the corpus callosum, below the cingulate sulcus. It may be divided into an anterior part around the genu of the corpus callosum, a horizontal part relative to the body and a posterior part sweeping around the splenium and extending towards the parahippocampal gyrus. Its fibers link the cortex of the frontal, parietal, temporal and occipital lobes (neocerebrum) with the limbic lobe. The precuneus receives a consistent amount of these fibers (Elze 1929) (Fig. 3.75).
2. The superior fronto-occipital fasciculus is found in the angle between the corpus callosum and the superolateral border of the lateral ventricle and the adjacent caudate nucleus. It was described by Déjerine (1895) and was presumed to be homologous to the bulky fiber bundles observed in cases of agenesis of the corpus callosum (Onufrowicz 1887; Kaufman 1887) (Fig. 3.76). It interconnects the frontal to the occipital cortices (Chusid et al. 1948). Both the identity and the role of this bundle are still debated. It is lesioned after frontal lobotomy (McLardy 1950).
3. The superior longitudinal fasciculus, is a long association tract situated dorsal to the upper border of the insula. It conveys impulses posteriorly from the frontal lobe to the associative regions of the parietal and occipital lobes. Lesions in the dominant hemisphere of the superior longitudinal fasciculus impair the capability to identify objects or to understand spoken or written sentences (Figs. 3.77, 3.78, 3.79).
4. The arcuate fasciculus is found dorsal to the insula around which it sweeps, interconnecting portions of the frontal to the temporal lobes. Zenker (1985) reported that the associative fibers interconnect the middle and inferior gyri of the frontal lobe with the middle and inferior gyri of the temporal lobe. This could represent a component of the superior longitudinal fasciculus.
5. The inferior fronto-occipital fasciculus, located more deeply than the uncinate fasciculus, is presumed to interconnect parts of the frontal and occipital lobes (Figs. 3.78–3.79).
6. The uncinate fasciculus interconnects the fronto-orbital lobe and parts of the middle and inferior frontal gyri, with the anterior temporal lobe and pole, coursing along the floor of the sylvian fissure. This fasciculus is found coursing through the anterior inferior border of the external capsule and the inferior aspect of the claustrum (Schnopfhagen 1890). It may also pass through the extreme capsule according to Landau (1919) (Figs. 3.77–3.79).
7. The inferior longitudinal fasciculus of Burdach is a long association fiber bundle situated contiguous to the lateral aspect of the inferior horn of the lateral ventricle, in the temporo-occipital lobe. It extends from the occipital to the temporal pole.

Fig. 3.74A–G. Dissection of the brain showing the subgyral medullary white matter and the short association fibers. **A,B** ▷ Lateral aspect. *1*, Sulcus intraparietalis; *2*, sulcus postcentralis; *3*, sulcus lateralis; *4*, sulcus postcentralis; *5*, sulcus centralis; *6*, sulcus praecentralis; *7*, sulcus centralis; *8*, sulcus praecentralis; *9*, sulcus frontalis inferior; *10*, sulcus frontalis medius; *11*, sulcus frontalis superior; *12*, sulcus lateralis, ramus anterior; *13*, sulcus lateralis, ramus ascendens; *14*, sulcus temporalis medius; *15*, sulcus temporalis superior; *16*, sulcus temporalis medius. **C,D** Superior aspect. *1*, Gyrus frontalis inferior; *2*, gyrus frontalis superior; *3*, gyrus frontalis medius; *4*, gyrus praecentralis; *5*, sulcus centralis; *6*, gyrus postcentralis; *7*, sulcus intraparietalis; *8*, lobulus parietalis superior. **E,F** Mesial aspect. *1*, Gyrus frontalis superior; *2*, gyrus cinguli; *3*, septum pellucidum; *4*, fornix; *5*, corpus callosum; *6*, stria medullaris thalami; *7*, lobulus paracentralis; *8*, ramus marginalis sulci cinguli; *9*, praecunens; *10*, sulcus parieto-occipitalis; *11*, cuneus; *12*, Sulcus calcarinus; *13*, Isthmus gyri cinguli; *14*, corpus pineale; *15*, gyrus parahippocampalis; *16*, aquaeductus cerebri; *17*, uncus; *18*, corpus mamillare; *19*, adhaesio interthalamica; *20*, commissura anterior; *21*, foramen interventriculare. **G,H** Inferior aspect. *1*, bulbus olfactorius; *2*, tractus olfactorius; *3*, gyrus rectus; *4*, trigonium olfactorium; *5*, nervus opticus; *6*, substantia perforata; *7*, chiasma opticum; *8*, tractus opticus; *9*, corpus mamillare; *10*, crus cerebri; *11*, substantia nigra; *12*, tectum mesencephali; *13*, aquaeductus cerebri; *14*, pulvinar; *15*, splenium corporis callosi; *16*, Isthmus gyri cinguli; *17*, pars communis sulcorium parieto-occipitalis, calcarini; *18*, sulcus temporalis inferior; *19*, sulcus collateralis; *20*, gyrus occipitotemporalis lateralis; *21*, gyrus parahippocampalis; *22*, sulcus rhinicus; *23*, polas temporalis; *24*, gyri orbitales; *25*, sulcus olfactorius. (By Klingler. From Ludwig and Klingler 1956, Tables 1–4)

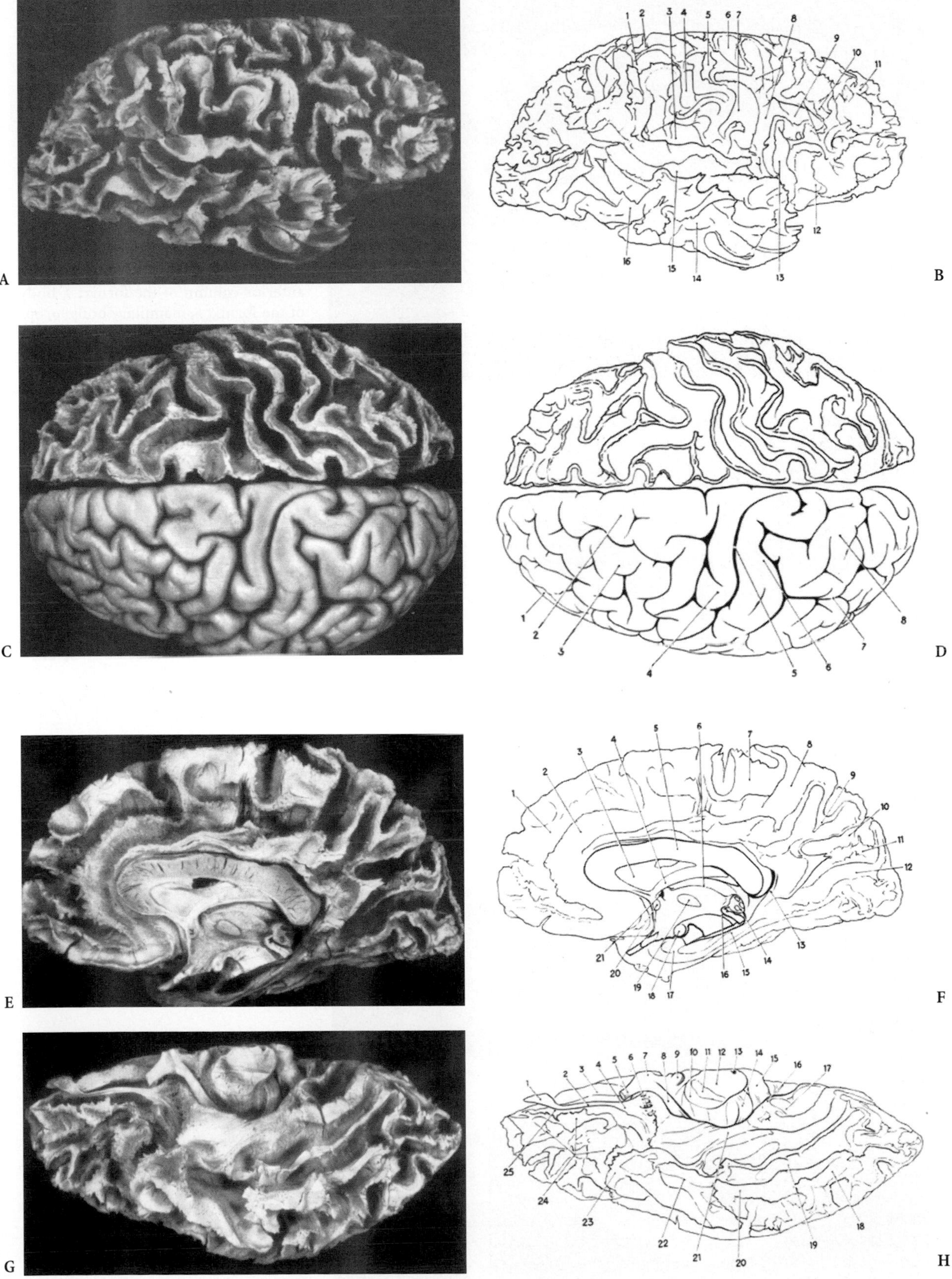
A
B
C
D
E
F
G
H

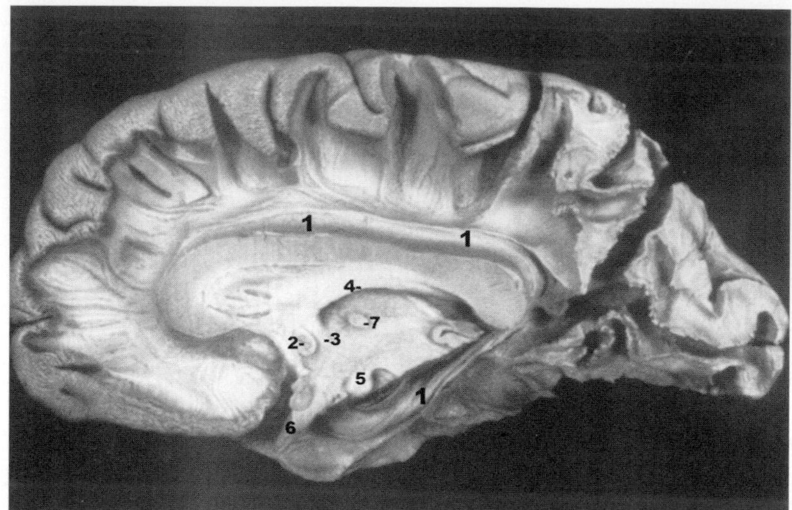

Fig. 3.75. Dissection of the brain disclosing the major association fiber bundles and showing the cingulum. *1*, Cingulum; *2*, anterior commissure; *3*, anterior column of the fornix; *4*, body of the fornix; *5*, mamillary body; *6*, optic chiasm; *7*, interthalamic adhesion. (By Klingler. From Ludwig and Klingler 1956, Table 9)

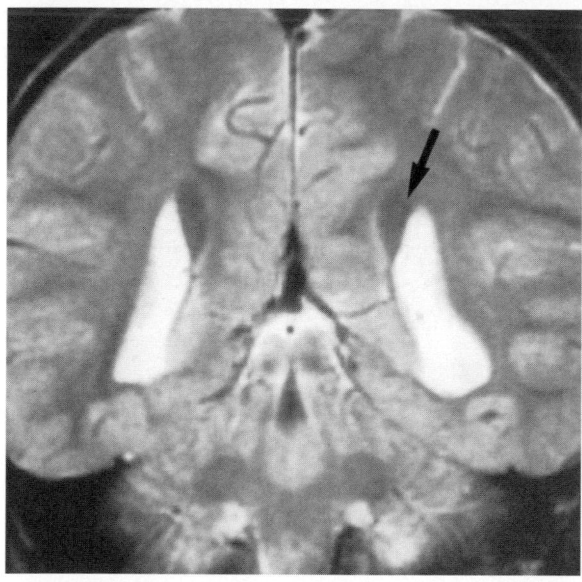

Fig. 3.76. Coronal MR cut (T2-ω) showing the Probst bundles (*arrow*) in a case of agenesis of the corpus callosum

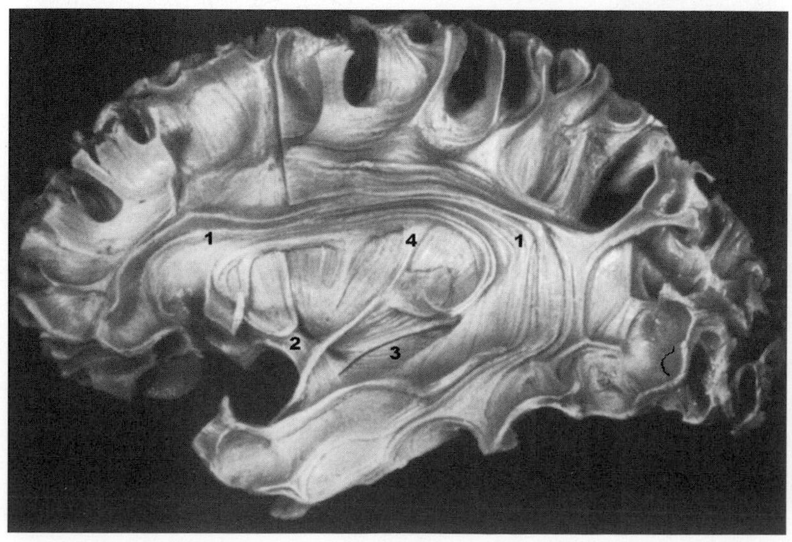

Fig. 3.77. Dissection of the brain disclosing the major association fiber bundles, showing the superior longitudinal fasciculus. *1*, Superior longitudinal fasciculus; *2*, uncinate fasciculus; *3*, inferior longitudinal fasciculus; *4*, medullary substance of the insula. (By Klingler. From Ludwig and Klingler 1956, Table 6)

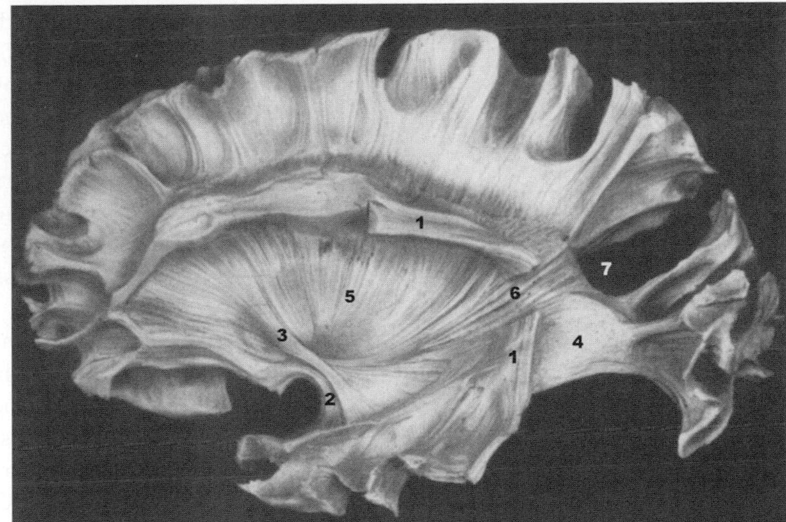

Fig. 3.78. Dissection of the brain disclosing the major association fiber bundles, showing the uncinate fasciculus and the external capsule. *1*, Superior longitudinal fasciculus; *2*, uncinate fasciculus; *3*, inferior fronto-occipital fasciculus; *4*, sagittal stratum; *5*, external capsule; *6*, splenium fibers; *7*, parieto-occipital sulcus. (By Klingler. From Ludwig and Klingler 1956, Table 8)

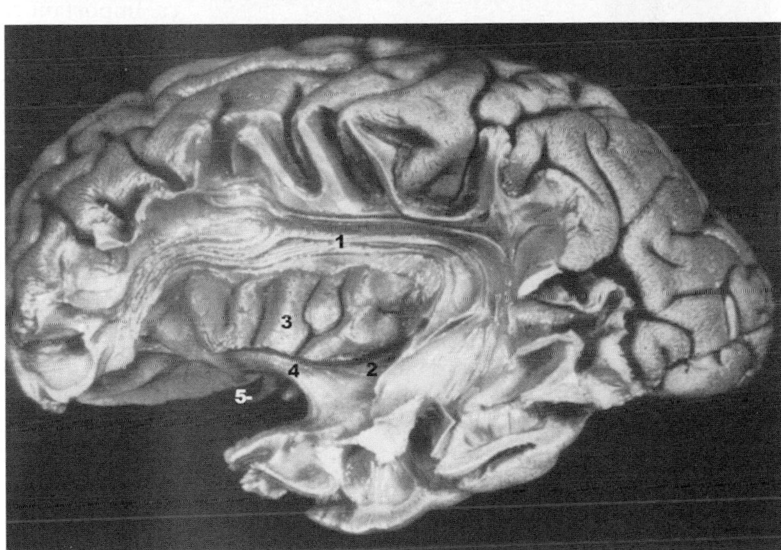

Fig. 3.79. Dissection of the brain disclosing the major association fiber bundles at the level of the insula. *1*, Superior longitudinal fasciculus; *2*, inferior fronto-occipital fasciculus; *3*, insula; *4*, uncinate fasciculus; *5*, optic chiasm. (By Klingler. From Ludwig and Klingler 1956, Table 5)

III Vascular Supply of the Brain

A The Arterial Supply of the Brain

The brain is supplied by the internal carotid arteries and the vertebral arteries (Fig. 3.80). The common carotid artery arises on the left side directly from the aortic arch. On the right side it arises from the bifurcation of the brachiocephalic artery (innominate artery). The common carotid arteries bifurcate at the upper level of the thyroid cartilage corresponding to the upper margin of the fourth cervical vertebra to form the internal and external carotid arteries. The vertebral artery originates in the neck as the third branch of the subclavian artery on each side. The vertebral arteries enter the transverse foramen of the C6 cervical vertebra and ascend in the transverse foramina until they reach the C2. At this level the vertebral arteries proceed laterally, penetrating the transverse foramen of the atlas. The arteries then proceed upward and medially, and pierce the atlanto-occipital membrane and dura as they enter the foramen magnum. The left and right vertebral arteries unite to constitute the basilar artery, usually at the lower border of the pons (Fig. 3.81).

1 The Internal Carotid Artery

The internal carotid artery may be divided into four segments: the cervical, intrapetrosal, intracavernous

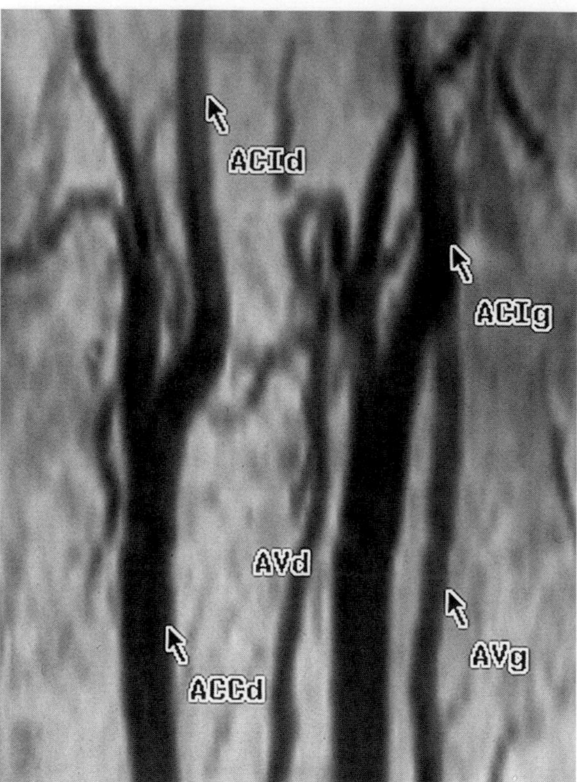

Fig. 3.80. MR angiography of the carotid and vertebral vessels, using 2D time of flight pulse sequence and a neck surface coil. *ACId*, Right internal carotid artery; *ACIg*, left internal carotid artery; *ACCd*, right common carotid artery; *AVd*, right vertebral artery; *AVg*, left vertebral artery

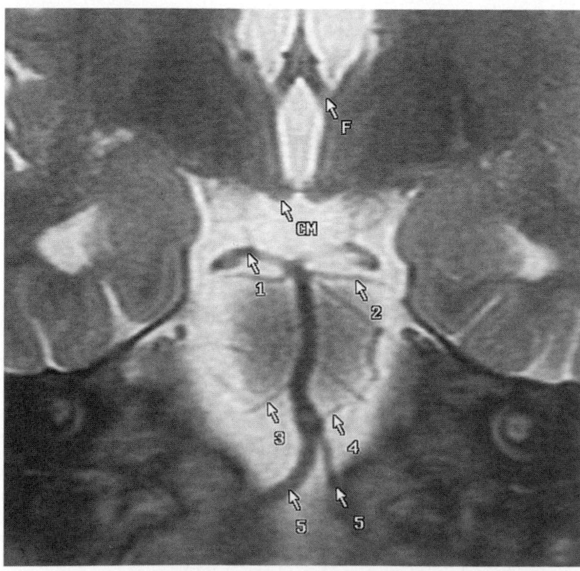

Fig. 3.81. The vertebral basilar system and major branches using FSE T2 weighted MR in the coronal plane. *1*, Posterior cerebral artery; *2*, superior cerebellar artery; *3*, middle cerebellary artery; *4*, posterior inferior cerebellar artery; *5*, vertebral artery. *F*, fornix; *CM*, Mammillary body (corpus mamillare)

and supraclinoid. The intracavernous and the supraclinoid segments are referred to as the "carotid siphon" because of their characteristic shape.

The cervical segment arises from the bifurcation of the common carotid, has no branches and ends as the artery enters the carotid canal in the petrous bone. This segment of the artery corresponds to the intrapetrosal portion where the carotid artery is contained for a short distance in a canal surrounded extradurally by areolar tissue. The intracavernous segment contained within the cavernous sinus lies near its the medial wall. Note that as it enters the cavernous sinus, the artery may show a circular constriction which should not be confused with abnormal narrowing on MR angiographs. In the cavernous sinus, the carotid artery courses roughly horizontally, at the level or just above the floor of the sella turcica. Important relationships to the cranial nerves III, IV, VI and V2, which are located along the wall of the sinus, can be identified. The abducens nerve (VI) is located within the cavernous sinus adjacent to the carotid artery. The supraclinoid segment begins as the artery emerges from the cavernous sinus and projects medially to the anterior clinoid process, becoming intradural, extending upward and backward to its bifurcation and giving rise to all its major branches.

The major branches of the internal carotid artery are the ophthalmic artery, the posterior communicating artery, the anterior choroidal artery, the anterior cerebral artery and the middle cerebral artery (Fig. 3.82).

a The Ophthalmic Artery

The ophthalmic artery arises from the carotid artery immediately after the latter leaves the cavernous sinus. It enters the orbit through the optic foramen, ventral and lateral to the optic nerve (II), then turns upward and medially to pass over the nerve in the orbital cavity. The ophthalmic artery yields several branches, including the lacrimal, supraorbital, ethmoidal and palpebral branches as well as the central retinal artery. It may originate from the middle meningeal artery. The branches of the ophthalmic artery anastomose profusely with those of the external carotid artery.

b The Posterior Communicating Artery

The posterior communicating artery originates from the dorsal aspect of the carotid siphon proceeding medially and posteriorly to join the posterior cerebral artery approximately 10 mm distal to the bifurcation of the basilar artery (Fig. 3.82). At its junction with the carotid siphon a slight dilatation may be observed which should not be confused with an ectasia. The posterior communicating artery may be continuous with the parieto-occipital branch of the posterior cerebral artery, the posterior temporal branch arising from the carotid siphon.

c The Anterior Choroidal Artery

The anterior choroidal artery arises distal to the origin of the posterior communicating artery in 75% of cases, and passes backward across the cisternal space and the optic tract. It then extends laterally to reach the medial surface of the temporal lobe before entering through the choroidal fissure in the temporal horn to supply the choroid plexus. The anterior choroidal artery also supplies the hippocampal formation and part of the basal ganglia. Its usual length is about 30 mm.

d The Anterior Cerebral Artery

The anterior cerebral artery arises at the bifurcation of the internal carotid artery, lateral to the optic chiasm, as one of the two terminal branches of the internal carotid artery(Fig. 3.83). It is subdivided into a horizontal and a vertical segment. The horizontal (A1) portion runs medially and forward above the cisternal optic nerve to the anterior communicating artery. At this level, the artery bends sharply and the vertical segment (A2) ascends along the interhemispheric fissure. At the junction between the rostrum and the genu of the corpus callosum, the anterior cerebral artery turns dorsally forming a so-called arterial "knee" (A3), then continues backward above and along the corpus callosum (A4 and A5). The anterior cerebral artery gives rise to the medial striate artery or recurrent artery of Hubner, an orbital artery, a frontopolar artery, a callosomarginal artery and a pericallosal artery.

The medial striate artery arises usually distal (80% of cases) to the anterior communicating artery but may also arise proximal to it or even at the same level. This recurrent artery courses caudally and laterally and branches many times before entering the anterior perforated substance to partially supply the striatum and internal capsule. It may give rise to branches supplying the inferior aspect of the frontal lobe (Perlmutter and Rhoton 1976).

The orbital artery, consisting sometimes of two or three branches, arises from the ascending portion of the anterior cerebral artery. It extends forward and downward to supply the orbital and medial surfaces of the frontal lobe.

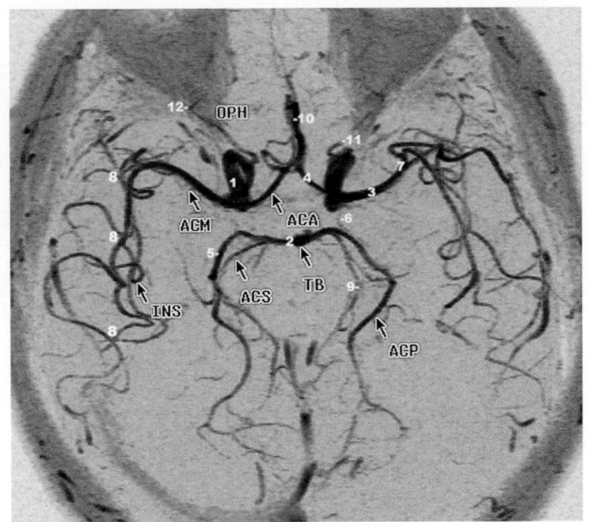

Fig. 3.82. The circle of Willis (MR angiography using 3D time of flight pulse sequence). *1*, Internal carotid artery; *2*, basilar artery; *3*, proximal segment of middle cerebral artery; *4*, proximal segment of anterior cerebral artery; *5*, proximal segment of posterior cerebral artery; *6*, posterior communicating artery; *7*, bifurcation of middle cerebral artery; *8*, insular branches of middle cerebral artery; *9*, perimesencephalic segment of superior cerebellar artery; *10*, pericallosal artery; *11*, ophthalmic artery; *12*, perioptic loop of ophthalmic artery; *OPH*, ophthalmic artery; *ACA*, anterior cerebral artery; *ACM*, middle cerebral artery; *INS*, insular branches of middle cerebral artery; *TB*, basilar artery; *ACP*, posterior cerebral artery; *ACS*, superior cerebellar artery

The callosomarginal artery is the major branch of the anterior cerebral artery. It arises from the knee of the anterior cerebral artery, distal to the origin of the frontopolar artery, around the genu of the corpus callosum. It gives an anterior, a middle and a posterior internal frontal branch, and may terminate as a paracentral branch. When the internal frontal and the paracentral branches reach the upper margin of the cerebral hemisphere, they anastomose with the pre- and postcentral branches of the middle cerebral artery. The branches of this artery supply the paracentral lobule and parts of the cingulate gyrus (Lazorthes et al. 1976).

The pericallosal artery, also called the terminal branch of the anterior cerebral artery, is usually located close to the upper surface of the corpus callosum giving rise to the paracentral branch, which may alternatively arise from the callosomarginal artery. It terminates as the precuneal branch which supplies the medial surface of the parietal lobe, including the precuneus. A posterior callosal branch supplies the corpus callosum and anastomoses with

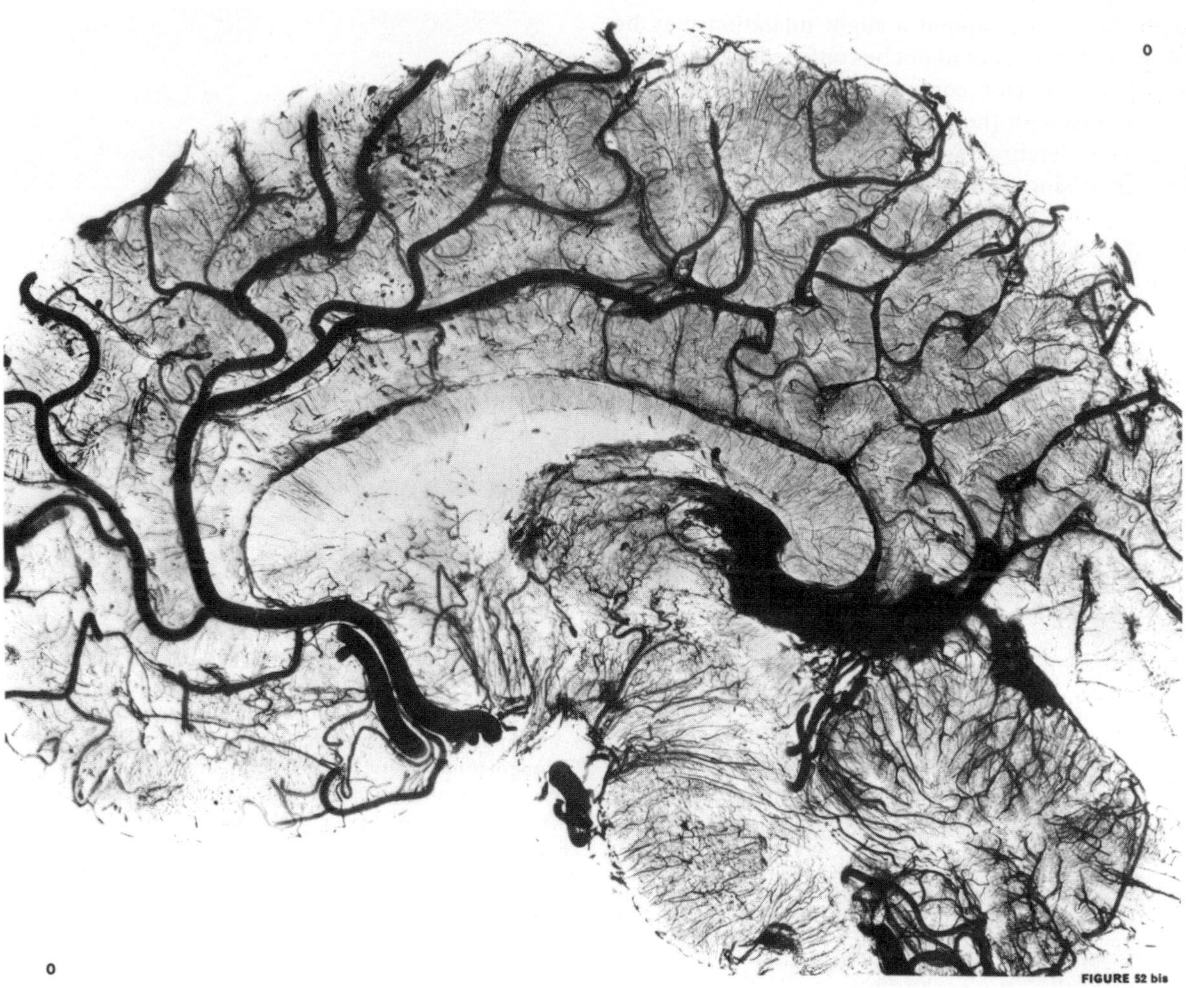

A

FIGURE 52 bis

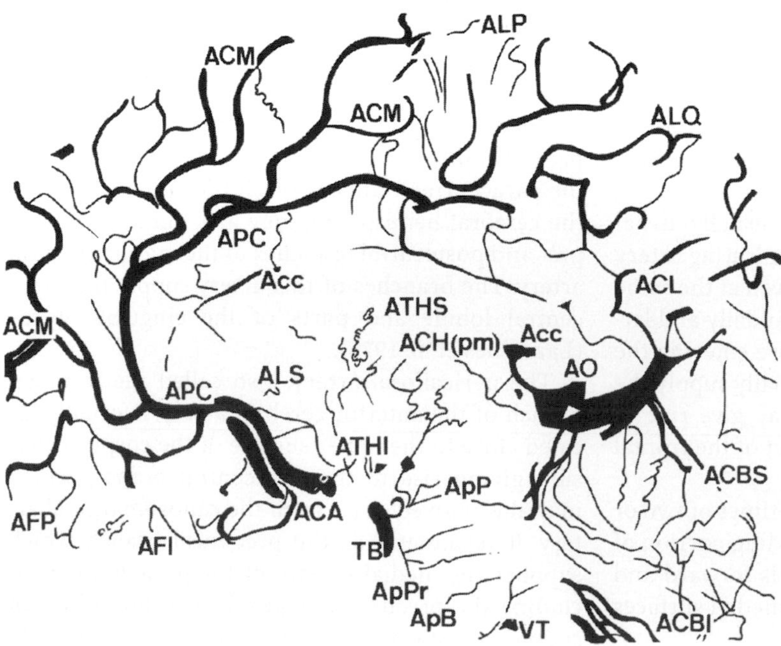

B

Fig. 3.83A,B. The anterior cerebral artery (*ACA*) and its cortical branches. **A** Macroscopic cut and corresponding diagram (**B**) of a brain specimen showing the disposition of the arterial branches. *ACA*, Anterior cerebral artery; *ACBI*, posterior inferior cerebellar artery; *ACBS*, superior cerebellar artery; *Acc*, arteries of the corpus callosum; *ACH*, medial posterior choroidal arteries; *ACL*, calcarine artery; *ACM*, callosomarginal artery; *AFI*, orbitofrontal artery; *AFP*, frontopolar artery; *ALQ*, artery of the precuneus; *ALP*, artery of the paracentral lobule; *ALS*, lenticulostriate arteries; *AO*, occipital artery; *ApB*, perforating medullary arteries; *APC*, pericallosal artery; *ApP*, peduncular branches; *ApPr*, pontine arteries; *ATHI*, inferior thalamic arteries; *ATHS*, superior thalamic arteries; *TB*, basilar trunk; *VT*, vertebral artery. (From Salamon 1971)

a branch of the posterior cerebral artery. Anatomic variants of the anterior cerebral artery occur in about 25% of brains including a hypoplastic horizontal portion or, more rarely, a total absence of this segment.

e The Middle Cerebral Artery

The middle cerebral artery is larger than the anterior artery and is regarded as the direct continuation of the internal carotid artery or its main branch. It is normally never absent. The proximal portion of the middle cerebral artery is nearly horizontal (M1) coursing laterally over the anterior perforated substance to enter the lateral cerebral fossa between the temporal lobe and the lower aspect of the insula (Figs. 3.84, 3.85). Turning around the lower part of the insula, the middle cerebral artery passes upward and backward in the deepest portion of the lateral fissure forming a number of large branches. Variations of two or three, in the number of branches formed at the end of M1 segment, are the rule (Figs. 3.84, 3.85).

In the insular area, the middle cerebral artery gives rise to five to eight branches. The most posterior branch emerging from the lateral fissure corresponds to the sylvian point. The branches of the middle cerebral artery emerge from the lateral fissure and are distributed over the lateral aspect of the cerebral hemisphere (Fig. 3.86).

Before giving rise to the cortical branches, the horizontal segment of the middle cerebral artery forms the striate arteries, represented by two groups of three to six small arteries named the medial and lateral striate arteries, which penetrate the brain through the anterior perforated substance. These small perforating arteries tend to rise at nearly right angles from the main vessels (Fig. 3.87).

Before describing the cortical branches, it is important to consider the anatomy of these middle cerebral arterial branches as they course through the sylvian fissure and form the so-called "sylvian triangle" (Schlesinger 1953). The inferior side of the sylvian triangle, as shown on a lateral cut or projection, is formed by the line starting at the posterior point of the lateral fissure, called the angiographic sylvian point, and extending to the anterior extremity of the middle cerebral artery. The anterior superior aspect of the triangle corresponds to the top of the first identifiable opercular branch. The actual position of the sylvian or lateral fissure may be placed on lateral angiograms as the line joining the points where the opercular vessels turn to leave the lateral fissure after having descended. On frontal views the sylvian point, which corresponds to the most medial extent of the last branch of the middle cerebral artery before it emerges from the fissure, is centered between the roof of the orbit and the horizontal line tangential to the inner table of the skull vertex (Vlahovitch et al. 1964, 1965, 1970).

The orbitofrontal artery found on the orbitofrontal cortex may anastomose with the frontopolar branch of the anterior cerebral artery. The remaining branches of the cerebral artery are ascending on the lateral aspect of the frontoparietal lobe including the precentral branches, a central or rolandic artery, a postcentral artery and a posterior parietal branch. A posterior temporal branch supplies the lateral aspect of the occipital lobe. The angular artery, or angular branches, form the terminal segment of the middle cerebral artery supplying the angular gyrus. The middle cerebral artery, which is the major artery of the lateral aspect of the cerebral hemisphere, supplies an extensive and functionally important region of the cerebral cortex including the central and motor areas, the somesthetic and the auditory areas, as well as large regions of the associative cortex (Figs. 3.86, 3.88).

2 The Arterial Circle of Willis

Described by Willis (1664), this anastomotic arterial circle is a constant anatomic structure located at the basal surface of the brain in the chiasmal cistern encircling the optic chiasm, the tuber cinereum and the interpeduncular fossa (Fig. 3.82). It is formed by anastomotic branches of the internal carotid artery and the basilar artery, as well as by the anterior and posterior communicating arteries and the proximal segments of the anterior, middle and posterior cerebral arteries. Several variants are observed and it is common to find asymmetrical development of the various components. A symmetrical circle is observed in about 20% of cases.

From the arterial circle of Willis and the main cerebral arteries arise the central and cortical branches. The small central arteries arise from the circle of Willis and the proximal segments of the anterior, middle and posterior cerebral arteries. These arteries penetrate perpendicularly into the basal brain substance to supply the basal ganglia, the internal capsule and the diencephalon. The cortical or circumferential arteries, branches of the three major cerebral arteries, course on the lateral and medial aspects of the cerebral hemispheres. From these cortical branches arise smaller terminal arteries which penetrate the brain substance at right angles, some

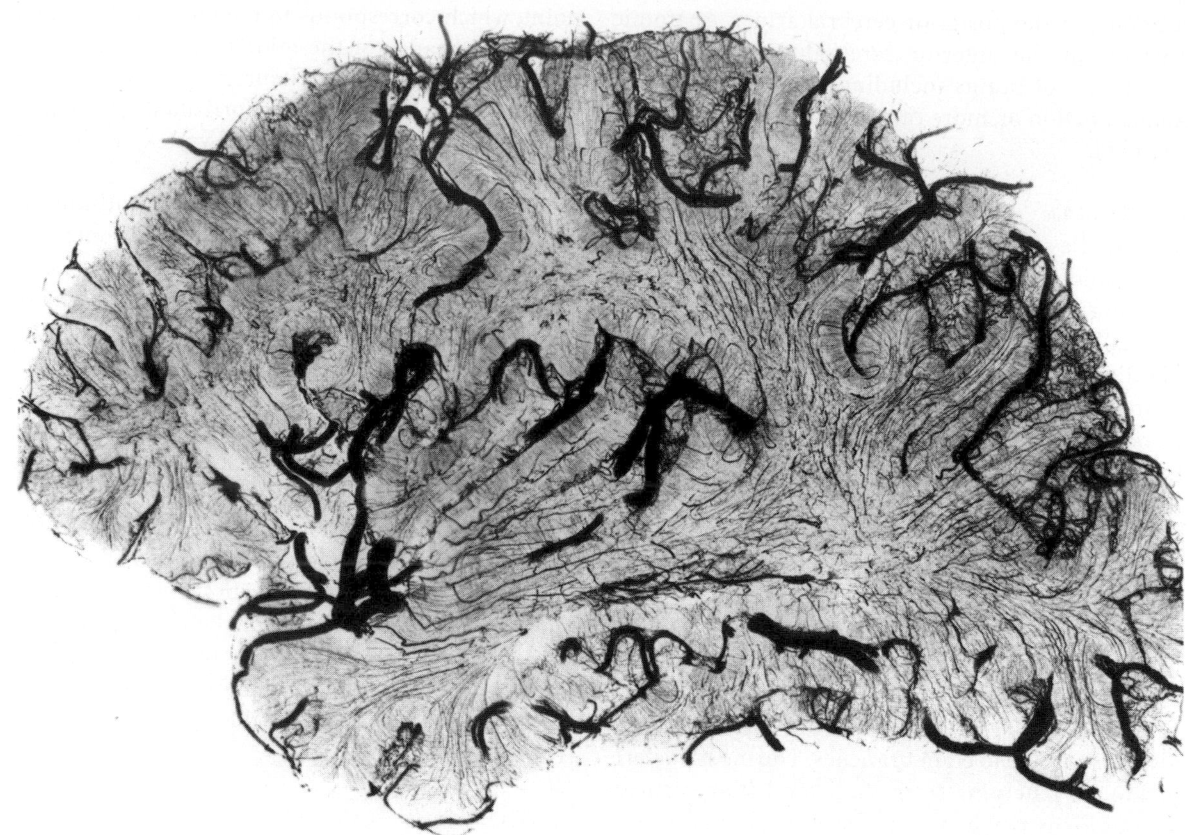

A

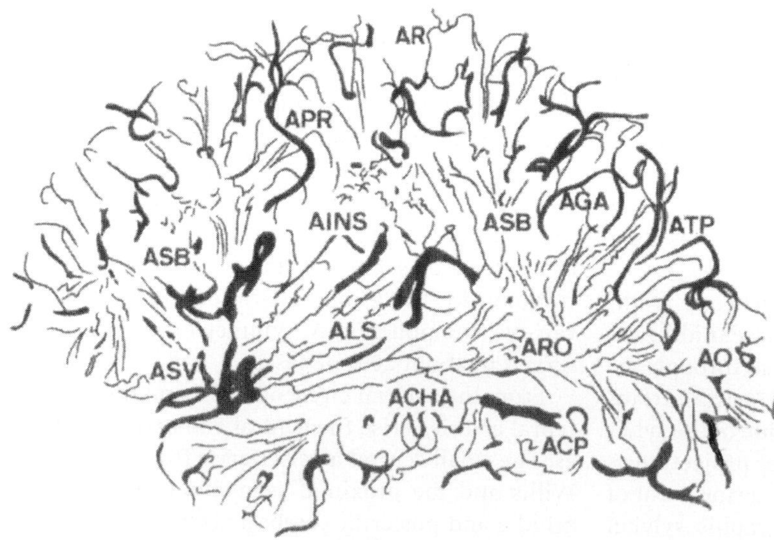

B

Fig. 3.84A,B. The insular branches of the middle cerebral artery (*MCA*) and the cortical branches. **A** Macroscopic cut and corresponding diagram (**B**) of a brain specimen showing the disposition of the arterial branches. *ACHA*, Anterior choroidal artery; *ACP*, posterior cerebral artery; *AGA*, artery of the angular gyrus; *AINS*, insular artery; *ALS*, lenticulostriate arteries; *AO*, occipital artery; *APR*, prerolandic artery; *AR*, rolandic artery; *ARO*, arteries of the optic radiation; *ASB*, arteries of the white matter; *ASV*, sylvian artery; *ATP*, posterior temporal artery. (From Salamon 1971)

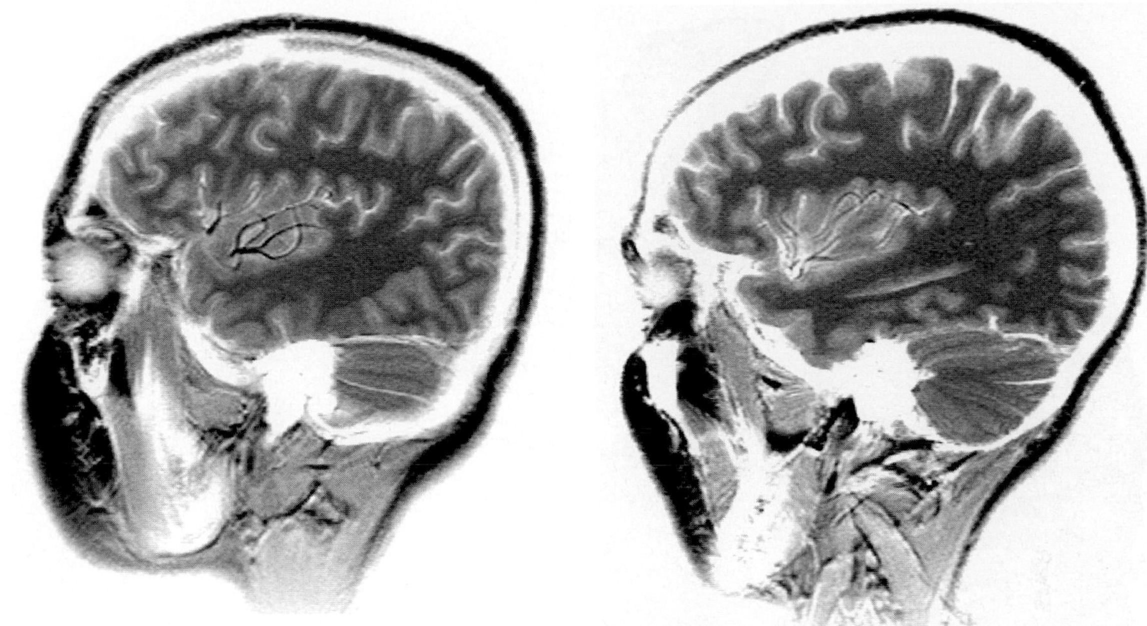

Fig. 3.85A,B. Parasagittal MR cuts showing the variable branching of the insular branches of the middle cerebral artery

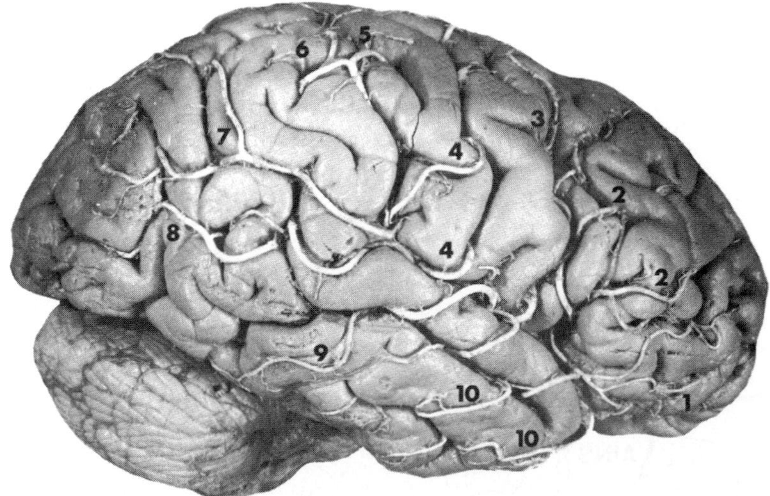

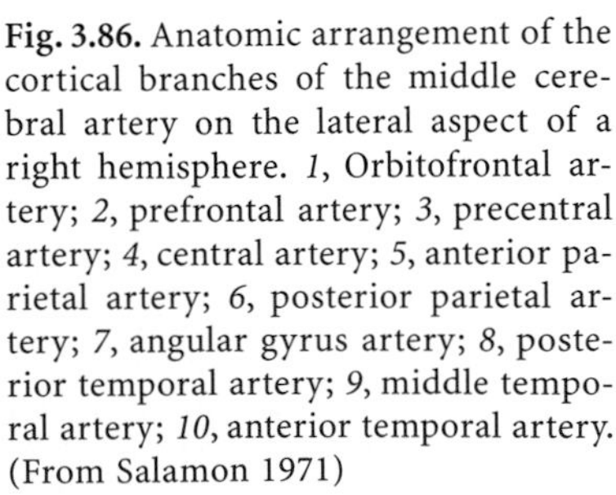

Fig. 3.86. Anatomic arrangement of the cortical branches of the middle cerebral artery on the lateral aspect of a right hemisphere. *1*, Orbitofrontal artery; *2*, prefrontal artery; *3*, precentral artery; *4*, central artery; *5*, anterior parietal artery; *6*, posterior parietal artery; *7*, angular gyrus artery; *8*, posterior temporal artery; *9*, middle temporal artery; *10*, anterior temporal artery. (From Salamon 1971)

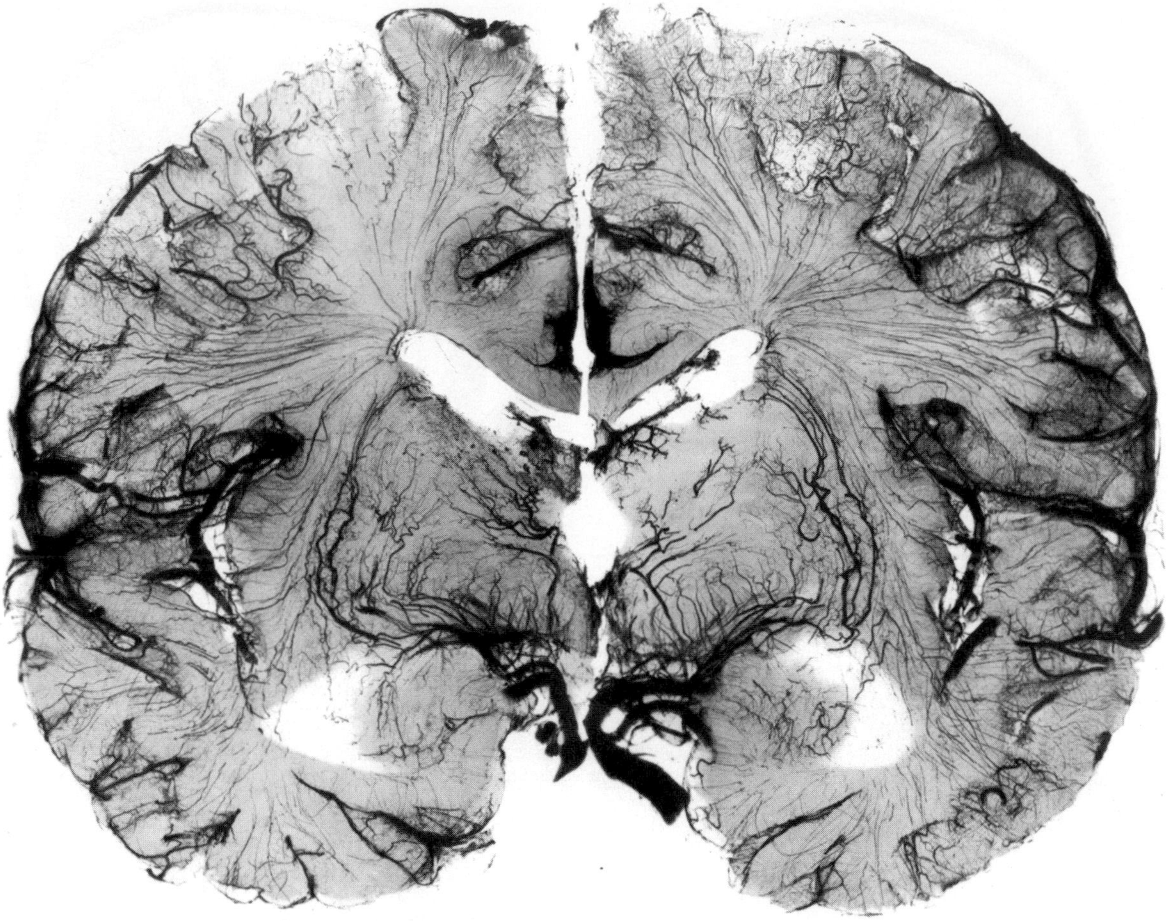

A

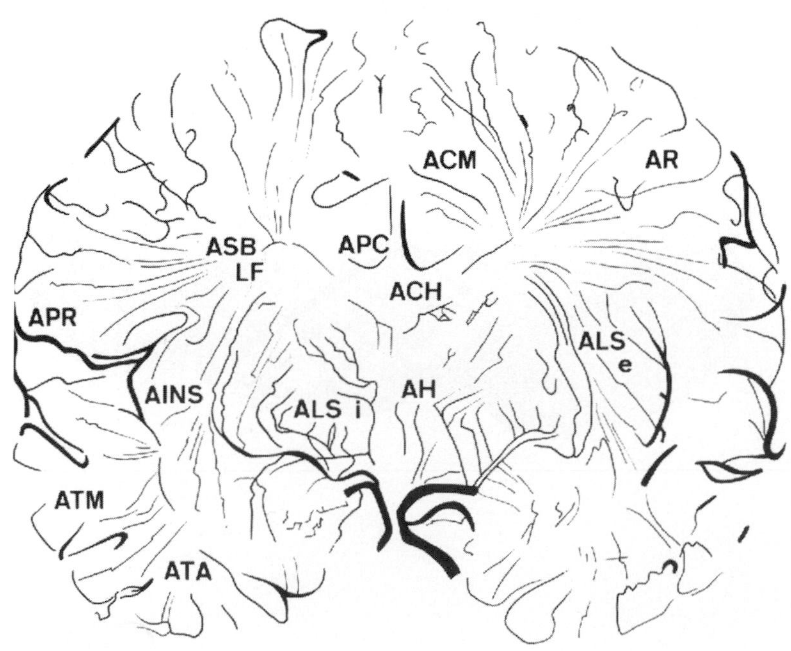

B

Fig. 3.87A,B. The striate arteries of the interbrain structures. **A** Macroscopic section and corresponding diagram (**B**) of a brain specimen and correlated angiogram. *ACH*, choroidal arteries (superior group); *ACM*, callosomarginal artery; *AH*, artery of Heubner; *AINS*, insular arteries; *ALS*, lenticulostriate arteries; *e*, external striate; *i*, internal striate; *APC*, pericallosal artery; *APR*, prerolandic artery; *AR*, rolandic artery; *ASB*, arteries of the white matter (*LF*) of the frontal lobe; *AYA*, anterior temporal artery; *ATM*, middle temporal artery. (From Salamon 1971)

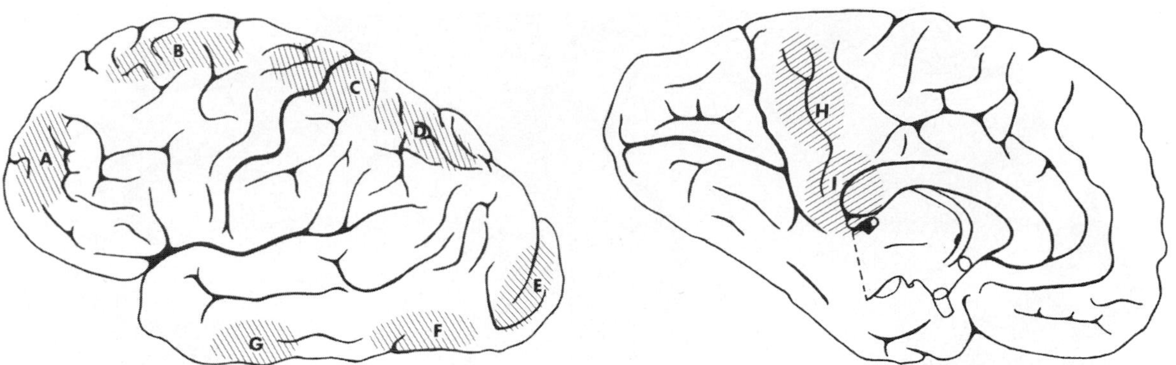

Fig. 3.88. A Areas of anastomoses (*hatched*) between the terminal branches of the major cerebral arteries (lateral aspect of the hemisphere). *A*, Orbital branches of ACA and MCA; *B*, callosomarginal (ACA) and operculofrontal (MCA) branches; *C*, central (MCA) and pericentral (ACA) branches; *D*, posterior parietal branches (MCA) and PCA; *E*, posterior temporal branches (MCA) and calcarine (PCA); *F*, posterior temporal branches (MCA) and posterior cerebral branches (PCA); *G*, anterior temporal branches (MCA and PCA). **B** Areas of anastomoses (*hatched*) between the terminal branches of the major cerebral arteries (mesial aspect of the hemisphere). *H*, Precuneal branches (ACA) and parieto-occipital (PCA); *I*, pericallosal branch (ACA) and posterior callosal ramus of PCA. (From Gillilan 1974)

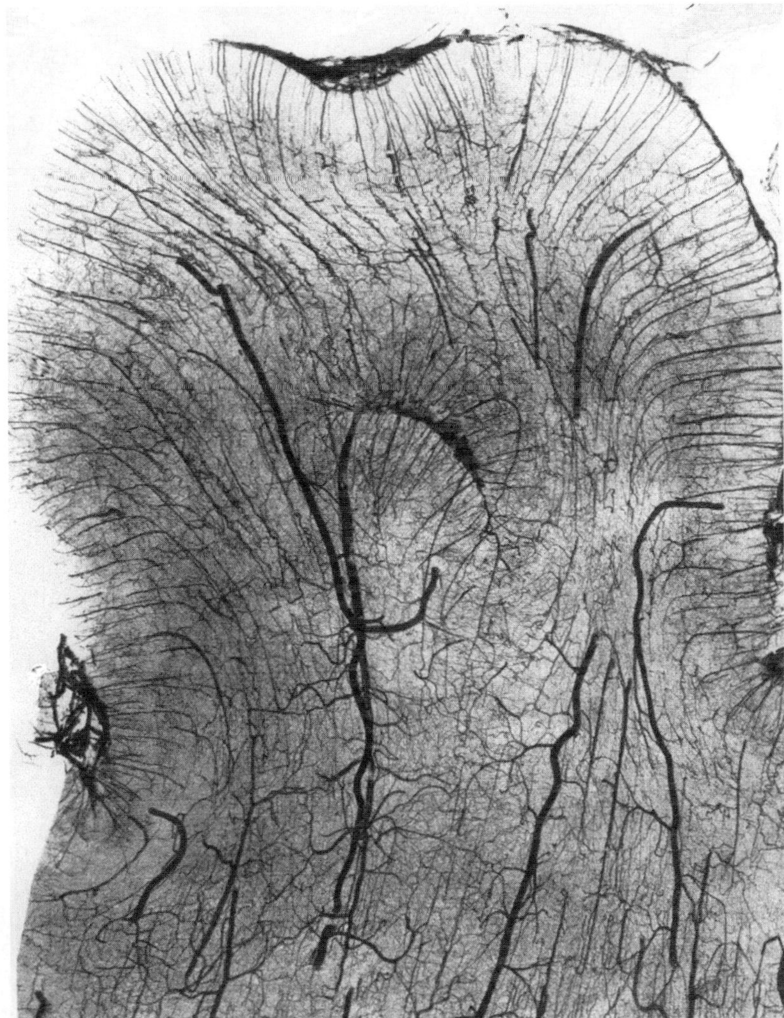

Fig. 3.89. Perforating arteries of the central cortex of the cerebral hemisphere, corresponding to the smaller terminal arteries penetrating the brain substance at right angles which supply the cortical mantle and the subcortical white matter. (From Salamon 1971) +100

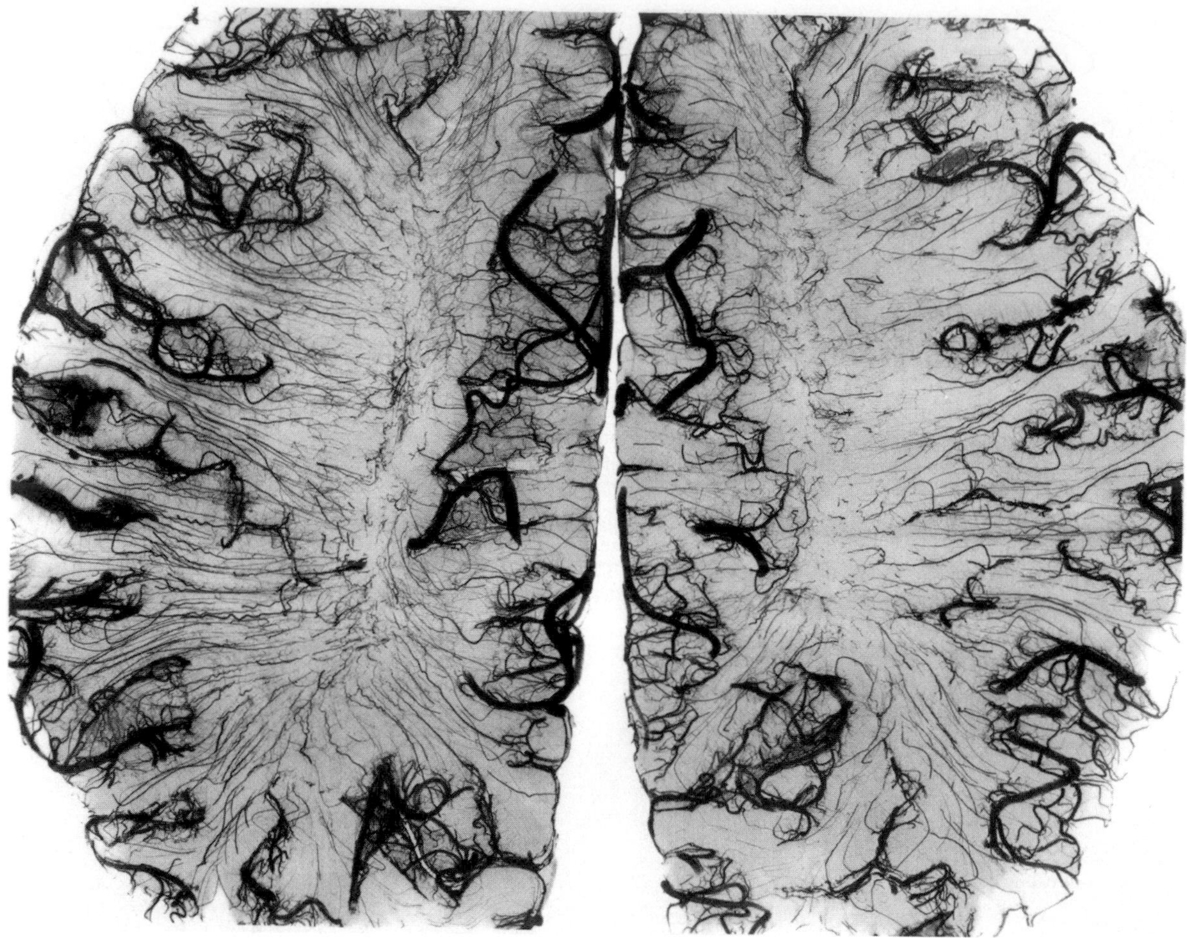

Fig. 3.90. The watershed junctional zones in the deep white matter, showing a roughly symmetrical disposition, as seen on the axial cut through the centrum semiovale. (From Salamon 1971)

of which arborize in the cortex while the longer ones supply the subcortical deep white matter (Fig. 3.89). These cortical branches are not end arteries and show anastomoses which may compensate to a variable extent the occlusion of one of these vessels with the blood supply from adjacent branches. The watershed zones, which may show ischemia in the case of hypotension, correspond to the areas of the cerebral cortex, the basal ganglia and the internal capsule situated between the territorial distributions of two of the primary arteries (Fig. 3.87,3.90).

B Vascular Supply of the Posterior Fossa

The vascular supply of the posterior fossa is provided by two vertebral arteries, which join at the level of the pontomedullary junction to form the basilar artery. Branches of the vertebral and basilar arteries can be classified into three types: the penetrating arteries, which penetrate the brainstem in its ventral aspect at the midline; The short circumferential and the long circumferential arteries. At each level of the brain stem, one circumferential artery is markedly developed and provides the blood supply for that portion of the brain stem and cerebellum. At the level of the medulla, the posterior inferior cerebellar artery supplies part of the medulla and the suboccipital surface of the cerebellum. The pons and petrosal surface of the cerebellum are supplied by the anterior inferior cerebellar artery, and the midbrain and tentorial surface of the cerebellum are supplied by the superior cerebellar artery.

1 The Posterior Inferior Cerebellar Artery

The posterior inferior cerebellar artery (PICA) is the largest branch of the vertebral artery, arising most commonly from its intradural segment. The PICA is divided into five segments according to Rhoton: an anterior medullary segment, beginning at the origin of the PICA and terminating at the level of the inferior olive, continues with the second or lateral medullary segment which ends at the level of the lower cranial nerves. The third, or tonsilomedullary, segment is closely related to the tonsils, forming a caudal loop. The fourth, or retrotonsilar, segment starts at the midlevel of the tonsil and ends where the artery exits to become hemispheric. The last segment, the hemispheric segment, supplies the occipital surface of the vermis and cerebellar hemisphere.

The vascular territory of the PICA is highly variable and reflects the high degree of variability of this artery. It appears to be in balance with other major vessels in the posterior fossa. It supplies the lateral medullary area in 50% of cases. Its cerebellar territory includes the globose and emboliform nuclei.

2 The Anterior Inferior Cerebellar Artery

The anterior inferior cerebellar artery (AICA) originates from the basilar artery at the level of the pontomedullary sulcus and curves in a caudal direction around the pons towards the cerebellopontine angle. At this level it divides into superior and inferior trunks. The inferior trunk passes below the flocculus and vascularizes the inferior portion of the petrosal surface of the cerebellar hemisphere. The superior trunk has an upward curve and anastomoses with the superior cerebellar artery.

3 The Superior Cerebellar Artery

The superior cerebellar artery (SCA) originates from the superior segment of the basilar artery, usually a few millimeters before it divides into the posterior cerebral arteries. Duplication of the SCA is common and noted in 80% of cases. The course of the SCA is parallel to the postcerebral artery and is separated from the latter by the third nerve. Both arteries sweep around the brain stem towards the quadrigeminal plates. There, the SCA makes a sharp upward turn to reach the cerebellar hemisphere. It supplies the lower midbrain, upper pons, the dentate nucleus and the tentorial surface of the cerebellar hemisphere.

C The Cerebral Venous System

The cerebral venous system comprises the superficial cerebral veins and the deep cerebral veins, all of which, like dural sinuses, are devoid of valves. These two venous systems are very richly anastomosed (Fig. 3.91). The superficial cerebral veins are extremely variable, most running upward to end in the superior longitudinal sinus. In general, these veins drain the blood from the cortex and subcortical white matter to the superior sagittal sinus or the basal sinuses. The deep cerebral veins drain the choroid plexus, the diencephalon, the basal ganglia and the periventricular and deep white matter into the internal cerebral veins and the great cerebral vein.

The superficial cerebral veins form a network in the pia mater and then converge to form larger confluents which empty into the dural sinuses. These veins drain the blood from the lateral and medial aspects of the cerebral hemisphere into the superior sagittal sinus. There are about 10 to 15 superficial cerebral veins, the locations of which are extremely variable, most of them running upward before entering the superior sagittal sinus against the flow of the blood stream. Some of the veins of the medial hemispheric surface may drain into the inferior sagittal sinus. The largest of these veins is the superior anastomotic vein, or vein of Trolard, which anastomoses with the inferior anastomotic vein, or vein of Labbé. Both are variable in position, size and configuration. These two veins connect the superficial middle cerebral vein with the superior sagittal and transverse sinuses. The middle cerebral vein courses downward and forward in the lateral fissure before ending in the sphenoparietal or the cavernous sinus. The inferior aspect of the brain shows extensive venous plexus draining into the basal sinuses. The veins originating from the anterior temporal lobe and interpeduncular fossa drain into the cavernous and sphenoparietal sinuses. The orbital region may drain into the sagittal sinuses. The transverse and the petrosal sinuses collect the venous flow from the tentorium cerebelli. Note that the cortical regions of the medial and inferior aspects of the hemispheres may drain through anastomotic channels into the deep cerebral venous system.

The deep cerebral veins, angiographically more important than the superficial veins, comprise the insular and striate veins, the internal cerebral veins, the basal vein of Rosenthal and the great cerebral vein of Galen.

The insular veins present a similar configuration to the arterial branches of the middle cerebral artery even assuming a similar triangular configuration, “the venous sylvian triangle”. These veins drain into the deep middle cerebral vein, which in turn drains into the basal cerebral vein or the sphenoparietal sinus. The striate veins and veins originating from the

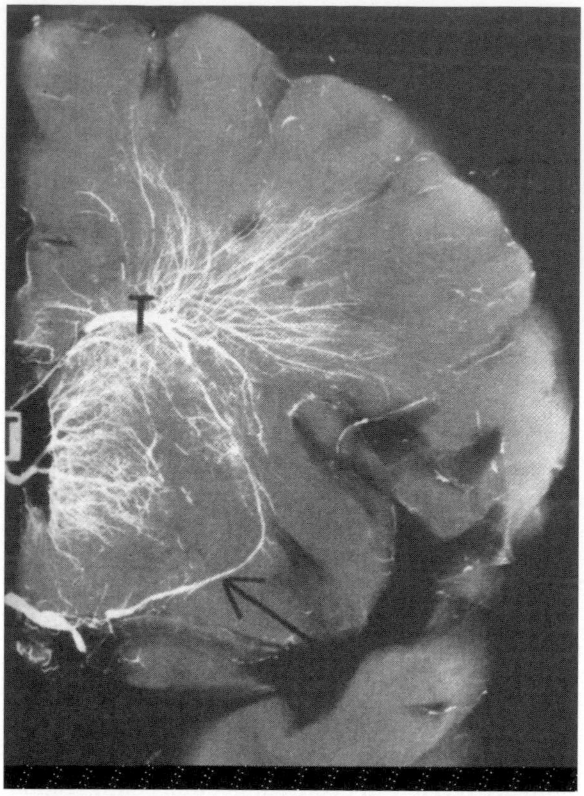

A

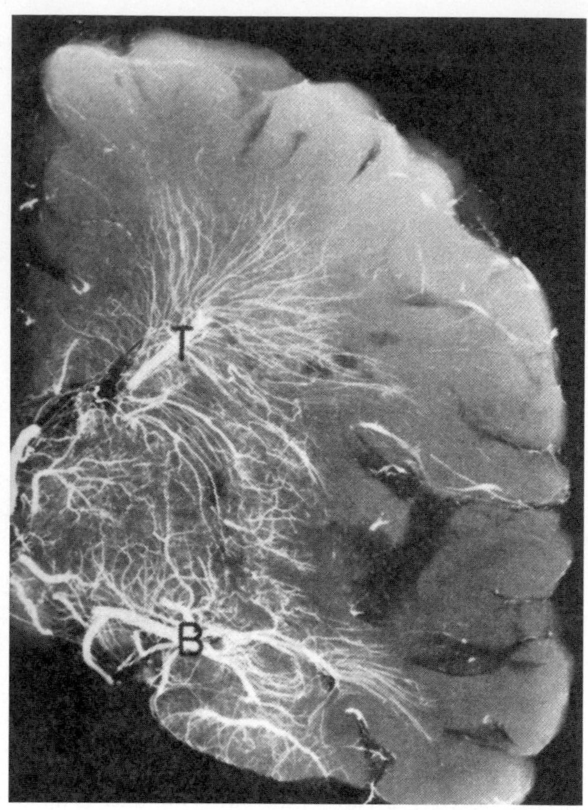

B

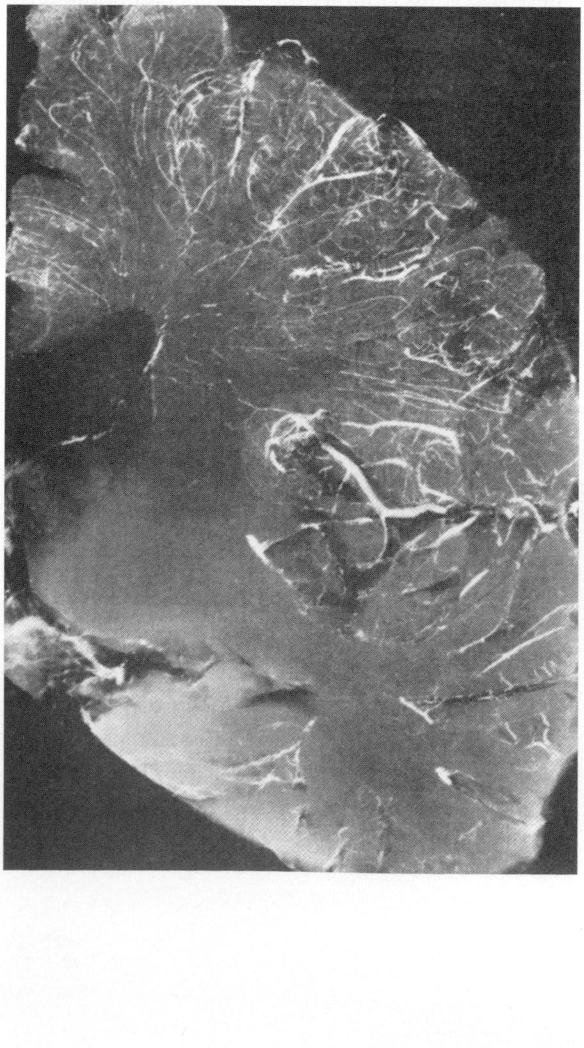

C

Fig. 3.91 A–C. Coronal cuts of 1 cm thickness through head of the caudate (**A**) and the thalamus (**B**). *B*, basal vein; *T*, terminal vein; *I*, internal cerebral vein. **C** Coronal cut of 1 cm thickness through the posterior thalamus after contrast injection into the superior longitudinal sinus. (From Hassler 1966)

inferior aspect of the frontal lobe are also drained through the deep middle cerebral vein. An uncal vein coursing from the medial aspect of the temporal lobe drains into the sphenoparietal or cavernous sinus.

The paired internal cerebral veins, located just off the midline in the tela choroidea of the roof of the third ventricle, extend from the interventricular foramina of Monro over the superior and internal aspect of the thalamus to reach the upper portion of the quadrigeminal cistern. There they join to form the great cerebral vein of Galen. The latter follows a concave upward curve and ends in the straight sinus. The main tributary of the internal cerebral veins are: (1) the thalamostriate vein, which runs forward in the groove formed by the caudate nucleus and the thalamus; (2) the choroidal vein, which courses along the lateral border of the choroid plexus extending to the inferior horn of the lateral ventricle and draining the choroid plexus and the adjacent hippocampal regions; (3) the septal vein, which drains the rostral portion of the corpus callosum and the septum lucidum before joining the internal cerebral vein at the interventricular foramen; and (4) the epithalamic vein, which drains the dorsal portion of the diencephalon before joining the internal cerebral vein. The ventral portions of the diencephalon are drained into the pial venous plexus of the interpeduncular region. The lateral ventricular vein runs over the posterior superior aspect of the thalamus and joins the internal cerebral vein.

The basal vein of Rosenthal originates from the medial aspect of the anterior portion of the temporal lobe. It receives a small anterior cerebral vein which accompanies the anterior cerebral artery and drains the orbitofrontal region, the anterior corpus callosum and corresponding portions of the cingulate gyrus. The deep middle cerebral vein, situated in the depth of the lateral fissure, drains the insula and the opercular cortex. The inferior striate veins leave the striatum through the anterior perforated substance to drain into the deep middle cerebral vein. All these veins join the basal vein which passes backward around the brainstem to join the great cerebral vein of Galen.

The great cerebral vein of Galen is formed by the union of the paired internal cerebral veins, the paired basal veins, the paired occipital veins, which drain the internal and inferior aspects of the occipital lobes and the adjacent parietal lobes, and the posterior callosal vein, which drains the splenium and the adjacent internal brain areas. The great cerebral vein is a short vein located beneath the splenium of the corpus callosum. It drains into the rectus sinus.

References

Aresu M (1914) La superficie cerebrale nell'uomo. Arch Ital Anat Embr 12:380–433

Ariens Kappers CU (1947) Anatomie comparée du système nerveux. Masson and Cie, Paris (with the collaboration of E.H. Strasburger)

Ariens Kappers CU, Huber GC, Crosby EC (1936) Comparative anatomy of the central nervous system of vertebrates, including man, vols 1 and 2. Macmillan, New York

Bailey P (1948) Concerning the organization of the cerebral cortex. Tex Rep Biol Med 6:34–56

Bailey P, von Bonin G, Mc Culloch WS (1950) The isocortex of the chimpanzee. University of Illinois Press, Urbana, Ill

Bailey P, von Bonin G (1951) The isocortex of man. University of Illinois Press, Urbana, Ill

Baillarger JGF (1840) Recherches sur la structure dela couche corticale des circonvolutions du cerveau. Mem Acad R Med 8:149–183

Beccari N (1911) La superficie degli emisferi cerebrali dell'uomo nelle regioni prossime al rinecefalo. Arch Ital Anat Embr 10:482–543

Benedikt M (1906) Aus meinem Leben. Stulpnagel, Vienna

Betz W (1874) Anatomischer Nachweis zweier Gehirnzentra. Centr Med Wissensch 12:578–580, 595–599

Brissaud E (1893) Anatomie du cerveau de l'homme. Masson, Paris

Broca P (1878) Nomenclature cérébrale. Rev Anthropol 2:3

Brodmann K (1909) Vergleichende Lokalisationslehre der Großhirnrinde. Barth, Leipzig

Cabanis EA, Doyon D, Halimi PH, Iba-Zizen MT, Sigal R, Tamraz J (1988) Atlas d'IRM de l'encéphale et de la moëlle. Masson, Paris

Calori L (1870) Del cervello nei due tipi brachicefalo. zzz

Campbell AW (1905) Histological studies on the localization of cerebral function. Cambridge University Press, Cambridge

Chi T, Chang C (1941) The sulcal pattern of the Chinese brain. Am J Phys Anthropol 28:167–209

Chi JG, Dooling ED, Gilles FH (1977) Gyral development of the human brain. Ann Neurol 1:86

Chusid TG, Sugar O, French JD (1948) Corticocortical connections of the cerebral cortex lying within the arcuate and lunate sulci of the monkey (Macaca mulatta). J Neuropathol Exp Neurol 439–446

Comair Y, Hong SC, Bleasel A (1996a) Invasive investigation and surgery of the supplementary motor area. In: Lüders HO (ed) Advances in neurology, vol 70. Lippincott-Raven, Philadelphia

Comair YG, Choi HY, Tamraz J (1996b) Cortical anatomy: sulcal and gyral patterns. In: Wyllie E (ed) The treatment of epilepsy: principles and practice, 2nd edn. Lea and Febiger, Philadelphia

Connolly CJ (1950) External morphology of the primate brain. Thomas, Springfield, Ill

Cunningham DJ (1890) The intraparietal sulcus of the brain. J Anat Physiol 24:137–155

Cunningham DJ, Horsley V (1892) Contribution to the surface anatomy of the cerebral hemispheres. Royal Irish Academy, Dublin

Déjerine J (1895) Anatomie des centres nerveux, vol 1 and 2. Rueff, Paris

Delmas A, Pertuiset B (1959) Topométrie crânio-encéphalique chez l'homme. Masson, Paris

Duvernoy H, Cabanis EA, Iba-Zizen MT, Tamraz J, Guyot J (1991) The human brain surface three-dimensional sectional anatomy and MRI. Springer, Vienna New York

Eberstaller O (1884) Zur Oberflächen-Anatomie der Grosshirn-Hemisphären. Wien Med Bl 7:644–646

Eberstaller O (1890) Das Stirnhirn. Ein Beitrag zur Anatomie des Oberfläche des Großhirns. Urban and Schwarzenberg, Vienna

Ecker A (1869) Die Hirnwindungen des Menschen. Vieweg, Braunschweig

Elze K (1929) Einige Fasersysteme des menschlichen Grosshirns mit der Abfaserungs-methode untersucht. Z Anat Entwicklungsgesch 88:166–178

Filimonoff IN (1947) A rational subdivision of the cerebral cortex. Arch Neurol Psychiatr 58:296–311

Flechsig P (1898) Neue Untersuchungen über die Markbildung in den menschlichen Grosshirnlappen. Neurol Centrlbl 17:977–996

Giacomini C (1878) Guida allo studio delle circonvoluzioni cerebrali dell'uomo. Camilla e Bertolero, Turin, pp 96

Gillilan (1974) Potential collateral circulation to the human cerebral cortex. Neurology 24:941–948

Geyer H (1940) Über Hirnwindungen bei Zwillingen. Z Morphol Anthropol 38:51–55

Gratiolet P (1854) Mémoire sur les plis cérébraux de l'homme et des primates. Bertrand, Paris

Hassler H (1966) Deep cerebral venous system in man. Neurology 16:505–511

Henneberg R (1910) Messung der Oberflächenausdehnung der Grosshirnrinde. J Psychol Neurol 17:144–158

Heschl RL (1878) Über die vordere quere Schläfenwindung des menschlichen Grosshirns. Braumuller, Vienna

Higeta K (1940) Morphologische Untersuchungen des Gehirns bei den japanischen Zwillingsfeten. Okajimas Fol Anat Jpn 19:239–284

His W (1904) Die Entwicklung des menschlichen Gehirns während der ersten Monate. Hirzel, Leipzig

Holl M (1908) Die Insel des Menschen und Affenhirns in ihren Beziehung zum Schlafenlappen. Sitz Berl Akad Wissensch Wien Math Naturw Kl 117(3):365–410

Huang CC (1991) Sonographic cerebral sulcal development in premature newborns. Brain Dev 13:27

Huxley TH (1861) On the brain of Ateles paniscus. Proc Zool Soc Lond pp 247–260

Jaeger R (1914) Inhaltsberechnungen der Rinden und Marksubstanz des Grosshirns durch planimetrishce Messungen. Arch Psychiatr Nervenkrankh 54:261–272

Jefferson G (1913) The morphology of the sulcus interparietalis. J Anat Physiol 47:365–380

Jensen J (1870) Die Furchen und Windungen der menschlichen Grosshirnhemispharen. Allg Z Psychiatr 27:473–515

Jensen J (1875) Untersuchungen uber die Beziehungen zwischen Grosshirn und Geistesstörung an sechs Gehirnen geisteskranker Individuen. Arch Psychiatr Nervenkrankh. 5:587–757

Kanai T (1938) Über die Furchen und Windungen der Orbitalfläche des Stirnhirns bei Japanern. Okajimas Fol Anat Jpn 18:229–306

Karplus JP (1905) Über Familienähnlichkeiten an den Grosshirnfurchen des Menschen. Arb Neurol Inst Wien Univ 12:1–58

Karplus JP (1921) Zur Kenntnis der Variabilität und Vererbung am Zentralnervensystem des Menschen und einiger Sauger, 2nd edn. Deuticke, Leipzig

Kaufman E (1887) Über Mängel des Balkens im menschlichen Gehirn. Arch Psychiatr Nervenkrankh 18:769

Klingler J (1935) Erleichterung der makroskopischen Präparation des Gehirns durch den Gefrierprozess. Schw Arch Neurol Psychiatr 36:247–256

Kohlbrugge JHF (1906) Die Grosshirrfurchen der Javanen. Verh K Akad Wetens, Sect II, Amsterdam Deel 12(4):195 (9 plates)

Kraus WM, Davison C, Weil A (1928) The measurement of cerebral and cerebellar surfaces. Arch Neurol Psychiatr 19:454–477

Kükenthal W, Ziehen T (1895) Untersuchungen über die Grosshirnfurchen der Primaten. Jen Z Naturwiss 29:1–122

Landau E (1910) Über die Orbitalfurchen bei den Esten. Z Morphol Anthropol 12:341–352

Landau E (1911) Über die Grosshirnfurchen am basalen Teile des temporooccipitalen Feldes bei den Esten. Z Morphol Anthropol 13:423–438

Landau E (1914) Über die Furchen an der Lateralfläche des Grosshirns bei den Esten. Z Morphol Anthropol 16:239–279

Landau E (1919) The comparative anatomy of the nucleus amygdalae, the claustrum and the insular cortex. J Anat 53:351–360

Larroche J-C, Feess-Higgins A (1987) Development of the human foetal brain. An anatomical atlas. Editions INSERM. Masson, Paris

Lazorthes G, Gouazé A, Salamon G (1976) Vascularisation et circulation cérébrales. Masson, Paris

Leboucq G (1929) Le rapport entre le poids et la surface de l'hemisphere cerebral chez l'homme et les singes. Mem Acad R Belge Cl Sc 10(9):57

Leuret F, Gratiolet P (1839) Anatomie comparée du système nerveux, considérée dans ses rapports avec l'intelligence, vol 1 and 2. Baillière, Paris. Atlas. Masson, Paris

Lorente de No R (1933) Studies on the structure of the cerebral cortex. I. The area endorhinalis. J Psychol Neurol 45:381–438

Ludwig E, Klingler J (1956) Atlas cerebri humani. Karger, Basel

Marchand F (1895) Die Morphologie des Stirnlappens und der Insel der Anthropomorphen. Arb Pathol Inst Marb 2:1–108

McLardy T (1950) Uraemic and trophic deaths following leucotomy: neuro-anatomical findings. J Neurol Neurosurg Psychiatry 13:106–114

Meynert T (1867/1868) Der Bau der Grosshirnrinde und seine örtlichen Verschiedenheiten, nebst einem pathologisch-anatomischen Corollarium. Vierteljahrsch Psychiatr 1:77–93, 125–217, 381–403; 2:88–113

Meynert T (1877) Neue Studien über die Associationsbundel des Hirnmantels. Sitz Berl K Akad Wiss Wien Kl 101(3):361–380

Naidich P, Valavanis G, Kubik S (1995) Anatomic relationships along the low-middle convexity. I. Normal specimens and magnetic resonance imaging. Neurosurgery 36(3):517–531

Nieuwenhuys R, Voogd J, Van Huijzen C (1988) The human central nervous system. A synopsis and atlas, 3rd edn. Springer, Berlin Heidelberg New York

Ono N, Kubik S, Abernathy DG (1990) Atlas of the cerebral sulci. Thieme, Stuttgart

Onufrowicz W (1887) Das balkenlose Mikrocephalengehirn Hofmann. Arch Psychiatr Nervenkrankh 18:305–328

Paturet G (1964) Traité d'anatomie humaine, vol 4: système nerveux. Masson, Paris

Perlmutter D, Rhoton AL Jr (1976) Microsurgical anatomy of the anterior cerebral-anterior communicating-recurrent artery complex. J Neurosurg 45(3):259–272

Pfeifer RA (1936) Pathologie der Hörstrahlung und der corticale Hörsphäre. In: Foerster O (ed) Handbuch der Neurologie, vol 6. Springer, Berlin, pp 533–626

Ramon y Cajal S (1911) Histologie du système nerveux de l'homme et des vertébrés, vol II. (translated by L. Azoulay) Maloine, Paris

Retzius G (1896) Das Menschenhirn. Studien in der makroskopischen Morphologie, vol 1. Norstedt, Stockholm

Rose M (1926) Über das histogenetische Prinzip der Einteilung der Grosshirnrinde. J Psychol Neurol 32:97–158

Rössle R (1937) Zur Frage der Ähnlichkeit des Windungsbildes an Gehirnen von Blutsverwandten, besonders von Zwillingen. Sitz Ber Preuss Akad Wissensch pp 146–68

Salamon G (1971) Atlas of the arteries of the human brain. Sandoz, Paris

Salamon G, Raynaud C, Regis J et al (1990) Magnetic resonance imaging of the pediatric brain. An anatomical atlas. Raven, New York

Sano F (1916) The convolutional pattern of the brains of identical twins. Philos Trans R Soc Lond B 208:37–61

Schlesinger B (1953) The insulo-opercular arteries of the brain, with special reference to the angiography of striothalamic tumors. Am J Roentgenol 70:555–563

Schnopfhagen F (1890) Die Entstehung der Windungen des Grosshirns. J Psychiatr 9:197–318

Shellshear JL (1926) The occipital lobe in the brain of the Chinese with special reference to the sulcus lunatus. J Anat 61:1–13

Slome I (1932) The bushman brain. J Anat 67:47–58

Symington J, Crymble PT (1913) The central fissure of the cerebrum. J Anat 47:321–39

Szikla G, Bouvier G, Hori T, Petrov V (1977) Angiography of the human brain cortex: atlas of vascular patterns and stereotactic cortical localization. Springer, Berlin Heidelberg New York

Talairach J, Szikla G, Tournoux P, Prossalentis A, Bordas-Ferrer M, Covello L, Iacob M, Mempel E (1967) Atlas d'anatomie stéréotaxique du télencéphale. Masson, Paris

Tamraz J (1983) Atlas d'anatomie céphalique dans le plan neuro-oculaire (PNO). MD Thesis, Schering, Paris (1986)

Tamraz J (1991) Morphometrie de l'encephale par resonance magnetique: application à la pathologie chromosomique humaine, à l'anatomie comparée et à la teratologie. These Doct Sci Paris V, Paris

Tamraz J, Rethoré M-O, Iba-Zizen M-T, Lejeune J, Cabanis EA (1987) Contribution of magnetic resonance imaging to the knowledge of CNS malformations related to chromosomal aberrations. Hum Genet 76:265–273

Tamraz J, Saban R, Reperant J, Cabanis EA (1990) Définition d'un plan de référence céphalique en imagerie par résonance magnétique: le plan chiasmato-commissural. CR Acad Sci Paris 311(III):115–121

Tamraz J, Saban R, Reperant J, Cabanis EA (1991) A new cephalic reference plane for use with magnetic resonance imaging: the chiasmato-commissural plane. Surg Radiol Anat 13:197–201

Tamraz J, Rethoré M-O, Lejeune J, Outin C, Goepel R, Stievenart JL, Iba-Zizen M-T, Cabanis EA (1993) Morphométrie encéphalique en IRM dans la maladie du cri du chat. A propos de sept patients, avec revue de la littérature. Ann Génét 2:75–87

Testut L, Latarjet A (1948) Traité d'anatomie humaine. Tome 2: système nerveux central, 9th edn. Doin, Paris

Turner OA (1948) Growth and development of the cerebral cortical pattern in man. Arch Neurol Psychiatr 59:1–12

Turner OA (1950) Some data concerning the growth and development of the cerebral cortex in man II. Postnatal Psychiatr (Chic) 64:378–385

Turner W (1891) The convolutions of the brain. J Anat Physiol 25:105–153

van Bork-Feltkamp AJ (1930) Utkomsten van een onderzoek van een 60-tal hersenen van chineezen. Versluis Uitgevers-Maatschappij, Amsterdam

Vint FW (1934) The brain of the Kenya native. J Anat 68:216–223

Vlahovitch B, Gros C, Fernandez-Serrats A, Adib-Yazdi IS, Billet M (1964) Repérage du sillon insulaire supérieur dans l'angiographie carotidienne de profil. Neurochirurgie 10:91–99

Vlahovitch B, Gros C, Fernandez-Serrats A (1965) Les repères de l'insula dans la partique de l'angiographie carotidienne. Expansion Scientifique Française, Paris

Vlahovitch B, Frerebeau P, Kuhner A, Billet M, Gros C (1970) Etude des lignes supra et infra-insulaires dans l'angiographie carotidienne normale et pathologique. Neurochirurgie 16:127–183

Vogt C, Vogt O (1919) Allgemeinere Ergbnisse unserer Hirnforschung. J Psychol Neurol (Lpz) 25:279–461

von Bonin G, Bailey P (1947) The neocortex of macaca mulatta. University of Illinois Press,Urbana, Ill (Illinois Monographs in the Medical Sciences, vol V, no 4)

von Economo C (1927) L'architecture cellulaire normale de l'ecorce cerebrale. Masson, Paris

von Economo C (1929) The cytoarchitectonics of the human cerebral cortex. Oxford University Press, London

von Economo C, Koskinas GN (1925) Die Cytoarchitektonik der Hirnrinde des erwachsenen Menschen. Textband und Atlas. Springer, Vienna New York

Wagner H (1864) Massbestimmungen der Oberfläche des Gehrins. Wigand, Cassel

Weinberg R (1905) Die Gehirnform der Polen. Ztschr Morphol Anthropol 8:123–214; 279–424

Wernicke C (1876) Das Urwindungsstystem des menschlichen Gehirns. Arch Psychiatr Nervenkr 6:298–326

Wernicke C (1881–83) Lehrbuch der Gehirnkrankheiten, vol 1–3. Fischer, Kassel

Wilder BC (1886) The paroccipital. A newly recognized fissural integer. J Nerv Ment Dis 8:301–315

Willis T (1664) Cerebri anatome, cui accessit nervorum descriptio et usus. Martyn and Allestry, London

Zenker W (1985) Benninghoff Makroskopische und mikroskopische Anatomie des Menschen. Nervensystem. Urban and Schwarzenberg, Munich

Zernov D (1877) The individual types of the brain sinuosity. University of Moscow, Moscow

Zuckerkandl E (1906) Zur Anatomie der Fissura calcarina. Arb Neurol Inst Wien Univ 13:25-61

4 Central Region and Motor Cortex

The excitability of the sensorimotor cortex was described in 1870 by two groups working independently. Hughling Jackson (1870) hypothesized that the cerebral cortex is excitable particularly in the motor area, based on the clinical phenomenology of observed seizures. Fritsch and Hitzig (1870) based their observations on experimental grounds. In 1876, Ferrier performed regional ablations of the motor cortex and described the deficits produced (Ferrier 1876a,b). Dusser de Barenne, in 1924, described the sensory cortex.

Numerous authors subsequently added to these observations. Most illustrious of these authors are Foerster (1936) and Wilder Penfield and his colleagues (1950, 1954), who produced detailed maps of the sensorimotor cortex and described the supplementary motor area, the second sensory area and the localization of speech.

II Embryology of the Sensorimotor Cortex

Understanding of the sulcal development is the key to precise localization of the sensorimotor cortex. The sensory motor cortex is usually divided into the primary sensorimotor area, a premotor area and a supplementary motor area (Fig. 4.1A–D).

The central sulcus makes its appearance at 26 weeks of gestation, almost at the same time as the cingulate sulcus, and the superior temporal sulcus. It is preceded by the calcarine and the parieto-occipital sulci. The temporalization process is nearly completed by then. The central sulcus assumes an oblique backward orientation and, at this stage, it is well developed inferiorly. A sulcus located in the midfrontal convexity is seen, which has been labeled by some authors (Larroche 1987; Feess-Higgins and Larroche 1987) as the precentral sulcus. Contrary to its development in other primates, the human central sulcus does not appear to arise from two anlages which unite to form a single sulcus. This explains the rare interruption of the central sulcus which occurs in only 1% of human brains studied (Eberstaller 1890; Waterston 1907; Ono et al. 1990).

By the 28th week of gestation, the central sulcus has covered the entire convexity, and it is still a straight line, which has notched the superior hemispheric border. The postcentral sulcus has made its appearance as the ascending portion of the intraparietal sulcus.

The development of the precentral sulcus is more complex and appears to arise from the posterior extension of the superior and inferior frontal sulci. These sulci branch posteriorly to form the inferior precentral and the superior precentral sulci. These two sulci do not unit but leave a gap in the mid portion of the convexity making the middle frontal gyrus readily accessible with the rolandic cortex.

As previously mentioned in Chap. 3, the inferior frontal sulcus is a deep sulcus that extends towards the insula. Similarly, the inferior precentral sulcus is a continuous sulcus extending deep into the frontal opercular area. The superior precentral sulcus has a variable depth and extent. It rarely reaches the superior hemispheric border and in this region the supplementary motor area blends into the rolandic cortex.

With further brain growth, the central sulcus deepens and becomes convoluted, assuming a near mature appearance at 36–37 weeks of gestation.

III Morphology and Imaging

A The Central Sulcus

The central sulcus is a deep sulcus extending throughout the convexity. It is characterized by two knees or bends: a superior and an inferior bend (Figs. 4.2–4.6). These are convex anteriorly with an intervening concave bend, according to Symington and Crymble (1913). These bends are likely due to

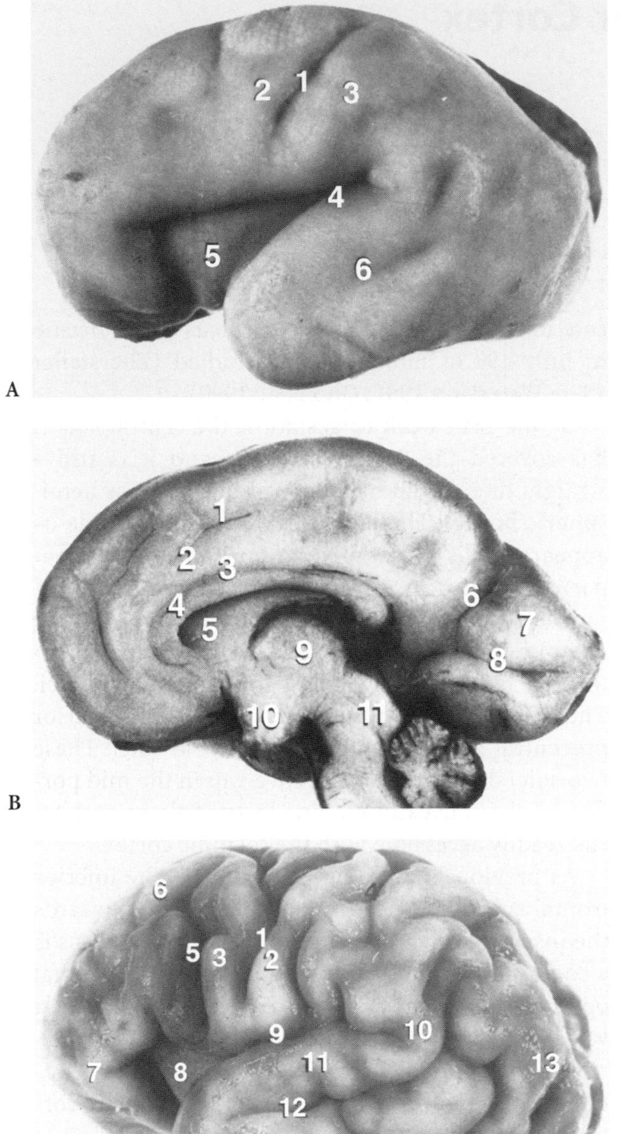

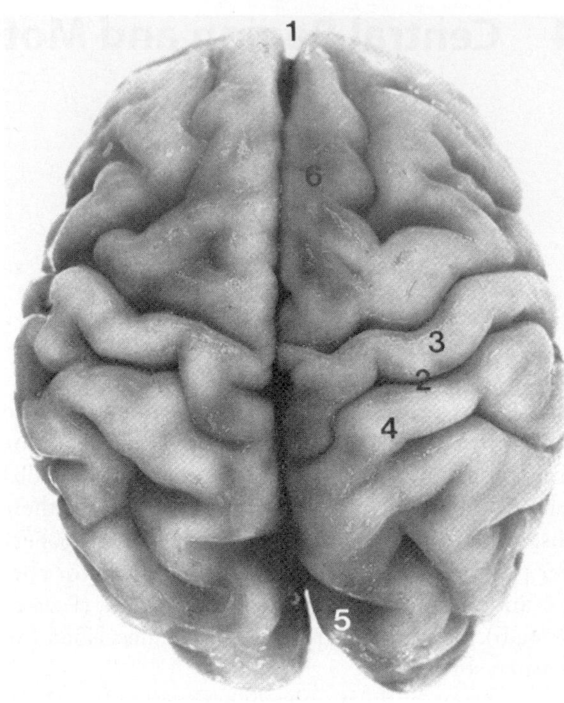

Fig. 4.1A–D. Developmental anatomy of the sensorimotor region. **A** Lateral view of the cerebral hemisphere at 25–26 weeks: *1*, central sulcus; *2*, precentral area; *3*, postcentral area; *4*, lateral fissure; *5*, insula; *6*, superior temporal sulcus. **B** Midsagittal view of the cerebral hemisphere at 25–26 weeks: *1*, cingulate sulcus; *2*, cingulate gyrus; *3*, callosal sulcus; *4*, corpus callosum; *5*, cavum septi pellucidi; *6*, parieto-occipital sulcus; *7*, cuneus; *8*, calcarine sulcus; *9*, thalamus; *10*, hypothalamus; *11*, tectal plate. **C** Lateral view of the cerebral hemisphere at 32–33 weeks: *1*, central sulcus; *2*, postcentral gyrus; *3*, precentral gyrus; *4*, postcentral sulcus; *5*, precentral sulcus; *6*, superior frontal gyrus; *7*, inferior frontal gyrus; *8*, insula; *9*, lateral fissure; *10*, supramarginal gyrus; *11*, superior temporal gyrus; *12*, parallel sulcus; *13*, occipital lobe. **D** Superior view of the cerebral hemispheres at 32–33 weeks: *1*, interhemispheric fissure; *2*, central fissure; *3*, precentral gyrus; *4*, postcentral gyrus; *5*, parieto-occipital sulcus; *6*, superior frontal gyrus (Modified from Larroche 1987)

one or two buttresses occurring in the anterior wall. Smaller spurs cutting into the adjacent gyri are noted. In addition, two submerged or annectant gyri are noted, one at the superior and one at the inferior end, of the central sulcus. The straight length of the sulcus is 9.1 cm ±0.6 cm, and when the central sulcus is measured along its bends, it measures 10.2 cm ±0.7 cm (Bailey and von Bonin 1951). At its inferior end, the central sulcus ends above the sylvian fissure in the majority of cases, leaving a frontoparietal operculum or "pli de passage fronto-rolandique". At the level of the sylvian fissure, a small sulcus originating from the latter is seen, the sulcus subcentralis anterior. At this time, the small sulcus unites with the lower end of the central sulcus or, frequently, with the precentral sulcus (Eberstaller 1890; Symington and Crymble 1913). The superior end of the sulcus bends on the superior aspect of the hemisphere, giving the appearance of a comma or, in French, the "crochet rolandique" (Broca 1878; Testut and Latarjet 1948).

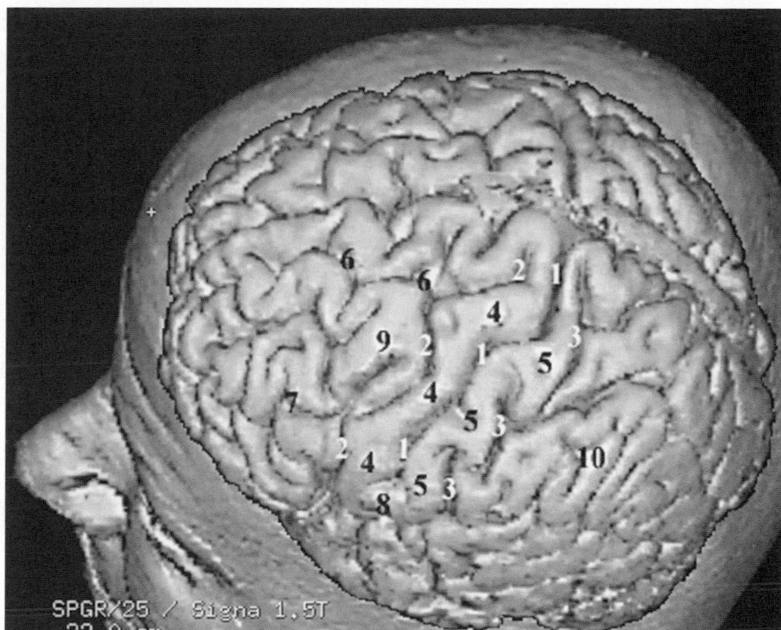

Fig. 4.2. The central sulcus. *1*, Central sulcus; *2*, precentral sulci; *3*, postcentral sulci; *4*, precentral gyrus; *5*, postcentral gyrus; *6*, superior frontal sulcus; *7*, inferior frontal sulcus; *8*, central operculum; *9*, middle frontal sulcus; *10*, inferior parietal lobule

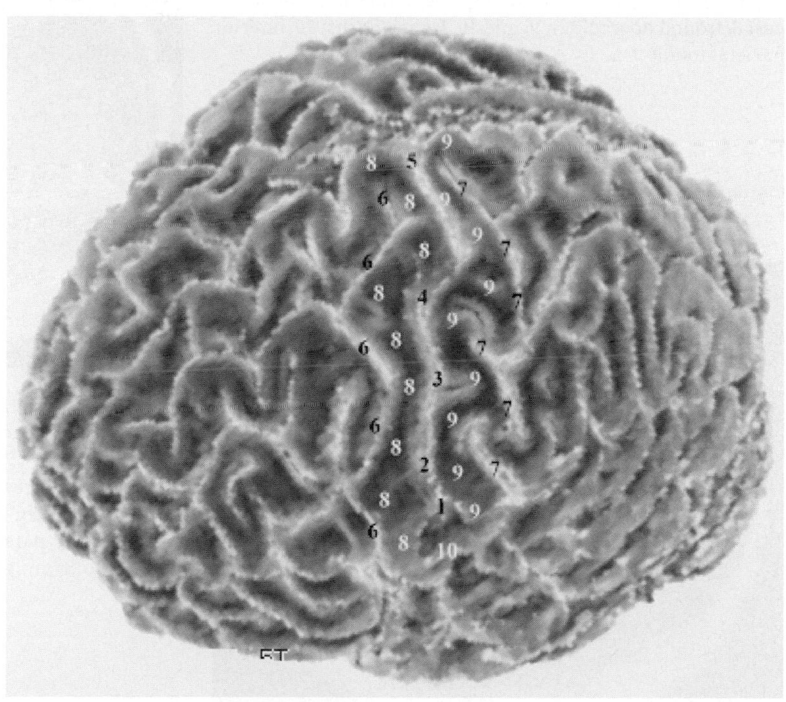

Fig. 4.3. The central sulcus and sensorimotor cortex. *1*, Inferior end of central sulcus; *2*, inferior genu of central sulcus; *3*, middle genu of central sulcus; *4*, superior genu of central sulcus; *5*, superior end of central sulcus; *6*, precentral sulcus; *7*, postcentral sulcus; *8*, precentral gyrus; *9*, postcentral gyrus; *10*, central operculum ("pli de passage" frontoparietal)

Two atypical patterns are noted: an additional buttress or genu is found in the middle of the central sulcus and another even rarer variation is seen superiorly close to the interhemispheric fissure.

The depth of the central sulcus is variable along its extent. It is deepest at the level of the hand-arm representation, corresponding roughly to its mid-portion. At the level of the face, corresponding to its first 3 cm, it is slightly less deep, averaging 15 mm. At the level of the trunk, the recurrence of the annectant gyrus reduces its depth to 12 mm. In the interhemispheric leg portion it reaches, at most, 13 mm (Figs. 4.5, 4.6).

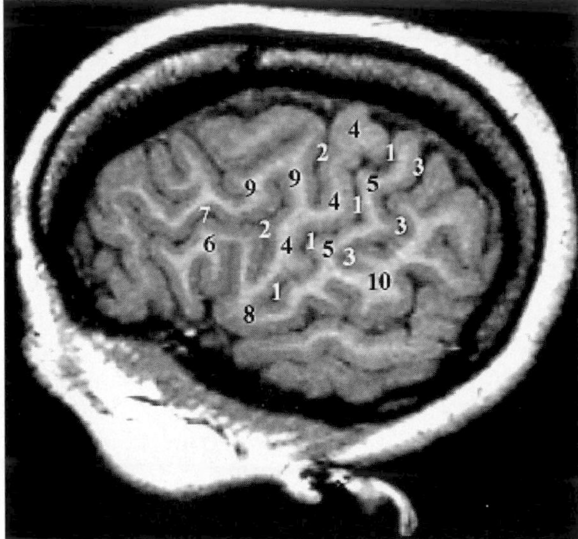

Fig. 4.4. MR oblique reformatted cut (2 mm) parallel to the forniceal reference plane (see Sect. 10.III), displaying the central area and the frontal region. *1*, Central sulcus; *2*, precentral sulcus; *3*, postcentral sulcus; *4*, precentral gyrus; *5*, postcentral gyrus; *6*, inferior frontal gyrus; *7*, inferior frontal sulcus; *8*, frontal operculum; *9*, middle frontal gyrus; *10*, inferior parietal lobule

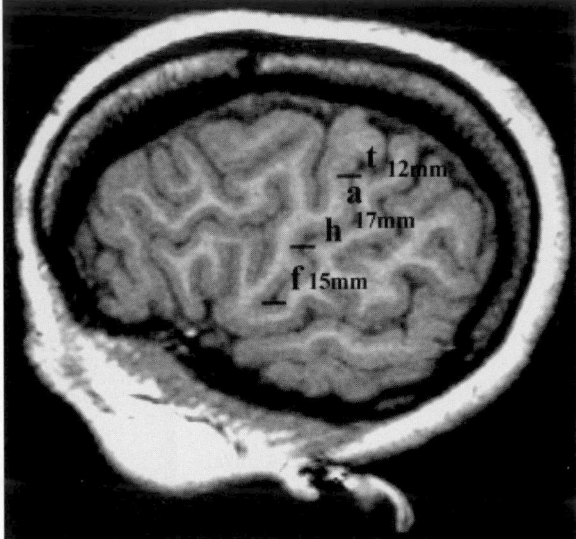

A

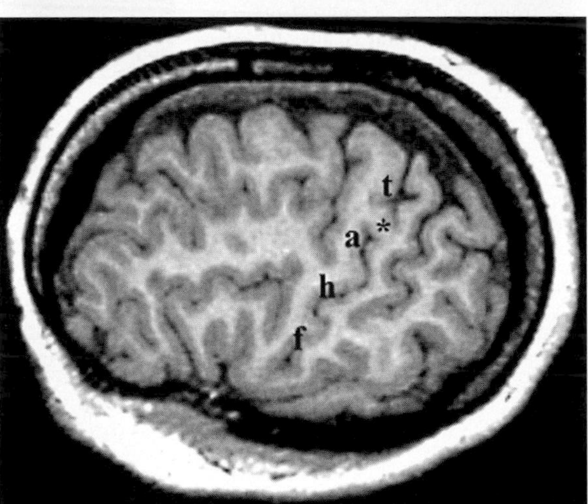

B

Fig. 4.6A,B. Variations of the depth of the central sulcus. Regional variations on the lateral aspect of the cerebral hemisphere. Face (*f*): 15 mm; hand and arm: 17 mm; trunk: 12 mm. Note the presence of an annectant gyrus (marked by an *asterisk*) in B. The leg region is not shown as it is on the mesial aspect, in the paracentral lobule (depth about 13 mm). (According to Symington and Crymble 1913)

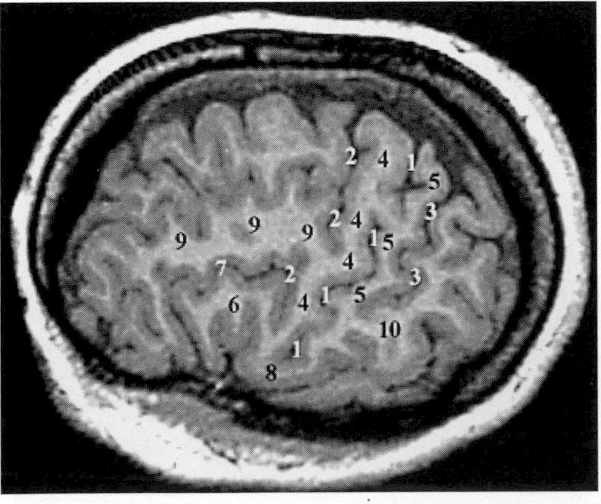

Fig. 4.5. MR oblique reformatted cut (2 mm) parallel to the forniceal reference plane (see Sect. 10.III), displaying the central area and the frontal, mainly inferior, region. *1*, Central sulcus; *2*, precentral sulcus; *3*, postcentral sulcus; *4*, precentral gyrus; *5*, postcentral gyrus; *6*, inferior frontal gyrus; *7*, inferior frontal sulcus; *8*, frontal operculum; *9*, middle frontal gyrus; *10*, inferior parietal lobule

B The Precentral Sulcus

As discussed previously, the precentral sulcus derives from the posterior extension of the superior frontal sulci. It is most commonly composed of two segments, the superior and inferior precentral sulci (Figs. 4.4, 4.5). These two segments are interrupted by the middle frontal convolution, the latter extending into the rolandic motor cortex. The significance of this constant interruption is unknown.

The inferior precentral sulcus terminates inferiorly at the level of the sylvian fissure. There is usually a direct termination or, at times, through an intercalated sulcus the anterior subcentral sulcus branching up from the sylvian fissure (Ebeling et al. 1989) (Figs. 4.4, 4.5).

The superior precentral sulcus has a complex relationship with the rolandic motor cortex. It rarely reaches the superior hemispheric border where it can be replaced by one or two sulci: (1) a horizontal sulcus running parallel to the interhemispheric fissure, above the first frontal sulcus, which is the marginal precentral sulcus (Cunningham and Horsley 1892), and is easily distinguishable from the first frontal sulcus, given its shallower depth; and (2) the medial precentral sulcus, a vertical sulcus situated most frequently anterior to the precentral sulcus and cutting the interhemispheric border (Eberstaller 1890). Therefore, in this region there is no clear sulcal demarcation between the supplementary motor area and the primary motor cortex (Figs. 4.7, 4.8).

C The Postcentral Sulcus

The postcentral sulcus is the ascending branch of the intraparietal sulcus, showing wide variations (Jefferson 1912). This sulcus has been discussed in detail in Chap. 3. It is frequently a deeper sulcus than the central. In its horizontal segment it is one of the deepest sulci of the lateral aspect of the hemisphere reaching 20 cm in depth.

D Topographical and Functional Anatomy and Imaging

1 The Primary Sensorimotor Cortex or Central Cortex

The primary motor and sensory cortices (PMSC) include the precentral and postcentral gyri. The primary motor cortex extends from the bottom of the precentral sulcus to the bottom of the central sulcus, and the primary sensory area extends from the bottom of the central sulcus to the bottom of the postcentral sulcus (Figs. 4.2–4.5).

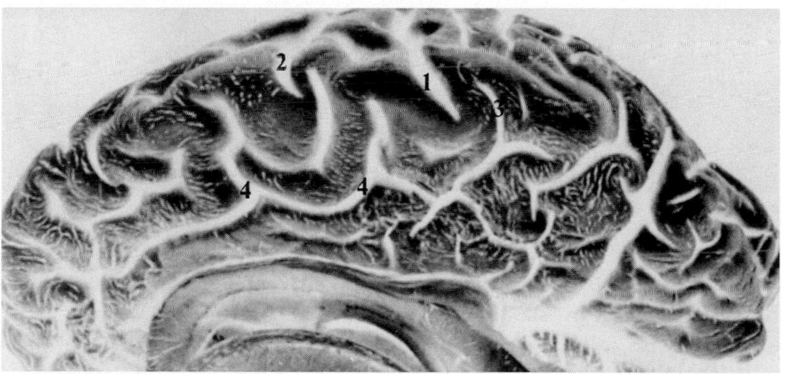

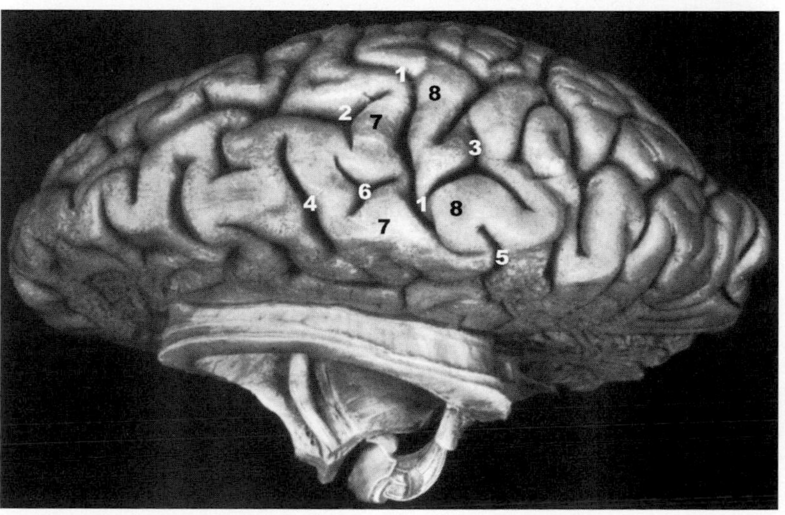

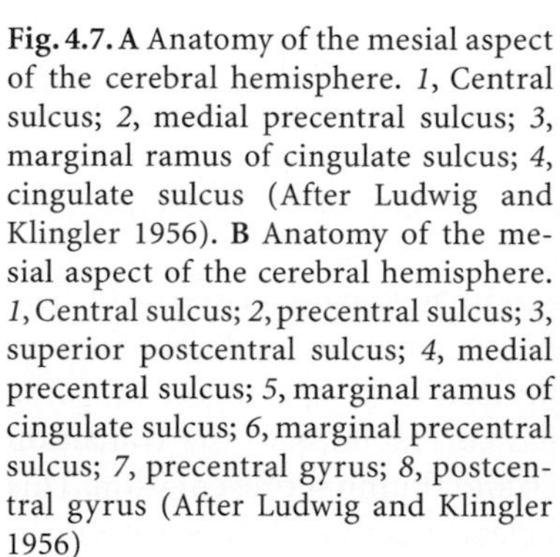

Fig. 4.7. A Anatomy of the mesial aspect of the cerebral hemisphere. *1*, Central sulcus; *2*, medial precentral sulcus; *3*, marginal ramus of cingulate sulcus; *4*, cingulate sulcus (After Ludwig and Klingler 1956). **B** Anatomy of the mesial aspect of the cerebral hemisphere. *1*, Central sulcus; *2*, precentral sulcus; *3*, superior postcentral sulcus; *4*, medial precentral sulcus; *5*, marginal ramus of cingulate sulcus; *6*, marginal precentral sulcus; *7*, precentral gyrus; *8*, postcentral gyrus (After Ludwig and Klingler 1956)

A 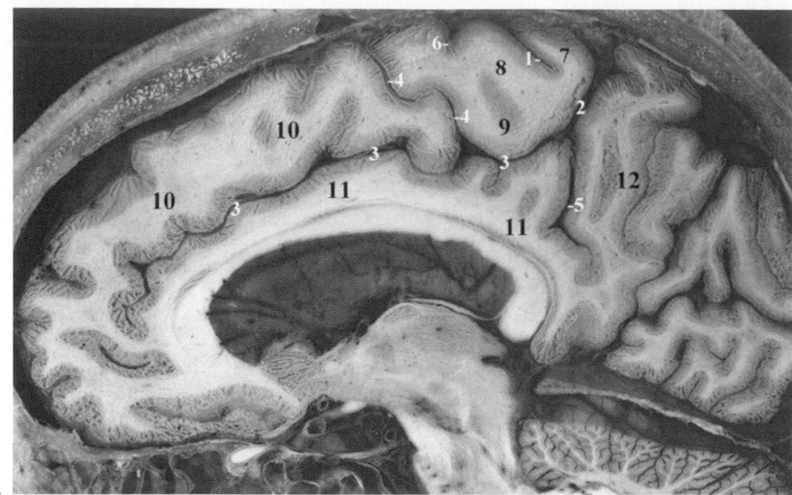

B 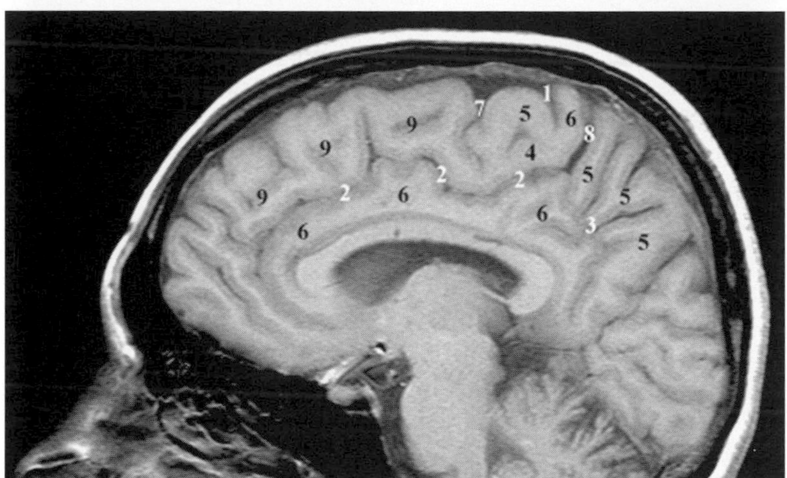

Fig. 4.8. A Parasagittal anatomical cut of the paracentral lobule. *1*, Central sulcus, mesial extension; *2*, marginal ramus of cingulate sulcus; *3*, cingulate sulcus; *4*, paracentral sulcus; *5*, subparietal sulcus; *6*, medial precentral sulcus; *7*, postcentral gyrus; *8*, precentral gyrus; *9*, paracentral lobule; *10*, medial frontal gyrus; *11*, cingulate gyrus; *12*, precuneus. **B** Superior end of central sulcus on a parasagittal MR cut. *1*, Central sulcus; superior end; *2*, cingulate sulcus; *3*, subparietal sulcus; *4*, paracentral lobule; *5*, precuneus; *6*, cingulate gyrus; *7*, medial precentral sulcus; *8*, marginal ramus of cingulate sulcus; *9*, medial frontal gyrus

The extent of the PMSC was defined mostly on the basis of stimulation studies performed under local anesthesia by several workers in the field. Penfield defines the precentral gyrus as "primarily a motor organ that is indispensable for certain forms of voluntary motor action" and the postcentral gyrus as "a sensory organ that is indispensable for the appreciation of discriminative tactile and proprioceptive sensation". This same author concludes that "taken together these two organs form a sensorimotor functional unit". This definition was later extended to the concept of a central lobe by Rasmussen (1969).

a The Primary Motor Cortex or Precentral Gyrus

The cytoarchitecture of the precentral gyrus is not homogeneous. It includes agranular cortex, represented in areas 4 and 6 of Brodmann, area 4 being characterized by the presence of giant pyramidal or Betz cells in layer V (Fig. 4.9A–C). The cells possess the longest and largest axons in the body. In addition, the cortex in this region is particularly thick. This can be useful for the localization of the motor cortex.

Anatomically, the precentral gyrus can be divided into four segments, defined by its three bends in addition to the paracentral lobule:

1 The inferior segment is convex anteriorly, and it is close to the sylvian fissure which makes its inferior boundary (Figs. 4.4, 4.5). It commonly communicates with the postcentral gyrus, forming the central operculum. Medially it reaches the insula. Frequently, the inferior segment communicates with the pars opercularis of the frontal lobe (Figs. 4.10,4.11).
2 The middle segment is convex posteriorly. The junction between the inferior and middle segments is characterized by a tapering or thinning of the gyri, which corresponds to the transition area between face and thumb representation. This segment has no clearly defined limits anteriorly,

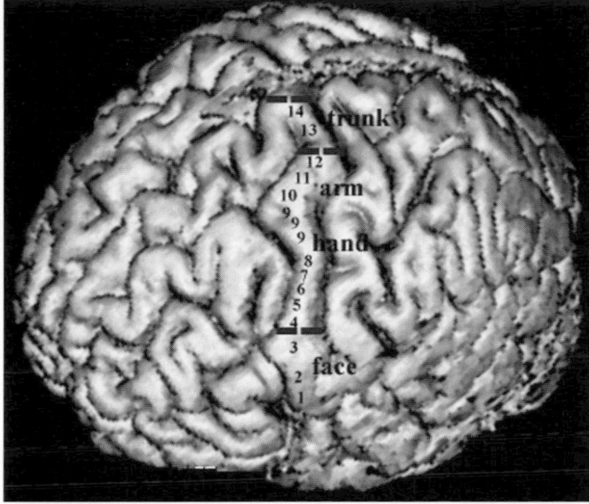

A

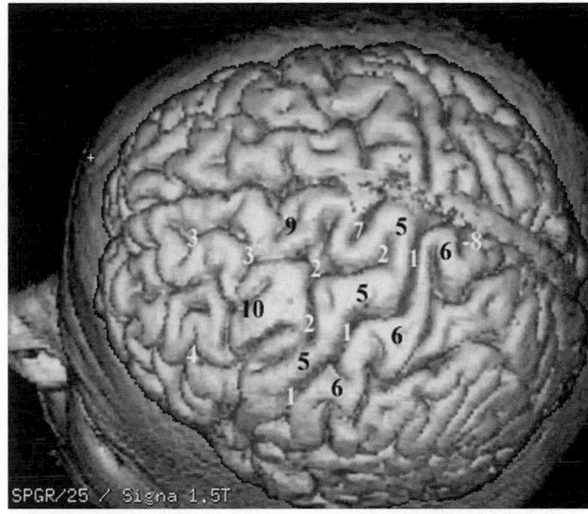

B

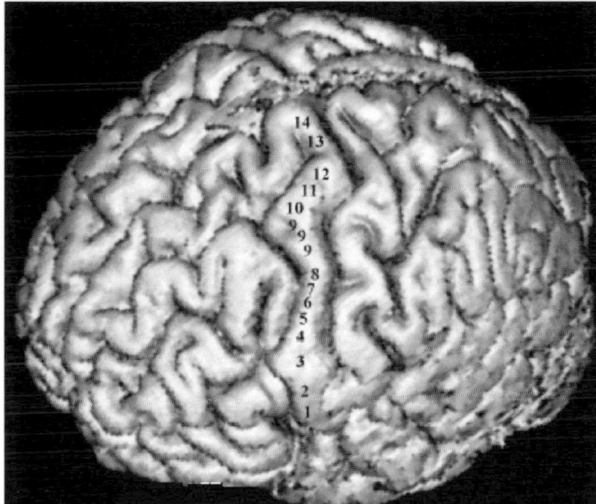

C

Fig. 4.9. A The precentral gyrus and its functional subdivision into four segments. Inferior: functional unit of the face; middle: functional unit of the hand and arm; superior: functional unit of the trunk; and paracentral on the mesial aspect of the hemisphere: functional unit of the leg. *1*, Tongue; *2*, lips; *3*, face; *4*, thumb; *5*, index finger; *6*, middle finger; *7*, ring finger; *8*, little finger; *9*, hand; *10*, wrist; *11*, elbow; *12*, shoulder; *13*, trunk; *14*, proximal leg. **B** Superior end of central sulcus on the lateral 3D MR view of the hemisphere. *1*, Central sulcus; *2*, superior precentral sulcus; *3*, superior frontal sulcus; *4*, inferior frontal sulcus; *5*, precentral gyrus (5' superior end); *6*, postcentral gyrus; *7*, medial precentral sulcus; *8*, marginal ramus; *9*, superior frontal gyrus; *10*, middle frontal gyrus. **C** The precentral gyrus (the homunculus). *1*, Tongue; *2*, lips; *3*, face; *4*, thumb; *5*, index finger; *6*, middle finger; *7*, ring finger; *8*, little finger; *9*, hand; *10*, wrist; *11*, elbow; *12*, shoulder; *13*, trunk; *14*, proximal leg

as it extends into the premotor area, due to the interruption of the precentral sulcus in this region. Posteriorly, it is sharply bound by the central sulcus and medially by the corona radiata, fanning towards the internal capsule. This segment assumes an oblique posterior course. (Figs. 4.4, 4.5, 4.11, 4.12, 4.13).

3 The superior segment is convex anteriorly. In its initial segment it is sharply distinct from the premotor cortex. Towards the interhemispheric fissure, these boundaries become difficult to define given the presence of embryologically variable sulci, which result in a communication of this gyrus with the supplementary motor area (SMA). It is sharply bound posteriorly by the central sulcus, and superiorly by the interhemispheric fissure. Medially this segment is bound by the corona radiata. The direction of the superior segment assumes a less oblique course than that of the middle segment, as the fiber tract arising

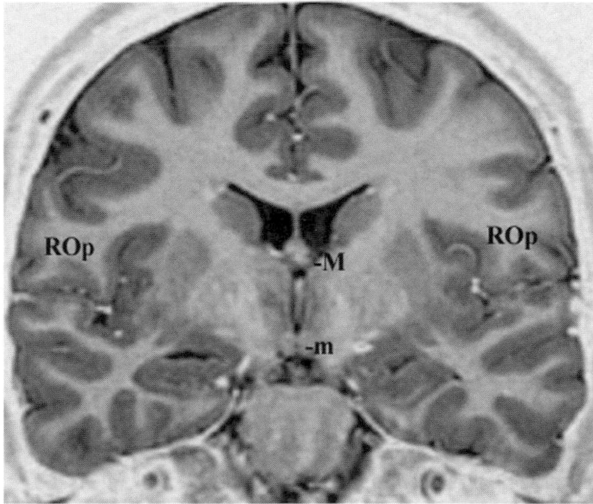

Fig. 4.10. Coronal Monro-mamillary MR cut of the brain, parallel to PC-OB reference plane, and passing through the inferior opercular end of the central region. *ROp*, Rolandic (central) operculum; *M*, interventricular foramen of Monro; *m*, mamillary body

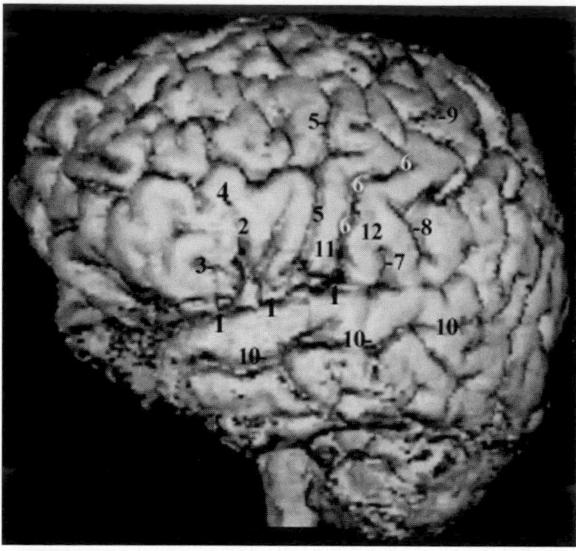

Fig. 4.11. Inferior frontal gyri and inferior end of precentral gyrus. *1*, Lateral fissure; *2*, inferior frontal gyrus; *3*, horizontal ramus of lateral fissure; *4*, vertical ramus of lateral fissure; *5*, inferior precentral sulcus; *6*, central sulcus; *7*, posterior subcentral sulcus; *8*, inferior postcentral sulcus; *9*, superior postcentral sulcus; *10*, superior temporal (parallel) sulcus; *11*, precentral gyrus; *12*, postcentral gyrus

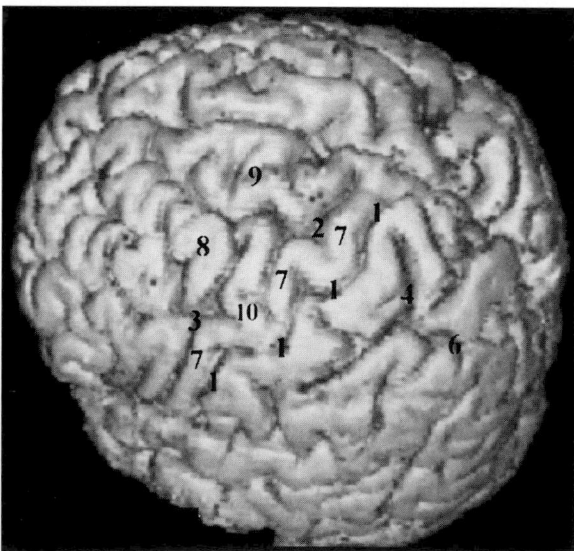

Fig. 4.12. Connection of the middle frontal gyrus with the middle genu of the precentral gyrus. *1*, Central sulcus; *2*, superior precentral sulcus; *3*, inferior precentral sulcus; *4*, superior postcentral sulcus; *5*, inferior postcentral sulcus; *6*, intraparietal sulcus; *7*, precentral gyrus; *8*, middle frontal gyrus; *9*, superior frontal gyrus; *10*, middle frontal gyrus

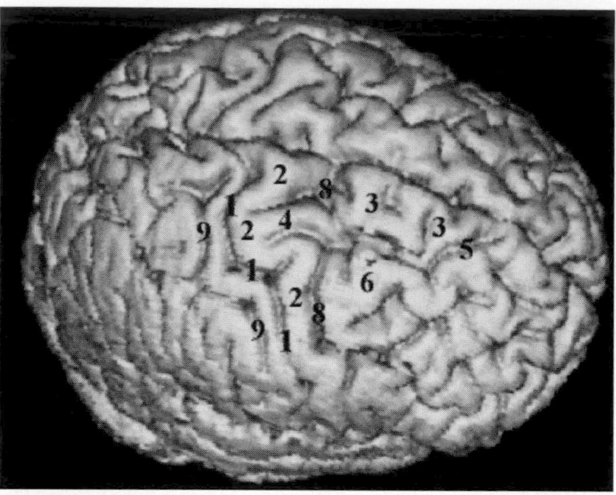

Fig. 4.13. Unusual connection of the superior frontal gyrus with the precentral gyrus. *1*, Central sulcus; *2*, precentral gyrus; *3*, superior frontal gyrus; *4*, extension of F1 into precentral gyrus; *5*, superior frontal sulcus; *6*, middle frontal gyrus; *7*, superior precentral sulcus; *8*, inferior precentral sulcus; *9*, postcentral sulcus

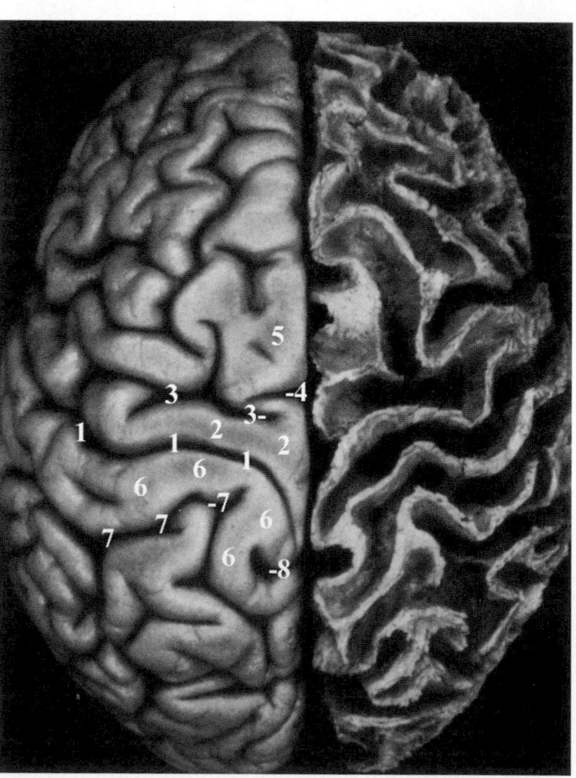

Fig. 4.14. Superior view of the cerebral hemispheres. *1*, Central sulcus; *2*, precentral gyrus; *3*, superior precentral sulcus; *4*, medial precentral sulcus; *5*, superior frontal sulcus; *6*, postcentral gyrus; *7*, superior postcentral sulcus; *8*, marginal ramus of cingulate sulcus (after Ludwig and Klingler 1956)

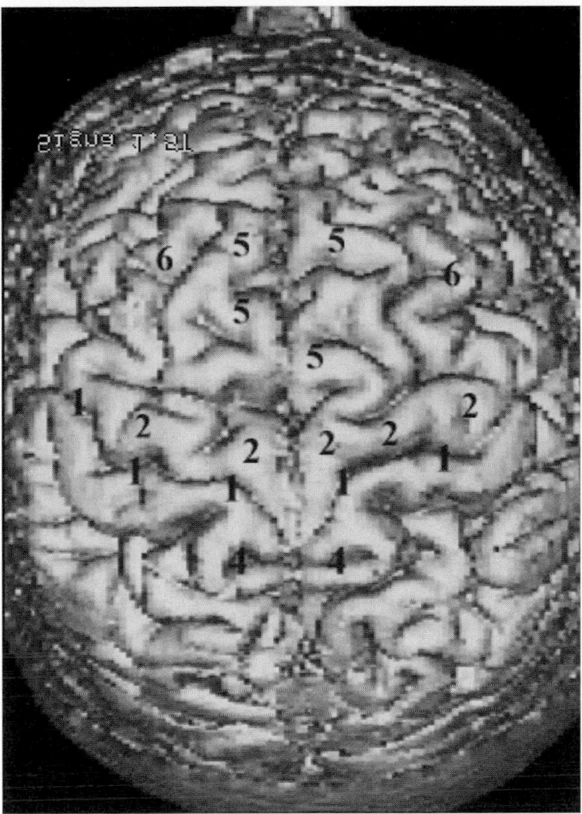

Fig. 4.15. Superior view of the cerebral hemispheres. *1*, Central sulcus; *2*, precentral gyrus; *3*, postcentral gyrus; *4*, marginal ramus of cingulate sulcus; *5*, superior frontal gyrus; *6*, middle frontal gyrus

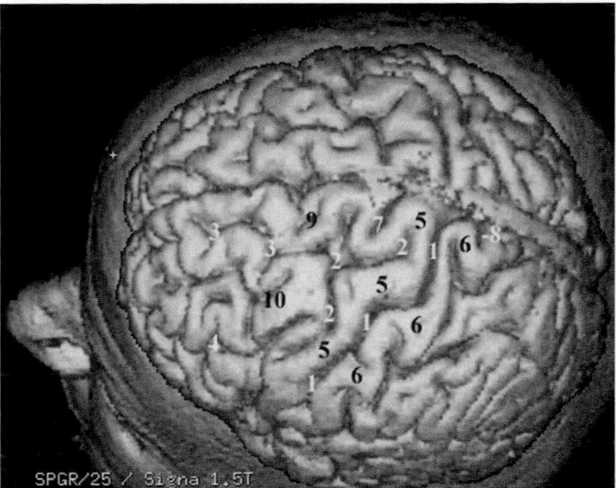

Fig. 4.16. Superior end of precentral gyrus on a lateral 3D MR aspect of the hemisphere. *1*, Central sulcus; *2*, superior precentral sulcus; *3*, superior frontal sulcus; *4*, inferior frontal sulcus; *5*, precentral gyrus (*5'*, superior end); *6*, postcentral gyrus; *7*, medial precentral sulcus; *8*, marginal ramus; *9*, superior frontal gyrus; *10*, middle frontal gyrus

from this segment is deflected by the fibers crossing from the corpus callosum. (Figs. 4.14–4.17).

4 The paracentral segment: the sulcal variations seen in this segment are most likely the result of the simultaneous development of the central sulcus, the superior frontal sulcus and the cingulate sulcus. It occupies the posterior extent of the paracentral lobule. There are no sharp anterior boundaries to this segment. The marginal precentral and mesial precentral sulci, which at times constitute its anterior limit, are shallow. Posteriorly it is bound for a short distance by the central sulcus. Thus, in the paracentral lobule another communication with the primary sensory area exists (Figs. 4.7, 4.8). Inferiorly its supposed limit is the cingulate sulcus as defined cytoarchitecturally in the Brodmann map. However, most stimulation studies do not corroborate this finding, as primary motor and sensory responses are not elicited in the inferior portion of the paracentral lobule.

b The Postcentral Gyrus

The postcentral gyrus can also be divided into four segments (Figs. 4.2, 4.3, 4.5, 4.18). Its configuration closely resembles the precentral gyrus. Inferiorly, in the opercular region, it is wider and thicker than its motor counterpart. The middle and superior segments are thinner and more sharply defined by the postcentral sulcus. Superiorly, since the postcentral sulcus terminates caudal to the marginal ramus of the cingulate sulcus, the primary sensory area of the leg extends beyond the paracentral lobule.

c Motor and Sensory Representation in the Primary Sensorimotor Cortex

Although there is evidence for a functional overlap in the representation of specific body areas (Penfield and Jasper 1954), an orderly sequence of responses is elicited in the primary motor sensory cortex. This is represented in the homunculus of Penfield and Rasmussen (1950). Penfield observed that the responses obtained were the same if the stimulation was elicited in the depth of the central sulcus towards the crown of the gyrus or close to the precentral sulcus. He hypothesized that the motor sensory units were arranged in horizontal strips extending from precentral to postcentral sulci, through the central sulcus. This observation was later confirmed in animal experiments (Murphy et al. 1978). Thus, the sensorimotor cortex can be divided from inferior to superior position into four functional units: (1) the

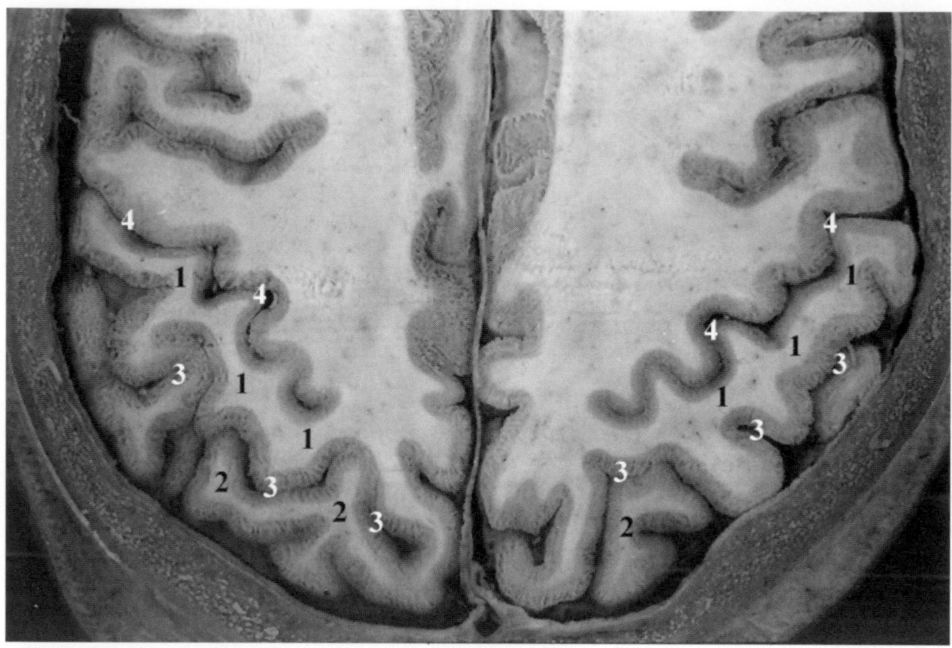

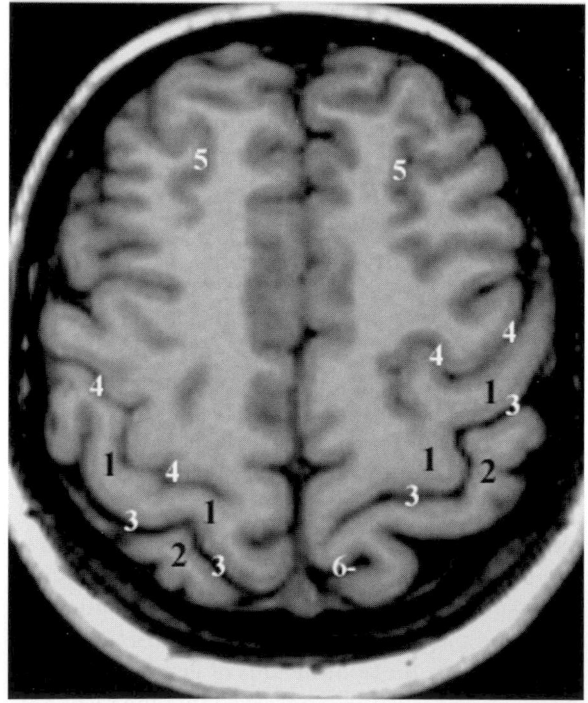

Fig. 4.17. **A** Horizontal supraventricular anatomical cut, showing the posterior topography of the central region as compared to the more oblique bicommissural orientation (see Chap. 2); note the relative difference in cortical thickness of the precentral and postcentral gyri that could help to differentiate the central sulcus from the precentral and postcentral sulci on high contrast resolution MRI. The mean ratio between pre- versus postcentral sulci averages 1.5, corresponding with the cytoarchitectonic data. *1*, Precentral gyrus; *2*, postcentral gyrus; *3*, central sulcus; *4*, precentral sulcus. **B** Horizontal supraventricular MR cut, showing the posterior topography of the central region as compared to the more oblique bicommissural orientation (see Chap. 2). *1*, Precentral gyrus; *2*, Postcentral gyrus; *3*, Central sulcus; *4*, Superior precentral sulcus; *5*, Superior frontal sulcus; *6*, Marginal ramus of cingulate sulcus

face functional unit, extending from the sylvian fissure up approximately 3 cm; (2) the hand-arm functional unit, starting with the thumb motor sensory representation and corresponding to inferior genu, and ending at the shoulder area; (3) the trunk functional unit, bordering on the interhemispheric fissure; (4) the leg-foot functional unit located at the mesial aspect of the hemisphere within the paracentral lobule (Figs. 4.9A,C, 4.19–4.21).

2 The Premotor Cortex

The premotor cortex is a transitional area located between the polar aspect of the frontal lobe and the primary motor cortex. Cytoarchitecturally, it is composed of dysgranular cortex, the polar aspect of the frontal lobe being composed of granular cortex. The boundaries of the premotor cortex in humans are not defined and are variable. The anterior boundary

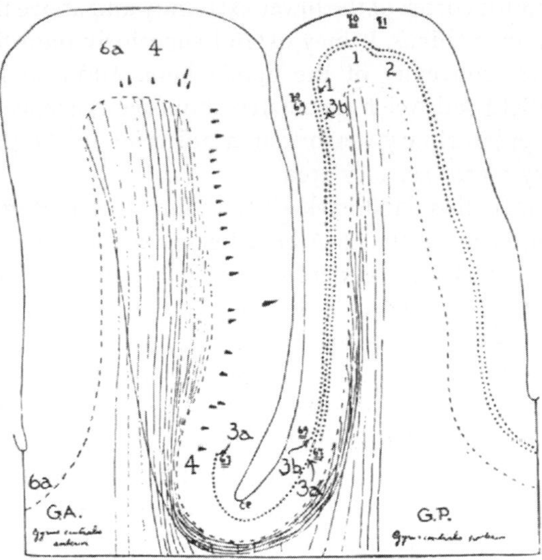

Fig. 4.18. Transverse section through the precentral (*GA*) and the postcentral (*GP*) gyri, showing the first myelinated fibers to appear (*4*) in the area gigantopyramidalis (After Vogt and Vogt 1919; Vogt 1928; from Penfield and Jasper 1954)

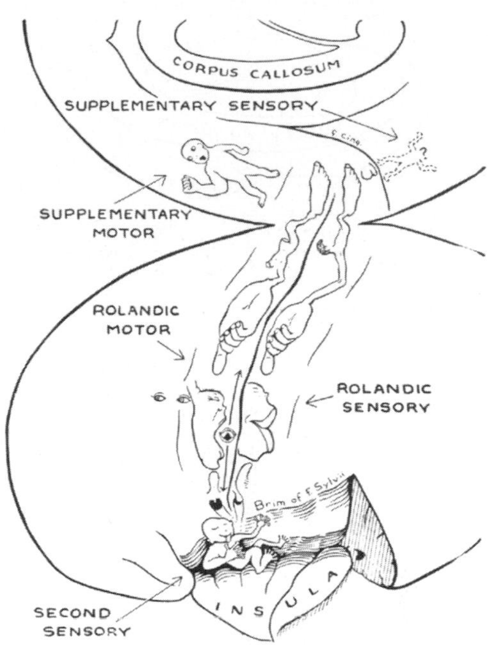

Fig. 4.19. The homunculus of Penfield: figurines drawn on the left hemisphere (Penfield and Jasper 1954)

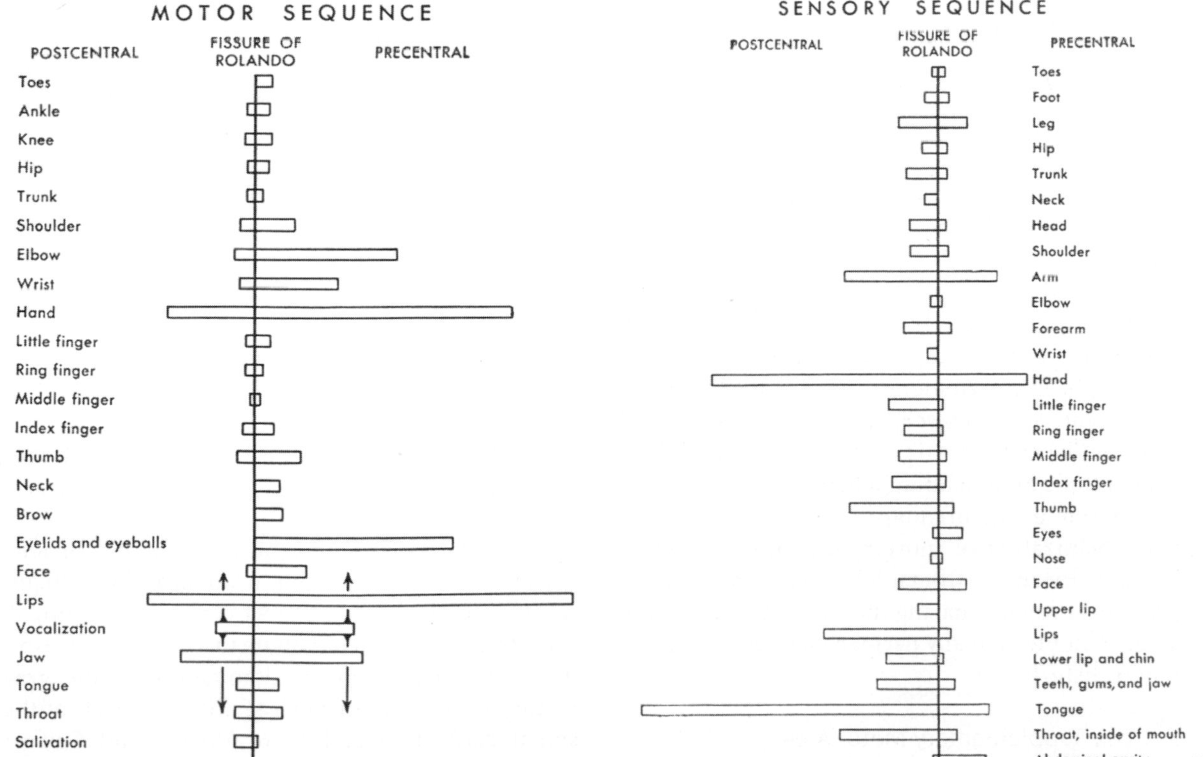

Fig. 4.20. A Motor sequence as drawn on the right hemisphere according to Penfield and Rasmussen (1950, From Penfield and Jasper 1954). **B** Sensory sequence as drawn on the right hemisphere according to Penfield and Rasmussen (1950, From Penfield and Jasper 1954)

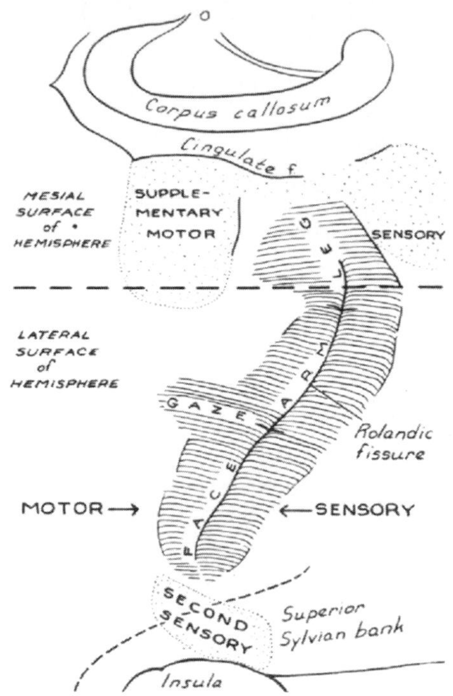

Fig. 4.21. Map of somatic rolandic sensorimotor and supplementary areas (after Penfield and Jasper 1954)

is arbitrarily defined as a line joining the anterior extent of the supplementary motor area with the cortical eye fields. Posteriorly, the premotor cortex extends to the depth of the pre central sulcus.

The role of the premotor cortex is not completely understood. Inputs to the premotor cortex include the cerebellum via the ventrolateral nucleus of the thalamus. Its output is destined to the rostral spinal segments; distal spinal terminations are unlikely. Another major output is the corticofugal projections via the pyramidal tract to the medullary reticular formation. The premotor cortex is activated during movement, requiring sensory clues, particularly visual. Unlike the primary motor cortex, there is no somatotopic organization in man.

The role of the premotor cortex in the planning and organization of movement appears limited in humans. Extensive frontal lobe resections up to the precentral sulcus, sparing the supplementary motor area, do not lead to any permanent or even transient motor disturbance.

3 The Supplementary Motor Area

The SMA, as described by Penfield and Welch (1951), is of variable extent and located in the mesial aspect of the first frontal convolution, anterior to the primary motor cortex of the lower extremity and above the cingulate sulcus. It may extend superiorly onto the lateral convexity of the hemisphere. Additionally, Penfield and Welch speculated about the existence of a supplementary sensory area posterior to the primary motor sensory area.

Since this landmark description, the anatomic boundaries of the SMA have been a subject of considerable debate (Luders 1996). Van Buren and Fedio (1976) described complex sensory responses from stimulation of the cingulate gyrus, concluding that the SMA extends inferiorly into the cingulum. Similarly, Talairach et al. (1973) obtained motor responses from stimulation of the same area. The anterior extent of the SMA was defined by Talairach and Bancaud (1966) as a line perpendicular to the AC-PC line, passing by the anterior-most extent of the genu of the corpus callosum. Because, in these studies, a correlation between the variable gyral anatomy and stimulation results has not been performed, the anatomic boundaries of the SMA remain to be defined. It is imperative that in future studies the marked sulcal and gyral variations of the mesial frontal and parietal lobes be taken into account.

The relationship of the paracentral lobule to the central area is shown in Fig. 4.8A,B. The mesial precentral sulcus anteriorly limits the extent of the primary motor area. SMA-type responses are frequently noted on stimulation in the anterior portion of the paracentral lobule, since this sulcus is posterior to the paracentral sulcus and does not extend down to the cingulate. Similarly, because of the multiple interruptions along the course of the cingulate sulcus, the SMA invaginates into the cingulum and SMA-type responses can occur from stimulation of this area. The mesial extent of the primary sensory area is consistently posterior to the marginal ramus. Primary sensory responses are thus noted beyond the limits of the paracentral lobule.

The SMA is closely connected with the contralateral SMA through the corpus callosum. These fibers occupy a large portion of the body of the callosum and explain the rapid spread of a stimulus or ictal discharge, which may result in lateralization difficulties of ictal discharges. Direct corticospinal projections from the SMA contribute to a direct corticospinal tract terminating predominantly in the gray matter of the anterior horn at different levels of the spinal cord (Bertrand 1956; Murray and Coulter 1981). Trunk and proximal limb responses can be obtained on stimulation of the SMA, even following resection of the central area (Penfield and Welch 1951).

V The Pyramidal Tract

The pyramidal tract has been described as a "brain highway used by a variety of corticofugal fiber traffic" (Kuypers 1987). In humans it is composed of approximately 1 million myelinated fibers and an undetermined number of unmyelinated fibers. The myelinated fibers destined for motor neural control originate mostly from Betz cells in area 4 according to Brodmann.

Although the pyramidal tract is present at birth, it undergoes several modifications postnatally. Firstly, there is pruning of its fibers as they initially originate from widespread cortical areas. This progressive decrease in the fiber numbers is coupled with an increase in the distribution of the fibers to target areas in the spinal cord, correlating with the acquisition of motor skills.

The pyramidal tract in adults appears to arise from areas 4, 3a, and 3b with an additional input from area 6 and the parietal association cortex (Figs. 4.22–4.28). The contribution of the supplementary motor area to the pyramidal tract is an important one. There is evidence that the SMA contributes mostly to the homolateral direct pyramidal tract destined for proximal limb control. The fibers converge towards the coronal radiata occupying a central position in this structure. In the internal capsule,

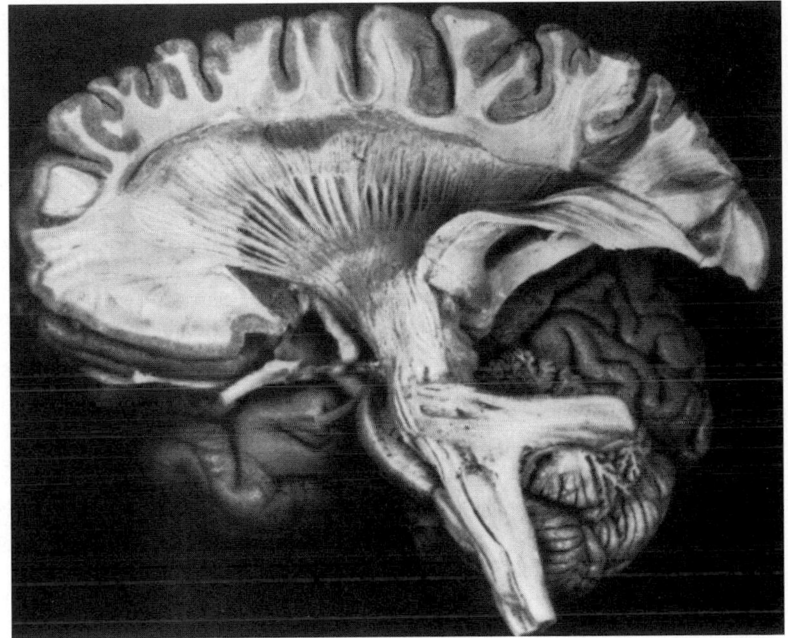

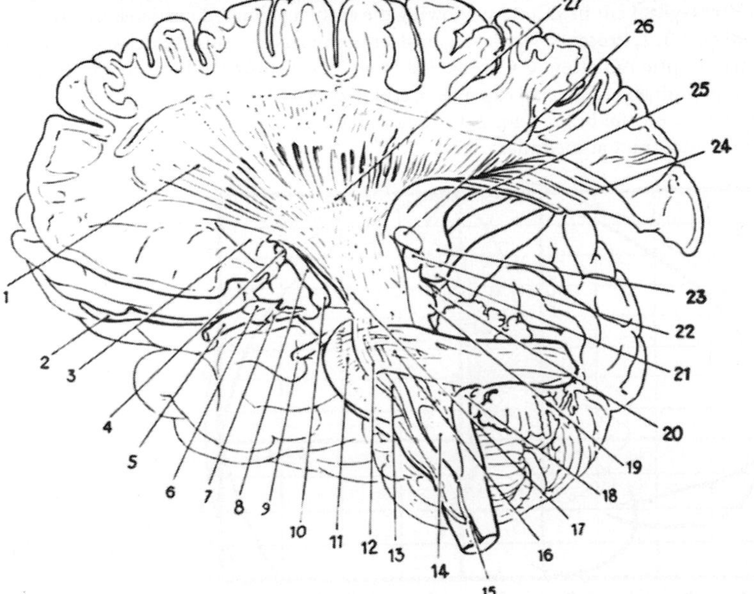

Fig. 4.22A,B. Dissection of the corticospinal tract (From Ludwig and Klingler 1956)

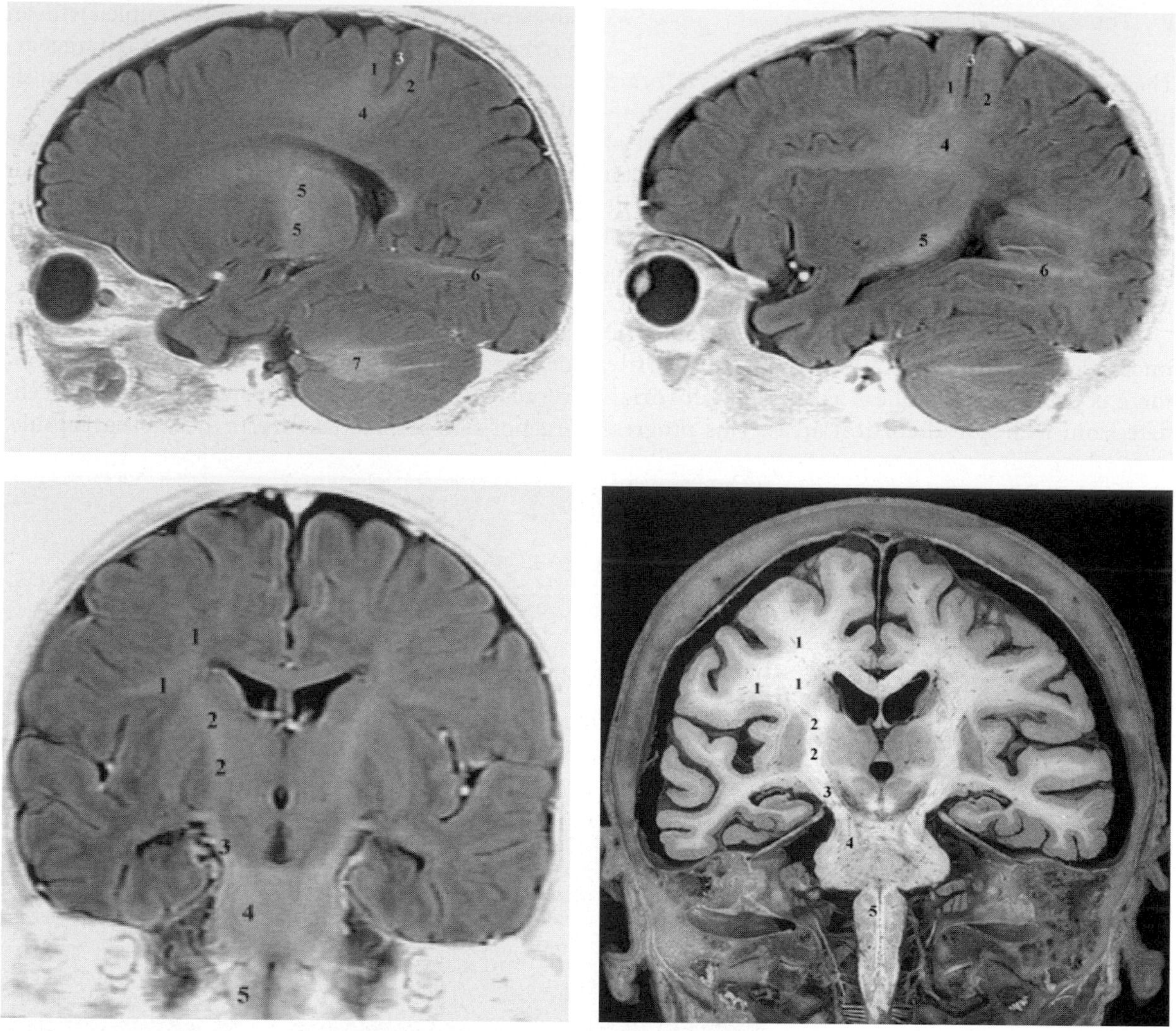

Fig. 4.23. A Parasagittal cut in an infant, showing the early myelinated corticospinal tract at the level of central sulcus (*3*), in the corona radiata (*4*) and in the posterior limb of the internal capsule (*5*). *1*, Precentral gyrus; *2*, postcentral gyrus; *3*, central sulcus; *4*, corticospinal tract in corona radiata; *5*, internal capsule, posterior limb; *6*, optic radiations; *7*, cerebellar white matter. **B** Parasagittal cut in an infant showing the early myelinated corticospinal tract at the level of central sulcus (*3*), in the corona radiata (*4*). *1*, Precentral gyrus; *2*, postcentral gyrus; *3*, central sulcus; *4*, corticospinal tract; *5*, internal capsule, sublenticular part; *6*, optic radiation. **C** Coronal cut in an infant showing the early myelinated corticospinal tract. *1*, Corticospinal tract in corona radiata; *2*, internal capsule; *3*, crus cerebri; *4*, corticospinal tract in basis pontis; *5*, pyramid of medulla. **D** Coronal cut of brain and the brainstem. *1*, Corona radiata; *2*, internal capsule; *3*, crus cerebri; *4*, corticospinal tract at pontine level; *5*, pyramidal tract at medullary level

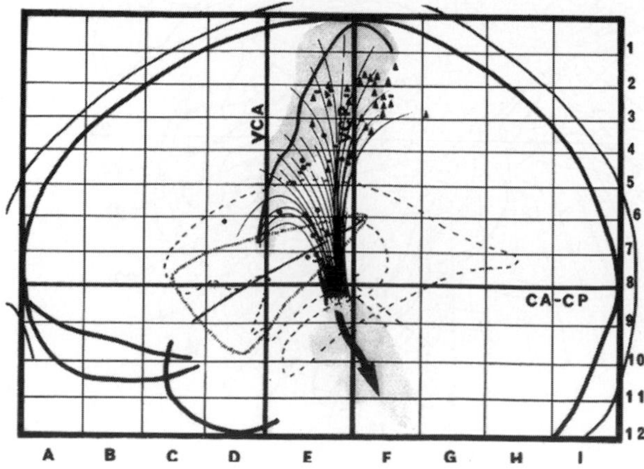

Fig. 4.24. The central sulcus and the corticospinal tract according to the bicommissural coordinates (From Szickla et al. 1977)

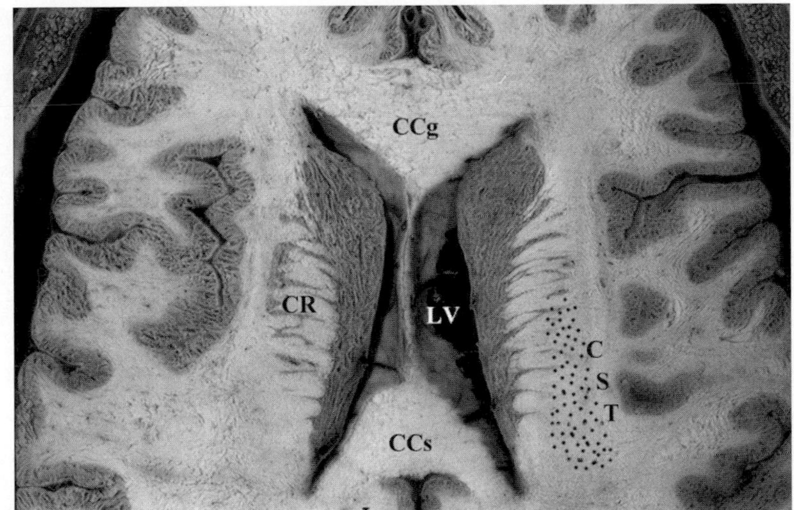

Fig. 4.25. Localization of the corticospinal pyramidal tract in the corona radiata. *CCg*, genu of corpus callosum; *CCs*, splenium of corpus callosum; *CN*, caudate nucleus; *CR*, corona radiata; *CST*, corticospinal tract (*dotted area*); *LV*, lateral ventricle. (Modified from Ross 1980)

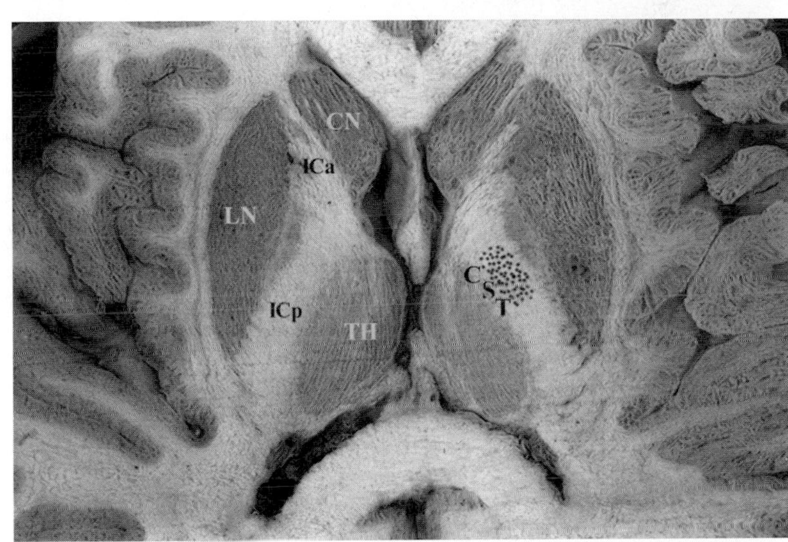

Fig. 4.26. Localization of the corticospinal pyramidal tract in the internal capsule (upper level). *CN*, caudate nucleus; *CST*, corticospinal tract (*dotted area*); *ICa*, anterior limb of internal capsule; *ICp*, posterior limb of internal capsule; *LN*, lenticular nucleus; *LV*, lateral ventricle; *TH*, thalamus. (Modified after Ross 1980)

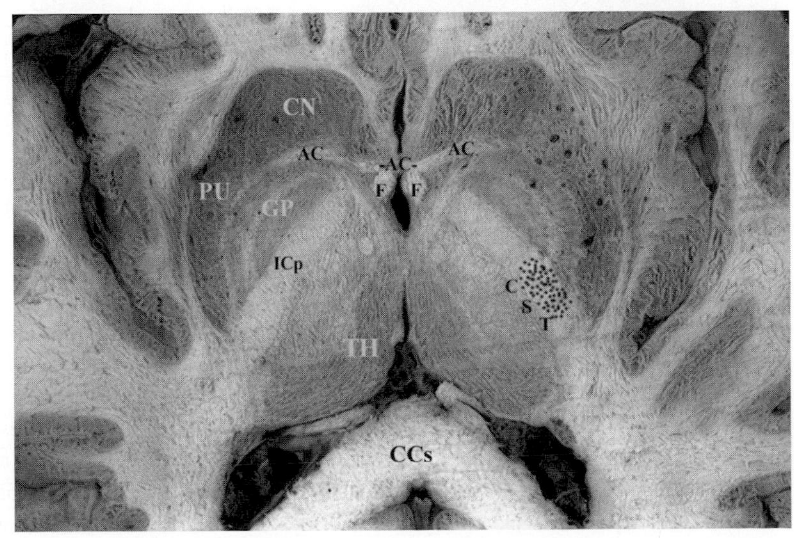

Fig. 4.27. Localization of the corticospinal pyramidal tract in the internal capsule (lower level). *AC*, anterior commissure; *CCs*, splenium of corpus callosum; *CN*, caudate nucleus; *CST*, corticospinal tract (*dotted area*); *F*, fornix; *GP*, globus pallidus; *ICp*, posterior limb of internal capsule; *LN*, lenticular nucleus; *LV*, lateral ventricle; *PU*, putamen; *TH*, thalamus. (Modified after Ross 1980)

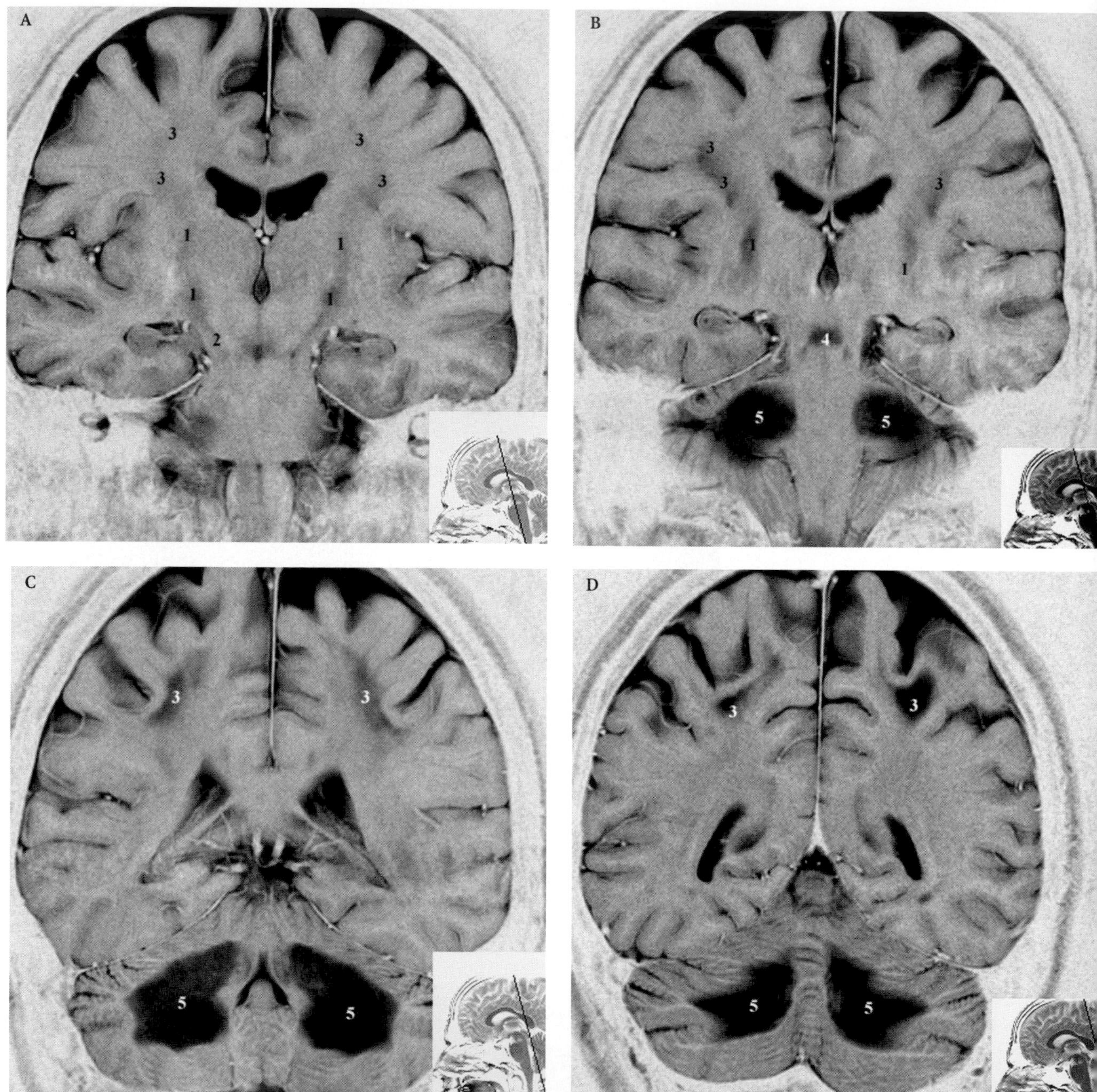

Fig. 4.28. A–D The corticospinal pathway: toxic opioid Wallerian degeneration as shown on T2 weighted MR (inverted), in the coronal plane parallel to the PC-OB reference (**B**), and in the axial plane parallel to the sylvian orientation/CH-PC reference (**E**), as compared to the bicommissural AC-PC reference plane (**F**)

the position of the pyramidal tract fiber shifts from anterior to posterior, initially located in the junction of the anterior and mid-third portion of the posterior limb of the internal capsule and progressively shifting backwards between the mid- and the posterior third of the internal capsule at a low thalamic level (Déjerine 1895; Bucy 1944; Ross 1980; Denny-Brown 1982; Davidoff 1990, Uchino et al. 1990; Orita et al. 1991; Yagishita et al. 1994; Meyer et al. 1996).

Three arteries supply the pyramidal tract. The middle cerebral artery provides blood to the corona radiata with a contribution from the lenticulostriate arteries at the level of the internal capsule. The len-

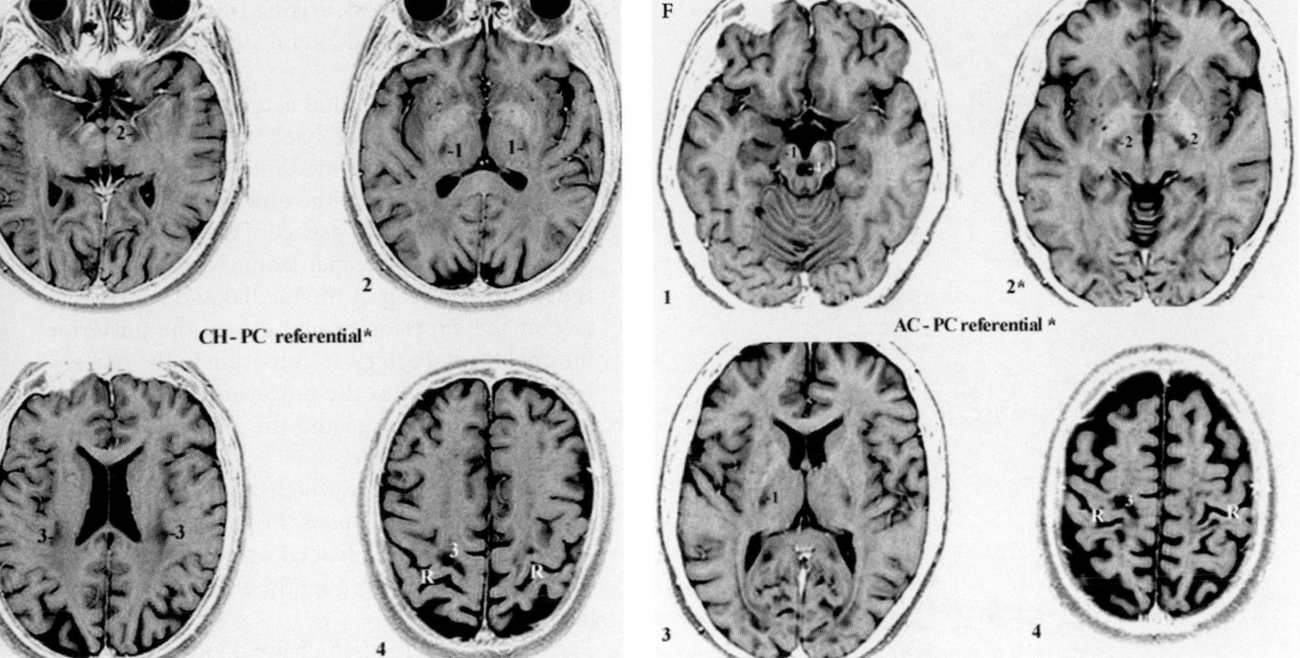

Fig. 4.28. A–D The corticospinal pathway: toxic opioid Wallerian degeneration as shown on T2 weighted MR (inverted), in the coronal plane parallel to the PC-OB reference (B), and in the axial plane parallel to the sylvian orientation/CH-PC reference (E), as compared to the bicommissural AC-PC reference plane (F)

ticulostriate arteries and the anterior choroidal artery share the supply to this structure. There is considerable overlap in the supply of each artery, explaining the variable clinical picture noted following occlusion of one of these branches (Manelfe et al. 1981).

VI Vascular Supply of the Sensorimotor Cortex

A Arterial Supply of the Sensorimotor Cortex

1 Arterial Supply of the Lateral Aspect of the Hemisphere

The vascular supply of the central area has received much attention given the functional importance of this region and since, prior to the advent of MRI, it was an essential part of the localization process. Adequate visualization of the arteries and veins of this region is essential in the planning and execution of neurosurgical procedures (Fig. 4.29).

Two arteries provide blood supply to the central area: the anterior cerebral artery and the middle cerebral artery. Bailey described a prerolandic and rolandic branch (Bailey 1933) and Testut and Latarjet (1948) described the artery of the rolandic fissure, this artery reaching at times beyond the upper margin of the hemisphere.

Salamon and Huang (1976) described the arteries supplying the lateral surface of the central area: the prerolandic, the rolandic and the anterior parietal artery (Fig. 4.29). A detailed description of these arteries is found in Szikla's monumental work from the Sainte-Anne school. This work demonstrates the essential role of stereo-angiography in understanding the relationship of arteries to their respective gyral territory (Szikla et al. 1977).

The vascular territory of the central group of arteries was examined by Gibo et al. (1981). The precentral branch of the middle cerebral artery supplies the inferior and middle portions of the precentral gyrus and extends to the posterior half of the pars opercularis and the middle frontal gyrus. The central branch supplies the superior part of the precentral gyrus and the inferior half of the postcentral gyrus. The postcentral branch supplies the upper central sulcus, the superior postcentral gyrus, the anterior part of the inferior parietal lobule and the antero-inferior region of the superior parietal lobule.

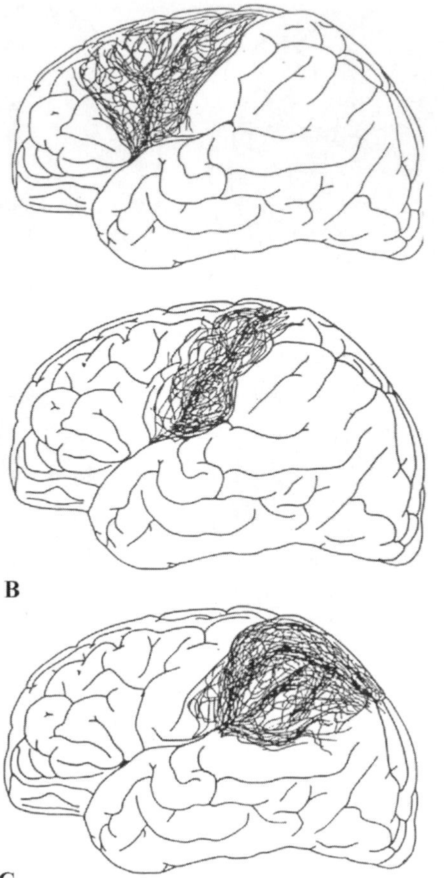

Fig. 4.29A–C. Vascular supply to the central region by the prerolandic artery (**A**), the rolandic artery (**B**) and the parietal artery (**C**). (After Salamon and Huang 1976)

2 Arterial Supply to the Mesial Aspect of the Hemisphere

The anterior cerebral artery provides the arterial supply of the mesial part of the hemisphere. There is considerable variation in its cortical branches. The most constant is the pericallosal artery, which begins distal to the anterior communicating artery and courses in the callosal cistern. The callosal marginal artery is usually the largest branch of the pericallosal artery. It is present in 82% of examined brains (Perlmutter and Rhoton 1978). It courses in the cingulate sulcus and has an inverse size relationship with the pericallosal artery. Any branch of the callosal marginal artery can also have its origin in the pericallosal artery.

Eight cortical branches of the anterior cerebral artery are usually encountered. These are as follows, from anterior to posterior:

1. The orbital frontal artery, most commonly arising from A-2 and supplying the gyrus rectus.
2. The frontopolar artery, arising from A-2 and supplying the medial and lateral surface of the frontal pole.
3. The three internal frontal arteries, supplying the superior frontal gyrus back to the paracentral lobule. These are separated into anterior, middle, and posterior arteries: the anterior frontal arteries supply the anterior aspect of the mesial frontal lobe; the middle internal frontal artery supplies the middle portion of the medial and lateral surface of the superior frontal gyrus; the posterior internal frontal artery, terminating in the precentral fissure, supplies the posterior portion of the superior frontal gyrus and the anterior aspect of the paracentral lobule.
4. The paracentral artery, which courses in the paracentral sulcus and supplies the paracentral lobule. The middle internal frontal and paracentral arteries arise most frequently from the callosal marginal artery.
5. The parietal arteries, which are divided into superior and inferior groups: the superior parietal artery supplies the superior portion of the precuneus and courses in the marginal limb of the cingulate sulcus; the inferior parietal artery, which is the last cortical branch of the anterior cerebral artery, supplies the inferior portion of the precuneus and cuneus.

B Venous Drainage of the SensorimotorCortex

1 The Lateral Venous Drainage System

Two venous systems drain the hemisphere, one mesial and one lateral. The lateral venous drainage system can be divided into three groups: anterior, central, and posterior convexity ascending systems. Three veins drain the anterior convexity: the frontopolar, anterior frontal, and middle frontal veins. They arise at the junction between the third and second frontal convolution and course anteriorly. They enter the subpolar space prior to joining the superior sagittal sinus in the direction of flow.

The central venous drainage system is comprised of the posterofrontal, precentral, central, and postcentral veins. The precentral, central, and postcentral veins run in their respective sulci in an almost vertical fashion. Superiorly, they exit the subarachnoid space lateral to the venous lacuna and then course in the subdural space below the venous lacuna prior to entering the sagittal sinus in a direction opposite to flow. The central vein is usually the smallest. The postcentral is usually the largest and frequently constitutes the anastomotic vein of Trolard.

Three veins constitute the posterior convexity group: (1) the anterior parietal vein, which arises from the supramarginal and angular gyri and drains superiorly in the postcentral vein or in the superior sagittal sinus; (2) the posterior parietal vein, which arises from the inferoposterior part of the parietal lobule and courses in the intraparietal sulcus, and then runs posteriorly on the convexity for a few centimeters, parallel to the superior sagittal sinus, prior to entering it; (3) the lateral occipital vein, which drains the lateral portion of the occipital lobe and is located near the parieto-occipital sulcus. It then comes forward a few centimeters in the subdural space prior to entering the superior sagittal sinus.

Two areas devoid of tributaries are noted. The first is between the anterior and the central convexity group. This area contains few or no ascending veins and is frequently used to access the anterior interhemispheric fissure. Posteriorly, since the lateral occipital vein is directed anteriorly, no large vein enters the superior sagittal sinus for a distance of 4–5 cm proximal to the torcula.

2 The Mesial Venous Drainage System

This system is divided into an ascending group, draining into the superior sagittal sinus, and a descending group, draining into the inferior sagittal sinus or the basal vein of Rosenthal. Both assume a similar distribution as their lateral counterpart. Those coursing superiorly frequently join the convexity group to enter the superior sagittal sinus.

VII Imaging Approaches for the Localization of the Central Sulcus

Three approaches are used for the localization of the central sulcus. An indirect approach has relied on skull landmarks and, subsequently, on brain reference coordinates (Horsley 1892; Taylor and Haughton 1900; Rowland and Mettler 1948; Matsui et al. 1977; Takase et al. 1977; Tokunaga et al. 1977; Salamon and Lecaque 1978; Taylor et al. 1980; Kido et al. 1980; Vanier et al. 1985; Bergvall et al. 1988). These approaches are reviewed in Chap. 2. Two widely used indirect methods are the Talairach method based on the AC-PC reference plane (Talairach et al. 1952, 1967; Szikla and Talairach 1965; Szikla et al. 1975; Talairach and Tournoux 1988; Rumeau et al. 1988; Missir et al. 1989), and the Olivier method based on the callosal reference plane (Olivier et al. 1987; Villemure et al. 1987; Devaux et al. 1996).

The direct approach relies on identification of the central sulcus with modern imaging modalities. Various authors have described landmarks for the localization of the central sulcus. These landmarks are visible on axial and sagittal CT and MR scans (Naidich et al. 1995, 1996). All these methods suffer from the inability to visualize the full extent of the central sulcus from superior to inferior. For this reason, 3D MR has been used as a more realistic alternative. This approach, however, is complex due to technical difficulties (Stievenart et al. 1993) and lack of display of the finer details, as secondary and tertiary sulci are difficult to depict with this approach.

Using an oblique 2D approach (Fig. 4.30) obtained parallel to the ventricular reference plane (or even parallel to the forniceal reference plane as described in Chap. 6), we believe the pericentral anatomy can be easily and precisely displayed, including the finer morphological details. This approach is easily obtainable on nearly all available imaging equipment, rapidly and reliably. Because the whole extent of the central sulcus is displayed, we think that this approach might be useful for functional techniques (refer to figures in Sect. 10.II).

The third approach relies on identification of the sensorimotor cortex, using functional activation techniques by PET or functional MRI. Discussion of the reliability of these methods is beyond the scope of this book. The reader is referred to selected papers and reviews on the subject (Berger et al. 1990; Orrison 1990; Connelly et al. 1993; Rao et al. 1993; Jack et al. 1994; Hammecke et al. 1994; Yousry et al. 1995; Yetkin et al. 1995, 1997; Kahn et al. 1996; Kim et al. 1996; Mattay et al. 1996; Dassonville et al. 1997; Roberts and Rowley 1997; Yetkin et al. 1997; Yoshiura et al. 1997; Posner and Raichle 1998).

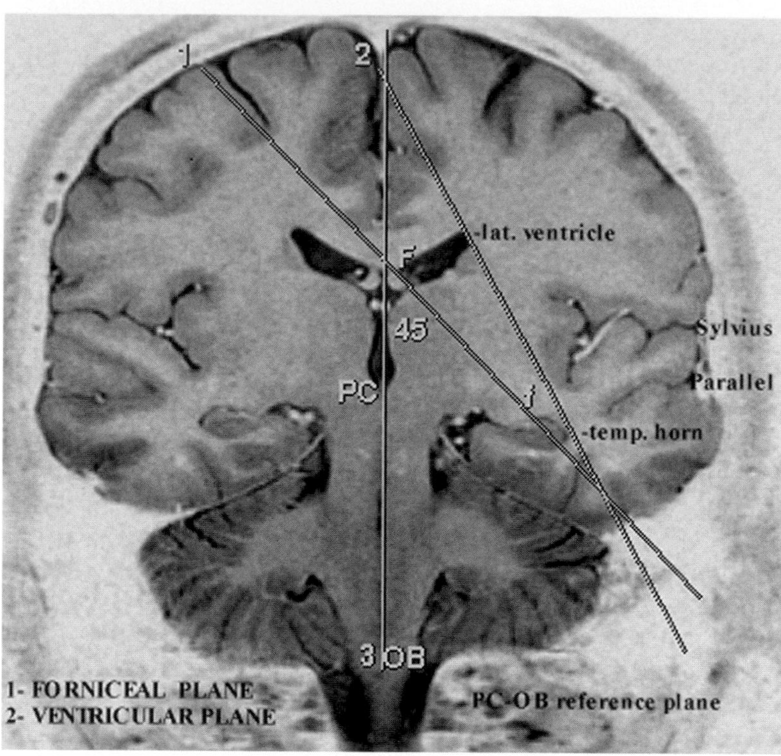

Fig. 4.30. Topogram showing the oblique references projected onto the coronal PC-OB reference plane. *1*, The "forniceal (*Ff*) plane" (see Figs. 4.4 and 4.5) and *2*, the "ventricular" plane (see

References

Bailey P (1933) Intracranial tumors. Thomas, Springfield, Ill

Bailey P, von Bonin G (1951) The isocortex of man. University of Illinois Press, Urbana, Ill

Berger MS, Cohen WA, Ojemann GA (1990) Correlation of motor cortex brain mapping data with magnetic resonance imaging. J Neurosurg 72:383–387

Bergvall U, Rumeau C, Van Bunnen Y, Corbaz JM, Morel M (1988) External references of the bicommissural plane. In: Gouaze A, Salamon G (eds) Brain anatomy and magnetic resonance imaging. Springer, Berlin Heidelberg New York, pp 2–11

Bertrand G (1956) Spinal efferent pathways from the supplementary motor area . Brain 79:461–473

Broca P (1878) Nomenclature cerebrale. Rev Anthropol Ser 2:3

Bucy PC (1944) The precentral motor cortex. University of Illinois Press, Urbana, Ill

Connelly A, Jackson GD, Frackowiak RSJ, Belliveau JW, Vargha-Khadem F, Gadian D (1993) Functional mapping of activated human primary cortex with a clinical MR imaging system. Radiology 188:125–130

Cunningham DJ, Horsley V (1892) Contribution to the surface anatomy of the cerebral hemispheres. Royal Irish Acad, Dublin

Dassonville P, Zhu XH, Ugurbil K, Kim SG, Ashe J (1997) Functional activation in motor cortex reflects the direction and the degree of handedness. Proc Natl Acad Sci USA 94:14015–14018

Davidoff RA (1990) The pyramidal tract. Neurology 40:332–339

Déjerine J (1895) Anatomie des centres nerveux, vol 1 and 2. Rueff, Paris

Denny-Brown D (1982) Relations and functions of the pyramidal tract. In: Schaltenbrand G, Walker AE (eds) Stereotaxy of the human brain, 2nd edn. Thieme, Stuttgart, pp 131–139

Devaux B, Meder JF, Missir O, Turak B, Dilouya A, Merienne L, Chodkiewicz JP, Fredy D (1996) La ligne rolandique: une ligne de base simple pour le repérage de la région centrale. J Neuroradiol 23:6–18

Dusser de Barenne (1924) Experimental researches on sensory localization in the cerebral cortex of the monkey (macacus). Proc R Soc Lond 96B:272–291

Ebeling U, Steinmetz H, Huang Y, Kahn T (1989) Topography and identification of the inferior precentral sulcus in MR imaging. AJNR 10:937–942

Eberstaller O (1890) Das Stirnhirn. Ein Beitrag zur Anatomie der Oberfläche des Großhirns. Urban and Schwarzenberg, Vienna

Feess-Higgins A, Larroche JC (1987) Le developpement du cerveau foetal humain: atlas anatomique. INSERM/CNRS, Masson, Paris

Ferrier D (1876a) The localization of functions in the brain. Proc R Soc 22:229–232

Ferrier D (1876b) The function of the brain. Smith Elder, London

Foerster O (1936) The motor cortex in man in the light of Hughling Jackson's doctrines. Brain 59:135–159

Fritsch G, Hitzig E (1870) Über die elektrische Erregbarkeit des Grosshirns. Arch Anat Physiol Wiss Med 37:300–332

Gibo H, Carver CC, Rhoton AL, Lenkey C, Mitchell RJ (1981) Microsurgical anatomy of the middle cerebral artery. J Neurosurg 54:151–169

Hammeke TA, Yetkin FZ, Mueller WM, Morris GL, Haughton VM, Rao SM, Binder JR (1994) Functional magnetic resonance imaging of somatosensory stimulation. Neurosurgery 35(4):677–681

Horsley V (1892) On the topographical relations of the cranium and surface of the cerebrum. In: Cunningham DJ (eds) Contribution to the surface anatomy of the cerebral hemispheres. Academy House, Dublin, pp 306–355

Jack CR, Thompson R, Butts RK, Sharbrough FW, Kelly PJ, Hanson DP, Rieder SJ, Ehman RL, Hangiandreou NJ, Cascino GD (1994) Sensory motor cortex: correlation of presurgical mapping with functional MR imaging and invasive cortical mapping. Radiology 190:85–92

Jackson JH (1870) A study of convulsions. Trans St Andrews Med Grad Assoc 3:162–207 (selected writings 1:8–36)

Jefferson G (1912) The morphology of the sulcus interparietalis. J Anat Physiol 47:365–380

Kahn T, Schwabe B, Bettag M, Harth T, Ulrich F, Rassek M, Schwarzmaier HJ, Mödder U (1996) Mapping of the cortical motor hand area with functional MR imaging and MR imaging-guided laser-induced interstitial thermotherapy of brain tumors. Radiology 200:149–157

Kido DK, LeMay M, Levinson AW, Benson WE (1980) Computed tomographic localization of the precentral gyrus. Radiology 135:373–377

Kim JH, Shin T, Kim JS, Kim HJ, Chung SH (1996) MR Imaging of cerebral activation performed with a gradient echo technique at 1.5 T: sources of activation signals. AJNR 167:1277–1281

Kuypers HGJM (1987) Pyramidal tract. In: Adelman G (ed) The encyclopedia of science, vol 2. Birkhäuser, Basel

Larroche JC (1987) Le developpement du cerveau foetal humain. Atlas anatomique. INSERM/CNRS, Masson, Paris

Li A, Yetkin Z, Cox R, Haughton VM (1996) Ipsilateral hemisphere activation during motor and sensory tasks. AJNR 17:651–655

Luders HO (1996) The supplementary sensorymotor area: an overview. In: Luders HO (ed) Supplementary sensorimotor area. Lippincott-Raven, Philadelphia, pp 1–16 (Advances in neurology, vol 70)

Ludwig E, Klingler J (1956) Atlas cerebri humani. Karger, Basel

Manelfe C, Clanet M, Gigaud M, Bonafe A, Guiraud B, Rascol A (1981) Internal capsule: anatomy and ischemic changes demonstrated by computed tomography. Am J Neuroradiol 2:149–155

Matsui T, Kawamoto K, Labarre L, Imai T, Tamotsu O, Hirano A (1977) Anatomical and pathological study of the brain by CT scanner. II. Anatomical study of the normal brain at various angles. Multiple angle examination. Comput Tomogr 2:1–16

Mattay VS, Frank JA, Santha AK, Pekar JJ, Duyn JH, McLaughlin AC, Weinberger DR (1996) Whole-brain functional mapping with isotropic MR imaging. Radiology 201:399–404

Meyer JR, Roychowdhury S, Russel E, Callahan C, Gitelman D, Mesulam M (1996) Location of the central sulcus via cortical thickness of the precentral and postcentral gyri on MR. Am J Neuroradiol 17:1699–1706

Missir O, Dutheil-Desclers C, Meder JF, Musolino A, Fredy D (1989) Aspect du sillon central en IRM. J Neuroradiol 16:133–144

Murphy JT, Kwan HC, Mackay WA, Wong YC (1978) Spatial organization of the precentral cortex in awake primates. III. Input-output coupling. J Neurophysiol 41:1132–1139

Murray EA, Coulter JD (1981) Organization of corticospinal neurons in the monkey. J Comp Neurol 195:339–365

Naidich T, Brightbill TC (1996) Systems for localizing fronto-parietal gyri and sulci on axial CT and MRI. Int J Neuroradiol 4:313–338

Naidich P, Valavanis G, Kubik S (1995) Anatomic relationships along the low-middle convexity: part I. Normal specimens and magnetic resonance imaging. Neurosurgery 36(3):517–531

Olivier A, Peters TM, Clark JA, Marchand E, Mawko G, Bertrand G, Vanier M, Ethier R, Tyler J, de Lotbinière A (1987) Intégration de l'angiographie numérique, de la résonance magnétique, de la tomodensitométrie et de la tomotroencephalogr. Neurophysiol Clin 17:25–43

Ono N, Kubik S, Abernathy DG (1990) Atlas of the cerebral sulci. Thieme, Stuttgart

Orita T, Tsurutani T, Izumihara A, Matsunaga T (1991). Coronal MR imaging for visualisation of wallerian degeneration of the pyramidal tract. J Comput Assist Tomogr 15(5):802 804

Orrison WW, Davis LE, Sullivan GW, Mettler FA, Flynn ER (1990) Anatomic localisation of cerebral cortical function by magnetoencephalography combined with MR imaging and CT. AJNR 11:713–716

Penfield W, Jasper H (1954) Epilepsy and the functional anatomy of the human brain. Little Brown, Boston

Penfield W, Rasmussen T (1950) The cerebral cortex of man. A clinical study of localization of function. Macmillan, New York

Penfield W, Welch K (1951) The supplementary motor area of the cerebral cortex. A clinical and experimental study. Arch Neurol Psychiatr 66:289–317

Perlmutter D, Rhoton AL (1978) Microsurgical anatomy of the distal anterior cerebral artery. J Neurosurg 49:204–208

Posner MI, Raichle ME (1998) The neuroimaging of human brain function. Proc Natl Acad Sci USA 95:763–764 (colloquium paper)

Rao SM, Binder JR, Bandettini PA, Hammeke TA, Yetkin FZ, Jesmanowicz A, Lisk LM, Morris GL, Mueller WM, Estowski LD, Wong EC, Haughton VM, Hyde JS (1993) Functional magnetic resonance imaging of complex human movements. Neurology 43:2311–2318

Rassmussen T (1969) The neurosurgical treatment of focal epilepsy. In: Niedermeyer E (ed) Epilepsy, recent views on its therapy, diagnosis and treatment. Karger, Basel (Moderns problems of pharmacopsychiatry, vol 4)

Roberts TPL, Rowley HA (1997) Mapping of the sensorimotor cortex: functional MR and magnetic source imaging. AJNR 18:871–880

Ross ED (1980) Localization of the pyramidal tract in the internal capsule by whole brain dissection. Neurology 30:59–64

Rowland LP, Mettler FA (1948) Relation between the coronal suture and cerebrum. J Comp Neurol 89:21–40

Rumeau C, Gouaze A, Salamon G, Laffont J, Gelbert F, Einseidel H, Jiddane M, Farnarier P, Habib M, Perot S

(1988) Identification of cortical sulci and gyri using magnetic resonance imaging: a preliminary study. In: Gouaze A, Salamon G (eds) Brain anatomy and magnetic resonance imaging. Springer, Berlin Heidelberg New York, pp 11–32

Salamon G, Huang YP (1976) Radiologic anatomy of the brain. Springer, Berlin Heidelberg New York

Salamon G, Lecaque G (1978) Choice of the plane of incidence for computed tomography of the cerebral cortex. J Comput Assist Tomogr 2:93–97

Stievenart JL, Cabanis EA, Menart P, Knoplioch J, Lopez A, Tamraz J, Iba-Zizen MT, Philippe B, Prevost G, Bertrand JC (1993) A survey of different high resolution visualization modes of a volumetric object with applications. Surg Radiol Anat 15(1):47–54

Szikla G, Talairach J (1965) Coordinates of the Rolandic sulcus and topography of cortical and subcortical motor responses to low frequency stimulation in a proportional stereotactic system. Confin Neurol (Basel) 26: 474–475

Szikla G, Bouvier G, Hori T (1975) In vivo localization of brain sulci by arteriography: a stereotactic anatomoradiological study. Brain Res 95:497–502

Szikla G, Bouvier G, Hori T, Petrov V (1977) Angiography of the human brain cortex. Springer, Berlin Heidelberg New York

Symington J, Crymble PT (1913) The central fissure of the cerebrum. J Anat Physiol 47:321–339

Takase M, Tokunaga A, Otani K, Horie T (1977) Atlas of the human brain for computed tomography based on the glabella-inion line. Neuroradiology 14:73–79

Talairach J, Bancaud J (1966) The supplementary motor area in man. Anatomic functional findings by stereotactic encephalography in epilepsy. Int J Neurol 5:330–347

Talairach J, Tournoux P (1988) Co-planar stereotaxic atlas of the human brain. 3-dimensional proportional system: an approach to cerebral imaging. Thieme, Stuttgart

Talairach J, De Ajuriaguerra J, David M (1952) Etudes stéréotaxiques des structures encéphaliques chez l'homme. Presse Med 28:605–609

Talairach J, Szikla G, Tournoux P, Prossalentis A, Bordas-Ferrer M, Covello L, Iacob M, Mempel E (1967) Atlas d'anatomie stéréotaxique du télencéphale. Masson, Paris

Talairach J, Bancaud J, Seier S, Bordas-Ferrer M, Bonis A, Szikla G, Rusu M (1973) The cingulate gyrus and human behavior. Electroencephalogr Clin Neurophysiol 34:45–52

Taylor EH, Haughton WS (1900) Some recent researches on the topography of the convolutions and fissures of the brain. Trans R Acad Ireland 18:511–522

Taylor AJ, Haughton VM, Syvertsen A, Ho KC (1980) Taylor-Haughton line revisited. AJNR 1:55–56

Testut L, Latarjet A (1948) Traité d'anatomie humaine, vol 2: Angiologie, système nerveux central, 9th edn. Doin, Paris

Tokunaga A, Takase M, Otani K (1977) The glabella-inion line as a baseline for CT scanning of the brain. Neuroradiology 14:67–71

Uchino A, Imada H, Ohno M (1990) MR imaging of Wallerian degeneration in the humain brain stem after ictus. Neuroradiology. Springer, Berlin Heidelberg New York

Van Buren JM, Fedio P (1976) Functional representation on the medial aspect of the frontal lobes in man. J Neurosurg 44:275–289

Vanier M, Roch Lecours A, Ethier R, Habib M, Poncet M, Milette PC, Salamon G (1985) Proportional localization system for anatomical interpretation of cerebral computed tomograms. J Comput Assist Tomogr 9 (4):715–724

Villemure JG, Marchand E, Peters TM, Leroux G, Olivier A (1987) Magnetic resonance imaging stereotaxy: recognition and utilization of the commissures. Appl Neurophysiol 50:57–62

Waterston D (1907) Complete bilateral interruption of the fissure of Rolando. J Anat 41:143–146

Yagishita A, Nakano I, Oda M, Hirano A (1994) Location of the corticospinal tract in the internal capsule at MR imaging. Radiology 191:455–460

Yetkin FZ, Papke RA, Leighton PM, Daniels DL, Mueller WM, Haughton VM (1995) Location of the sensorimotor cortex: functional and conventional MR compared. AJNR 16:2109–2113

Yetkin FZ, Mueller WM, Morris GL, Mcauliffe TL, Ulmer JL, Cox RW, Daniels DL, Haughton VM (1997) Functional MR activation correlated with intraoperative cortical mapping. AJNR 18:1311–1315

Yoshiura T, Hasuo K, Mihara F, Masuda K, Morioka T, Fukui M (1997) Increased activity of the ipsilateral motor cortex during a hand motor task in patients with brain tumor and paresis. AJNR 18:865–869

Yousry TA, Schmid Urs D, Jassoy AG, Schmidt D, Eisner WE, Reulen HJ, Reiser MF, Lissner J (1995) Topography of the cortical motor hand area: prospective study with functional MR imaging and direct motor mapping at surgery. Radiology 195:23–29

5 Perisylvian Cognitive Region

I The Lateral Fissure and the Perisylvian Opercula

The lateral fissure or fissure of Sylvius is the major sulcal landmark on the lateral surface of the brain. It is the most important and constant of the cerebral sulci. It is the only true fissure of the lateral aspect of the cerebral hemisphere, developing initially as a shallow vertical depression between the frontal and temporal lobes at the 14th week of gestation (Chi et al. 1977). During later embryonic stages it assumes a horizontal course due to the dramatic expanse of the frontoparietal and temporal opercula over the insula (Cunningham 1892).

The lateral fissure is divided into three segments: the first is the hidden stem segment, extending from the lateral border of the anterior perforated substance and coursing over the limen insulae before ending at the falciform sulcus. The second, or the horizontal segment, is the longest and the deepest segment, coursing on the lateral surface of the hemisphere. The third segment is limited anteriorly by the transverse supratemporal sulcus, or Bailey's (1951) "sulcus supratemporalis transversus posterior," separating Heschl's gyri from the planum temporale and cutting into the superior temporal gyrus. This last segment is complex, asymmetrical and appears to correlate with hemispheric dominance.

Several branches are distinguished on the horizontal segment. Two sulci of almost similar length (2–3 cm) are noted, cutting into the inferior frontal gyrus: the horizontal ramus and the vertical ramus. These rami diverge from the sylvian fissure separately or from a common trunk in one third of cases. The terminal segment usually bifurcates at its end, in about 80% of the cases (Witelson and Kigar 1992), as a long terminal ascending branch and a short descending branch, more frequently (70%) found on the right. The terminal ascending branch is the true continuation of the lateral or sylvian fissure. The short descending branch is inconsistent and shallower, seen mostly over the right hemisphere and represents a "processus acuminis," resulting from the sharp bending of the ascending branch (Welker 1990) (Figs. 5.1–5.8).

The cortical regions adjacent to the lateral sulcus are the frontal, parietal and temporal opercula, or lids, covering the insular lobe (see Chap. 3).

II The Insula of Reil

Lying in the depth of the horizontal segment of the sylvian fissure is the insular lobe of Reil. It is the smallest of the cerebral lobes and has a pyramidal shape. It is distinguished by a triangular base, with the apex of the triangle anterior and inferior. The boundaries of the insula are the anterior limiting sulcus rostrally, dorsally the superior limiting sulcus and ventrocaudally the inferior limiting sulcus. Since limiting sulci are circular and continuous, they are together called the circular sulcus. The insula is continuous anteriorly with the preinsular area and posteriorly with the retroinsular region (Figs. 5.9–5.14, 5.28).

A The Preinsular Area

The preinsular area corresponds to a cortical ribbon made by the confluence of the frontal lateral and the temporopolar cortex. This area surrounds the falciform sulcus of Broca. This is a short and deep sulcus rudimentary in humans and well developed in animals. This fold forms an edge with its mesial aspect corresponding to the stem of the sylvian fissure and a lateral aspect which is the base of the apex of the insula.

B The Insular Lobe

The insular lobe is a preeminence with a triangular base. The apex of this triangle is directed anteriorly and inferiorly and overhangs the falciform sulcus

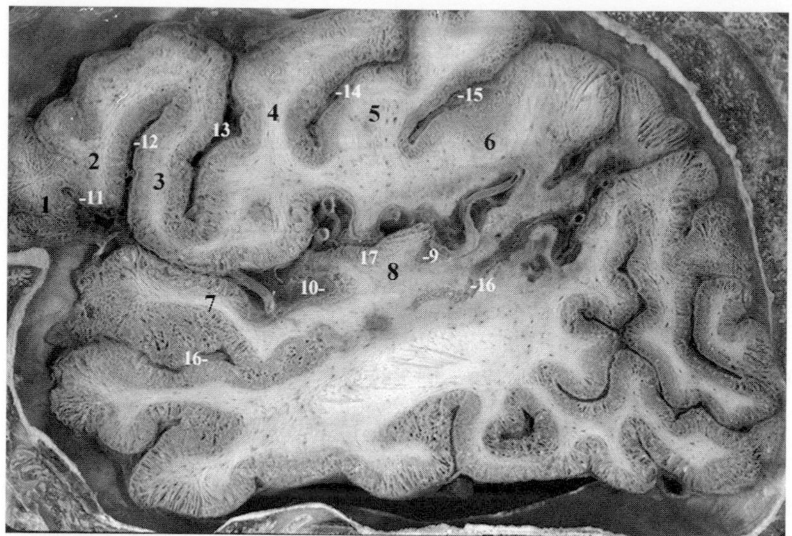

Fig. 5.1. Anatomy of the lateral aspect of the cerebral hemisphere showing the lateral fissure and the surrounding opercula. *1*, Inferior frontal gyrus, pars orbitalis; *2*, inferior frontal gyrus, pars triangularis; *3*, inferior frontal gyrus, pars opercularis; *4*, precentral gyrus; *5*, postcentral gyrus; *6*, inferior parietal lobule; *7*, superior temporal gyrus; *8*, transverse temporal gyri; *9*, posterior transverse temporal sulcus; *10*, anterior transverse temporal sulcus; *11*, horizontal ramus of lateral fissure; *12*, ascending ramus of lateral fissure; *13*, inferior precentral sulcus; *14*, central sulcus; *15*, inferior postcentral sulcus; *16*, parallel sulcus; 17, intermediate transverse temporal sulcus. (Modified from Tamraz 1983)

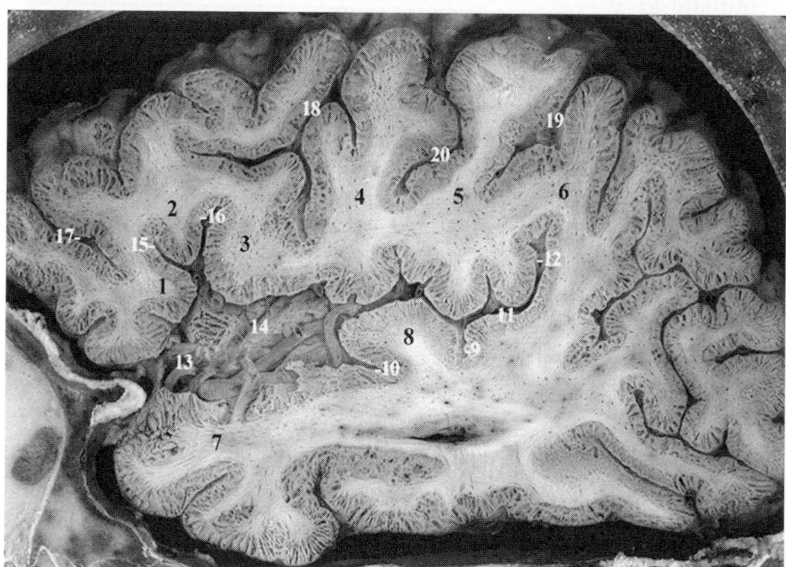

Fig. 5.2. Anatomical cut of the cerebral hemisphere passing through the lateral surface of the insula and showing the branches of the posterior ramus of the lateral fissure. *1*, Inferior frontal gyrus, pars orbitalis; *2*, inferior frontal gyrus, pars triangularis; *3*, inferior frontal gyrus, pars opercularis; *4*, precentral gyrus, inferior end; *5*, postcentral gyrus; *6*, supramarginal gyrus; *7*, superior temporal gyrus; *8*, transverse temporal gyrus; *9*, posterior transverse temporal sulcus; *10*, anterior transverse temporal sulcus; *11*, planum temporale; *12*, terminal ascending branch of lateral fissure; *13*, limen insulae; *14*, insula; *15*, horizontal ramus of lateral fissure; *16*, vertical ramus of lateral fissure; *17*, lateral orbital sulcus; *18*, inferior precentral sulcus; *19*, inferior postcentral sulcus; *20*, central sulcus. (Modified from Tamraz 1983)

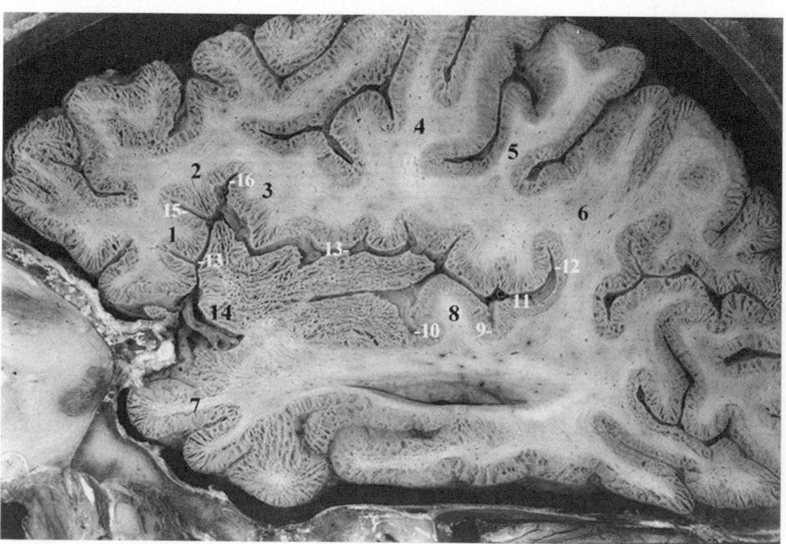

Fig. 5.3. Anatomical cut of the brain passing through the insular lobe and displaying the inferior frontal-parietal and the superior temporal lobes. *1*, Inferior frontal gyrus, pars orbitalis; *2*, inferior frontal gyrus, pars triangularis; *3*, inferior frontal gyrus, pars triangularis; *4*, precentral gyrus; *5*, postcentral gyrus; *6*, supramarginal gyrus; *7*, superior temporal gyrus; *8*, transverse temporal gyrus; *9*, posterior transverse temporal sulcus; *10*, anterior transverse temporal sulcus; *11*, planum temporale; *12*, terminal ascending branch of lateral fissure; *13*, circular sulcus of insula; *14*, limen insulae; *15*, horizontal branch of lateral fissure; *16*, vertical ascending branch of lateral sulcus. (Modified from Tamraz 1983)

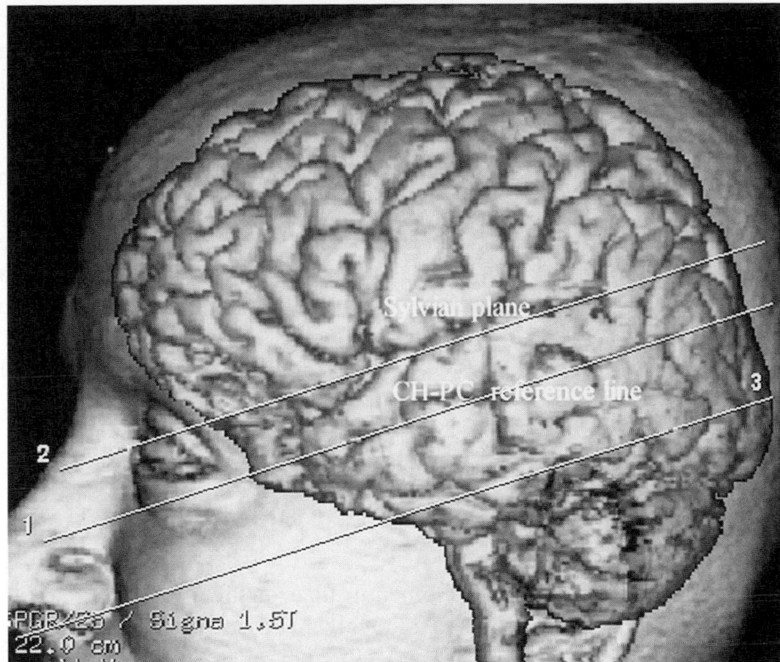

Fig. 5.4. Lateral aspect of the brain showing the lateral projection of the chiasmatico-commissural reference plane (CH-PC) and its close parallelism to the parallel sulcus (*1*) and therefore to the sylvian or lateral fissure orientation plane (*2*). Note that the CH-PC reference plane is roughly parallel to the cutaneous reference (*3*), joining the subnasal point to the superior otobasion, and paralleling the inferior aspect of the temporal lobe

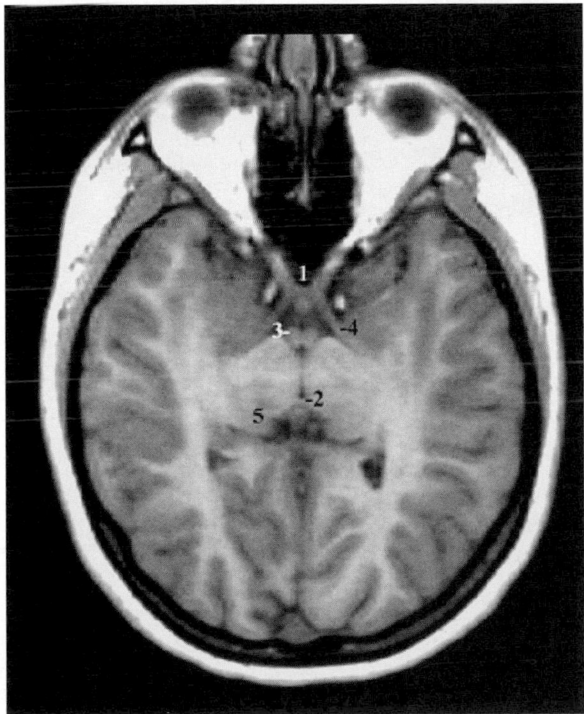

Fig. 5.5. Horizontal MR cut through the chiasmatico-commissural (CH-PC) reference plane. This cut shows the major anatomic landmarks as contained in the slice passing through the parallel sulcus on the lateral aspect of the cerebral hemisphere: *1*, chiasmal point; *2*, posterior commissure; *3*, mamillary bodies; *4*, cisternal optic tracts; *5*, the pulvinar thalami, and laterally, the lateral geniculate bodies. All of these anatomic structures are highly consistent topographically, validating the accuracy of this reference

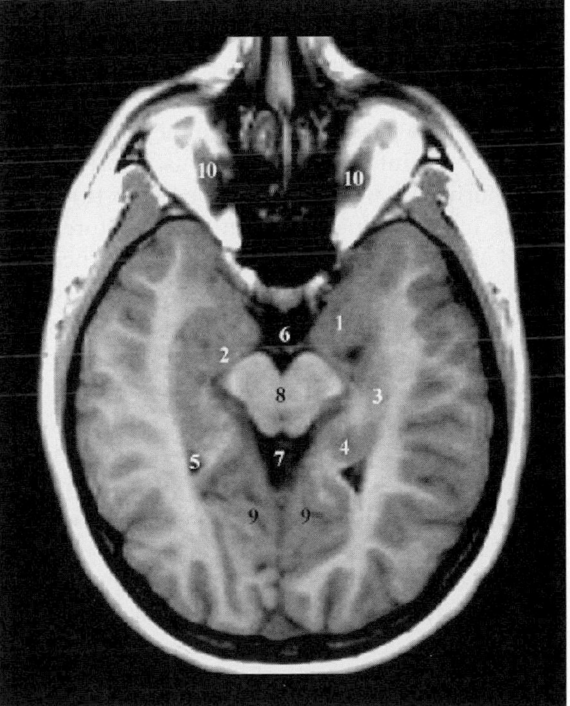

Fig. 5.6. Horizontal MR cut parallel to the chiasmatico-commissural reference plane (CH-PC), passing through the amygdala-hippocampal complex and the inferior horns of the lateral ventricles, found at the level of the inferior recti orbital muscles. *1*, Amygdala; *2*, hippocampal head; *3*, hippocampal body; *4*, hippocampal tail; *5*, inferior horn of the lateral ventricle; *6*, chiasmal cistern; *7*, ambient cistern; *8*, mesencephalon; *9*, calcarine sulcus; *10*, inferior recti muscles

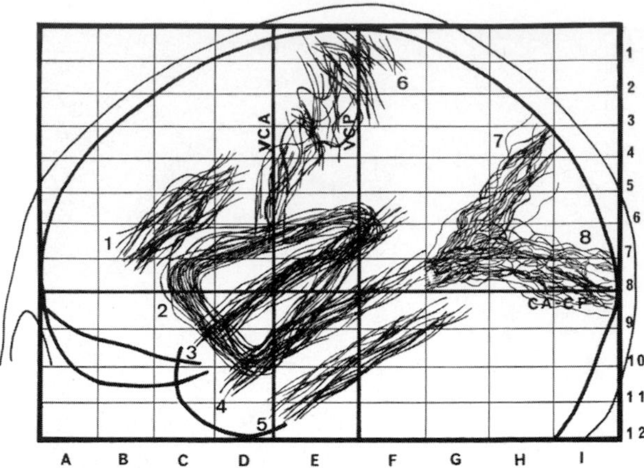

Fig. 5.7. Lateral projections of the lateral fissure and the surrounding major parallel sulci of frontotemporal lobes, as localized using the proportional system according to Szikla. (From Szikla et al. 1977)

and the preinsular region. The limen insulae, or the "seuil de l'insula," although used frequently in neurosurgery textbooks, is not clearly defined. French anatomists define it as corresponding to the preinsular region.

The anterior and inferior limiting sulci of the circular sulcus of the insula are frequently interrupted in the region of the falciform sulcus by a communication ("pli de passage") between the pole of the insula and the inferior frontal gyrus anteriorly and posteriorly with the temporal lobe (Fig. 5.10).

The insula proper is a fan-like structure composed of the anterior and posterior lobes. These two lobes are almost always separated by the well developed central sulcus of the insula. This sulcus is the deepest and longest of the insular sulci. It originates from the superior limiting sulcus and is directed obliquely towards the falciform sulcus.

The anterior lobe is triangular in shape with a superior base and is made of three short gyri, the gyri breves. The anterior, middle and the posterior gyri are separated by two short sulci, the sulci breves. The apical region is the reunion of the three gyri.

The posterior lobe is smaller than its anterior counterpart. It is composed of two long gyri obliquely oriented and originating from a common stem inferiorly. They are separated by a long sulcus and are continuous with the temporal pole.

The size of the insula has been studied by several authors. Kodama (1934) showed that the length of the insula on the sagittal plane is about 56.04±0.64 mm on the left and 52.8±0.52 mm on the right side. The height is 38.1±0.45 mm on the left and 37.5±0.38 mm on the right. Thus the overall surface of the left insula is larger than the right.

Anatomic variations of the insula have been rarely reported, with additional sulci found in the anterior or the posterior lobe (Kodama 1934).

C The Anatomic Relationships of the Insula

The insular lobe covers the lentiform nucleus, separated from it laterally to mesially by the extreme capsule, the claustrum, and the external capsule.

The uncinate fasciculus, running in the polar aspect of the insula, is covered laterally by the orbitofrontal operculum anteriorly, and the frontoparietal

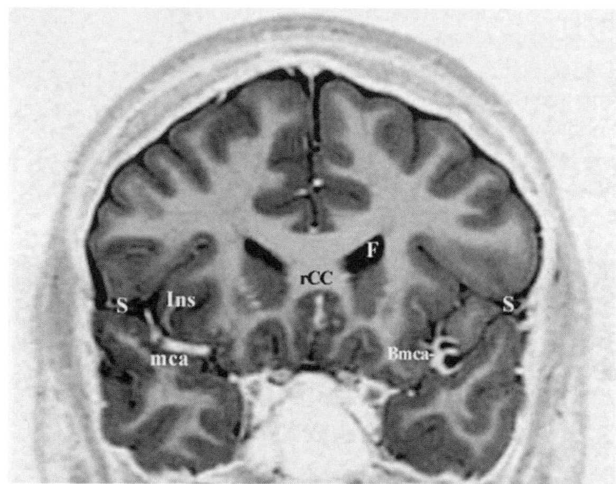

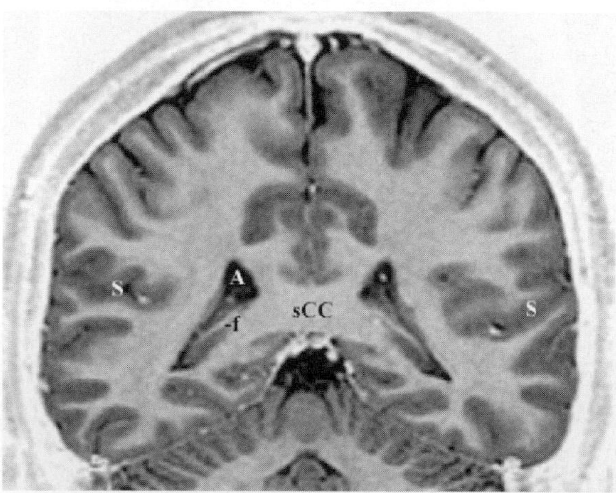

Fig. 5.8A,B. Coronal MR cuts parallel to the commissural-obex reference plane (PC-OB), passing through the anterior aspect (A) and the posterior end (B) of the posterior ramus of the lateral fissure, involving the rostrum and the splenium of the corpus callosum, respectively. *A*, Atrium of the lateral ventricle; *Bmca*, bifurcation of the middle cerebral artery into insular branches; *F*, frontal horn of the lateral ventricle; *f*, crus of fornix; *Ins*, insula; *mca*: middle cerebral artery; *rCC*, rostrum of corpus callosum; *S*, sylvian or lateral fissure; *sCC*, splenium of corpus callosum

operculum superiorly, and the temporal operculum inferiorly.

The sulci of the insula bear a relatively constant relationship with the overlying cortical sulci. The central rolandic sulcus appears to be continuous with the central sulcus of the insula, interrupted at the level of the hidden central operculum. The precentral rolandic gyrus covers part of the anterior lobe of the insula and the postcentral rolandic gyri covers the posterior insular lobe.

The relationship of the anterior speech area with the insula is interesting. The vertical ramus of the sylvian fissure extends through the operculum to reach the superior limiting sulcus. The horizontal ramus when present also extends from the operculum to the circular sulcus (Fig. 5.9).

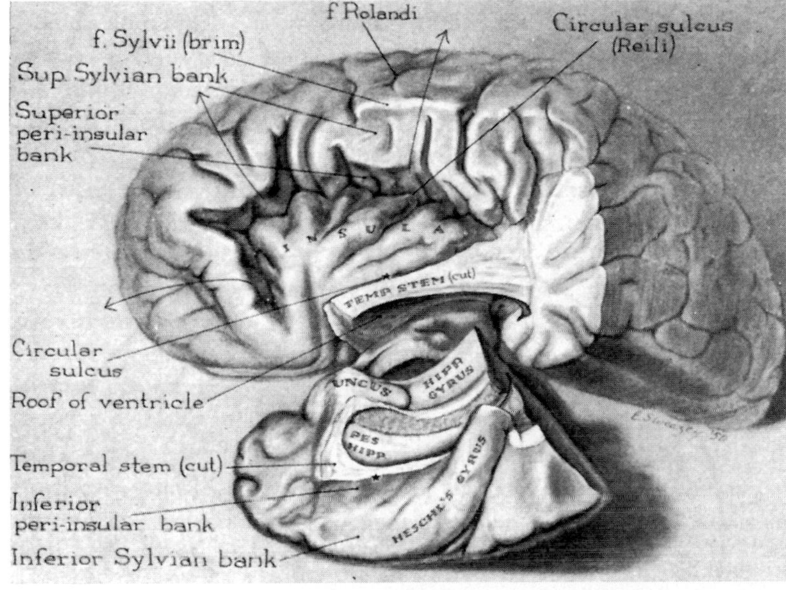

Fig. 5.9. Anatomy of the insula and its relationship with the sulci of the inferior frontal lobe, as disclosed in the depth of the lateral fissure. The topographical anatomy of the temporal stem is also shown. (From Penfield and Jasper 1954)

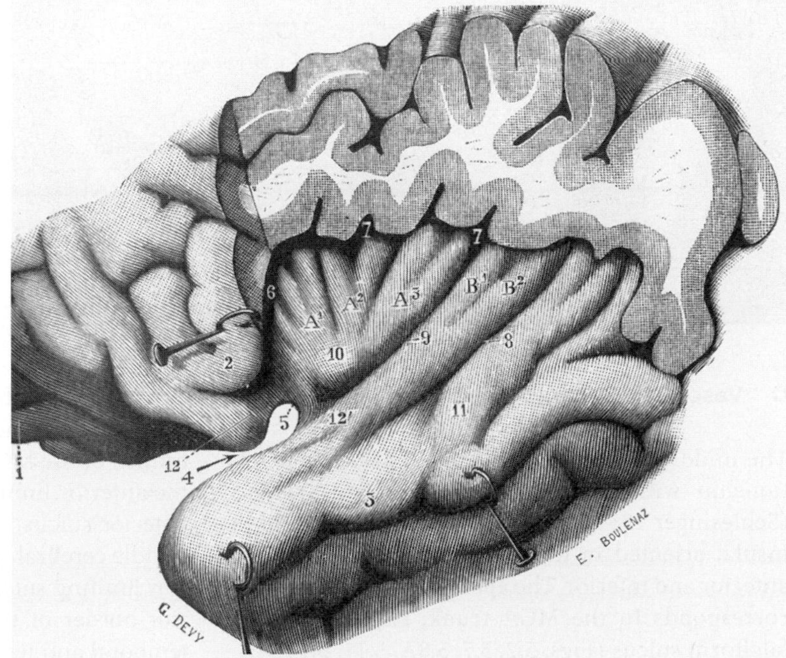

Fig. 5.10. Anatomy of the insula, the supratemporal, and the retroinsular regions. *1*, Fronto-orbital lobe; *2*, inferior frontal lobe, pars triangularis ("cap"); *3*, superior temporal gyrus; *4*, lateral fissure (Sylvius); *5*, falciform sulcus; *6*, circular sulcus of insula, anterior part; *7*, circular sulcus of insula, superior part; *8*, circular sulcus of insula, posterior part; *9*, central sulcus of insula; *10*, insular pole; *11*, temporoparietal "pli de passage"; *12*, *12'*, interruption of the circular sulcus of insula; *A1*, *A2*, *A3*, first, second and third short gyri of the anterior insular lobule; *B1*, *B2*, first and second long gyri of the posterior insular lobule. (After Testut and Latarjet 1948)

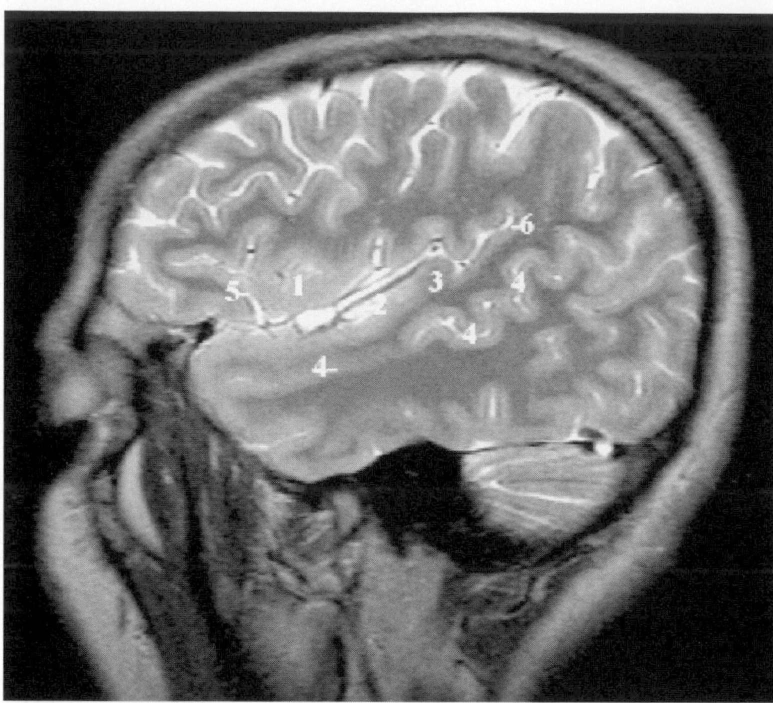

Fig. 5.11. Sagittal MR cut passing through the lateral fissure. *1*, Insula; *2*, middle cerebral artery; *3*, transverse temporal gyrus; *4*, parallel sulcus; *5*, common trunk of horizontal and vertical rami; *6*, terminal ascending ramus of lateral fissure

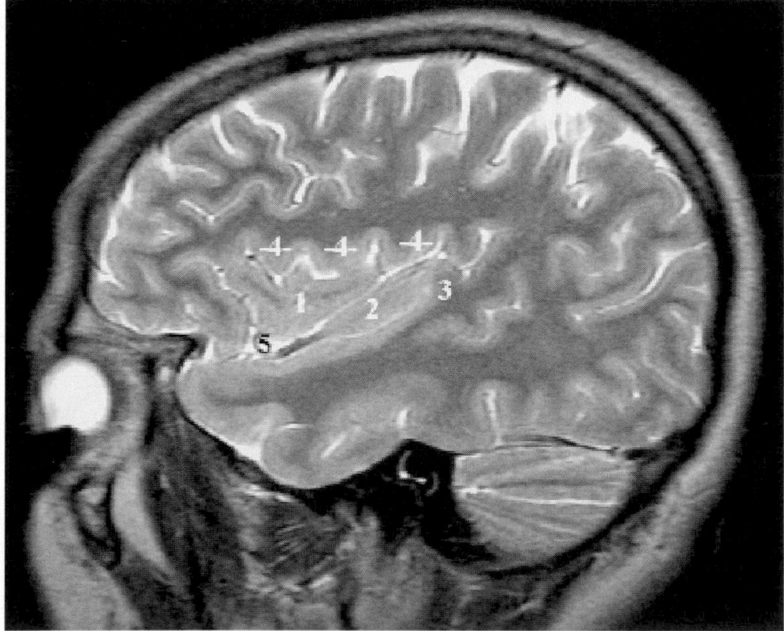

Fig. 5.12. Sagittal MR cut passing through the insula. *1*, Short gyri of insula; *2*, long gyri of insula; *3*, transverse temporal gyrus and auditory radiation; *4*, superior insular line; *5* falciform sul-

D Vascular Relationships of the Insula

The middle cerebral artery (MCA) has a close relationship with the insula. The "sylvian triangle" (Schlesinger 1953) is an angiographic marker of the insula, oriented in the same fashion with its apex anterior and inferior. The apex of the sylvian triangle corresponds to the MCA trunk, running into the falciform sulcus (Figs. 5.2, 5.7, 5.8A, 5.11, 5.13).

The anterior border of the triangle is at times difficult to trace and corresponds to the entire anterior branch of the MCA, coursing in the neighborhood of the anterior limiting sulcus. The superior part of the anterior sulcus, corresponding to the looping of the middle cerebral sulcus, branches as it leaves the superior limiting sulcus towards the operculum. The inferior border of the triangle is defined by the lowest temporal and temporo-parietal branches. It is curved

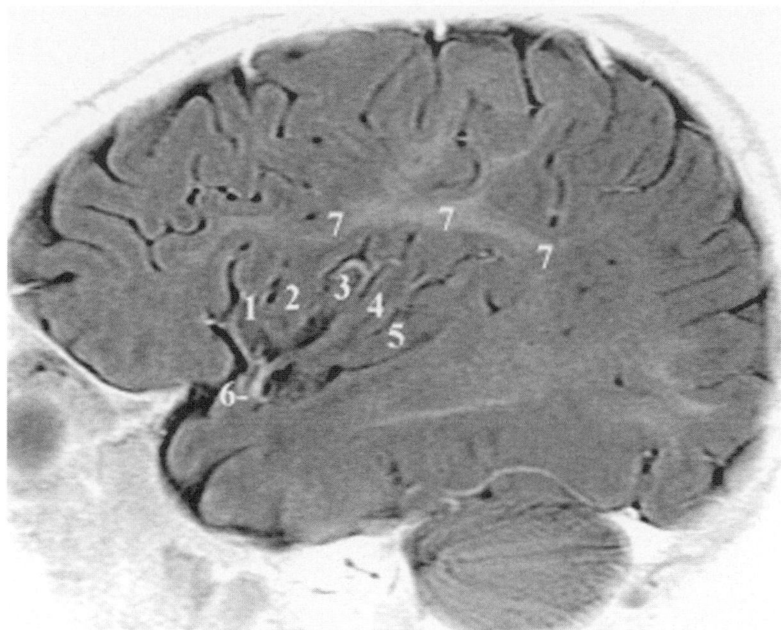

Fig. 5.13. Sagittal MR cut passing through the insula and showing the gyral anatomy of this hidden lobe. (See Fig. 5.10, anatomy of the insula). *1–3*, Short gyri of insula (anterior lobule); *4*, *5* long gyri of insula (posterior lobule); *6*, middle cerebral artery; *7*, myelinated arcuate fasciculus

slightly upward by the presence of Heschl's gyrus (Vlahovitch et al. 1964, 1965, 1970; Szikla et al. 1977).

The last loop of the superior insular line corresponds to Heschl's gyrus. This loop is best seen on axial MR slices oriented along the sylvian CH-PC plane.

E Function of the Insula

The precise role of the insula is unknown since its location does not easily allow cortical stimulation studies. Several reports have implicated the insula in a variety of visceral motor functions, including heart rate, olfaction and taste. A secondary somatosensory area has been described by Penfield and Jasper (1954). Recent evidence suggests that the insula can be functionally divided into an anterior precentral motor area and a posterior somatosensory area. The anterior motor area appears to be associated with motor planning of speech (Fronkers 1996). The posterior postcentral area appears to function as a second somatosensory processing area (Schneider et al. 1993).

III The Anterior Speech Region

The anterior speech region was defined by Broca (1861, 1863, 1865) as including the posterior third of the left inferior frontal gyrus. During his lecture given at the Societe d'Anthropologie de Paris (1863), Broca pointed out the importance of this anatomical region following his observation of motor aphasia subsequent to insults in the posterior extent of the left third frontal convolution in eight consecutive patients. (" *...Ainsi voilà huits faits où la lésion a siégé dans le tiers postérieur de la troisième circonvolution frontale. Ce chiffre me parait suffisant pour donner de fortes présomtions. Et, chose bien remarquable, chez tous ces malades la lésion existait du coté gauche...*").

Extensive cortical stimulation studies by Penfield and Roberts (1959), Penfield and Rasmussen (1950), and Ojemann et al. (1989) have shown marked individual variations in the anterior speech area. Rasmussen defines the speech area as including the pars triangularis and pars opercularis of the dominant frontal lobe. This is concordant with Broca's description. Cortical stimulation and functional imaging studies have shown anterior speech representation outside of the above defined Broca's area.

The anterior speech area includes cytoarchitecturally Brodmann's area 44 and 45. Area 44 is nonexistent in human primates. This speech area is anatomically limited anteriorly by the horizontal ramus of the sylvian fissure and posteriorly by the inferior segment of the precentral sulcus. Posteriorly and inferiorly it is limited by the posterior ramus of the sylvian fissure and superiorly by the inferior frontal sulcus of Broca. Two gyri thus constitute this area, the pars triangularis and the pars opercularis of the inferior frontal lobe (Figs. 5.15–5.19).

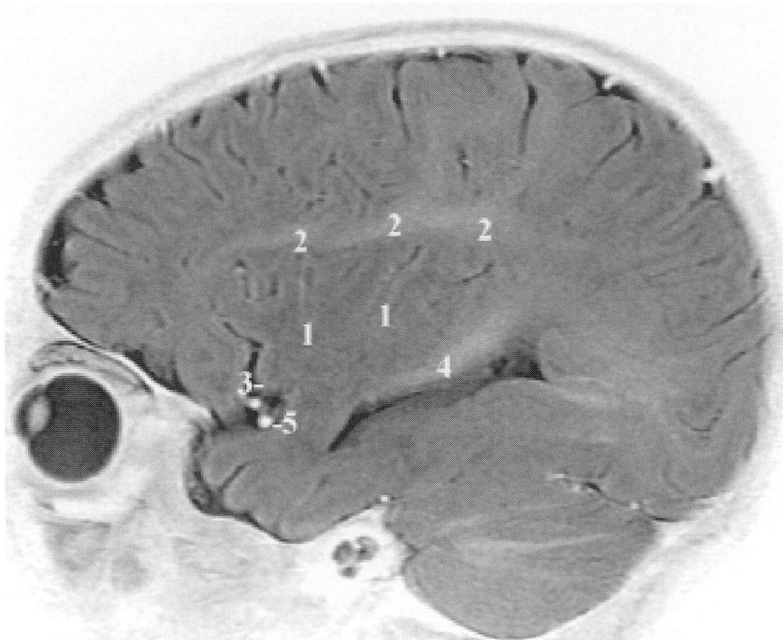

Fig. 5.14. Sagittal MR cut passing through the insula in an infant and showing the myelinated arcuate fasciculus as well as the optic radiation. *1*, Insular cortex; *2*, myelinated arcuate fasciculus; *3*, falciform sulcus; *4*, optic radiations; *5*, middle cerebral artery branches

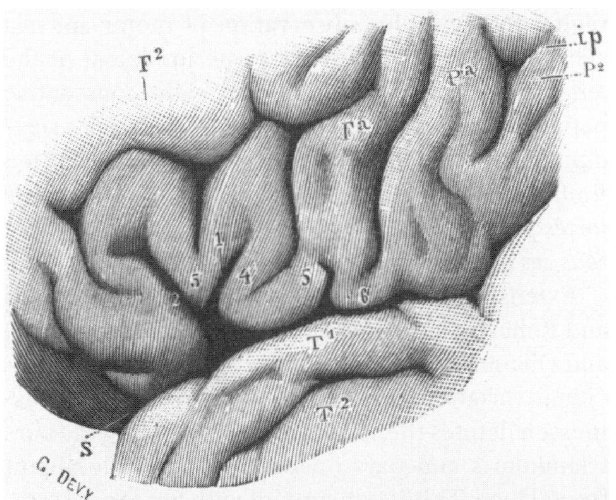

Fig. 5.15. Anatomical drawing of the inferior frontal lobe of the left cerebral hemisphere, showing Broca's area. *1*, Ascending ramus of lateral fissure; *2*, horizontal ramus of lateral fissure; *3*, inferior frontal gyrus, pars triangularis; *4*, inferior frontal gyrus, pars opercularis; *5*, anterior subcentral sulcus; *6*, central operculum (annectant gyrus); *Fa*, precentral gyrus ("frontale ascendante"); *F2*, middle frontal gyrus; *ip*, intraparietal sulcus; *Pa*, postcentral gyrus ("parietale ascendante); *P2*, inferior parietal lobule; *T1*, superior temporal gyrus; *T2*, middle temporal gyrus; *S*, sylvian or lateral fissure. (After Testut and Latarjet 1948)

A Sulcal Anatomy of the Anterior Speech Region

1 The Horizontal Ramus

The horizontal ramus is a deep sulcus originating from the sylvian fissure and cutting through the inferior frontal gyrus mesially, reaching the circular sulcus of the insula at its anterior border. Superiorly it does not reach the inferior frontal gyrus. This ramus is absent on the right in 8% and on the left in 16% of cases, according to Ono et al. (1990).

The horizontal ramus is the anterior border of the pars triangularis, which is limited posteriorly by the vertical ramus of the lateral fissure. In the absence of the horizontal ramus, the presence of a diagonal sulcus may mimic the usual triangular shape of the pars triangularis, however it will not extend to the level of the insula.

2 The Vertical Ramus

The vertical ramus is defined by its extension to the circular sulcus of the insula (Eberstaller 1890; Cunningham 1892). This ramus arises from the sylvian fissure as a separate sulcus and from a common trunk with the horizontal ramus in one third of the cases. It is a constant sulcus, absent in 3% of cases, according to Eberstaller (1890) and Ebeling et al. (1989), and superiorly it does not reach the inferior frontal sulcus.

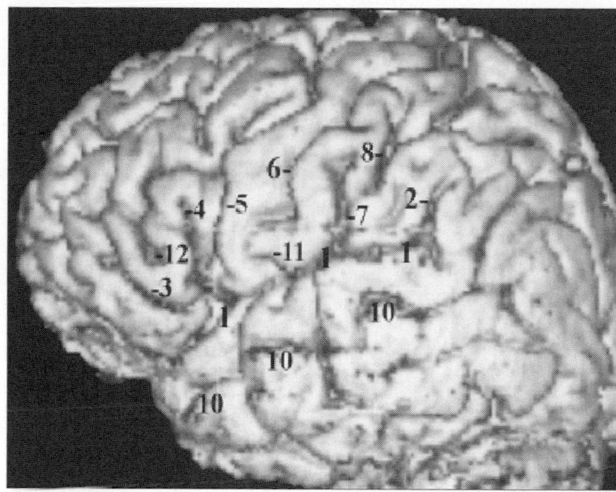

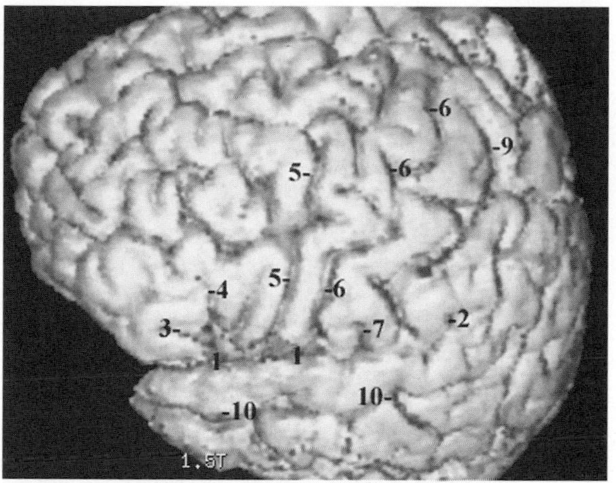

Fig. 5.16A,B. Three-dimensional MR of the lateral surface of the brain showing the sulcal and gyral anatomy of the anterior perisylvian region. *1*, Lateral fissure; *2*, ascending ramus of lateral fissure; *3*, horizontal ramus of lateral fissure; *4*, vertical ramus of lateral fissure; *5*, inferior precentral sulcus; *6*, central sulcus; *7*, posterior subcentral sulcus; *8*, inferior postcentral sulcus; *9*, superior postcentral sulcus; *10*, superior temporal or parallel sulcus

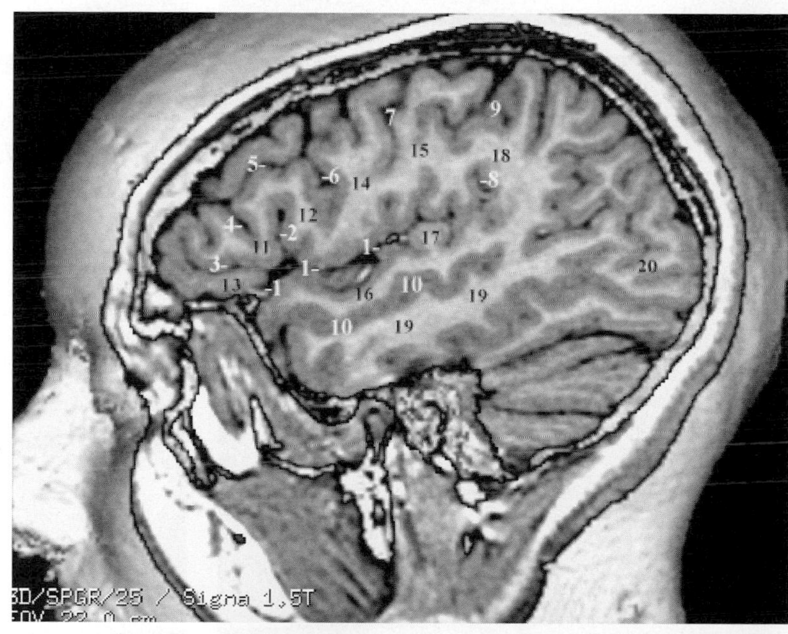

Fig. 5.17. Sagittal MR cut showing the anatomy of the inferior frontal region and Broca's area. *1*, Lateral fissure; *2*, ascending ramus of lateral fissure; *3*, horizontal ramus of lateral fissure; *4*, radiate sulcus; *5*, inferior frontal sulcus; *6*, inferior precentral sulcus; *7*, central sulcus; *8*, terminal ascending branch of lateral fissure; *9*, postcentral sulcus; *10*, parallel sulcus; *11*, inferior frontal gyrus, pars triangularis; *12*, inferior frontal gyrus, pars opercularis; *13*, inferior frontal gyrus, pars orbitalis; *14*, precentral gyrus; *15*, postcentral gyrus; *16*, superior temporal gyrus; *17*, transverse temporal gyrus; *18*, supramarginal gyrus; *19*, middle temporal gyrus; *20*, occipital lobe

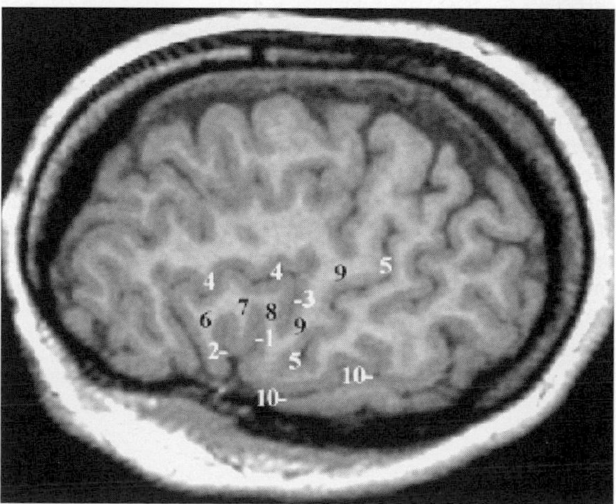

Fig. 5.18. Oblique MR cut, performed parallel to the "forniceal reference plane" displaying the detailed anatomy of the inferior frontal gyrus and Broca's area (7 and 8). *1*, Vertical ascending ramus of lateral fissure; *2*, horizontal ramus of lateral fissure; *3*, inferior precentral sulcus; *4*, inferior frontal sulcus; *5*, central sulcus; *6*, pars orbitalis; *7*, pars triangularis; *8*, pars opercularis; *9*, precentral gyrus; *10*, lateral fissure

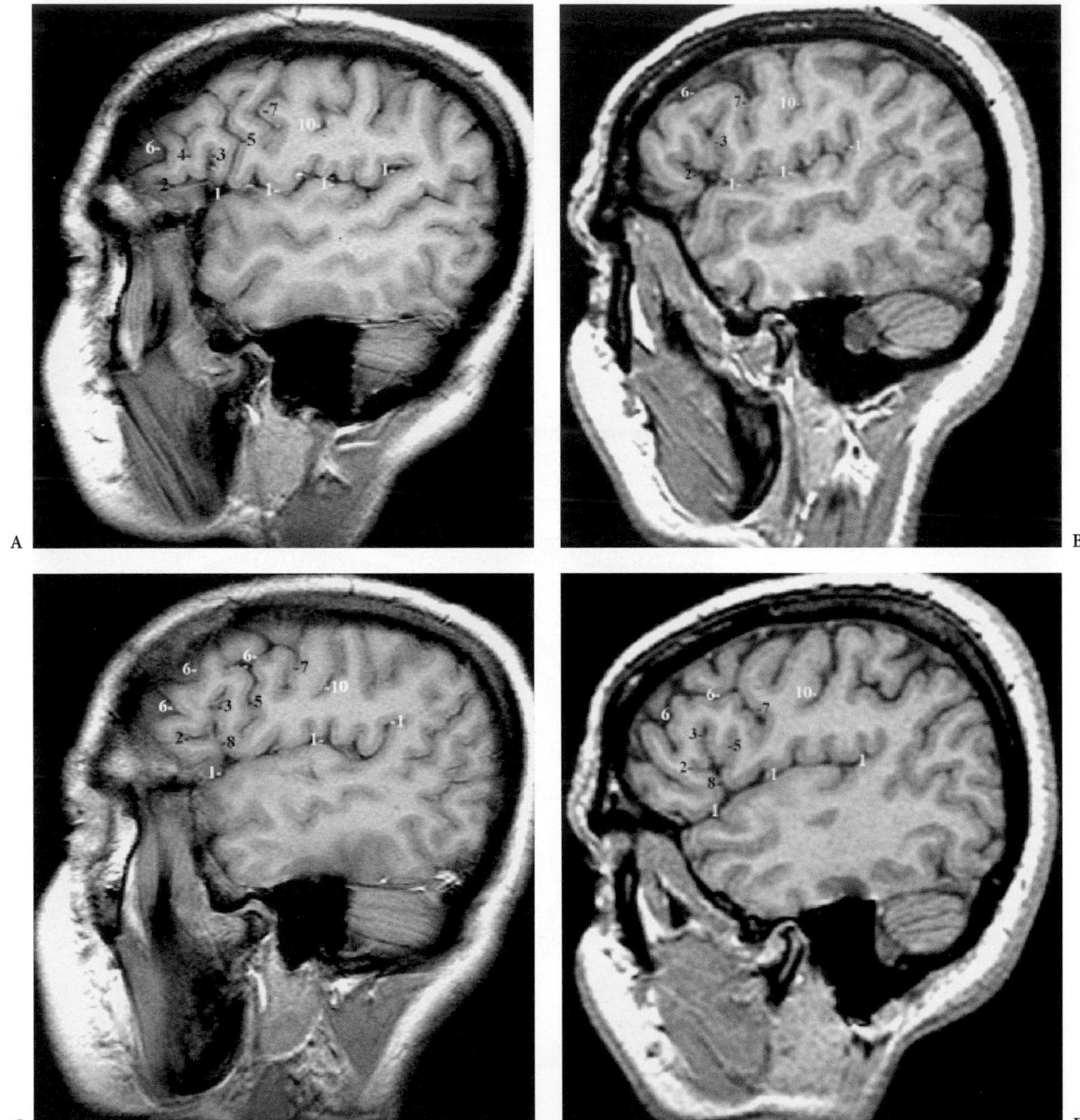

Fig. 5.19A–F. Sagittal MR cuts of the lateral aspect of the cerebral hemisphere showing some of the variations of the sulcal pattern of the inferior frontal region. *1*, Lateral fissure, posterior ramus; *2*, horizontal branch of lateral fissure; *3*, vertical ascending branch of lateral fissure; *4*, radiate sulcus; *5*, diagonal sulcus; *6*, inferior frontal sulcus; *7*, inferior precentral sulcus; *8*, common trunk of horizontal and ascending rami; *9*, anterior subcentral sulcus; *10*, central sulcus. **A** Radiate sulcus cutting into the pars triangularis as the incisura capitis, and diagonal sulcus connected with the posterior ramus of the lateral fissure; **B** bifid ending of both horizontal and vertical rami of the lateral fissure; **C** horizontal and vertical rami of the lateral fissure arising from a common trunk; **D** diagonal sulcus connected with the common trunk of the horizontal and vertical rami; **E** inferior precentral sulcus connected with the posterior ramus of the lateral fissure; **F** diagonal sulcus connected with the common trunk and inferior precentral sulcus connected with the lateral fissure

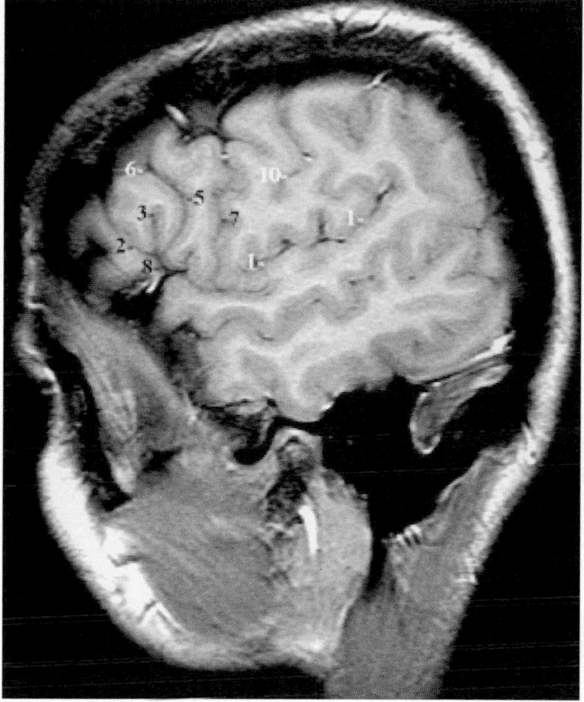

E

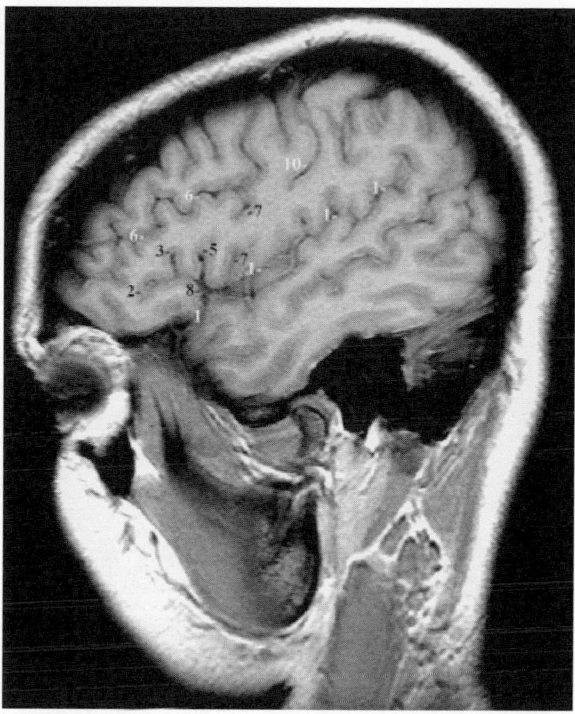

F

Fig. 5.19A–F. Sagittal MR cuts of the lateral aspect of the cerebral hemisphere showing some of the variations of the sulcal pattern of the inferior frontal region. *1*, Lateral fissure, posterior ramus; *2*, horizontal branch of lateral fissure; *3*, vertical ascending branch of lateral fissure; *4*, radiate sulcus; *5*, diagonal sulcus; *6*, inferior frontal sulcus; *7*, inferior precentral sulcus; *8*, common trunk of horizontal and ascending rami; *9*, anterior subcentral sulcus; *10*, central sulcus. **A** Radiate sulcus cutting into the pars triangularis as the incisura capitis, and diagonal sulcus connected with the posterior ramus of the lateral fissure; **B** bifid ending of both horizontal and vertical rami of the lateral fissure; **C** horizontal and vertical rami of the lateral fissure arising from a common trunk; **D** diagonal sulcus connected with the common trunk of the horizontal and vertical rami; **E** inferior precentral sulcus connected with the posterior ramus of the lateral fissure; **F** diagonal sulcus connected with the common trunk and inferior precentral sulcus connected with the lateral fissure

3 The Inferior Precentral Sulcus

The inferior precentral sulcus is an important landmark, representing an extension of the inferior frontal sulcus. This sulcus communicates with the inferior frontal sulcus in 15% of cases according to Cunningham (1892) and in 42% of cases according to Lang et al. (1981). The frequency reported by Ono et al. (1990) is around 25%.

B Gyral Anatomy of the Anterior Speech Region

1 The Pars Triangularis

The pars triangularis is limited anteriorly by the horizontal ramus and posteriorly by the vertical ramus of the sylvian fissure, corresponding to area 45 of Brodmann. It is characteristically U-shaped in the dominant hemisphere and Y-shaped in the nondominant hemisphere. It is traversed superiorly by the incisura capitis branch of the radiate sulcus. The pars triangularis extends deep into the third frontal convolution, reaching the level of the insula.

2 The Pars Opercularis

The pars opercularis is located in between the vertical ramus and the inferior precentral sulcus. It is limited inferiorly by the sylvian fissure, reaching the inferior frontal sulcus superiorly. It communicates with the pars triangularis superiorly and anteriorly. Posteriorly and inferiorly it can communicate with the precentral gyrus. It may be divided into two parts by the diagonal sulcus, as described by Eberstaller (1890). More frequently found on the left than over the right side (72% and 64%, respectively), the diagonal sulcus appears to almost always be connected to the sylvian fissure on the right and only infrequently on the left, according to Ono et al. (1990).

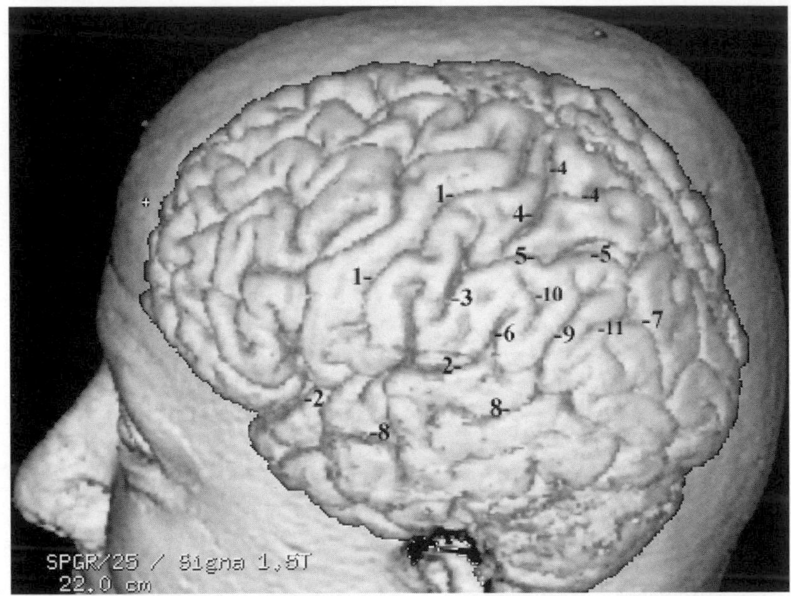

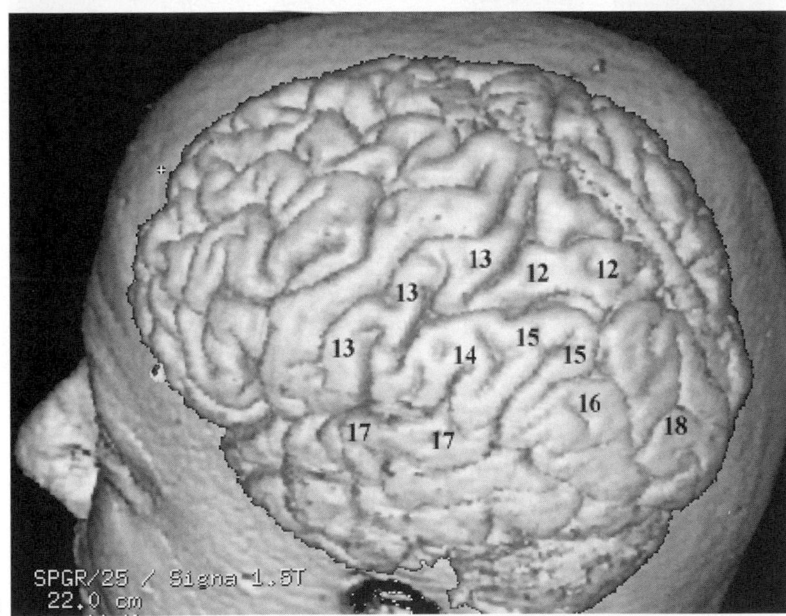

Fig. 5.20A,B. Three-dimensional MR surface rendering of the brain showing the sulcal (**A**) and the gyral (**B**) anatomy of the posterior perisylvian functional temporoparietal region. *1*, Central sulcus; *2*, lateral fissure; *3*, inferior postcentral sulcus, or ascending segment of intraparietal; *4*, superior postcentral sulcus; *5*, horizontal segment of intraparietal sulcus; *6*, terminal ascending branch of lateral fissure; *7*, occipital descending segment of intraparietal sulcus; *8*, parallel sulcus; *9*, terminal ascending branch of parallel sulcus; *10*, sulcus intermedius primus of Jensen; *11*, sulcus intermedius secundus; *12*, superior parietal lobule; *13*, postcentral gyrus; *14*, supramarginal gyrus; *15*, angular gyrus; *16*, posterior parietal gyrus; *17*, superior temporal gyrus; *18*, occipital lobe

Eberstaller (1890) reported that the diagonal sulcus is a shallow sulcus not reaching the entire depth of the gyrus and thus not apparent at the level of the insula.

IV The Posterior Speech Area

Because of its marked variability (Penfield and Roberts 1959), the anatomic localization and extent of the posterior speech area is difficult and can only be determined by cortical stimulation. Recent studies with functional MRI have contributed some insight into the organization and localization of speech (Figs. 5.20–5.25).

Numerous stimulation studies (Fig. 5.24), cortical excisions (Fig. 5.25), and pathological examinations have shown that the receptive speech area is most frequently infrasylvian and includes the posterior extent of the first temporal convolution and the mid- and posterior second temporal gyrus. Speech appears not to extend to the third temporal convolution and is, in some cases, exclusively suprasylvian. Thus it is localized to the supramarginal and angular gyri.

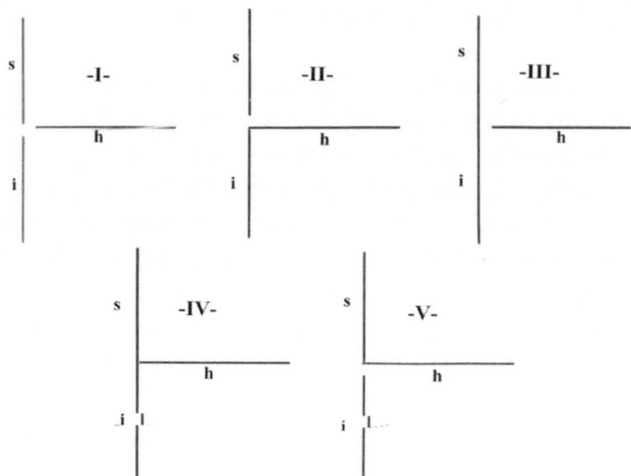

Fig. 5.21. Anatomical variations into five types (I–V) of the intraparietal sulcus (*s*, superior postcentral sulcus; *i*, inferior postcentral sulcus; *h*, horizontal segment of intraparietal sulcus) and their incidence according to Retzius (*R*), Cunningham (*C*) and Jefferson (*J*). *I*, interrupted three i, s, h sulci: R (9); C (6.3); J (35). *II*, Confluence of i and h sulci: R (11); C (19.1); J (26.3). *III*, Continuous postcentral i and s sulcus: R (17); C (11.1); J (25). *IV*, Confluence of the three i, s, h sulci: R (55); C (60.3); J (8.8); *V*, Confluence of s and h sulci: R (4); C (2); J (5). (Modified after Jefferson 1913)

Fig. 5.22. Sulcal patterns of the inferior parietal lobule as shown in four adult hemispheres; the inferior parietal sulcus separates throughout the supramarginal from the angular gyri. *1*, Lateral fissure; *2*, central fissure; *3*, parallel sulcus; *4*, inferior postcentral sulcus; *5*, superior postcentral sulcus; *6*, sulcus parietalis horizontalis (horizontal segment of intraparietal sulcus); *7*, sulcus parietalis inferior; *8*, sulcus parietalis superior; *9*, ascending terminal branch of parallel sulcus; *10*, marginal branch of cingulate sulcus; *11*, parieto-occipital incisure; *12*, sulcus paroccipitalis. (Modified after Jefferson 1913)

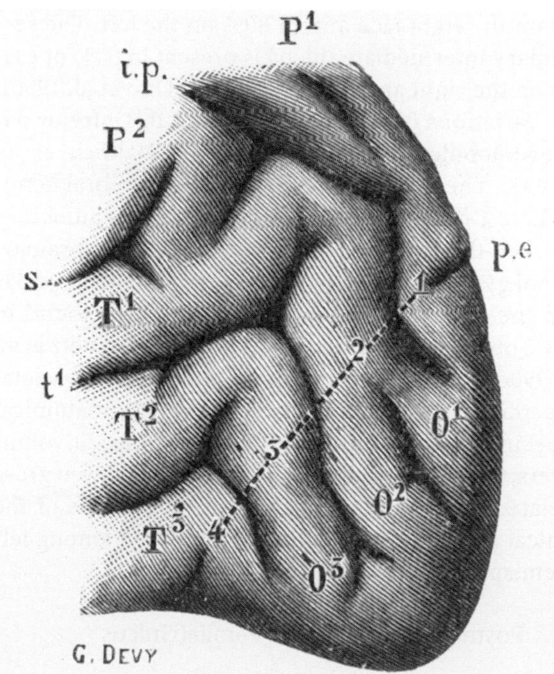

Fig. 5.23. Anatomy of the parieto-occipital region; the four "plis de passage" of Gratiolet. The *dotted line* indicates the direction of the lateral parieto-occipital sulcus (*p.e.*) at the parieto-occipital junction. This line is traversed by the first (*1*) and second (*2*) parieto-occipital "plis de passages" and by the third (*3*) and fourth (*4*) temporo-occipital plis de passages, as defined by Gratiolet. *i.p.*, intraparietal sulcus; S, lateral fissure (Sylvius); *t1*, parallel sulcus; *T1*, superior temporal gyrus; *T2*, middle temporal gyrus; *T3*, inferior temporal gyrus; *P1*, superior parietal lobule; *P2*, inferior parietal lobule; *O1*, superior occipital gyrus; *O2*, middle occipital gyrus; *O3*, inferior occipital gyrus. (After Testut and Latarjet 1948)

A Sulcal Anatomy of the Posterior Speech Area

The sulcal description of this area includes the third segment of the sylvian fissure, the inferior parietal sulci, and the posterior extent of the parallel sulcus.

1 The Third Segment of the Lateral Fissure

Originating at the transverse supratemporal sulcus, it extends to the end of the terminal ascending branch of the sylvian fissure. Included in this seg-

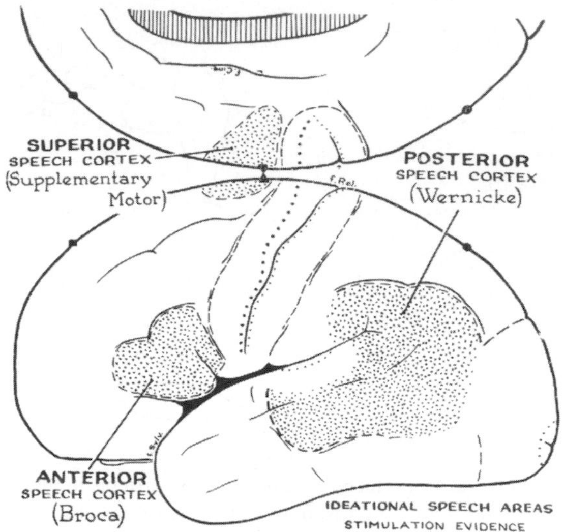

Fig. 5.24. Speech cortical areas: mapping derived from electrical stimulations. (From Penfield and Roberts 1959)

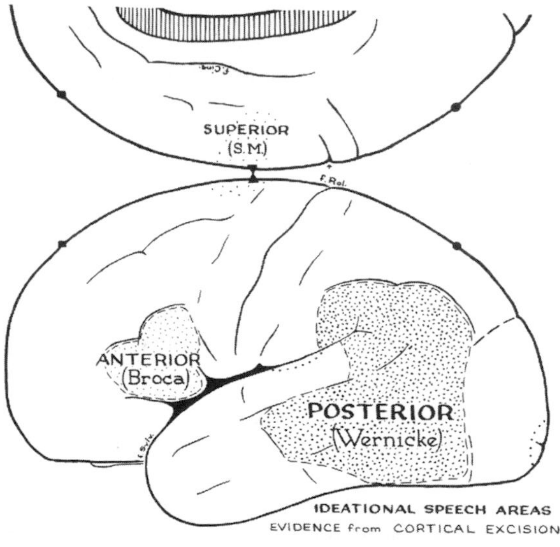

Fig. 5.25. Speech cortical areas: mapping derived from cortical excisions. (From Penfield and Roberts 1959)

ment is the short descending branch. The course and inclination of the third segment correlate with the existence and extent of the temporal planum (Figs. 5.1–5.3, 5.17).

This third segment assumes one of three configurations, described by Witelson and Kigar (1992): type I (H and V type) has a horizontal retrocentral part and an ascending vertical segment; type II (H type) is a horizontal prolongation of the second segment; type III (V type) is characterized by the absence of the horizontal part, the entire segment assuming an ascending direction.

2 The Inferior Parietal Sulci

The sulcal variations of the intraparietal sulcus, according to Jefferson (1913), are depicted in Fig. 5.22, with their respective incidence shown in Fig. 5.21. Recently, Ebeling and Steinmetz (1995), using MRI, found that the postcentral sulcus and the intraparietal joined each other in 77% of the 100 hemispheres studied. Four sulci are important to visualize in delineating this area: the ascending and horizontal parts of the intraparietal sulcus, the third segment of the sylvian fissure and the posterior extent of the parallel sulcus, and the sulcus intermedius primus of Jensen (1870) intervening between the two previously described sulci (refer to Chap. 3).

Eberstaller (1884) divided the inferior parietal lobule into three contiguous arciform convolutions: the supramarginal, the angular, and the posterior parietal, separated by two intermediate sulci. These sulci are not present during late embryonic development but are progressively present during postnatal development, according to Turner (1948). The primary intermediate sulcus (corresponding to Jensen's sulcus intermedius primus) is present in 24% of cases on the right side and in 80% on the left. The secondary intermediate sulcus is present in 64% of cases on the right and 72% on the left (Ono et al. 1990).

Variations of the gyral pattern of the inferior parietal lobule were pointed out by Naidich et al. (1995). These authors reported, in 50 cerebral hemispheres, the presence of accessory supernumerary gyri in the inferior parietal lobule: a presupramarginal gyrus, found in 16% of cases on the left and 4% on the right side, and a preangular gyrus found in 28% on the left and 16% on the right. Steinmetz et al. (1990d) focused on the sulcal pattern of the parietal opercular region. In their study of 80 anatomical specimens and sagittal MR images from 20 volunteers, they found that 38% of the brains showed gross related right-left asymmetry, with variations of the sulcal pattern more frequently observed among left hemispheres.

3 Posterior Extent of the Parallel Sulcus

The first temporal sulcus extends posteriorly past the sylvian fissure, with its terminal segment branching within the temporoparietal area into one or two or more branches. The superior temporal sulcus, or parallel sulcus, terminates in the inferior parietal lobule as the angular sulcus. This terminal ascending branch is the deepest branch, cutting into the inferior parietal lobule. The termination is ascending and

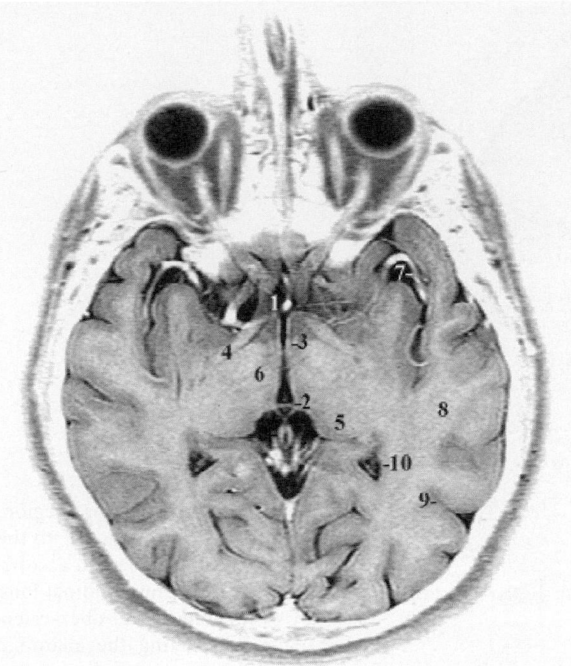

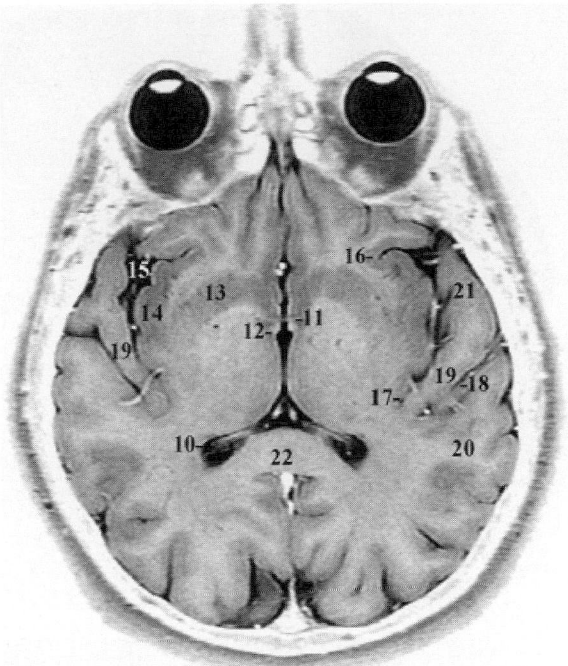

Fig. 5.26A,B. The supratemporal region. Axial MR cuts in the sylvian orientation (CH-PC plane), displaying the anatomic structures found at the reference level, paralleling the superior temporal sulcus (**A**), and at the level of the anterior commissure (**B**), paralleling the supratemporal plane, including the planum polare, Heschl's gyrus, and the planum temporale. *1*, Chiasmal point; *2*, posterior commissure; *3*, mamillary bodies; *4*, cisternal optic tracts; *5*, pulvinar; *6*, midbrain-diencephalic junction; *7*, middle cerebral artery in the sylvian fissure; *8*, superior temporal gyrus; *9*, superior temporal or parallel sulcus; *10*, atrium of lateral ventricle; *11*, anterior commissure; *12*, anterior column of fornix; *13*, striatum (putamen and caudate head); *14*, insula of Reil; *15*, sylvian or lateral fissure; *16*, anterior border of circular sulcus of insula; *17*, posterior of circular sulcus of insula; *18*, posterior transverse supratemporal sulcus (sulcus of Heschl); 19, transverse temporal gyrus or Heschl's gyrus; *20*, planum temporale

single in 56% of cases on the right side and 48% of cases on the left. A double ending is noted in 28% of cases on the right side and 24% of cases on the left side (Ono et al. 1990). When this variation is present, the superior ending is the angular sulcus and the inferior branch corresponds to the anterior occipital sulcus (refer to Chap. 3).

B Gyral Anatomy of the Posterior Speech Area

The posterior speech area includes: Heschl's gyrus, the temporal planum, the parietal operculum, and the parietal and temporal speech related gyri (Figs. 5.10, 5.23, 5.26–5.28).

1 Anatomy of Heschl's Gyrus

Heschl's gyrus is a hidden arch-like gyrus located entirely in the sylvian fissure. The posterior oblique orientation extends within the supratemporal plane from the level of the subcentral region laterally to the retroinsular level medially where it corresponds to the lateral wall of the ventricular atrium. This relationship is seen on axial MR cuts performed in the sylvian orientation, as obtained using the CH-PC reference plane (Tamraz et al. 1990, 1991).

Heschl's gyrus is limited anteriorly and posteriorly by transverse supratemporal sulci. Controversy exists regarding the terminology used by various authors in the denomination of the various sulci that cut the lateral temporal operculum. Holl's (1908) description included: (a) an anterior limiting sulcus separating Heschl's gyrus from the planum polare or the hidden surface of the temporal lobe anterior to Heschl's gyrus; (b) the transverse supratemporal sulcus or Heschl's sulcus separating Heschl's gyri from the planum temporale posteriorly. This sulcus is deep and cuts the lateral aspect of the first temporal convolutions in the anterior and inferior oblique directions. Holl also describes a transverse supratemporal sulcus that occasionally cuts the lateral surface

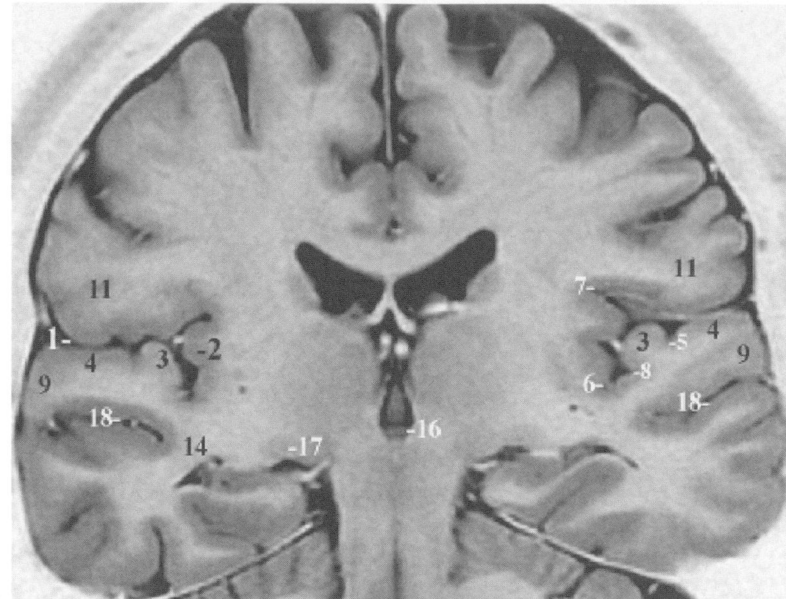

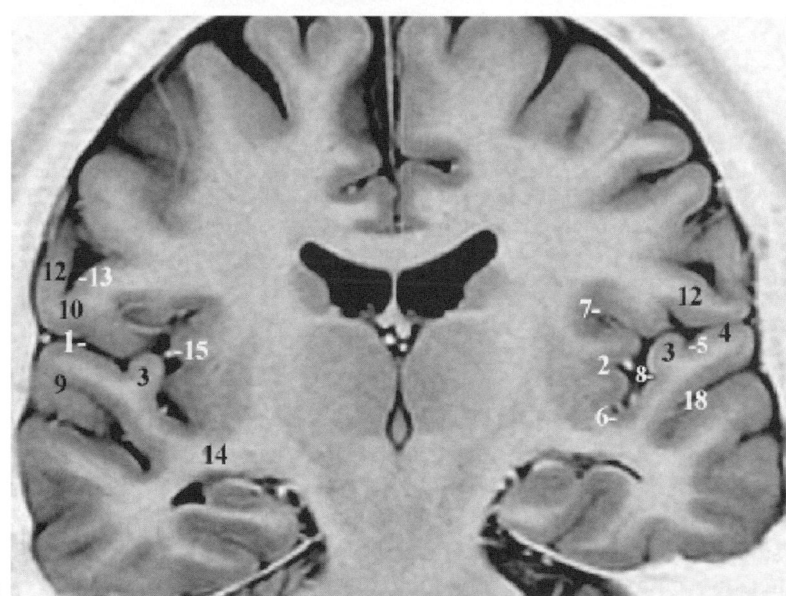

Fig. 5.27A,B. The supratemporal region. Coronal MR cuts, perpendicular to the sylvian fissure plane, oriented according to the brainstem longitudinal long axis (PC-OB, commissural-obex reference plane), displaying the anatomic structures of the retroinsular region, including Heschl's gyrus and temporal planum. **A** Cut through the reference plane; **B** cut anterior to the reference point passing through the whole brainstem. *1*, Sylvian fissure; *2*, insula; *3*, Heschl's gyrus; *4*, planum temporale; *5*, posterior transverse supratemporal sulcus (sulcus of Heschl); *6*, inferior border of circular sulcus of insula; *7*, superior border of circular sulcus of insula; *8*, anterior transverse supratemporal sulcus (anterior limiting sulcus of Holl); *9*, superior temporal gyrus; *10*, central operculum; *11*, inferior end of postcentral gyrus; *12*, inferior end of precentral gyrus; *13*, central sulcus; *14*, temporal stem; *15*, insular branches of middle cerebral artery; *16*, posterior commissure; *17*, lateral geniculate body; *18*, parallel sulcus

and separates the anterior from the posterior Heschl's gyri, when they do exist.

This terminology was, however, not universally used. Niessl Von Mayendorf (1911) described as "sulcus acusticus" any sulcus cutting through the lateral aspect of the temporal lobe in relation to the Heschl area. von Economo and Koskinas (1925) described the sulcus limiting Heschl's gyrus posteriorly as sulcus temporalis profundus secundus, with the sulcus profundus primus corresponding to the intermediate sulcus of Holl. Bailey and von Bonin (1951) adopted a terminology based on three transverse sulci: an anterior, intermediate, and a posterior transverse supratemporal sulci. Szikla et al. (1977), using the Parisiensa Nomina Anatomica, the international nomenclature revised in 1972, used the sulcus temporalis transversus as the posterior limiting sulcus of Heschl's gyrus. More recently, Duvernoy (1991) also adopted the international nomenclature. However, he designated the furrow originating from the parallel sulcus and cutting into the first temporal gyrus, approximately at the level of the central sulcus, as the sulcus acusticus. The Bailey and von Bonin terminology was used more recently by Ono et al.

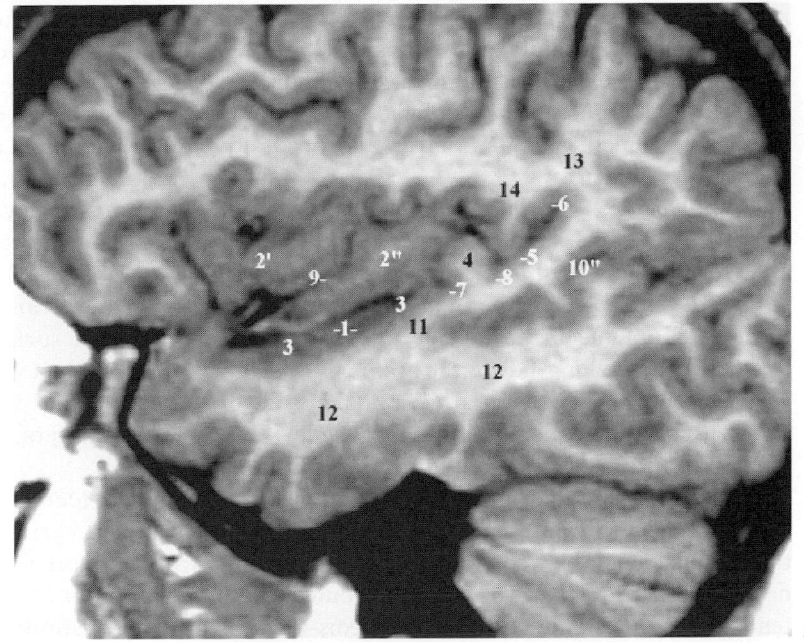

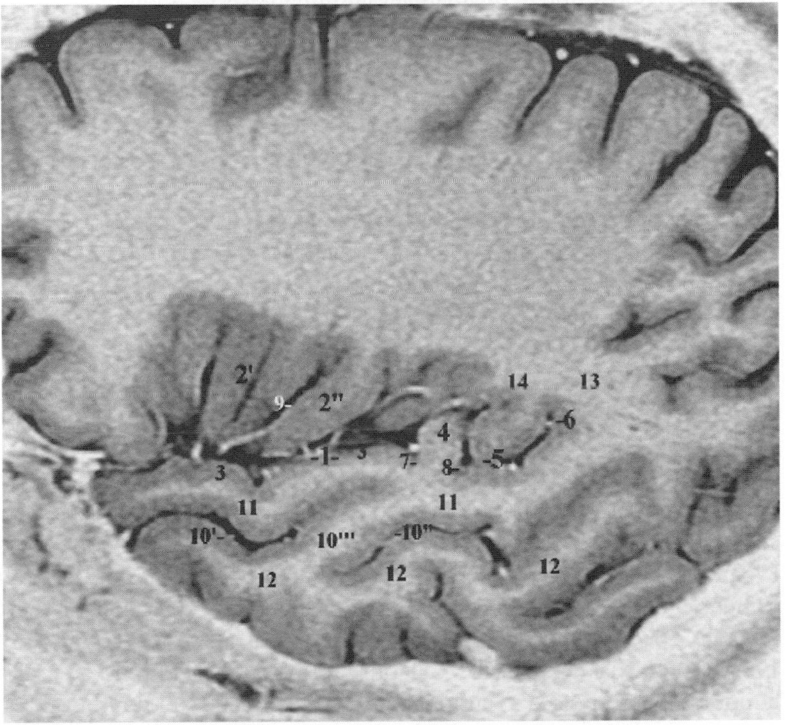

Fig. 5.28 A,B. The supratemporal region. Sagittal (**A**) and sagittal oblique (**B**) MR cuts parallel to the ventricular plane, displaying the regional anatomy of the supratemporal plane at the level of the insula. *1*, Supratemporal plane; *2*, insula; *2'*, anterior lobe (gyri breves); *2''*, posterior lobe (gyri longi); *3*, planum polare; *4*, Heschl's gyrus; *5*, planum temporale; *6*, terminal ascending branch of the lateral fissure; *7*, anterior transverse supratemporal sulcus (anterior limiting sulcus of Holl); *8*, posterior transverse supratemporal sulcus (sulcus of Heschl); *9*, central sulcus of the insula; *10*, parallel sulcus; *10'*, anterior segment; *10''*, posterior segment; *10'''*, "pli de passage"; *11*, superior temporal gyrus; *12*, middle temporal gyrus; *13*, supramarginal gyrus; *14*, angular gyrus

(1990). However, the authors did not define the respective relationship of the transverse temporal sulci to Heschl's gyri or the temporal planum.

In our opinion, the Bailey and von Bonin terminology should be used with the posterior transverse supratemporal sulcus as the most constant sulcus, since it is easily visualized on the lateral surface of the temporal lobe originating from the sylvian fissure with a distinct anterior oblique orientation. This sulcus is located in close proximity to the postcentral sulcus. It separates Heschl's gyri from the planum temporale. In addition, it reaches deep to the level of the insula. The anterior transverse temporal sulcus constitutes the anterior border of Heschl's gyrus. At times, it reaches the lateral aspect of the temporal lobe at the level of the central sulcus. The intermediate sulcus is inconstant and does exist when two Heschl's gyri (mainly on the right side) are noted (Pfeifer 1936). As Duvernoy suggested, in this text we described as sulcus acusticus the furrow which originates from the parallel sulcus and heads towards the Heschl area.

There have been few modern imaging studies of Heschl's gyri. Pfeifer (1936) as well as von Economo and Horn (1930) noted that this gyrus is frequently doubled, even tripled, on the right side and single on the left. It is oblique on the left side, whereas it is perpendicular to the long axis of the brain on the right. Tezner (1972) and Tezner et al. (1972), in a study of 100 anatomical specimens, showed that Heschl's gyri are larger and more obliquely oriented on the left side but shorter on the right side. Although it is assumed that the entire Heschl's gyrus corresponds to the primary auditory cortex, stimulation studies have elicited responses from its posteromedial extent close to the level of the insula (Liegeois-Chauvel et al. 1991). Activation in the primary auditory cortex using functional MR (Binder et al. 1994; Millen et al. 1995; Strainer et al. 1997; Zatorre 1997) seems promising and may increase our knowledge about the function of Heschl's gyri. Strainer et al. (1997), using pure tone activation, showed different tonotopic organization within Heschl's gyri, depending on the frequency of the auditory stimulus: responses elicited for tones in the lower frequencies (1000 Hz) predominated in the lateral transverse temporal gyrus, while those of higher frequencies (4000 Hz) appear localized in the medial transverse temporal gyrus.

2 Anatomy of the Temporal Planum

Studied initially by von Economo and Horn (1930) and subsequently by others (Pfeifer 1936; Geschwind and Levitsky 1968; Tezner et al. 1972; Witelson and Kigar 1992; Wada et al. 1975; Szikla et al. 1975; Rubens et al. 1976; Rubens 1977; Yeni-Komshian and Benson 1976; Galaburda et al. 1978a,b, Falzi et al. 1982, Galaburda et al. 1987, Galaburda 1993), the temporal planum is a triangular cortical surface, apparent as early as the 29th week of gestation (Larroche 1967). It is limited laterally by the sylvian fissure and anteriorly by the posterior transverse supratemporal sulcus, or Heschl's sulcus. Its posterior limit is not well defined. Habib et al. (1983a,b, 1984) and Steinmetz et al. (1989, 1990a,b) considered the terminal descending branch of the sylvian fissure as the posterior limit. In the absence of this branch, the temporal planum includes the entire supratemporal extent of the third division of the sylvian fissure. Because of the fusion of the posterior parietal operculum with the temporal planum, this posterior border is frequently curvilinear in shape. Cytoarchitecturally it corresponds to the posterior portion of area 22 of Brodmann and to area TA of von Economo and Koskinas (1925).

In most individuals, the left temporal planum is wider than its right-sided counterpart and is formed by several small gyri which assume a superior oblique orientation. The right-side planum has a smaller cortical surface and a flat surface (Szikla et al. 1977; Habib et al. 1984).

3 Imaging of the Posterior Speech Area

Imaging identification of the posterior speech area has been carried out extensively by Salamon and collaborators (Habib et al. 1984; Gelbert et al. 1986; Salamon et al. 1987; Rumeau et al. 1988) using the bicommissural AC-PC coordinates. The authors demonstrated that the perisylvian cortical speech area and the inferior parietal lobule may be reliably explored using a limited number of cuts (four slices, 5 mm thick), oriented parallel to the bicommissural plane, and performed at 45 and 50 mm above the reference line, to display the posterior part of the first and second temporal gyri, and at 60 and 70 mm, to explore the supramarginal and angular gyri (Salamon et al. 1987).

Using MRI, the temporal planum is best explored in the coronal plane perpendicular to the sylvian CH-PC reference as obtained using the PC-OB reference plane (See Chap. 2). This coronal approach permits identification of the sylvian fissure followed on more posterior sections on the left and located higher on the right. It also allows a direct evaluation of the entire depth of the planum as well as an easy depiction of Heschl's gyri, shown on both sides as the floor of the sylvian fissure. The axial cuts performed parallel to the CH-PC plane (Figs. 5.4; 5.5), which corresponds to the sylvian fissure orientation plane (Tamraz et al. 1990, 1991), best evaluate the supratemporal region displaying, from anterior to posterior, the gyral anatomy of the planum polare, the transverse temporal or Heschl's gyri, and posteriorly the temporal planum (Fig. 5.6,5.26).

V The Cerebral Asymmetries

Dominance of the left cerebral hemisphere for speech was noted early in the nineteenth century by

Marc Dax in 1836, promoter of the concept of speech localization in the left hemisphere (Dax 1865), followed by Paul Broca (1865) and Wernicke (1874), according to Alajouanine (1968).

Several attempts to correlate functional asymmetry of the human brain with morphological difference have been undertaken (Kakeshita 1925; von Economo and Horn 1930; Pfeifer 1936). Initial attempts focused on weight (Rey 1885; Charpy 1889; Moutier 1908; Broca 1875) and length (Charpy 1889; Cunningham 1892; Smith 1907; Inglessis 1919; Connolly 1950) differences between right and left hemispheres. Kakeshita initiated the study of opercular asymmetries in 1925. This work was largely ignored until the landmark contribution of Geschwind and Levitsky (1968).

- Ontogenesis of cerebral asymmetries: Asymmetric development of the hemispheres is apparent as early as the 29th week of gestation (Larroche 1967). Wada et al. (1975) demonstrated, in a study of 100 fetuses, that the left temporal planum was larger than the right in 67% of the specimens. Chi et al. (1977) showed that Heschl's gyrus developed 1 or 2 weeks earlier on the right side and was noted to be larger on the right in 54% of specimens.
- Asymmetries of speech related areas: The motor speech area of Broca is localized to the pars triangularis and opercularis of the third frontal convolution. Eberstaller (1884) noted that the pars opercularis was more frequently large on the left side. Wada et al. (1975), however, found a right-sided predominance. Falzi et al. (1892) found no asymmetry when measurements were taken on the outer hemispheric surface. However, planimetric studies of the total gyral surface showed a significant difference in volume, with the left being larger than the right. Recently, Comair et al. (1996) correlated speech dominance and MR based volumetric analysis of the Broca area. Left-sided speech dominance was associated with a larger pars opercularis on the same side. This asymmetry was not substantiated in patients with bilateral or right-sided speech dominance.

Sylvian fissure morphology and asymmetry was also investigated by Eberstaller (1890), who reported that the left sylvian fissure was 6.4 mm longer, on average, than the right. This was verified subsequently by Rubens (1977) and Witelson and Kigar (1992). These latter authors showed that there was strong correlation between the anatomy of the sylvian fissure in men and handedness. This correlation was, however, absent in women. The slope of the third segment of the sylvian fissure was noted as early as 1892 by Cunningham to be sharper on the right side. Multiple studies have again demonstrated this finding.

Since the temporal planum can be easily defined morphologically and radiologically using angiography (Le May and Gulebras 1972; Szikla et al. 1977), and MRI, this area has received much attention. Planimetric studies were initiated by von Economo and Horn (1930) and subsequently by Geschwind and Levitsky (1968), and others (Tezner et al. 1972; Witelson and Pallie 1973; Szikla et al. 1975; Wada et al. 1975; Rubens et al. 1976; Yeni-Komshian and Benson 1976; Rubens 1977; Kopp et al. 1977; Falzi et al. 1982; Jack et al. 1988). These authors have shown 60% (von Economo 1930) to 84% (Yeni-Komshian and Benson 1976) larger surface on the left as compared to the right side.

In vivo MRI of the planum temporale in musicians demonstrated a marked leftward asymmetry in individuals with musical ability (Schlaug et al. 1995). Neuroimaging studies showed global as well as regional brain pathologic findings in schizophrenic patients. Global abnormalities consisted of large lateral ventricles associated with enlargement of the subarachnoid spaces (Kelsoe et al. 1988; Gur et al. 1991). Regional morphometric studies of the brain disclosed more specific lobar or gyral abnormalities, such as a decreased volume of the temporal (Dauphinais et al. 1990) or the frontal lobe (Andreasen et al. 1986) and, more specifically, the medial limbic structures including the amygdala-hippocampal complex and the parahippocampal gyrus (Bogerts et al. 1990; Barta et al. 1990; Shenton et al. 1992). Barta et al. (1990) showed a correlation between a reduction in volume of the left superior temporal gyrus and the significance of auditory hallucinations, and Shenton et al. (1992) reported evidence of an anatomic clinical relationship between a decrease in volume of the posterior aspect of the left superior temporal gyrus and thought disorder. Asymmetrical anatomic findings were also reported by Turetsky et al. (1995), correlating a decrease in volume of the left temporal lobe with clinical negative symptoms in a study of 71 patients. MR morphometric study of 15 sets of monozygotic twins discordant for schizophrenia showed a smaller anterior hippocampus on the left side in 14 cases. The authors concluded that an anatomic, asymmetrical abnormality is a consistent pathologic feature of the disease (Suddath et al. 1990). Further data are needed to confirm the consistency of clinical imaging correlations and to evaluate more precisely the exact significance of the lateralized and focal anatomic abnormalities, as compared to the diffuse brain changes. Larger sample sizes, the use of high resolution MR imaging, and precise morphometric and methodological criteria may help in understanding the different findings.

References

Alajouanine T (1968) L'aphasie et le langage pathologique. Baillière, Paris

Andreasen NC, Nasrallah HA, Dunn V, Olson SC, Grove WM, Ehrhardt JC, Coffman JA, Crossett JHW (1986) Structural abnormalities in the frontal system in schizophrenia: a magnetic resonance imaging study. Arch Gen Psychiatry 43: 136–144

Bailey P, von Bonin G (1951) The isocortex of man. Univ. Illinois Press, Urbana, Ill

Barta PE, Pearlson GD, Powers RE, Richards SS, Tune LE (1990) Auditory hallucinations and smaller superior temporal gyral volume in schizophrenia Am J Psychiatry 147: 1457–1462

Binder JR, Rao SM, Mammeke TA, et al. (1994) Functional magnetic resonance imaging of human auditory cortex. Ann Neurol 35: 662–672

Binder JR, Rao SM, Hammeke TA, Frost JA, Bandettini PA, Jesmanowicz A, Hyde JS (1995) Lateralised human brain language systems demonstrated by task subtraction functional magnetic resonance imaging. Arch Neurol 52: 593–601

Binder JR, Swanson SJ, Hammeke TA, Morris GL, Mueller WM, Fischer M, Benbadis S, Frost JA, Rao SM, Haughton VM (1996) Determination of language dominance using functional MRI: a comparison with the Wada test. Neurology 46:978–984

Bogerts B, Ashtari M, Degreet G, Alvir JM, Bilder RM, Lieberman JA (1990) Reduced temporal limbic structure volumes on MRI in first episode schizophrenia Psychiatry Res Neuroimaging 35: 1–13

Broca P (1861a) Perte de la parole, ramollissement chronique et destruction partielle du lobe antérieur gauche du cerveau. Société d'Anthropologie. Bull SocAnthropol 11:235–238

Broca P (1861b) Remarques sur le siège de la faculté du language articulé, suivies d'une observation d'aphémie (perte de la parole) Bull Soc Anat 36: 330–357

Broca P (1861c) Nouvelle observation d'aphémie produite par une lésion de la moitié postérieure des deuxième et troisième circonvolutions frontales. Bull Soc Anat 6: 398–407

Broca P (1863) Localisation des fonctions cérébrales – siège du langage articulé. Bull Soc Anthropol Paris 4: 200–208

Broca P (1865) Du siège de la faculté du langage articulé dans l'hémisphère gauche du cerveau. Bull Soc Anthropol VI: 377–393

Broca P (1875) Instructions craniologiques et craniometriques de la Societe d'Anthropologie de Paris. Bull Soc Anthropol 16: 534–536

Charpy A (1889) Cours de splanchnologie. Les centres nerveux. Guillau, Montauban

Chen CY, Zimmerman RA, Faro S, Parrish B, Wang Z, Bilaniuk LT, and Chou TY (1995) MR of the cerebral operculum: topographic identification and measurement of interopercular distances in healthy infants and children. AJNR 16: 1677–1387

Chi Je G, Dooling EC, Gilles FH (1977) Gyral development of the human brain. Ann Neurol 1: 86–93

Choi H, Comair YG, Najm I, Chung C, Siemionow V, Luders H, Ruggieri P (1996) Non invasive method of hemispheric lateralization for language in patients with intractable epilepsy. Epilepsia 37 [Suppl] 5: 207

Connolly CJ (1950) External morphology of the primate brain. Thomas, Springfield, Ill

Dauphinais D, Delisi LE, Crow TJ, Alexandropoulos K, Colter N, Tuma I, Gershon ES (1990) Reduction in temporal lobe size in siblings with schizophrenia: a MRI study. Psychiatry Res Neuroimaging 35: 137–147

Dax M (1865) Lesions de la moitie gauche de l'encéphale coincidant avec l'oubli des signes de la pensee. Gazette Hebdo Med Chir 33: 259

Duvernoy H (1991) The human brain, surface, three dimensional sectional anatomy and MRI. Springer, Vienna

Eberstaller O (1884) Zur Oberflächenanatomie der Grosshirnhemisphären. Wien Med Bl 7

Eberstaller O (1890) Das Stirnhirn. Ein Beitrag zur Anatomie des Oberfläche des Großhirns. Urban and Schwarzenberg, Vienna

Ebeling U, Steinmetz H, Huang Y, Kahn T (1989) Topography and identification of the inferior precentral sulcus in MR imaging. AJNR 10: 937–942

Ebeling U, Steinmetz H (1995) Anatomy of the parietal lobe: mapping the individual pattern. Acta Neurochir Wien 136 (1–2): 8–11

Economo C von, Koskinas GN (1925) Die Cytoarchitektonik der Hirnrinde des erwachsenen Menschen. Springer, Vienna,

Economo C von, Horn L (1930) Ueber Windungsrelief, Masse und Rindenarchitektonik der Supratemporalfläche, ihre individuellen und ihre Seitenunterschiede. ZGes Neurol Psychiatrie 130: 678–757

Falzi G, Perrone P, Vignolo LA (1982) Right-left asymmetry in anterior speech region. Arch Neurol 39: 239–240

FitzGerald DB, Rees G, Cosgrove GR, Ronner S, Jiang H, Buchbinder BR, Beliveau JH, Rosen BR, and Benson RR (1997) Location of language in the cortex: a comparison between functional MR imaging and electrocortical stimulation. AJNR 18:1529–1539

Fronkers NF (1996) A new brain region for coordinating speech articulation. Nature 384: 159–160

Galaburda AM, Le May M, Kemper TL, Geschwind N (1978) Right-left asymmetries in the brain. Science 199: 852–856

Galaburda M, Sanides F, Geschwind N (1978) Human brain – cytoarchitectonic left-right asymmetries in the temporal speech region. Arch Neurol 35:3–7

Galaburda AM (1980) La région de Broca: Observations anatomiques faites un siècle après la mort de son découvreur. Rev Neurol 136:609–616

Galaburda AM (1993) The planum temporale. Arch Neurol 50: 457

Galaburda AM, Corsiglia J, Rosen GD, Sherman G F (1987) Planum temporale asymmetry: reappraisal since Geschwind and Levitsky. Neuropsychologia 25 (6): 853–868

Gelbert F, Bergvall U, Salamon G, Sobel D, Jiddane M, Corbaz JM, Morel M (1986) CT identification of cortical speech areas in the human brain. J Computer Assist Tomogr 10(1): 39–46

Geschwind N, Levitsky W (1968) Human brain: left-right asymmetries in temporal speech region. Science 161: 186–187

Gur RE, Mozley PD, Resnik SM, Shtasel D, Kohn M, Zimmerman R, Herman G, Atlas S, Grossman R, Erwin R, Gur RC (1991) MRI in schizophrenia. I Volumetric analysis of brain and cerebrospinal fluid. Arch Gen Psychiatry 48: 407–412

Habib M, Renucci RL, Corbaz JM, Salamon G, Gouaze A (1983a) Computed tomography localization of visual and auditory primary cortex. Otoneuroophtalmol 55:39–46

Habib M, Renucci RL, Corbaz JM, Salamon G, Gouaze A (1983b) Reperage en tomodensitométrie des aires corticales visuelle et auditive primaires. Rev Otoneuroophtalmol 55:39–46

Habib M, Renucci RL, Vanier M, Corbaz JM, Salamon G (1984) CT assessment of right-left asymmetries in the human cerebral cortex. J Comput Assist Tomogr 8(5):922–927

Hecaen H ,Albert ML (1978) Human neuropsychology. Wiley, New York

Hertz-Pannier L, Gaillard WD, Mott SH, Cuenod CA, Bookheimer SY, Weinstein S, Conry J, Papero PH, Schiff SJ, Le Bihan D, Theodore WH (1997) Noninvasive assessment of language dominance in children and adolescents with functional MRI: A preliminary study. Neurology 48: 1003–1012

Heschl RL (1878) Uber die vordere quere Schläfenwindung des menschlichen Grosshirns. Braumuller, Vienna

Holl M (1908) Die Insel des Menschen und Affenhirns in ihrer Beziehung zum Schläfenlappen. Sitz Ber D k Akad Wiessensch Wien, Math Naturw Kl 117:365–410

Inglessis M (1919) Einiges über Seitenventrikel und Hirnschwellung. Arch Psychiatrie 74:159–168

Jack CR, Gehring DG, Sharbrough FW, Felmlee JP, Forbes G, Hench VS, Zinsmeister AR (1988) Temporal lobe volume measurement from MR images. Accuracy and left-right asymmetry in normal persons. J Comput Assist Tomogr 12:21–29

Jefferson G (1913) The morphology of the sulcus interparietalis. J Anat Physiol 47:365–380

Jensen J (1870) Die Furchen und Windungen der menschlichen Grosshirnhemispharen. Allg Z Psychiatrie 27:473–515

Kakeshita T (1925) Zur anatomie der operkularen temporal region (Vergleichende Untersuchung der rechten und linken seite) Arbeiten aus dem Neurologischen Institut an der Wiener Universität, 27:292–326

Kelsoe JR, Cadet JL, Pickar D, Weinberger DR (1988) Quantitative neuroanatomy in schizophrenia: a controlled MRI study. Arch Gen Psychiatry 43:136–144

Kimura D (1983) Sex differences in cerebral organization for speech and praxic functions. Can J Psychol 37:19–35

Kodama K (1934) Beitrage zur Anatomie des Zentralnervensystems der Japaner. VIII. Insula Reilii. Fol Anat Japon 12:423–444

Kopp N, Michel F, Carrier H, Biron A, Duvillard P (1977) Etude de certaines asymetries hemispheriques du cerveau humain. J Neurol Sci 34:349–363

Lang J, Betz J (1981) Form und Masse der Gyri und Sulci an der Facies superolateralis und Facies inferior hemispherii. J Hirnforsch 22:517–533

Larroche JC (1967) Maturation morphologique du système nerveux central: ses rapports avec le développement pondéral de foetus et son âge gestationnel. In: Minkowski M (ed) Regional development of the brain in early life. Davis, Philadelphia, pp 247–256

Le May M, Gulebras A (1972) Human brain morphologic differences in the hemispheres demonstrable by carotid angiography. N Engl J Med 287:168–170

Liegeois-Chauvel C, Musolino A, Chauvel P (1991) Localization of the primary auditory area in man. Brain 114:139–153

Ludwig E, Klingler J (1956) Atlas cerebri humani. Karger, Basel

McGlone J (1978) Sex differences in functional brain asymmetry. Cortex 14:122–128

Millen SJ, Haughton VM, Yetkin Z (1995) Functional magnetic resonance imaging of the central auditory pathway following speech and pure-tone stimuli. Laryngoscope 105:1305–1310

Milner B, Branch C, Rasmussen T (1964) Observations on cerebral dominance. In: de Reuck AVS, O'Connor M (eds) Disorders of language. Churchill, London, pp 200–222

Milner B (1973) Hemispheric specialization: scope and limits. In: Schmitt FO, Worden FG (eds) The neurosciences: third study program. MIT Press, Boston

Moutier (1908) L'aphasie de Broca. Steinheil, Paris

Naidich P, Valavanis G, Kubik S (1995) Anatomic relationships along the low-middle convexity. I. Normal specimens and magnetic resonance imaging. Neurosurgery 36 (3):517–531

Niessl von Mayendorf E (1911) Die aphasischen Symptome und ihre corticale Lokalisation. Engelmann, Leipzig

Ojemann G, Ojemann J, Lettich E, Berger M (1989) Cortical language localization in left, dominant hemisphere: an electrical stimulation mapping investigation in 117 patients. J Neurosurg 71:316–326

Ono N, Kubik S, Abernathy DG (1990) Atlas of the cerebral sulci. Thieme, Stuttgart

Penfield W, Rasmussen T (1950) The cerebral cortex of man. Macmillan, New York

Penfield W, Jasper H (1954) Epilepsy and the functional anatomy of the human brain. Little, Brown, Boston

Penfield W, Roberts L (1959) Speech and brain – mechanisms. Princeton Univ. Press, Princeton, NJ

Pfeifer RA (1936) Pathologie der Hörstrahlung und der corticalen Hörsphäre. In: Bumke O, Foerster O (eds) Handbuch der Neurologie. vol 6. Springer, Berlin, p 533

Rey P (1885) Du poids des lobes cérébaux. Rev Anthropol 8:385–396

Rubens AB, Mahowald MW, Hutton JT (1976) Asymmetry of the lateral (sylvian) fissures in man. Neurology 22:620–624

Rubens AB (1977) Anatomical symmetries of human cerebral cortex. In: Harnard S, Doty RW, Jaynes J, Goldstein L, Krauthammer G (eds) Lateralization in the nervous system. Academic, New York, pp 329–336

Rumeau C, Gouaze A, Salamon G, Laffont J, Gelbert F, Einseidel H, Jiddane M, Farnarier P, Habib M, Perot S (1988) Identification of cortical sulci and gyri using magnetic resonance imaging: a preliminary study. In: Gouaze A, Salamon G (eds) Brain anatomy and magnetic resonance imaging. Springer, Berlin Heidelberg New York, pp 11–32

Salamon G, Gelbert F, Alicherif A, Poncet M, Khalil R, Sobel D, Von Einseidel O, Morel M, Corbaz JM (1987) Le repérage in vivo des aires corticales du langage. Rev Neurol (Paris) 143:8–9, 580–587

Schlaug G, Jancke L, Huang Y, Steinmetz H (1995) In vivo evidence of structural brain asymmetry in musicians. Science 267:699–701

Schlesinger B (1953) The insulo-opercular arteries of the brain with special reference to angiography of striothalamic tumor. Am J Roentgenol 70:555–563

Schneider R, Friedman DP, Mishkin M (1993) Brain Res 621:116–120

Shenton M, Kikinis R, Jolesz F, Pollak S, Lemay M, Wible C, Hokama H, Martin J, Metgale D, Coleman M, McCarley R (1992) Abnormalities of the left temporal lobe and thought disorder in schizophrenia. A quantitative MRI study. N Engl J Med 327: 604–612

Steinmetz H, Rademacher J, Huang Y, et al. (1989) Cerebral asymmetry: MR planimetry of the human planum temporale. J Comput Assist Tomogr 13:996–1005

Steinmetz H, Volkmann J, Janke L, Freund HJ (1990a) Anatomical left-right asymmetry of language-related temporal cortex is different in left and right handers. Ann Neurol 29:315–319

<referSteinmetz H, Rademacher J, Janke L, et al. (1990b) Total surface of temporoparietal intrasylvian cortex: diverging left-right asymmetries. Brain Lang 39:357–372

Steinmetz H, Fürst G, Freund H-J (1990c) Variation of perisylvian and calcarine anatomic landmarks within stereotaxic proportional coordinates. AJNR 11:1123–1130

Steinmetz H, Ebeling U, Huang YX, Kahn T (1990d) Sulcus topography of the parietal opercular region and MR study. Brain Lang 38(4):513–533

Strainer JC, Ulmer JL, Zerrin Yetkin F, Haughton VM, Daniels DL, Millen SJ (1997) Functional MR of the primary audi

Tamraz J, Saban R, Reperant J, Cabanis EA (1990). Definition d'un plan de référence céphalique en imagerie par résonance magnétique: le plan chiasmato-commissural. CR. Acad Sci Paris 311(III):115-121

6 Limbic Lobe and Mesial Temporal Region

I The Limbic Lobe or "Grand Lobe Limbique"

A Morphology and Topographical Anatomy

The limbic lobe, corresponding to the "grand lobe limbique" of Paul Broca, the French anthropologist and neurosurgeon who described it, includes anatomical structures bordering the diencephalon, as its name suggests (limbus meaning border in Latin). Phylogenetically, the anatomic structures which constitute the limbic lobe are very old. Ontogenetically, the arch convolution constituting the limbic lobe at the inferomedial aspect of the cerebral hemisphere is limited continuously by major primary sulci represented mainly by the cingulate sulcus or the "scissure limbique" of Broca (1978) dorsally and ventrally, the collateral sulcus posteriorly and the rhinal sulcus anteriorly. These sulci laterally limit the uncus and the parahippocampal gyrus, which curves posteriorly through the narrow isthmus around the splenium of the corpus callosum covering and surrounding it completely. It is separated from the corpus callosum by the callosal sulcus. Anteriorly, below the rostrum, it merges with the paraterminal gyrus, which corresponds to the prehippocampal rudiment, immediately in front of the lamina terminalis. Starting in the subcallosal region, the limbic lobe structures, which may be observed with MR (Fig. 6.1), encircle the upper brainstem and the corpus callosum as the subcallosal, cingulate, parahippocampal and hippocampal, and dentate gyri (Figs. 6.2–6.5).

Extensive research was triggered following the report by Papez (1937) of the important role of the limbic lobe in emotional behavior. The addition of anatomic structures functionally related to the limbic lobe led MacLean (1952) to propose in extenso the generic term of "limbic system". The structures include the septal nuclei, the hypothalamus, the epithalamus, various thalamic subnuclei, parts of the basal ganglia, and the rostral mesencephalon (Carpenter 1996). However, much controversy still remains concerning the concept of a limbic system (Kotter and Meyer 1992; Isaacson 1992). Despite the heterogeneity of these related structures, it is clear that they are to some extent involved in a neural circuitry subserving visceral, olfactory and memory, and learning functions.

B Imaging of the Limbic Lobe

The anatomic structures of this continuous limbic belt are mostly found on the paramedial aspect of both cerebral hemispheres, encircling and bordering the corpus callosum and the upper brainstem. The inferior arch of the limbic belt, comprising the hippocampal formation and the parahippocampal gyrus, is hidden by the brainstem.

Imaging of the limbic structures has dramatically improved with the advent of high resolution MRI. Despite the computing capabilities which make vol-

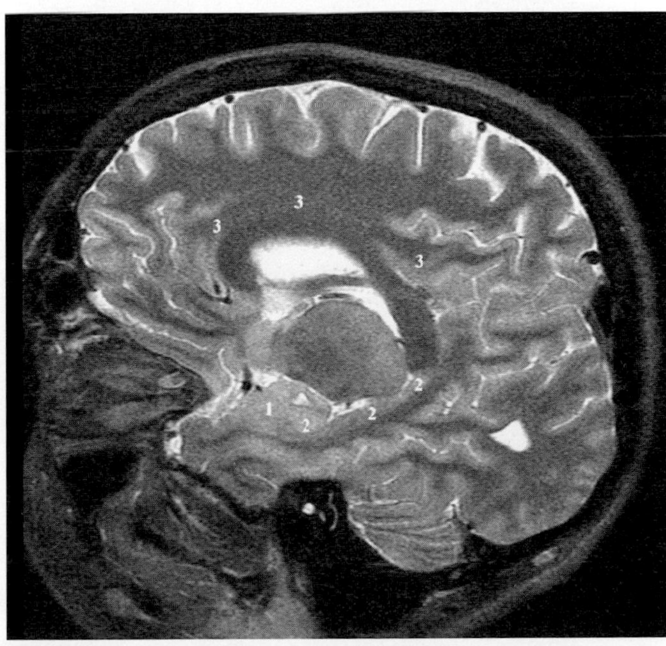

Fig. 6.1. The limbic lobe: MR oblique cut of the brain displaying the major anatomical components composing the limbic belt. *1*, Amygdala; *2*, hippocampus; *3*, cingulate gyrus

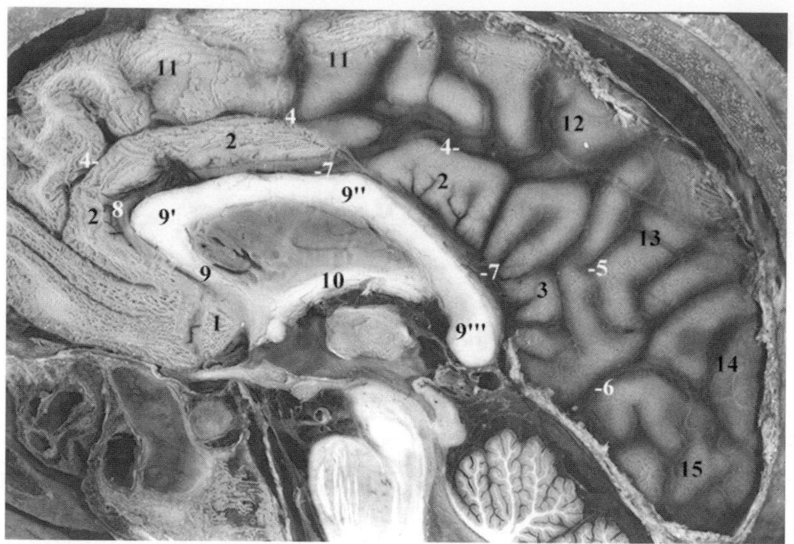

Fig. 6.2. Sagittal anatomical cut of the cerebral hemisphere. *1*, Subcallosal gyrus; *2*, cingulate gyrus; *3*, subparietal gyrus; *4*, cingulate sulcus; *5*, subparietal sulcus; *6*, anterior calcarine sulcus; *7*, callosal sulcus; *8*, pericallosal artery; *9*, corpus callosum, rostrum; 9', genu; 9'', body; 9''', splenium; *10*, fornix; *11*, medial frontal gyrus; *12*, paracentral lobule; *13*, precuneus; *14*, cuneus; *15*, lingual gyrus

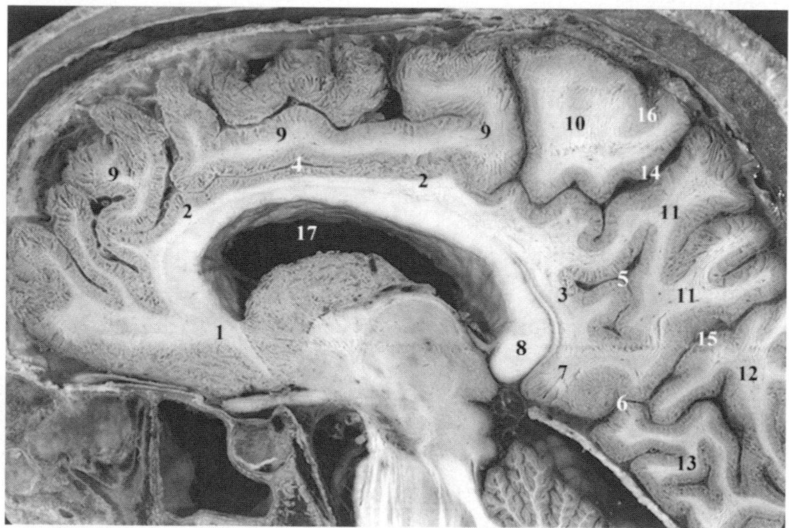

Fig. 6.3. Parasagittal anatomical cut of the cerebral hemisphere. *1*, Subcallosal gyrus; *2*, cingulate gyrus; *3*, subparietal gyrus; *4*, cingulate sulcus; *5*, subparietal sulcus; *6*, anterior calcarine sulcus; *7*, isthmus; *8*, splenium of corpus callosum; *9*, medial frontal gyrus; *10*, paracentral lobule; *11*, precuneus; *12*, cuneus; *13*, lingual gyrus; *14*, marginal ramus of cingulate sulcus; *15*, parieto-occipital sulcus; *16*, central sulcus; *17*, lateral ventricle

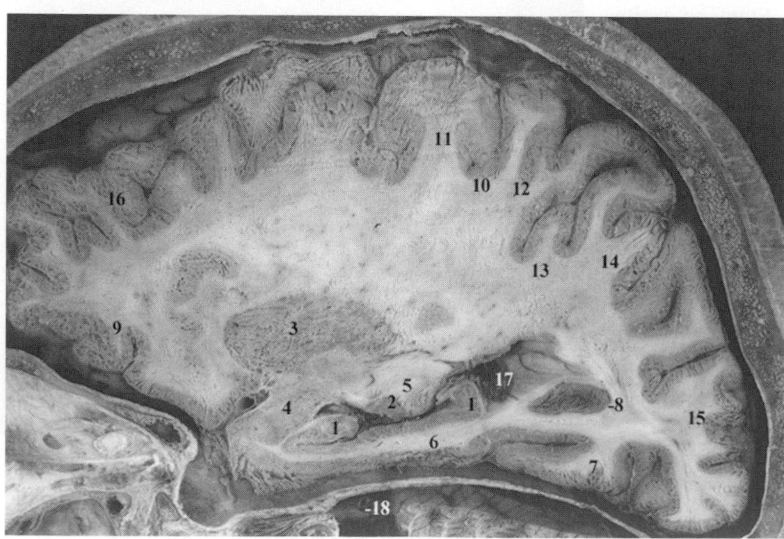

Fig. 6.4. Lateral sagittal anatomic cut of the cerebral hemisphere passing through the hippocampal formation and amygdala at the level of the lateral geniculate body. 1, Hippocampus; 2, lateral geniculate body; 3, lentiform nucleus; 4, amygdala; 5, area triangularis of Wernicke; 6, parahippocampal gyrus; 7, fusiform gyrus; 8, anterior calcarine sulcus; 9, medial orbital gyrus; 10, central sulcus; 11, precentral gyrus; 12, postcentral gyrus; 13, intraparietal sulcus; 14, inferior parietal lobule; 15, occipital lobe; 16, middle frontal gyrus; 17, atrium of lateral ventricle; 18, trigeminal nerve root

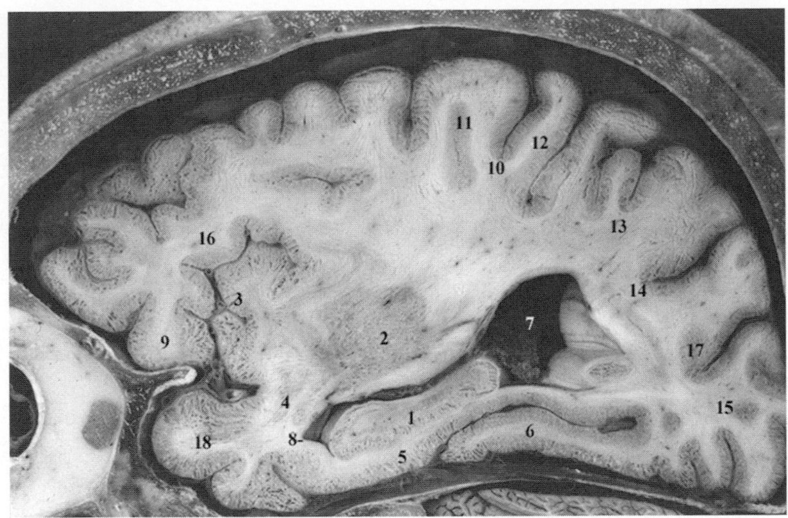

Fig. 6.5. Lateral sagittal anatomic cut of the cerebral hemisphere passing through the hippocampal formation and the temporal stem at the level of the inferior ventricular horn. 1, Hippocampus; 2, putamen; 3, insula; 4, temporal stem; 5, parahippocampal gyrus; 6, fusiform gyrus; 7, atrium of lateral ventricle; 8, temporal horn of lateral ventricle; 9, lateral orbital gyrus; 10, central sulcus; 11, precentral gyrus; 12, postcentral gyrus; 13, inferior parietal lobule; 14, intraparietal sulcus; 15, occipital lobe; 16, inferior frontal gyrus; 17, parieto-occipital sulcus; 18, temporal pole

umetric rendering widely available, this has not aided in the visualization of the limbic structures because of the low contrast resolution and the inability to extract the hippocampus and the core brain structures from the overlying anatomy.

Coronal slices performed according to the PC-OB reference plane (see Chap. 2) are essential for volumetric analysis of the amygdala-hippocampal complex.

1 The "Forniceal Plane"

Embryologically, the fornices together with the choroidal fissures develop along an oblique plane with a complex arciform course. This shape is focused on by temporalization of the brain. Since temporalization involves growth along multiple axes, the resulting shapes are less than ideally studied for the traditional axial, coronal, and sagittal imaging approaches.

Imaging along the "forniceal plane" was therefore attempted. This plane is defined as a line joining the lateral part of the fimbria fornix in the hippocampus with the lateral aspect of the crus fornicis. These structures are visualized on the coronal PC-OB reference plane (Fig. 6.6A–D).

Serial oblique section planes are then acquired or reformatted, parallel to the forniceal plane as defined above, to cover the entire mesial temporal lobe and extend to the convexity. Our protocol involves the successive acquisition of 30 2-mm contiguous slices on either side of the brain.

This reference plane appears especially interesting for the study of hippocampal, amygdala, and temporal polar cortex formation. In addition, the core brain structures are seen from mesial to lateral in the first 20 slices. These core structures are visualized along the plane of development. They include the choroidal fissure, thalamus, caudate, lenticular nucleus, insula, cingulate gyrus, and corpus callosum. The drawback of this plane of study is the visualization of part of the contralateral hemisphere in the same slice. In our series this was not, however, a marked inconvenience.

We have found the lateral slices particularly helpful for the study of the central brain region. These slices produce an unfolding of the complex sulcal geometry of this region. The frontal lobe perisylvian convolutions are well depicted, facilitating the understanding of the sulcal and gyral anatomy of this region (see Sect. 10.III). In our hands, the acquisition along the forniceal plane can replace the sagittal acquisition.

II Anatomy of the Mesial Temporal Region

The anatomy of this region is particularly complex and is composed of the temporal pole, the amygdala, the hippocampus, parahippocampal (Figs. 6.7, 6.8), and certain cortical areas related to these structures.

A The Temporal Polar Cortex

The temporal polar cortex (Fig. 6.9) corresponds to area 38 of Brodmann (1909), or area TG as defined by von Bonin and Bailey (1947). Its cytoarchitectural characteristics have been defined by Insausti (1998). Anatomically, this area corresponds to the temporal

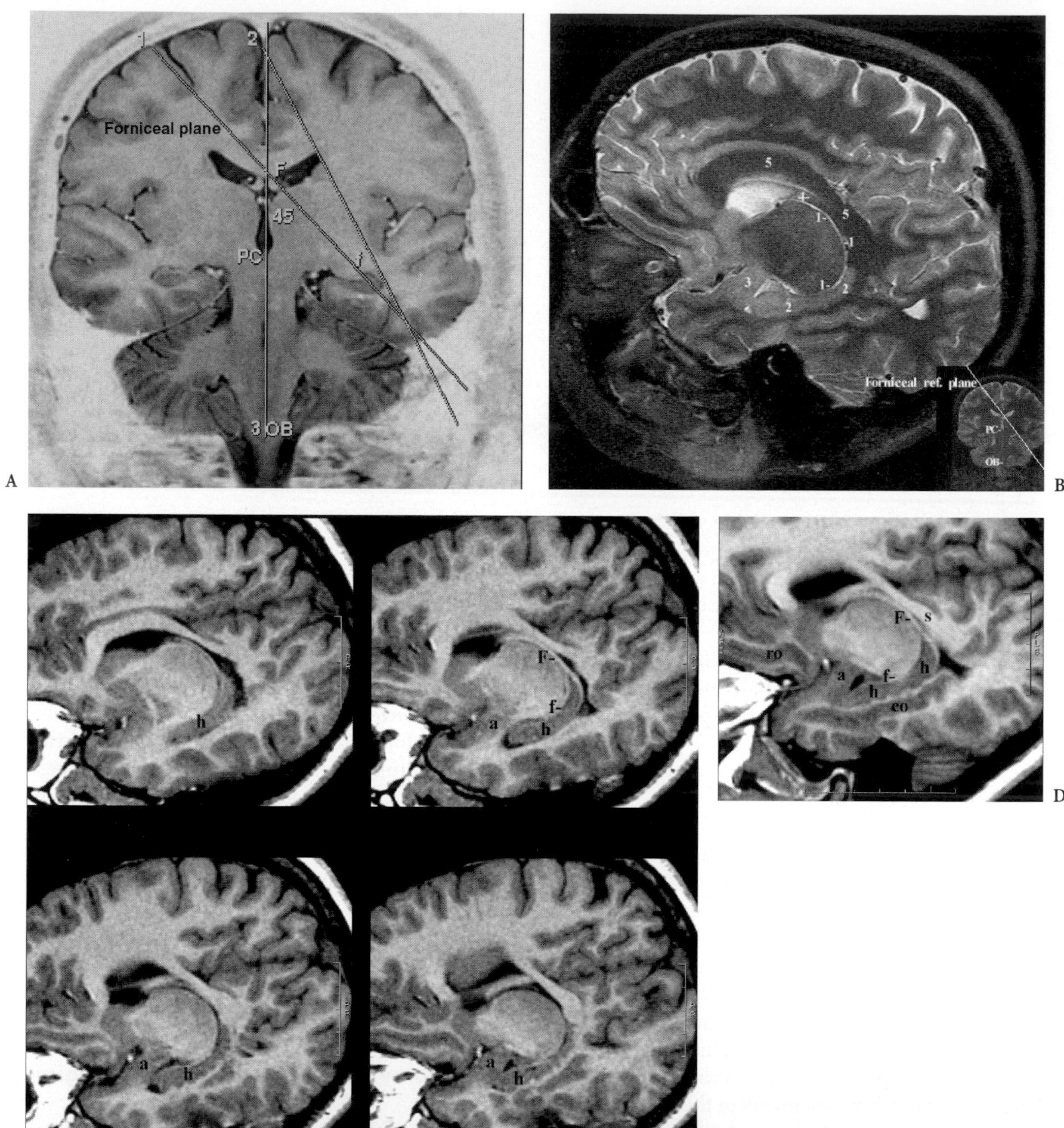

Fig. 6.6A–D. The forniceal plane. **A** Projection of the forniceal reference plane (*1*) on the PC-OB coronal reference plane. This plane is compared with another oblique plane tangential to the outer borders of the lateral ventricle (*2*) which is suitable for the study of the perisylvian cortex. **B** The forniceal plane; anatomic correlation using MR, displaying the choroidal fissure (STIR, T2 weighted sequence, 3 mm thick). **C** The forniceal plane; contiguous slices, showing the major anatomic structures of the limbic lobe, as displayed using this particular oblique orientation of the MR reformatted cuts (SPGR, T1 weighted, 2 mm thick). **D** The forniceal plane; the fimbria fornix continuum as well as the amygdala-hippocampal complex are nicely displayed in a single oblique cut (2 mm). F, crus fornicis; *f*, fimbria; *a*, amygdala; *h*, hippocampus; *co*, collateral sulcus; *ro*, rostral sulcus; *s*, splenium

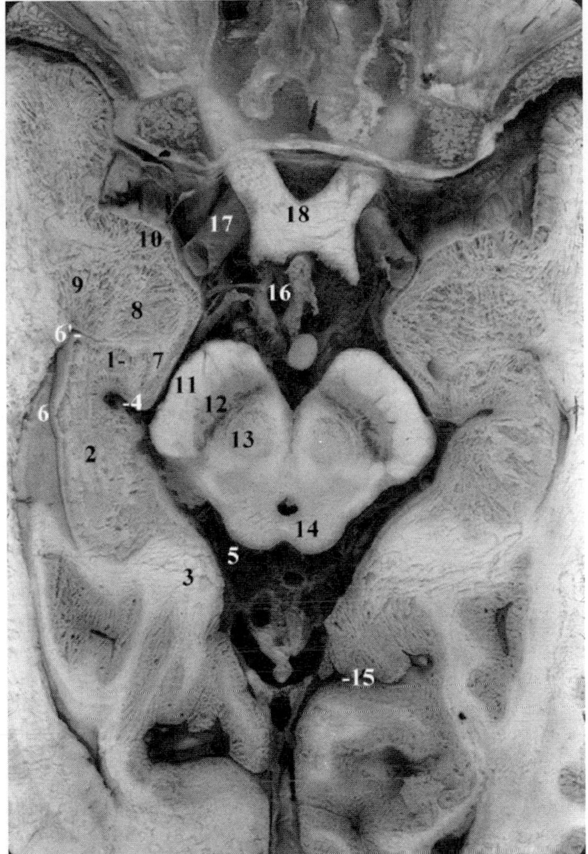

Fig. 6.7. Axial anatomic cut through the hippocampal formation and amygdala. *1*, Hippocampal head (digitations); *2*, hippocampal body; *3*, parahippocampal gyrus; *4*, hippocampal sulcus; *5*, ambient cistern; *6*, temporal horn; *6'*, uncal recess; *7*, gyrus uncinatus; *8*, basal nucleus of amygdala; *9*, lateral nucleus of amygdala; *10*, gyrus ambiens; *11*, crus cerebri; *12*, substantia nigra; *13*, red nucleus; *14*, superior colliculus; *15*, collateral sulcus; *16*, chiasmal cistern; *17*, internal carotid artery; *18*, optic chiasm

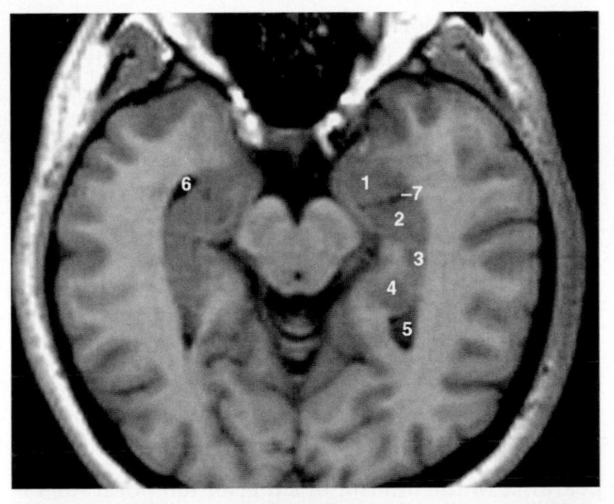

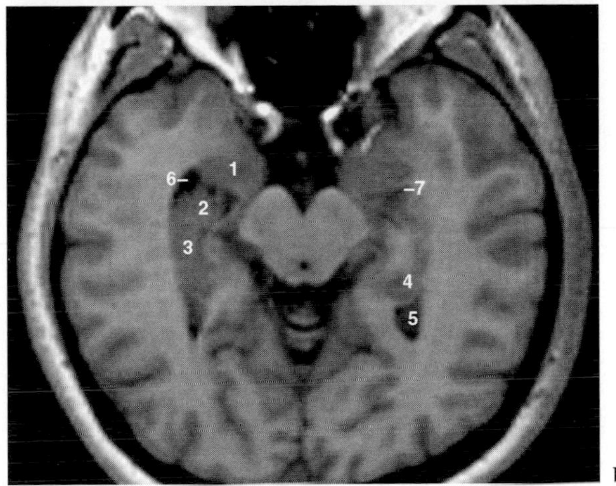

Fig. 6.8A,B. Axial MR cuts parallel to the CH-PC reference plane and passing through the hippocampus-amygdala complex (3D SPGR-T1 weighted, 3 mm thick). *1*, Amygdala; *2*, hippocampus, head; *3*, hippocampus, body; *4*, hippocampus, tail; *5*,atrium of lateral ventricle; *6*, temporal (inferior) horn of lateral ventricle

Fig. 6.9. Lateral sagittal anatomic cut through the hippocampus displaying its internal structure. *1*, Hippocampus; *1'*, cornu ammonis, hippocampal head; *1''*, cornu ammonis, hippocampal body; *1'''*, subiculum; *2*, gyrus dentatus, hippocampal head; *2'*, gyrus dentatus; hippocampal body; *3*, fimbria; *4*, optic radiations; *5*, putamen; *6*, claustrum; *7*, insula; *8*, endorhinal sulcus; *9*, amygdala, lateral nucleus; *10*, parahippocampal gyrus; *11*, fusiform gyrus; *12*, tail of caudate nucleus; *13*, collateral sulcus; *14*, atrium of lateral ventricle; *15*, calcar avis; *16*, lateral orbital gyrus; *17*, pterion; *18*, temporal fossa; *19*, internal capsule, retrolentiform part; *20*, choroid plexus; *21*, circular sulcus of insula; *22*, bifurcation and insular branches of middle cerebral artery; *23*, temporal horn of lateral ventricle; *24*, collateral trigone

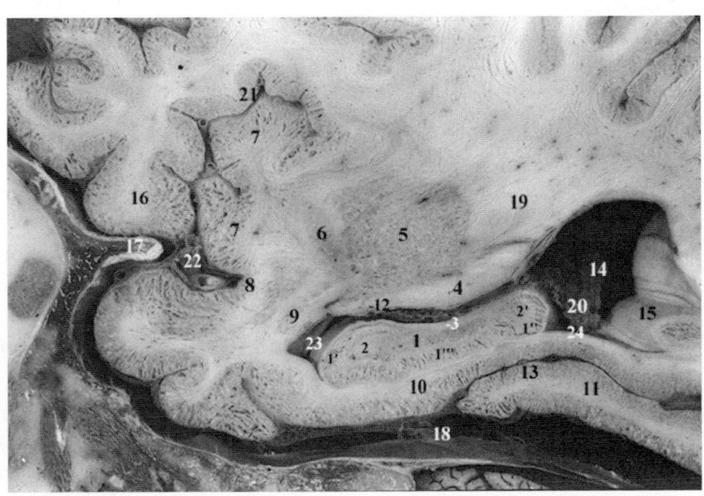

pole. The temporal pole, extending from the tip of the temporal lobe laterally and ventrolaterally to the level of the superior or inferior temporal gyri, is characterized by the appearance of the superior or inferior temporal sulci. Ventromedially, the temporal polar cortex blends with the perirhinal area and dorsally extends to the level of the limen insulae. The temporal pole displays three surfaces: dorsal, lateral, and mesial. One or two sulci, known as the transverse polar sulci, lie across the dorsal aspect in an anterior-posterior direction. They delineate one or two transverse temporal gyri, the gyri of Schwalbe. When it exists, the lateral polar gyrus separates the temporal polar cortex from the neocortex. Ventrally, the appearance of the inferior or superior temporal sulci is considered as a limit of the temporal polar cortex, the latter ending ventromedially at the level of the collateral sulcus.

B The Entorhinal Area

The entorhinal area occupies most of the anterior extent of the parahippocampal gyrus and extends dorsomedially to the peri-amygdaloid cortex (area 28 of Brodmann) (Figs. 6.10, 6.11). Caudomedially, it reaches the presubiculum and laterally extends into the medial bank of the collateral sulcus.

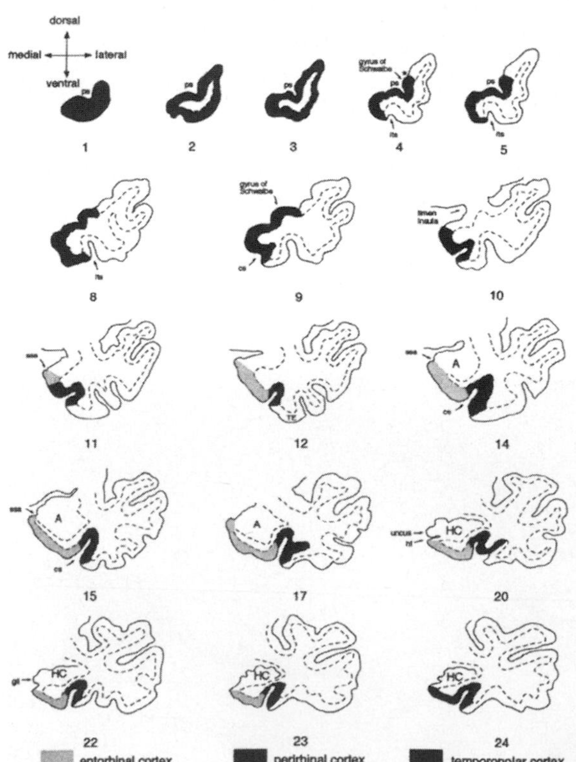

Fig. 6.10. The entorhinal, perirhinal and temporal polar cortex. (From Insausti et al. 1998)

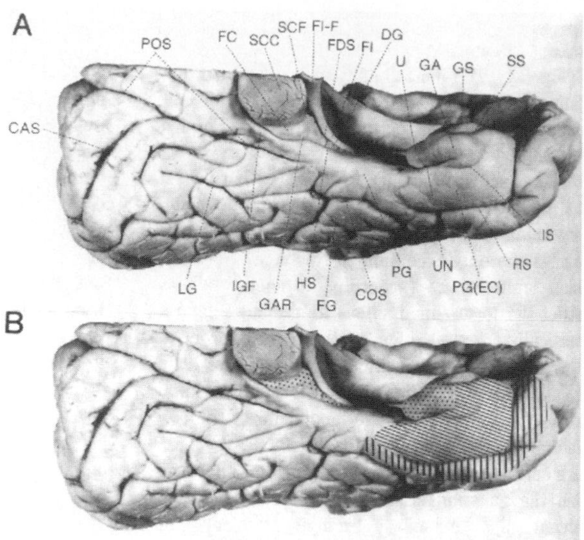

Fig. 6.11A Gyri and sulci of the left mesial temporal cortex. *CAS*, Calcarine sulcus; *COS*, Collateral sulcus; *DG*, Dentate gyrus; *FC*, Fasciola cinerea; *FDS*, Fimbrio-dentate sulcus; *FG*, fusiform gyrus; *FI*, fimbria; *FI-F*, fimbria-fornix transition; *GA*, gyrus ambiens; *GAR*, gyri of Andres Retzius; *GS*, gyrus semilunaris; *HS*, hippocampal sulcus; *IGF*, isthmus of gyrus fornicatus; *IS*, intrarhinal sulcus; *LG*, lingual gyrus; *PG*, parahippocampal gyrus; *PG(EC)*, parahippocampal gyrus (entorhinal cortex part); *POS*- parieto-occipital sulcus; *RS*, rhinal sulcus; *SCC*, splenium of corpus callosum; *SCF*, subcallosal flexure of dentate gyrus; *SS*, sulcus semiannularis; *U*, uncus; *UN*, uncal notch. **B** Components of the mesial temporal region: hippocampal cortex *(dotted)*, entorhinal cortex *(oblique hatching)* and perirhinal cortex *(vertical hatching)*. (from: Gloor, 1997, The temporal lobe and limbic system, Fig. 5-4, p. 330; Oxford University Press, New York)

The entorhinal area extends rostrally from the level of the limen insulae and medially to the peri-amygdaloid cortex. It is separated from the amygdala by the sulcus semiannularis. Its extension over the uncus includes the ambient gyrus and reaches laterally to the level of the collateral sulcus. According to Insausti et al. (1987), the rhinal sulcus has a limited value in defining the extent of the entorhinal area. At the level of the posteromedial uncus, its extent is limited by the hippocampal fissure. On coronal MRI sections of the entorhinal cortex extends one MR cut posterior to the gyrus intralimbicus.

C The Perirhinal Area

The perirhinal area corresponds to area 35 of Brodmann (1909) (Figs. 6.10, 6.11). It follows the collateral sulcus along its rostrocaudal extent, occupying its fundus and its medial bank. In addition, the perirhinal area comprises area 36. This area is medial to area 20 of Brodmann and anteriorly continues with area 38 defined as the TG of von Bonin and Bailey (1947). The perirhinal cortex constitutes the lateral border of the vestigial rhinal sulcus and, more caudally, the collateral sulcus. Recent work has replaced the term rhinal sulcus altogether by the collateral sulcus since the rostral extent of the collateral sulcus has a variable extent and depth and is usually anteriorly discontinuous and frequently doubled. When the two sulci are running in parallel, the collateral sulcus is identified at the point where all major sulci of the temporal lobe have made their appearance, e.g., the superior, inferior, lateral-occipito-temporal sulci.

The extent of the rhinal cortex is highly complex and variable and is in close correlation with the depth of the collateral sulcus. Insausti et al. (1998) classified the depth of the collateral sulcus as shallow when less than 1 cm, as regular when 1–1.5 cm and as deep when the tip is more that 1.5 cm. When the collateral sulcus is shallow, the perirhinal area extends from the depth of the sulcus to the midlevel of the crown of the fusiform gyrus. With the collateral sulcus at a regular depth, the perirhinal cortex extends from the midpoint of the medial border to its lateral edge. When the collateral sulcus is deep, it extends from its medial edge to the midpoint of its lateral bank. The posterior extent of the perirhinal cortex corresponds to the posterior extent of the

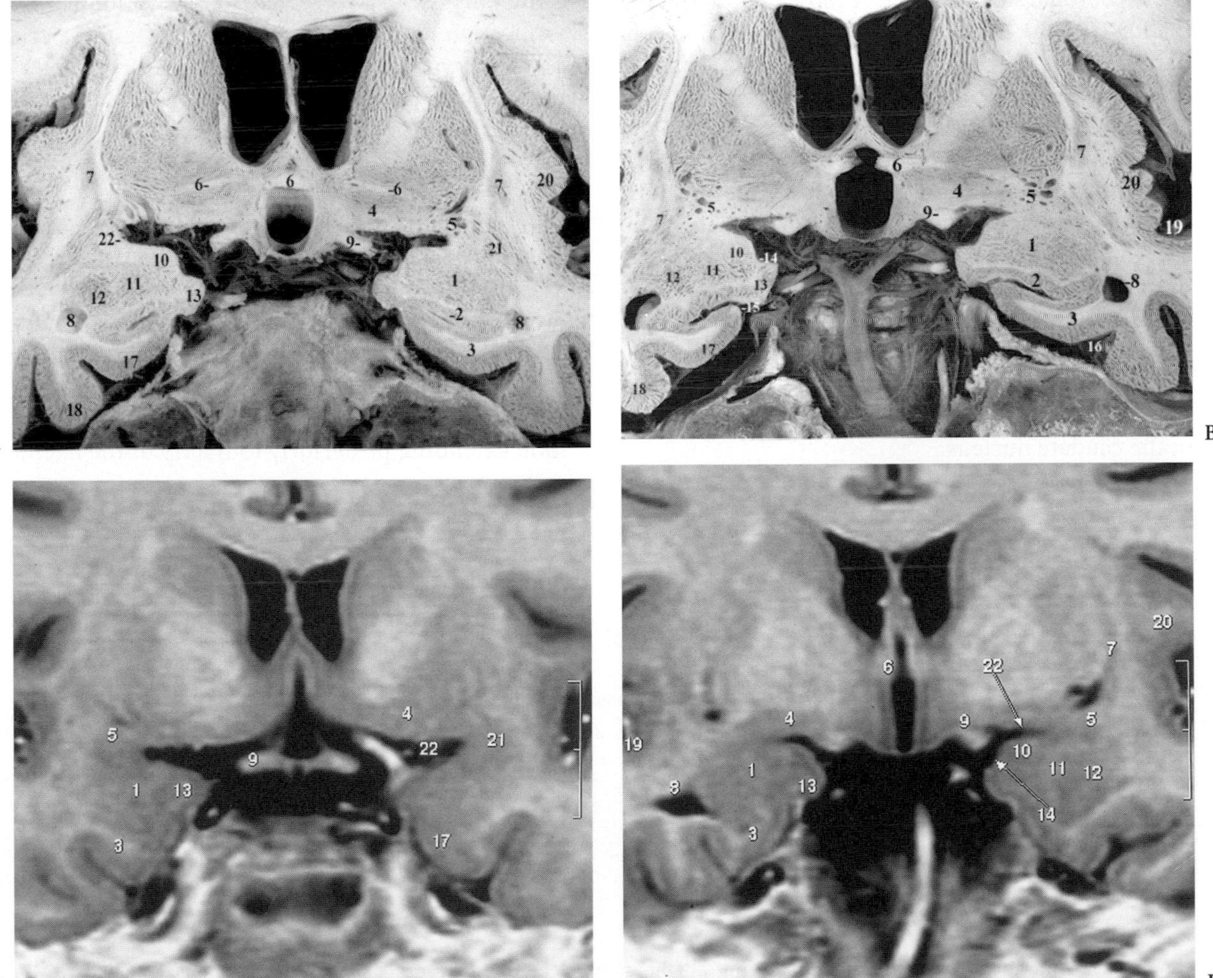

Fig. 6.12A–D. Contiguous coronal anatomic cuts through the amygdaloid nuclear complex at the level of the anterior commissure, as may be obtained using the PC-OB reference plane. *1*, Amygdala; *2*, hippocampus; *3*, parahippocampal gyrus; *4*, substantia innominata; *5*, anterior perforated substance; *6*, anterior commissure; *7*, claustrum; *8*, temporal horn; *9*, optic tract; *10*, cortical nucleus of amygdala; *11*, basal nucleus of amygdala; *12*, lateral nucleus of amygdala; *13*, gyrus ambiens; *14*, semiannular sulcus; *15*, uncal sulcus; *16*, collateral sulcus; *17*, entorhinal cortex; *18*, fusiform gyrus; *19*, inferior border of circular sulcus; *20*, insula; *21*, periamygdaloideum; *22*, endorhinal sulcus

intralimbic gyrus located on the caudal aspect of the uncus.

D The Amygdala

1 Morphology, Topographical Anatomy and Imaging of the Amygdala

The amygdala, or amygdaloid nuclear complex, received its name from its shape, which resembles that of an almond. It constitutes, along with the hippocampus, one of the two major telencephalic components of the limbic system (Figs. 6.12–6.15).

The topographical relationships of the amygdala are complex, and are best appreciated and evaluated on MR coronal sections such as those obtained using the PC-OB reference line. These coronal sections are parallel to the longitudinal axis of the brainstem and pass through the rostrum of the corpus callosum and the anterior commissure. They display the amygdaloid nuclear mass dorsal to the hippocampal formation and rostral to the tip of the inferior horn of the lateral ventricle. The superior aspect of the amygdala is shown partly continuous with the inferior margin of the claustrum, separated from the inferior aspect of the putamen and the pallidum by fibers of the external capsule and the ventral striatum, and found in close contact with the optic tract. At this level, the amygdala fuses with the tip of the tail of the caudate nucleus.

The amygdala is a corticonuclear transition area, located dorsomedially in the temporal lobe and forming the ventral superior and medial walls of the inferior horn of the lateral ventricle. Embryologically, it is derived from the medial division of the ganglionic hillock. Cells from this hillock are destined to form the paleocortex and the amygdaloid body. With development of the thalamus and the basal ganglia, the amygdala is pushed into the tip of the temporal lobe where it remains in a fixed position.

Numerous subdivisions of the amygdaloid have been reported. Humphrey (1968) has divided the amygdala into two large nuclei, the basolateral and corticomedial. Although there has been agreement regarding the terminology, there has been no universal agreement regarding the location of the nuclei. For the purpose of this review we have adopted the classification used by Gloor (1997). Using these criteria, the amygdala is divided into three large subnuclei: the basolateral, corticomedial, and central group of nuclei.

a *The Basolateral Group of Nuclei*

Phylogenetically, the basolateral group of nuclei is the younger group. It is, in addition, the largest group of nuclei in the amygdala. Volumetric studies have shown that the right side is larger than the left, with the lateral nucleus contributing most to this asymmetry. The basolateral group is divided into two parts:

1. The lateral nucleus occupies a ventrolateral position extending posteriorly to the tip of the lateral

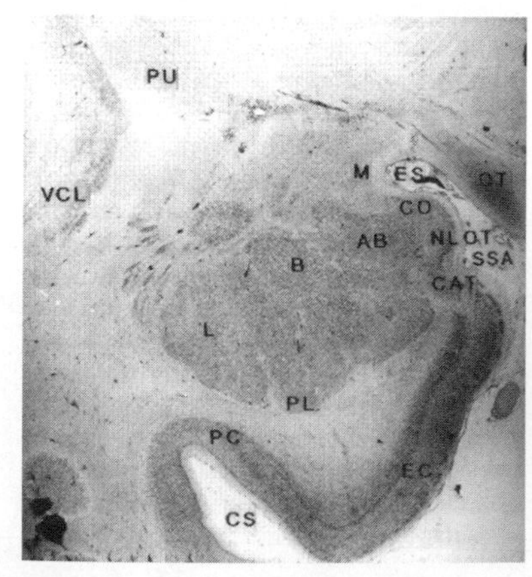

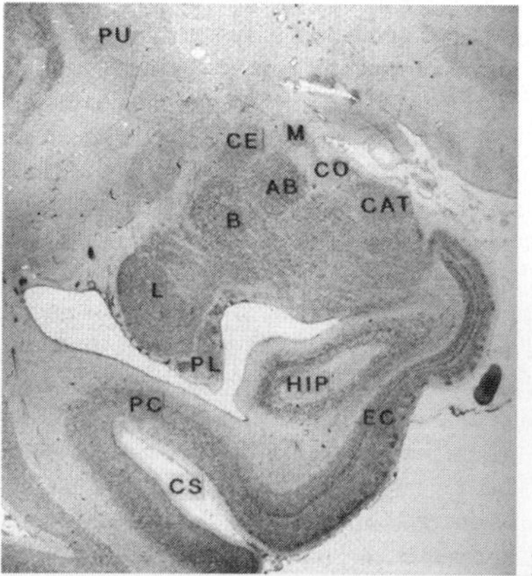

Fig. 6.13. A Anterior third of amygdala showing all the subnuclei. *AB*, accessory basal nucleus; *B*, basal nucleus; *CAT*, corticoamygdaloid transition area; *CO*, cortical nucleus; *CS*, collateral sulcus; *EC*, entorhinal cortex; *ES*, endorhinal sulcus; *L*, lateral nucleus; *M*, medial nucleus; *NLOT*, lateral nucleus of the olfactory tract; *OT*, optic tract; *PC*, perirhinal cortex; *PL*, paralaminar nucleus; *PU*, putamen; *SSA*, sulcus semiannularis. (from: Gloor, 1997, The temporal lobe and limbic system, Fig. 6-6, p. 604; Oxford University Press, New York) **B** Posterior third of amygdala *AB*, accessory basal nucleus; *B*, basal nucleus; *CAT*, periamygdaloid cortex; *CE*, central nucleus; *CO*, cortical nucleus; *CS*, collateral sulcus; *EC*, entorhinal cortex; *HIP*, hippocampus; *L*, lateral nucleus; *M*, medial nucleus; *PC*, perirhinal cortex; *PL*, paralaminar nucleus; *PU*, putamen;† (from: Gloor, 1997, The temporal lobe and limbic system, Fig. 6-8, p. 606, Oxford University Press; New York)

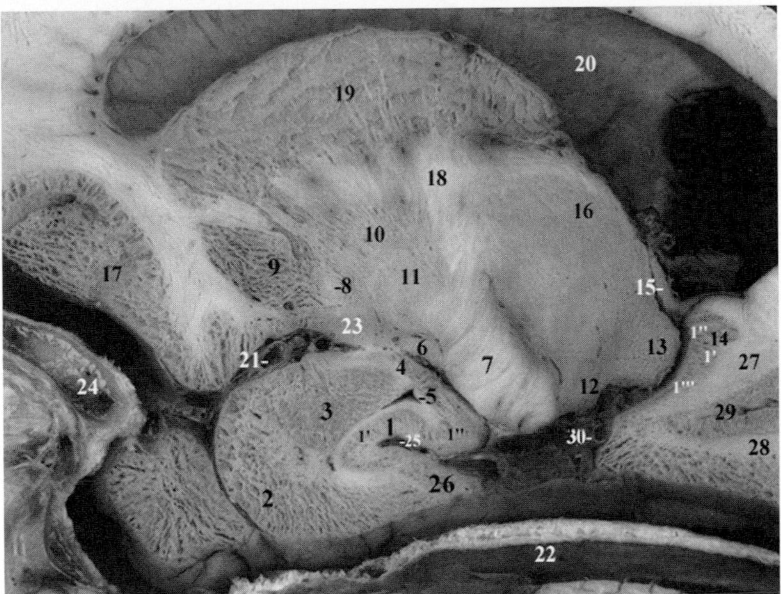

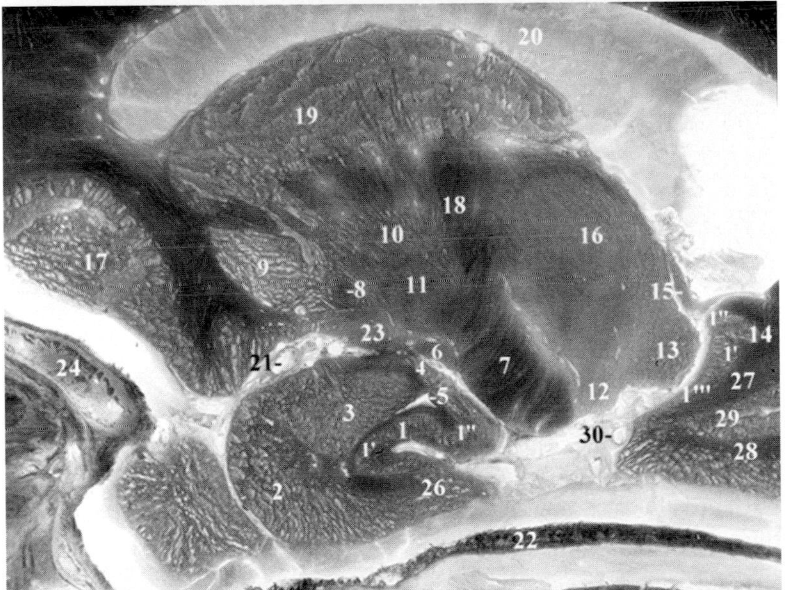

Fig. 6.14A,B. Parasagittal anatomic cut through the uncus and the amygdala (A and B are same cut with inverted contrast). *1*, Hippocampus; *1'*, cornu ammonis; *1''*, gyrus dentatus; *1'''*, subiculum; *2*, gyrus ambiens; *3*, amygdala, accessory basal nucleus; *4*, amygdala, cortical nucleus; *5*, temporal horn of lateral ventricle; *6*, optic tract; *7*, crus cerebri; *8*, anterior commissure; *9*, putamen; *10*, globus pallidus, lateral part; *11*, globus pallidus, medial part; *12*, medial geniculate body; *13*, pulvinar; *14*, hippocampal tail; *15*, crus fornicis; *16*, thalamus, lateral posterior nucleus; *17*, medial orbital gyrus; *18*, internal capsule; *19*, caudate; *20*, lateral ventricle; *21*, middle cerebral artery; *22*, tentorium cerebelli; *23*, anterior perforated substance; *24*, anterior clinoid process; *25*, uncal sulcus; *26*, parahippocampal gyrus; *27*, isthmus; *28*, lingual gyrus; *29*, anterior calcarine sulcus; *30*, posterior cerebral artery

horn and overlying the tip of the hippocampus. The AC fibers cross through its lateral border. Caudally and superiorly, this nucleus blends with the substriatal area; medially, the lateral medullary laminae are separated from the basal nucleus.

2. The basal nucleus is separated from the accessory basal nucleus by the medial limb of the intermediate medullary laminae. It is limited superiorly medially to laterally by the cortical nucleus of the amygdala, the central nucleus, and the subventricular area. Inferiorly, it is limited by the accessory nucleus and the roof of the temporal horn.

The accessory basal nucleus is located in the superomedial extent of the basal nucleus, being separated from the latter by the medullary laminae, and is dorsally bordered by the central nucleus. The paralaminar nucleus is a wide and thin nucleus wrapping the basal extent of the lateral nucleus.

b The Corticomedial Group of Nuclei

As their name indicates, the corticomedial group of nuclei is a much smaller group as compared to the basolateral group. It forms the cortical shell of the amygdaloid body and these nuclei are distributed ventrally to dorsally into the nucleus of the olfactory

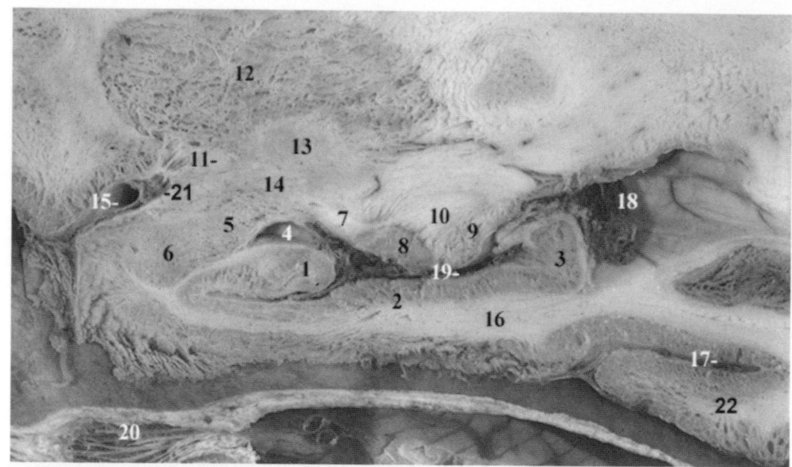

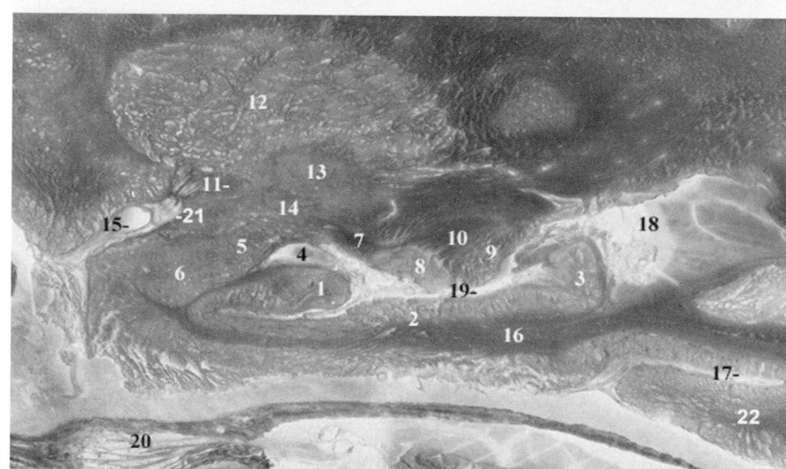

Fig. 6.15A,B. Parasagittal anatomic cut through the hippocampus and amygdala (A and B are same cut with inverted contrast). *1*, Hippocampus, head; *2*, presubiculum; *3*, hippocampus, tail; *4*, temporal horn; *5*, amygdala, basal nucleus; *6*, amygdala, lateral nucleus; *7*, optic tract; *8*, lateral geniculate body; *9*, pulvinar; *10*, area triangularis of Wernicke; *11*, anterior commissure; *12*, putamen; *13*, globus pallidus, lateral part; *14*, anterior perforated substance; *15*, middle cerebral artery; *16*, parahippocampal gyrus; *17*, collateral sulcus; *18*, atrium of lateral ventricle; *19*, choroidal fissure; *20*, Meckel's trigeminal cave; *21*, endorhinal sulcus; *22*, fusiform gyrus

tract, the nucleus of the accessory olfactory tract, the cortical nucleus, and the medial nucleus. The cortical nucleus forms the gyrus semilunaris. The medial nucleus is located lateral to the endorhinal sulcus at the level of the optic tract.

c The Central Group of Nuclei

The central nucleus is noted in the dorsocaudal aspect of the amygdala, tucked under the pallidum close to the bed of the stria terminalis. Some of its cells are continuous with the nucleus accumbens septi. This nucleus is sometimes included as part of the corticomedial group. Alhide and Heimer (1988) included it in the "extended amygdala" in addition to the bed nucleus of the stria terminalis, and the sublenticular portion of the substantia innominata. This superomedial extension is routinely visible on most anterior coronal MR cuts as well as on parasagittal cuts. It is related superiorly with the lateral expansion of the anterior commissure and bends towards the anterior temporal lobes.

Three other nuclei are noted: the interstitial nucleus of the stria terminalis, the small nuclei in the caudal aspect of the amygdala, and the anterior amygdalar nuclei.

d Boundaries of the Amygdaloid Bodies

The boundaries of the amygdala are difficult to precisely delineate on the MRI. For this reason, guidelines have been developed for determination of amygdala volume (Watson et al. 1992). These authors define the anteromedial extent of the amygdala at the start of the endorhinal sulcus.

The sulcus semiannularis is difficult to visualize on MRI, as the tentorial indentation lying just ventrally is considered as the ventromesial extent of the amygdala. Inferiorly and laterally, the borders are defined by the white matter of the temporal lobe. Superiorly, a line joins the endorhinal sulcus, or the superolateral extent of the optic tract, with the fundus of the circular sulcus of the insulae.

2 Functional and Clinical Considerations

The function of the amygdaloid nuclear complex has been largely underestimated in the past and still remains incompletely understood in humans. The amygdala is extensively connected with various regions of the brain.

The output of the amygdala is channeled through two efferent fiber systems, the stria terminalis and the ventral amygdalofugal pathway. The stria terminalis arises from the caudomedial aspect of the amygdaloid complex, and arches along the medial border of the caudate nucleus as the "stria semicircularis" to reach the level of the AC. There, it splits into its three components: a precommissural component, whose fibers descend anteriorly to the white commissure; a commissural part, which penetrates the anterior commissure; and a postcommissural component, which descends caudally to the commissure. As the stria reaches the anterior pole of the thalamus, it is associated with groups of neurons constituting the bed nucleus of the stria terminalis found lateral to the columns of the fornix and dorsal to the AC.

The second major efferent fiber bundle is the ventral amygdalofugal pathway, which originates from the dorsomedial aspect of the amygdala and courses medially through the sublenticular region of the substantia innominata and the anterior perforated substance beneath the lentiform nucleus. These fibers spread in the lateral preoptic-hypothalamic zone. Some of the fibers penetrate the inferior thalamic peduncle to terminate in the dorsomedial nucleus of the thalamus (Nauta 1969; Porrino et al. 1981; Cozan et al. 1965; Gloor 1955).

The stria terminalis and the ventral amygdalofugal pathways are not strictly independent, showing joined fibers. Efferent fibers arising from most of the amygdaloid nuclei course via both tracts (Amaral et al. 1992), which are mainly subcortical. Recent data from primates show that the amygdaloid nuclear complex is also connected with the neocortex via the internal capsule. The amygdalocortical projections are widely connected to unimodal sensory cortices.

Afferent fibers to the amygdaloid nuclear complex are mainly represented by convergent sensory fibers which transfer information mainly from numerous subcortical regions such as the hypothalamus, the ventral striatum, the basal forebrain, and autonomic centers in the brainstem. In view of these connections, the amygdala may be considered as an important relay center through which external inputs may modulate the emotional state (Aggleton 1973).

These projections comprise: (a) fibers originating from the olfactory bulb and the olfactory cortex, (b) fibers arising from the thalamus and the hypothalamus, (c) fibers originating from the basal forebrain, (d) afferents from the brainstem, (e) fibers from the cerebral cortex, and (f) fibers from the lateral parabrachial nucleus.

Fibers from the olfactory system are not dominated in primates by olfaction, even if these fibers originate in the olfactory bulb. These fibers terminate via the lateral olfactory tract in the corticomedial nuclear group. Actually, the role of the amygdala in olfaction seems unessential, considering that the amygdala is well developed in anosmic aquatic mammals and that bilateral destruction of this nuclear complex fails to impair olfactory discrimination (Allen 1941).

The basal nucleus of Meynert and the nucleus of the diagonal band project reciprocally to the amygdala along the ventral amygdalofugal pathway. The amygdala receives input from the dorsal and ventral thalamic regions which terminate mainly in the central amygdaloid nucleus. But hypothalamo-amygdaloid projections are not prominent.

Afferents from the brainstem also project to the central amygdaloid nucleus originating from the periaqueductal gray matter, the substantia nigra, the locus coeruleus, the dorsal raphe nucleus, the ventral tegmental area, and the nucleus of the solitary tract via the ventral amygdalofugal pathway.

The cortical projections to the amygdala originate from the anterior cingulate gyrus (area 24) and project to the basolateral nucleus, from the subiculum to the mediobasal and the cortical nuclei, and from the perirhinal cortex (areas 35 and 36) to the mediobasal nucleus. The neocortical afferents originate from the frontal lobe, the medial prefrontal (areas 11 and 12) and the caudal orbitofrontal cortex (area 13 and 14), and from the temporal lobe, mainly the auditory (area 22), the visual associative (areas 20 and 21), the temporal polar (area 38), and from the insular cortex. All these regions terminate in the lateral and basal amygdaloid nuclei. All wide cortical areas project to the central nucleus.

3 Clinical Considerations and Targeting

Stimulation of the amygdala in animals produces fear and defensive reactions, the intensity of the stimulus determining the level of the behavioral agonistic response (Davis 1992; Gloor 1960). Complete interruption of the ventral amygdalofugal pathway suppresses defense reaction. In humans, rage defensive responses are rarely observed with temporal lobe seizures, however, stimulation of the amygdala still produces fear, confusion and amnesia of the related event (Gloor 1972; Davis 1992; Feindel and Penfield 1954). The effect of bilateral lesions of the amygdaloid body in animals is associated with modifications of emotional behavior. In monkeys, the so-called Kluver-Bucy syndrome, in which the animals become placid with no fear or aggression reactions with a compulsion to explore objects orally, tactually or visually, is seen with bilateral amygdalar destruction (Kluver 1952; Kluver and Bucy 1939). A hypersexual behavior may also be observed. These experiments involved areas of the temporal lobe other than the amygdala. Such bilateral lesions in humans cause a decrease in aggressive behavior and a marked decrease in emotional excitation but no signs suggestive of the Kluver-Bucy syndrome (Lilly et al 1983; Terzian 1958; Narabayashi 1972).

The emotional component associated with Alzheimer's disease and its relation with the amygdala are of major interest in view of the marked volumetric decrease of the amygdaloid body present in this dementia (Scott et al. 1991). Emotional disturbances corresponding to a negative mood appear to be unrelated to the memory loss, which is related to the hippocampus. Similarly, the amygdala seems to be involved in the emotional modifications observed in schizophrenic patients based on the connections identified between the amygdala and the frontal cortex, the dysfunction of which has been considered as the primum movens of schizophrenia (Aggleton 1993). An increase in the activity of the mesolimbic dopaminergic system, which innervates the frontal cortex and the ventral striatum, is postulated to be the neurochemical feature of this disease. The role of the amygdala may be emphasized here, considering its reciprocal connections with the dopaminergic neurons of the midbrain which give rise to the mesolimbic pathway.

To summarize, the amygdaloid nuclear complex appears to play an important role in the initiation and integration of autonomic and somatic responses associated with affective behavior due to its wide-ranging cortico-amygdalo-tegmental and hypothalamic pathways.

E The Hippocampal Formation

As far as we know, the first description of the hippocampus was given by Arantius (1587) and J.G. Duvernoy provided the first illustrations in 1729 (H. Duvernoy 1988; Lewis 1923). Vicq d'Azyr (1786) presented an anatomic cut passing through the temporal lobes and the inferior horns, which appears oriented approximately in the CH-PC orientation, and shows the hippocampal formations protruding in the floor of the temporal horns and displayed throughout their anterior-posterior long axis. Reviews of the complex terminology may be found in Tilney (1939), Klingler (1948) and Meyer (1971). The hippocampus consists of two cortical lamina each interlocked with the other: Ammon's horn or the hippocampus proper, and the gyrus dentatus.

1 Embryology

The telencephalon enlarges markedly during development pushing the paleocortex or rhinencephalon basally into the mesial temporal lobe. The archicortex, which includes the hippocampal formation and the cingulum, initially consists of a thin cortical band located in the medial wall of the telencephalic vesicle. This cortical band extends cranially from the interventricular foramen to the posterior extent of the ventricular cavity. The increase in size of the hippocampus results in a bulging into the ventricle with a vascular supply being derived from the hippocampal sulcus. This sulcus originates from the medial wall of the ventricle and runs in parallel with the choroidal fissure.

As the cerebral hemispheres expand with formation of the temporal lobes, the hippocampal formation is displaced posteriorly and, finally, inferiorly into the temporal lobe (Fig. 6.16). The medial aspect of the hemisphere shows a longitudinal groove, the hippocampal fissure, oriented parallel to the choroidal fissure. The choroidal and hippocampal fissures arch from the region of the interventricular foramen to the tip of the inferior horn. The hippocampal arch does not show similar development. The upper portion of the hippocampal fissure is progressively invaded by the commissural fibers of the corpus callosum and undergoes little differentiation to form a very thin vestigial gyrus named the indusium griseum. With a forward growth of the temporal lobes, the inferior portion develops and differentiates into the hippocampal formation, which bulges deeply into the inferior horn with deepening of the hippocampal fissure. The lips of the hippocampal fissure give rise to the dentate gyrus and the parahippocampal gyrus. The superior portion of the parahippocampal gyrus, adjacent to the hippocampal fissure, is the subiculum. The progressive morphological modifi-

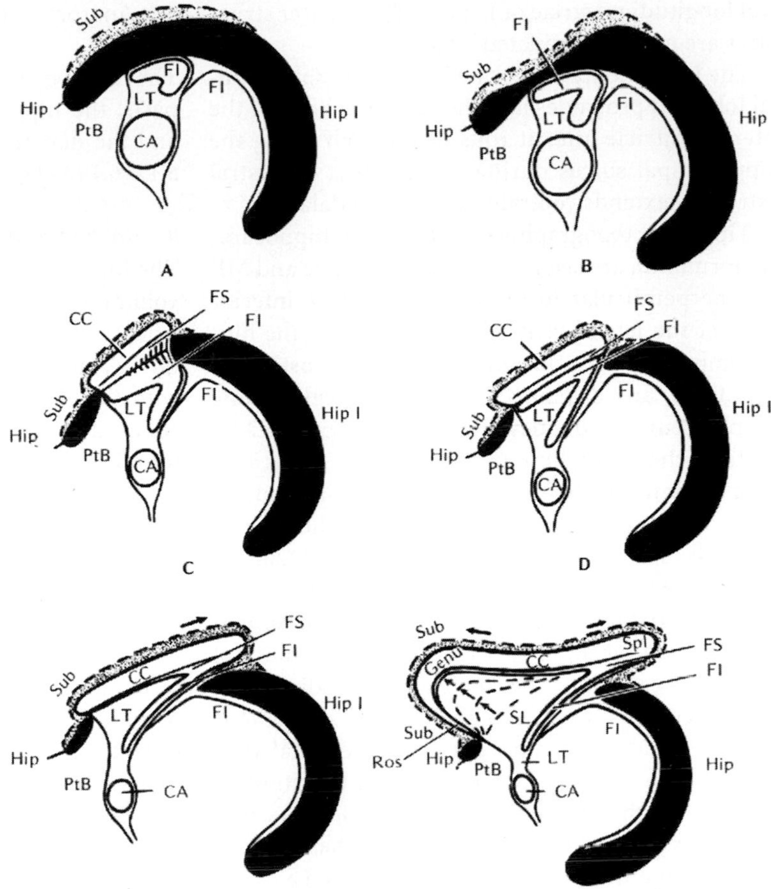

Fig. 6.16A–F. Phylogenesis and ontogenesis of the hippocampal formation and corpus callosum. **A** Monotremes; **B** intermediate stage; **C** hedgehog and bat; **D** small precommissural remnant of hippocampus; **E** rodents; **F** primates. *CA*, anterior commissure; *CC*, corpus callosum; *FI*, inferior fornix; *FS*, superior fornix; *LT*, lamina terminalis; *PtB*, paraterminal body; *Ros*, rostrum; *Spl*, splenium; *SL*, septum pellucidum; *Sub*, subiculum. (After Abbie 1939)

cations and folding of the hippocampus and related structures are easily visualized on coronal views, as schematically drawn by Warwick and Williams (1973, 1989).

a The Choroid Plexus, Tela, Taenia, and Lamina Affixa

The vascular matrix surrounding the developing brain invaginates into the ventricles forming the choroid plexus. This invagination has two edges: one free, called the tela choroidea connecting the choroid plexus with the original matrix, and one fixed, attached to the ventricular surface of the thalamus, known as the lamina affixa. The tenia choroidea is the tuft lifted into the ventricular cavity at the basis of the choroid plexus.

The development of the temporal horn pushes the choroid plexus posteriorly. With this rotation the choroid plexus position is reversed, becoming located on top off the hippocampal formation in the temporal horn. In addition, the position of the anchoring edges of the choroid plexus is reversed as compared to their position in the lateral ventricle.

2 Morphology and Imaging

Extensive and comprehensive works have been devoted to the topographic and functional anatomy of the hippocampal formation since the pioneering texts completed by Ramon Y. Cajal (1911) and Lorente De No (1934). These include the work of Gastaut and Lammers (1961), Crosby et al. (1962), Blackstaad and Flood (1963), Brodal (1969, 1981), Warwick and Williams (1973, 1989), Isaacson and Pribram (1975) and Carpenter (1976, 1996), to which the reader should refer.

The hippocampal formation may be subdivided morphologically into a precommissural, a supracommissural, and a retrocommissural portion. The retrocommissural portion represents the hippocampal formation, the other parts being vestigial anatomical structures. The precommissural portion occupies the caudal part of the area subcallosa. The supracommissural portion is represented by the indusium griseum or supracallosal gyrus which contains two white fiber bundles: the medial and the lateral longitudinal striae of Lancisi. These latter structures are not discriminated by MRI.

The hippocampus is located in the mesial temporal lobe and protrudes into the temporal horn of the lateral ventricle after it rolls in on itself along the hippocampal sulcus during ontogenesis. Its rostral extremity extends ventrally to the amygdala.

The major topographical structures of hippocampal formation are seen on coronal anatomic and MR cuts perpendicular to the long axis of the inferior horn of the lateral ventricle. The shape of the hippocampus and the localization of its constitutive structures are explained by the cortical folding which occurs during development. The external aspects of the subiculum and the dentate gyrus face each other in the depths of the hippocampal sulcus. When opening the hippocampal sulcus, the dentate gyrus is seen between the hippocampal sulcus, which is below, and the fimbria, which are above. The dentate gyrus may be followed backward accompanied by the fimbria until it reaches the splenium of the corpus callosum. The cortical zone medial to the dentate gyrus is the subiculum, which is contiguous with the parahippocampal gyrus or entorhinal area. The Ammon's horn, which is the third longitudinal structure of the hippocampal formation, is the hippocampus proper. In early development, the Ammon's horn and the dentate gyri are continuous. Later, for uncertain reasons, the dentate gyrus becomes concave and slips beneath the cornu ammonis to reach a final position in which both structures fit one into the other separated by the hippocampal sulcus.

The Ammon's horn and the dentate gyrus, as well as the subiculum, which may be subdivided into prosubiculum, subiculum, presubiculum, and parasubiculum, have an archicortical structure, while the pyriform cortex shows a paleocortical structure. The large inferior portion of the parahippocampal gyrus near the collateral sulcus is a transitional cortex resembling the isocortex with six layers. Actually, the cortex, extending on the parahippocampal gyrus through the parasubiculum, the presubiculum, the subiculum, and the prosubiculum to the hippocampus and the dentate gyrus, shows a progressive transition from a six-layered cortex to a three-layered cortex.

The hippocampal formation is covered by a lamina of whiter matter fibers, the alveus, which converges on the medial aspect of the hippocampus to form the fimbria, which constitutes the beginning portion of the fornix. Note that the alveus is a subependymal white matter tract which conveys fibers entering and leaving the hippocampus.

3 Anatomy of the Hippocampal Formation

The hippocampal formation is divided into two parts, the hippocampus proper or Ammon's horn, and the dentatus gyrus or the fascia dentata (Figs. 6.17–6.19A–D).

a The Hippocampus Proper

The hippocampus proper is a cylindrical structure, voluminous anteriorly, extending as much as 4–5 cm from the tip of the temporal horn to the splenium of the corpus callosum where it becomes continuous with the fornix. Its course assumes a strong inner concavity; the hippocampus commonly is divided into three parts: head, body, and tail.

b The Hippocampal Head

The hippocampal head is characterized by several digitations that are apparent on its ventricular surface, representing the foldings of the hippocampal formation (Figs. 6.20, 6.21). These are even more pronounced at the tip of the uncus. As discussed previously, these foldings result from excessive growth of the human hippocampus within a confined region.

The hippocampus and parahippocampal gyri bend backward to form the uncus. The location of

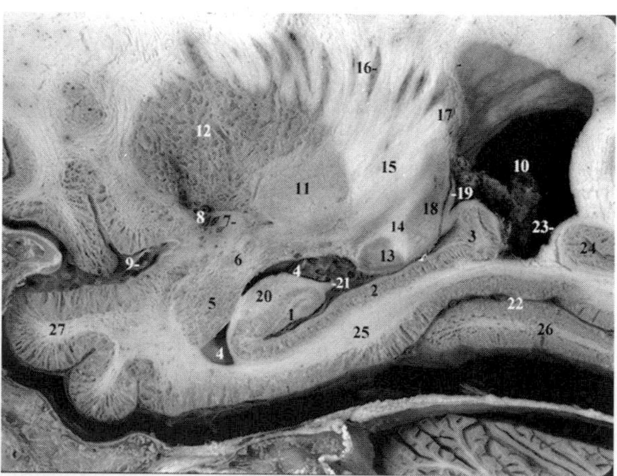

Fig. 6.17. The hippocampal formation (sagittal anatomic cut). *1*, Hippocampus, head; *2*, subiculum; *3*, hippocampus, tail; *4*, temporal horn of lateral ventricle; *5*, amygdala, lateral nucleus; *6*, amygdala, basal nucleus; *7*, anterior commissure; *8*, anterior perforated substance; *9*, middle cerebral artery; *10*, atrium of lateral ventricle; *11*, globus pallidus, lateral part; *12*, putamen; *13*, lateral geniculate body; *14*, area triangularis of Wernicke; *15*, internal capsule, pars retrolenticularis; *16*, gray striatal bridges; *17*, caudate nucleus; *18*, pulvinar; *19*, crus fornicis; *20*, alveus; *21*, fimbria; *22*, collateral sulcus; *23*, calcar avis; *24*, anterior calcarine sulcus; *25*, parahippocampal gyrus; *26*, fusiform gyrus; *27*, temporal pole

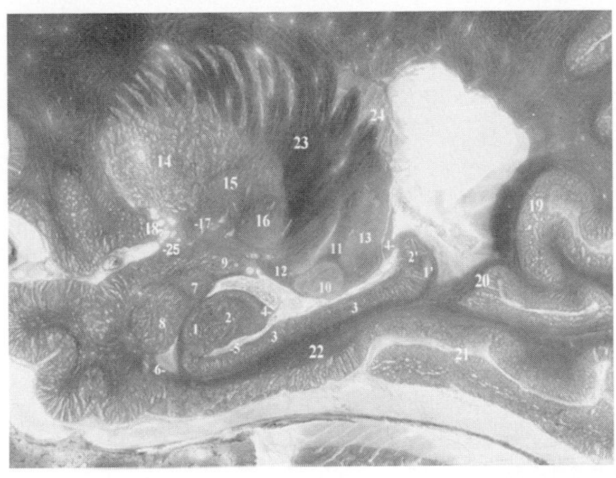

Fig. 6.18. The hippocampal formation (sagittal anatomic cut). 1, Hippocampal head, cornu ammonis; *1'*, hippocampal tail, cornu ammonis; 2, hippocampal head, gyrus dentatus; *2'*, hippocampal tail, gyrus dentatus; 3, subiculum; 4, fimbria; 5, hippocampal sulcus; 6, uncal recess of temporal horn; 7, amygdala, basal nucleus; 8, amygdala, lateral nucleus; 9, amygdala, cortical nucleus; *10*, lateral geniculate body; *11*, optic peduncle; *12*, optic tract; *13*, pulvinar; *14*, putamen; *15*, globus pallidus, lateral part; *16*, globus pallidus, medial part; *17*, anterior commissure; *18*, anterior perforated substance; *19*, calcar avis; *20*, collateral trigone; *21*, collateral sulcus; *22*, parahippocampal gyrus; *23*, internal capsule, posterior limb; *24*, caudate nucleus

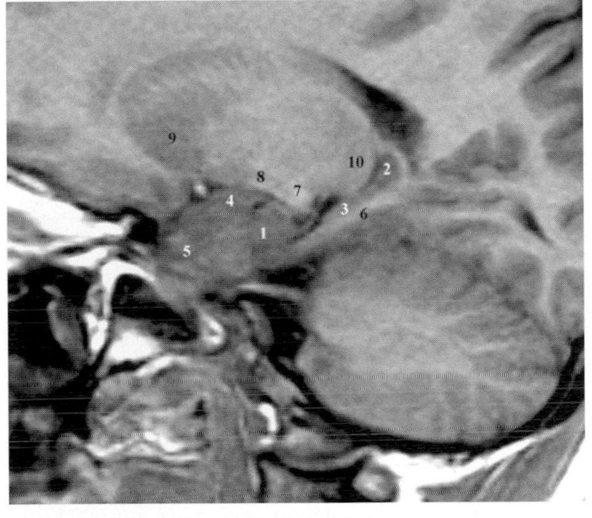

A

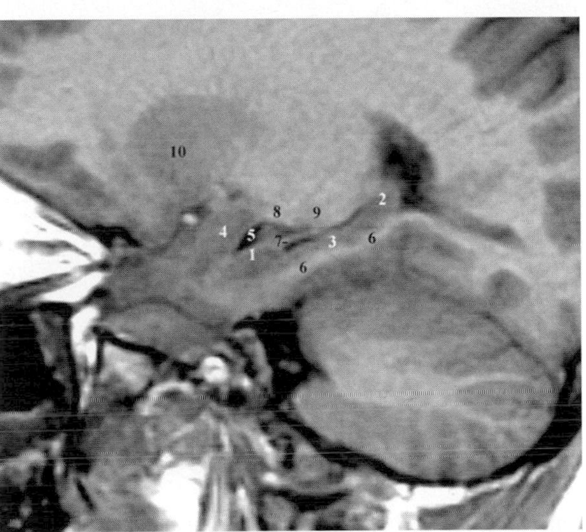

B

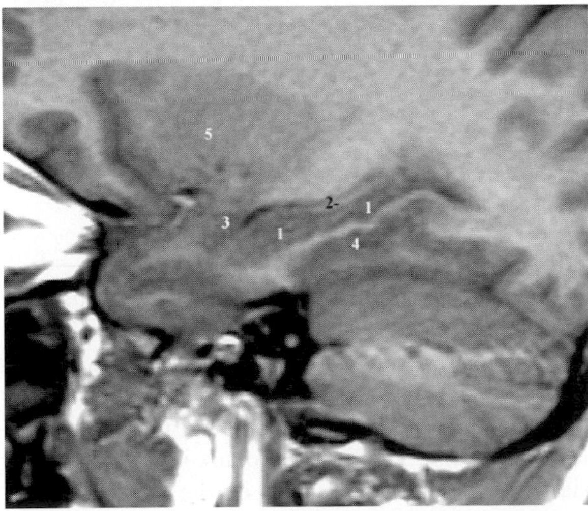

C

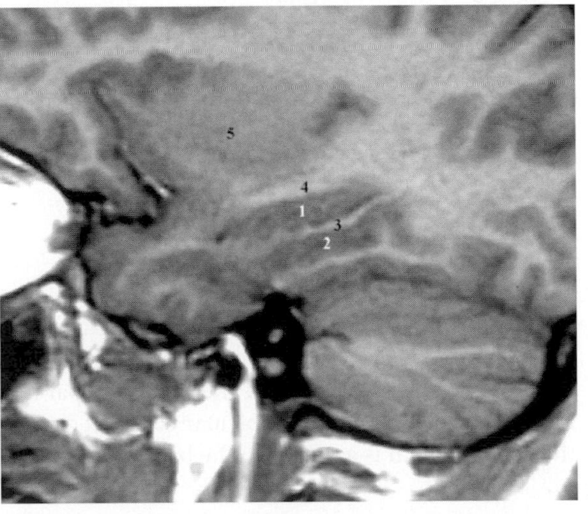

D

Fig. 6.19A–D. Sagittal MR contiguous cuts through the hippocampal formation (SPGR, T1 weighted, 4 mm thick). **A** *1*, Hippocampal head; *2*, hippocampal tail; *3*, presubiculum; *4*, amygdala; *5*, gyrus ambiens; *6*, parahippocampal gyrus; *7*, crus cerebri; *8*, optic tract; *9*, putamen; *10*, pulvinar. **B** *1*, Hippocampal head; *2*, hippocampal tail; *3*, presubiculum; *4*, amygdala; *5*, temporal horn of lateral ventricle; *6*, parahippocampal gyrus; *7*, fimbria; *8*, optic tract; *9*, lateral geniculate body; *10*, putamen. **C** 1, Hippocampus; *2*, fimbria; *3*, amygdala; *4*, collateral sulcus; *5*, putamen. **D** *1*, Hippocampus; *2*, collateral sulcus; *3*, parahippocampal gyrus; *4*, optic radiations; *5*, putamen

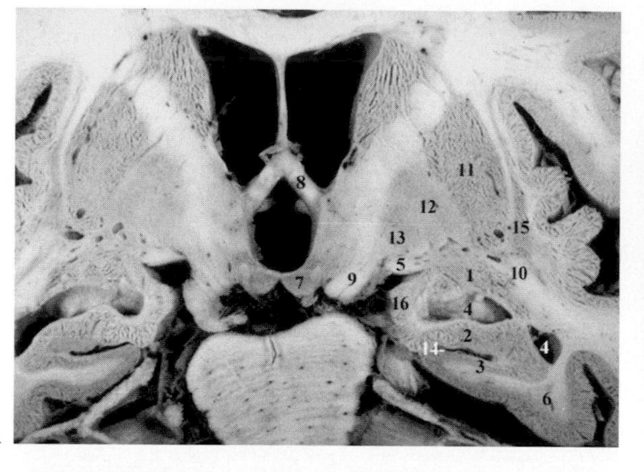

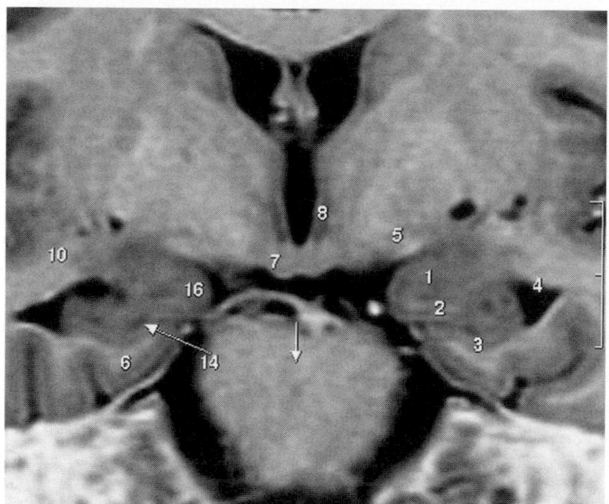

Fig. 6.20A,B. The hippocampal formation. Coronal anatomic cut through the hippocampal head, found at the level of the anterior columns of the fornix. *1*, Amygdala; *2*, hippocampus; *3*, subiculum; *4*, temporal horn; *5*, optic tract; *6*, parahippocampal gyrus; *7*, mamillary body; *8*, anterior column of fornix; *9*, crus cerebri; *10*, temporal stem; *11*, putamen; *12*, lateral pallidum; *13*, medial pallidum; *14*, uncal sulcus; *15*, claustrum; *16*, gyrus uncinatus

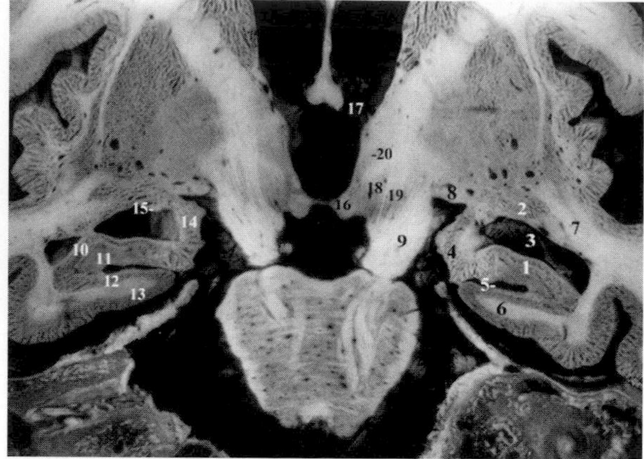

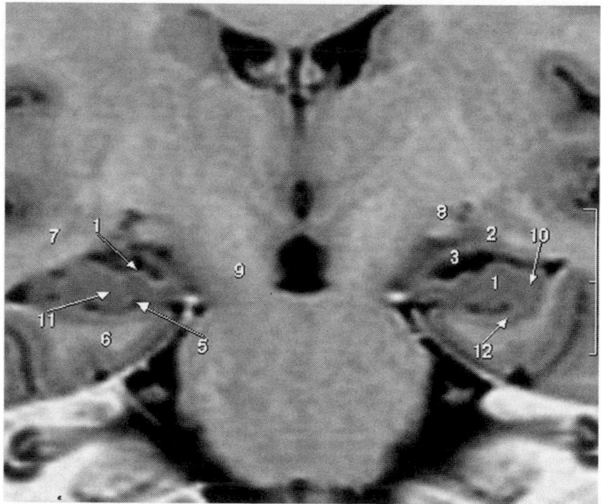

Fig. 6.21A,B. The hippocampal formation. Coronal anatomic section of the hippocampal head, at the level of the interventricular foramina of Monro. *1*, Hippocampal head, hippocampal digitations; *2*, amygdala, cortical nucleus; *3*, temporal horn; *4*, uncus; *5*, uncal sulcus; *6*, parahippocampal gyrus; *7*, temporal stem; *8*, optic tract, pericrural part; *9*, crus cerebri; *10*, cornu ammonis; *11*, gyrus dentatus; *12*, subiculum; *14*, entorhinal cortex; *14*, uncinate gyrus; *15*, stria terminalis; *16*, mamillary body; *17*, foramen interventriculare of Monro; *18*, subthalamic nucleus; *19*, comb; *20*, zona incerta

Ammon's horn in the uncus has been examined by several authors. Klingler (1948) and Duvernoy (1988) have shown that the intralimbic gyrus is occupied by areas C4 and C3 of the hippocampal formation. Area CA1 and the subicular complex occupy the region which is anterior to the band of Giacomini.

c *The Hippocampal Body*

At the level of the body, the hippocampal proper is limited laterally by the collateral eminence, a margin created in the temporal horn by the collateral sulcus. Its ventricular surface, the alveus, constitutes the output of the hippocampus, and is continuous with the fimbria fornix (Figs. 6.22–6.26). At the level of the body , the fimbria fornix is a thick white matter bundle, which assumes a U-shape with a lateral concavity directed towards the choroid plexus and the temporal horn. The fimbria fornix is separated mesially from the dentate gyrus by the fimbriomargodenticulate sulcus.

d *The Hippocampal Tail*

The anterior segment of the tail resembles the body of the hippocampus. It is, however, distinct due to a progressive thinning of the hippocampus proper and

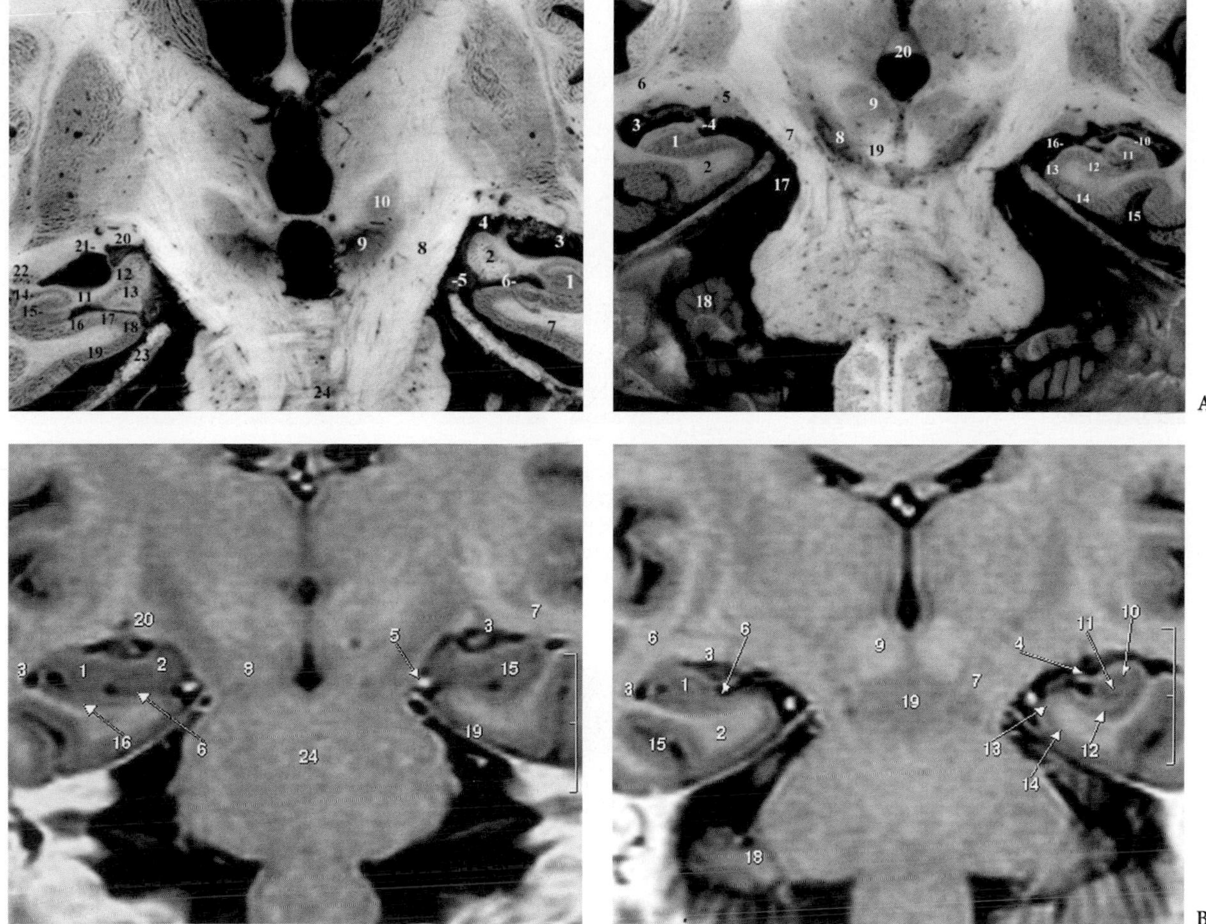

Fig. 6.22A,B. The hippocampal formation. Coronal anatomic section of the hippocampal body and the intralimbic gyrus, at the level of the subthalamic nucleus (*10*) and the cerebral peduncles (*8*). *1*, Hippocampus, body; *2*, intralimbic gyrus at uncal apex; *3*, temporal horn and choroid plexus; *4*, choroidal fissure; *5*, posterior cerebral artery; *6*, hippocampal sulcus between subiculum and dentate gyrus; *7*, parahippocampal gyrus; *8*, crus cerebri; *9*, substantia nigra; *10*, subthalamic nucleus; *11*, fimbria; *12*, hippocampal head, cornu ammonis; *13*, hippocampal head, gyrus dentatus; *14*, hippocampal body, cornu ammonis; *15*, hippocampal body, gyrus dentatus; *16*, subiculum; *17*, presubiculum; *18*, parasubiculum; *19*, entorhinal cortex; *20*, optic tract; *21*, stria terminalis; *22*, tail of caudate; *23*, tentorium cerebelli; *24*, pons

Fig. 6.23A,B. The hippocampal formation. Coronal anatomic sections of the hippocampal body, at the level of the flocculi at the advent of the cerebellum. *1*, Hippocampus; *2*, parahippocampal gyrus; *3*, temporal horn; *4*, fimbria; *5*, lateral geniculate body; *6*, temporal stem; *7*, crus cerebri; *8*, substantia nigra; *9*, red nucleus; *10*, hippocampal body, cornu ammonis; *11*, hippocampal body, gyrus dentatus; *12*, subiculum; *13*, parasubiculum; *14*, entorhinal cortex; *15*, collateral sulcus; *16*, transverse fissure, lateral wing; *17*, ambient cistern; *18*, flocculus of cerebellum; *19*, superior cerebellar peduncle; *20*, adhesio interthalamica

increase in size of the fimbria fornix (Fig. 6.26). The posterior aspect of the tail has a markedly different geometry as two important structures, the dentate gyrus and the fimbria fornix, assume divergent destinations. The dentate gyrus courses towards a supracallosal destination to become the indusium griseum, and the fornix, together with the rest of the body, moves towards an infracallosal course. This divergent course results in a widening of the fimbriodentate sulcus and exposure of the CA3 area of Ammon's horn; this region is named the gyrus fasciolaris.

4 Cytoarchitectonics and Intrinsic Circuitry

On the basis of intrinsic cellular architecture, the hippocampus and the parahippocampal cortex may be subdivided into sectors (Figs. 6.28–6.31). The cornu ammonis is subdivided into four sectors: CA1,

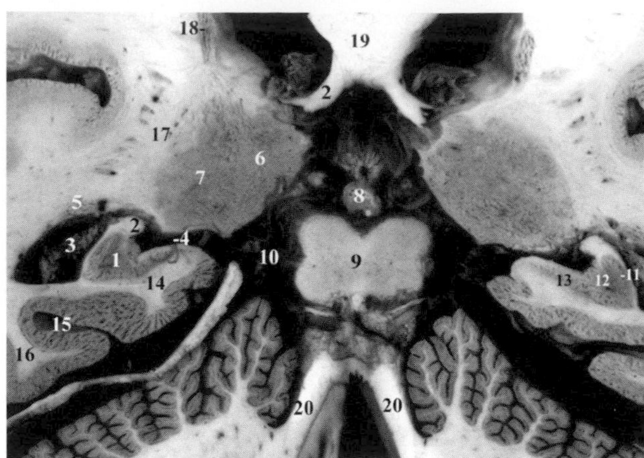

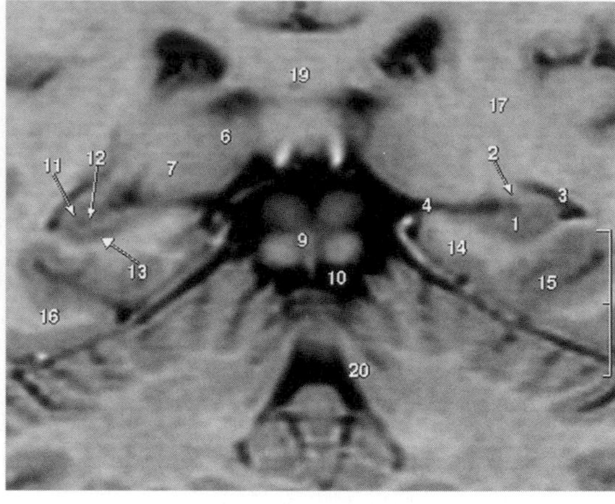

A B

Fig. 6.24A,B. The hippocampal formation. Coronal anatomic section of the hippocampal tail at the level of the pulvinar thalami and the quadrigeminal plate. *1*, Hippocampus, tail; *2*, crus of fornix; *3*, temporal horn and choroid plexus; *4*, transverse fissure, lateral wing; *5*, tail of caudate; *6*, medial pulvinar nucleus; *7*, lateral pulvinar nucleus; *8*, pineal body; *9*, quadrigeminal plate; *10*, quadrigeminal cistern; *11*, cornu ammonis; *12*, gyrus dentatus; *13*, subiculum; *14*, parahippocampal gyrus; *15*, collateral sulcus; *16*, fusiform gyrus; *17*, internal capsule, retrolentiform part; *18*, caudate nucleus; *19*, splenium of corpus callosum; *20*, superior cerebellar peduncle

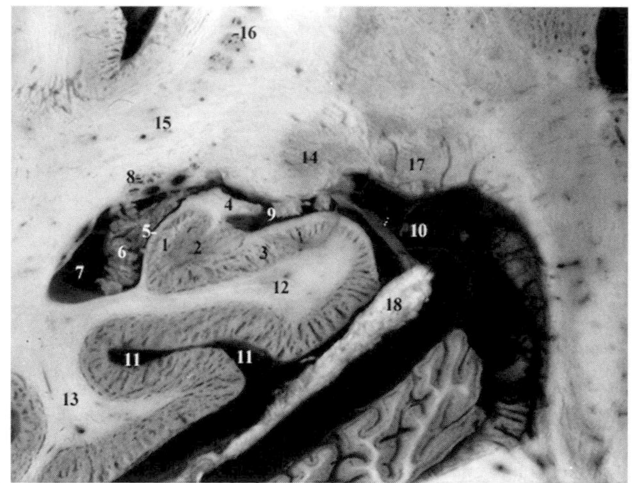

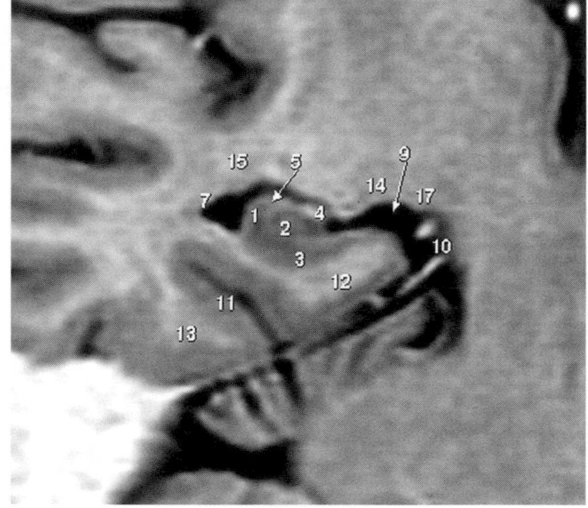

A B

Fig. 6.25A,B. Coronal anatomy of the hippocampus at the level of the lateral geniculate body, in the PC-OB reference plane. *1*, Cornu ammonis; *2*, gyrus dentatus; *3*, subiculum; *4*, fimbria; *5*, alveus; *6*, choroid plexus; *7*, temporal horn; *8*, tail of caudate; *9*, lateral wing of transverse fissure; *10*, ambient cistern; *11*, collateral sulcus; *12*, parahippocampal gyrus; *13*, fusiform gyrus; *14*, lateral geniculate body; *15*, temporal stem; *16*, putamen; *17*, medial geniculate body; *18*, tentorium cerebelli

CA2, CA3, and CA4 (Lorente De No 1934). The CA1 sector borders on the prosubiculum; the CA4 sector, often not recognized as a distinct entity, fills the hilus of the dentate gyrus; the CA2 and CA3 sectors are located between the first two. Another division of the hippocampus into sectors has been proposed by Rose (1927). The H1 field corresponds to CA1, extending into the prosubiculum; H2 and H3 correspond to CA2 and CA3, respectively; and H4 and H5 correspond to CA4, also contained in the hilus of the dentate gyrus. A simplification of this division has been proposed by Vogt and Vogt (1937) limiting the partition to three fields: H1 for CA1, H2 for CA2 and CA3, and H3 for CA4. Considering the difference in sensitivity to hypoxia of such fields, CA1 corresponds to the Sommer sector (Sommer 1880) which is the "vulnerable" sector, the CA3 sector being the resistant sector of Spilmeyer (Spilmeyer 1927). The CA4, a more or less vulnerable sector, is the Bratz sector (Bratz 1899).

Cytoarchitecturally, the hippocampus consists of three fundamental layers, the polymorphic, pyrami-

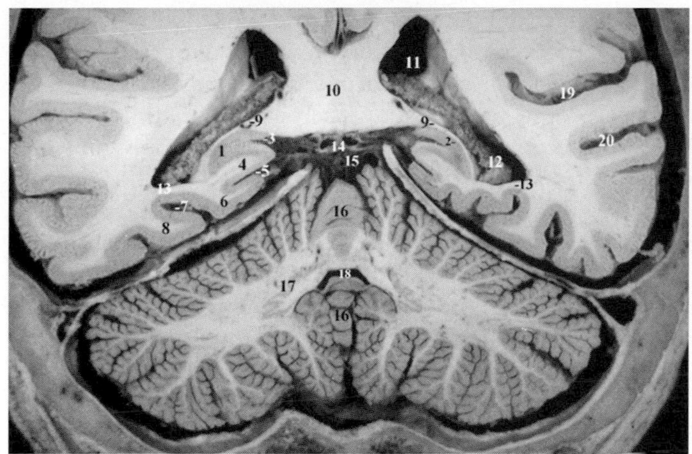

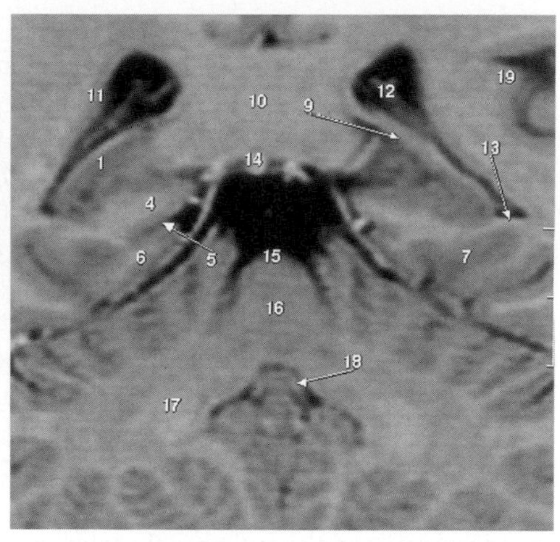

Fig. 6.26. The hippocampal formation. Coronal anatomic section of the hippocampal tail, at the level of the splenium of the corpus callosum. *1*, Hippocampal tail, subsplenial gyrus; *2*, cornu ammonis; *3*, gyrus fasciolaris; *4*, isthmus; *5*, anterior calcarine sulcus; *6*, parahippocampal gyrus; *7*, collateral sulcus; *8*, fusiform gyrus; *9*, crus of fornix; *10*, splenium of corpus callosum; *11*, atrium of lateral ventricle; *12*, choroid plexus; *13*, collateral trigone; *14*, internal cerebral veins; *15*, quadrigeminal cistern; *16*, vermis of cerebellum; *17*, dentate nucleus of cerebellum; *18*, fourth ventricle; *19*, lateral fissure; *20*, parallel sulcus

dal, and molecular layers. The most characteristic layer is the pyramidal layer which contains pyramidal cells, both large and small cells, and Golgi type II cells. Similarly, the dentate gyrus is organized into three layers: the molecular, the granular, and the polymorphic layers.

The intrinsic circuitry of the hippocampal formation, which is beyond the scope of this work, may be summarized by the following. Note that all the intrinsic connections are arranged transversely to the long axis of the hippocampal formation. A trisynaptic circuit characterizes these intrinsic connections. Projections from the entorhinal cortex (area 28) to the hippocampal formation follow two pathways: the perforant path, originating from the lateral portion of the entorhinal area and terminating in the outer two thirds of the dentate gyrus; and the alvear path, originating from the medial portion of the entorhinal cortex and terminating in the cornu ammonis. The dentate gyrus, in turn, gives rise to fibers which do not project outside of the hippocampal formation and end as mossy fibers in the CA3 sector. CA3 projects to the CA1 sector, which projects in turn to the subiculum. These successive projections constitute the classic trisynaptic circuit: entorhinal cortex-dentate gyrus, dentate gyrus-CA3 and CA3-CA1. From the CA1 sector, fibers are projected back to the subiculum and from the latter back to the entorhinal cortex (Amaral and Insausti 1990; Lorente De No 1934; Ramon y Cajal 1909; Witter et al. 1988, 1989; Ishizuka 1990; Brown and Zador 1990; Yeckel and Berger 1990). The entorhinal-hippocampal intrinsic projections are specifically organized although much remains to be learned about information processing inside the hippocampal formation, which is being extensively studied with respect to memory functions and learning.

5 Vascular Supply of the Mesial Temporal Region

The vascular supply of the mesial temporal region has attracted much interest recently. For a detailed review of the subject the reader is referred to the works of Erdem (1993), Yazargil (1985), Uchimura (1928), Nagata (1988), Duvernoy (1998), and Huther (1998).

The hippocampus derives its vascular supply from branches of the anterior choroidal artery and of the posterior cerebral artery. The anterior choroidal artery supplies parts of the uncus, while the posterior cerebral artery supplies, in addition to the uncus, the body and tail of the hippocampus. The amygdala is supplied by branches of the M1 segment of the middle cerebral artery and of the anterior choroidal artery. Terminal branches of the internal carotid artery supply the medial and lateral segments of the amygdala. The posterior cerebral artery rarely contributes branches to the amygdala. The parahippocampal gyrus is supplied through P2 segments of the posterior cerebral artery.

6 Functional and Clinical Considerations

The major afferents presumed to influence this intrinsic circuitry originate from:

1. The cerebral cortex, which sends cortico-hippocampal projections that terminate mainly in the entorhinal area and originate more precisely from the orbitofrontal (areas 12 and 13), the insular, the anterior cingulate (areas 23 and 24), the temporal polar (area 38), the intralimbic (area 25), as well as from the primary somesthetic, auditory, and visual cortices; thus, from all sensory modalities including the olfactory inputs originating from the olfactory bulb (Van Hoesen and Pandia 1975; Van Hoesen et al. 1975, 1979; Crettek and Price 1977; Van Hoesen 1982; Room and Gronewegen 1986; Vitter et al. 1986; Insausti et al. 1987)
2. The amygdala, which projects fibers to the hippocampus and the entorhinal cortex, mainly from its basolateral amygdaloid nuclei (Crettek and Price 1974, 1977; Room and Gronewegen 1986)
3. The medial septal nucleus and the nucleus of the diagonal band, which project massively to the hippocampus mainly via the fornix but may also project through the cingulum or the medial forebrain bundle. These projections explain the presence of cholinergic fibers in the hippocampal formation and may constitute the anatomical substratum of the characteristic slow theta rhythm of the hippocampus (Domesick 1976; Camper 1976; Meibach and Siegel 1977; Alonso and Cohler 1984; Amaral and Kurz 1985)
4. The anterior and midline nuclei of the thalamus, which project to the hippocampal and parahippocampal region via the cingulate bundle. This projection constitutes a portion of the circuit of Papez (Domesick 1970; Robertson and Kaitz 1981; Yanagihara 1985)
5. Noradrenergic and serotoninergic fibers arising from the locus coeruleus and the mesencephalic raphe nuclei, respectively, which project to the hippocampus mainly via the fornix (Nauta and Kuypers 1958; Pearson et al. 1990; Tork and Hornung 1990)

The main efferent fiber bundle of the hippocampal formation is represented by the fornix, which contains the axons of cells of the subiculum as well as of the pyramidal cells of the hippocampus, estimated as averaging 1.2 million fibers in humans (Powell et al. 1957) as compared to 500,000 in monkeys (Daitz and Powell 1954). These projections form the alveus and converge upon the medial border of the ventricular surface of the hippocampus to form the fimbria. The fimbriae are flattened bands of whiter fibers lying superior to the dentate gyrus, which increase in thickness as they proceed backward and form the inferior boundary of the choroidal fissure. Posteriorly, the fimbriae ascend towards and arch under the splenium of the corpus callosum, constituting the crura of the fornix. Closely applied to the inferior aspect of the corpus callosum, the crura are connected to each other by a number of fibers forming the hippocampal commissure or psalterium. This structure is poorly developed in humans. The crura join to form the body of the fornix, attached to the inferior border of the septum pellucidum, which overlies the superomedial aspect of the thalamus to reach its rostral extremity. At this level, the body of the fornix diverges again above the interventricular foramina as the anterior columns curve inferiorly caudal to the AC. At that level, each anterior column divides into two components: a precommissural fornix which proceeds rostrally to the AC and a major postcommissural fornix which continues inferoposteriorly, traversing the hypothalamic region in the lateral wall of the third ventricle, before ending in the mamillary nuclei (Daitz and Powelll 1954; Powelll et al. 1957; Meibach and Siegel 1977).

The precommissural fornix transfers fibers originating from the Ammon's horn and the subiculum and projects them mainly to the lateral septal nucleus, known to project, as previously mentioned, to the medial septal nucleus and the nucleus of the diagonal band, from which afferents to the hippocampal formation arise. Fibers from the cornu ammonis may be glutamatergic. The fibers arising from the subiculum also project to the nucleus accumbens, the medial portion of the frontal cortex, the gyrus rectus, and the anterior olfactory nucleus (Meibach and Siegel 1977; Rosen and Van Hoesen 1977; Swanson and Cowan 1977). The connections with the nucleus accumbens linked to the ventral pallidum and the mesencephalon may explain the influence of the hippocampus on the somatomotor activities.

The postcommissural fornical fibers originate from the subicular cortex to end in the mamillary body. Some of the fibers leave the postcommissural fornix and are distributed to the anterior thalamic nucleus, which receives the same amount of fibers as from the mamillothalamic tract, and to the lateral septal nuclei, the ventromedial hypothalamic nucleus and the bed nucleus of the stria terminalis (Guillery 1956; Nauta 1956; Powell et al. 1957; Swanson and Cowan 1975, 1977; Meibach and Siegel 1977; Krayniak et al. 1979). Some of the postcommissural fibers project caudally to the midbrain tegmentum and are joined by fibers originating in the septal nuclei to constitute a massive component of the medial forebrain bundle (Guillery 1956).

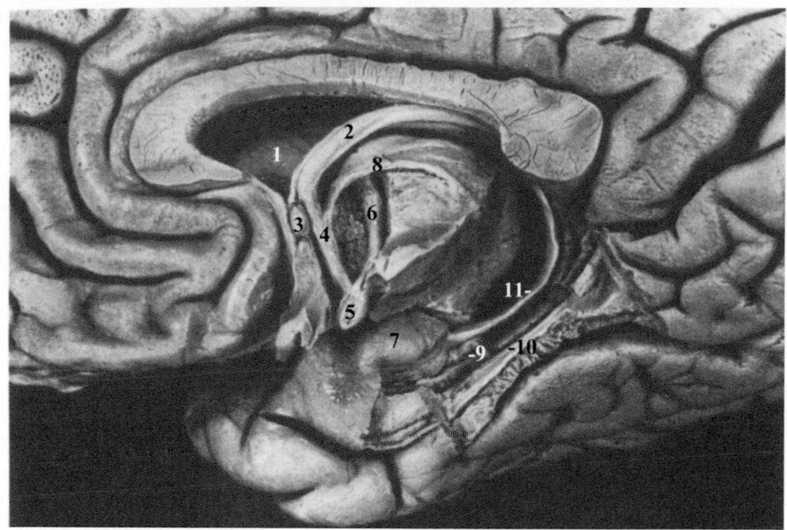

Fig. 6.27. Anatomic dissection of the major limbic pathways. *1*, Caudate nucleus; *2*, body of fornix; *3*, anterior commissure; *4*, column of fornix; *5*, mamillary body; *6*, mamillothalamic fasciculus; *7*, uncus; *8*, stria medullaris thalami; *9*, hippocampal sulcus; *10*, parahippocampal gyrus, medullary lamina; *11*, crus of fornix. (After Ludwig and Klingler 1956)

Some nonfornical fibers arise also from the subicular complex and project to the adjacent entorhinal cortex. These constitute part of the reciprocal projections connecting the subiculum and the entorhinal area (Beckstead 1978; Sorensen and Schipley 1979; Vitter and Groenewegen 1986; Van Groen et al. 1986). Efferents to the cerebral cortex terminate in the posterior cingulate cortex (area 23) and the retrosplenial cortex (areas 29 and 30) according to Irle and Markowitsch (1982). Projections to the amygdaloid nuclear complex have also been traced (Rosen and Van Hoesen 1977).

Anatomical data indicate that the hippocampal formation is interconnected via direct or indirect projections with the septal nuclei, the thalamus and hypothalamus, the midbrain reticular formation and widespread cortical areas, mainly sensory-specific and multimodal association areas (Swanson 1982). These cortical connections explain the functional role of the hippocampal formation in memory and learning mechanisms (Hyman et al. 1984; Duyckaerts et al. 1985; Volpe and Petito 1985).

7 Clinical Considerations

Several functions have been attributed to the hippocampus. The seminal work of Milner of the Montreal school (1973) has demonstrated the essential role of the hippocampal formation in memory and learning. In addition, the hippocampus participates, together with the amygdala, in the elaboration of emotional behavior. Several disease states result from damage to the hippocampal formation and its circuitry. The reader is referred to the following monographs (Gloor 1997; Mesulam 1985; Brodal 1981; Nieuwenhuys 1980; Carpenter 1996).

F The Uncus

The uncus includes parts of the amygdala, hippocampus and piriform cortex. It is posteriorly continuous with the parahippocampal gyrus and its posterolateral extent is separated from this latter structure by the uncal sulcus.

The amygdala produces a characteristic protrusion on the surface of the uncus, the semilunar gyrus. The semilunar gyrus is separated from the entorhinal cortex by the semiannular, or amygdaloid, sulcus. Anteriorly, the amygdala or rhinal cortex blends with the prepiriform cortex, the lateral olfactory striae and is separated from the perforated substance by the endorhinal sulcus. Posteromedially it is bordered by the optic tract. The posterior aspect of the uncus is occupied by parts of the head of the hippocampal formation.

Reerences

Abbie A (1939) J Comp Neurol 70: 12–44

Aggleton JP (1986) A description of the amygdalo-hippocampal interconnections in the macaque monkey. Exp Brain Res 16: 515–526

Aggleton JP (1992) The amygdala: neurobiological aspects of emotion, memory, and mental dysfunction. Wiley-Liss, New York

Alonso A, Kohler C (1984) A study of the reciprocal connections between the septum and the entorhinal area using anterograde and retrograde axonal transport methods in the rat brain. J Comp Neurol 225: 327–343

Alheid GF, Heimer L (1988) New perspectives in basal forebrain organization of special relevance for neuropsychiatric disorders and corticopetal components of substantia innominata. 27: 1–39

Allen WF (1941) Effect of ablating the pyriform amygdaloid areas and hippocampi on positive and negative olfactory conditioned reflexes and on conditioned olfactory differentiation. Am J Physiol 132: 81–92

Amaral DG, Insaust R (1990) Hippocampal formation . In: Paxinos G (ed) The human nervous system, Chap 21. Academic, New York, pp 711–755

Amaral DG, Kurz J (1985). An analysis of the origins of the cholinergic and noncholinergic septal projections to the hippocampal formation of the rat. J Comp Neurol 240: 37–59

Amaral DG, Price JL, Pitkanene A, Carmichael ST (1992) Anatomical organization of the primate amygdaloid complex. In: Aggleton JP (ed) The amygdala: neurobiological aspects of emotion, memory, and mental dysfunction. Wiley-Liss, New York, pp 1–66

Baulac M, Vitte E, Dormont D, Hasboun D, Chiras J, Sarcy JJ, Bories J, Signoret JL (1988) The limbic system: identification of its structures on brain slices. In: Gouaze A, Salamon G (eds) Brain anatomy and magnetic resonance imaging. Springer, Berlin Heidelberg New York, pp 140–150

Bhatia S, Bookheimer SY, Gaillard WD, Theodore WH (1993) Measurement of whole temporal lobe and hippocampus for MR volumetry: normative data. Neurology 43: 2006–2010

Brodal A (1981, 1969) Neurological anatomy in relation to clinical medicine, 3rd edn, Oxford University Press, New York, p 1053

Brodmann K (1909) Vergleichende Lokalisationslehre der Grosshirnrinde. Barth, Leipzig

Bronen RA, Cheung G (1991) MRI of the normal hippocampus. Magn Reson Imaging 9: 497–500

Bronen R. A. Cheung G. (1991) Relationship of hippocampus and amygdala to coronal MRI landmarks. Magn Reson Imaging 9: 449–457

Carpenter MB (1976, 1996) Human neuroanatomy. Williams and Wilkins, Baltimore, pp 521–545

Clifford RJ (1988) Temporal lobe volume measurement from MR images: accuracy and left-right asymmetry in normal persons. J Comput Assist Tomogr 12: 21–29

Cowan WM, Raisman G, Powelll TPS (1965).The connexions of the amygdala. J Neurol Neurosurg Psych 28: 137–151

Crosby EC, Humphrey T, Lauer EW (1962). Correlative anatomy of the nervous system. Macmillan, New York

Daitz HM, Powelll TPS (1954). Studies of the connections of the fornix system. J.Neurol Neurosurg Psych 17: 75–82

Davis M (1992) The role of the amygdala in fear and anxiety. Annu Rev Neurosci 15: 353–375

Domesick VB (1970) The fasciculus cinguli in the rat. Brain Res 20: 19–32

Domesick VB (1976) Projections of the nucleus of the diagonal band of Broca in the rat. Anat Rec 184: 391–392

Duyckaerts C, Derouesne C, Signoret JL, Gray F, Escourolle R, Castaigne P (1985) Bilateral and limited amygdalohippocampal lesions causing a pure amnesic syndrome. Ann Neurol 18: 314–319

Duvernoy H (1988) The human hippocampus. An atlas of applied anatomy. Bergmann, Munich

Duvernoy H (1998) The human hippocampus, 2nd edn. Springer, Berlin Heidelberg New York

Erdem A, Yazargil G, Roth P (1993) Microsurgical anatomy of hippocampal arteries. J Neurosurgery 79: 256–265

Feindel W, Penfield W (1954) Localization of discharge in temporal lobe automatism. Arch Neurol Psychiatry 72: 605–639

Gloor P (1972) Temporal lobe epilepsy: its possible contribution to the understanding of the functional significance of the amygdala and of its interaction with neocortical temporal mechanisms. In: Eleftheriou BE (ed) The neurobiology of the amygdala. Plenum, New York, pp 423–457

Gloor P (1997) The temporal lobe and the limbic system. Oxford University Press, London

Guillery RW (1956) Degeneration in the posterior commissural fornix and the mammillary peduncle of the rat. J Anat 90: 350–370

Honeycut N, Smith CD (1995) Hippocampal volume measurements using magnetic resonance imaging in young normal adults. J Neuroimaging 5: 95–100

Humphrey T (1968) The development of the human amygdala during early embryonic life. J Comp Neurol 132:135–166

Huther G, Dorfl J, Van der Loos H, Jeanmonod D (1998) Microanatomic and vascular aspects of the temporomesial region. Neurosurgery 43: 1118–1136

Hyman BT, Van Hoesen GW, Damasio AR, Barnes CL (1984) Alzheimer's disease: cell-specific pathology isolates the hippocampal formation. Science 225: 1168–1170

Insausti R, Amaral DG, Cowan WM (1987) The entorhinal cortex of the monkey. II. Cortical afferents. J Comp Neurol 264: 396–408

Insausti R, Juottonen K, Soininen H, Insausti AM, Partanen K, Vainio P, Laakso M, Pitkanen A (1998) MR volumetric analysis of the human entorhinal, perirhinal and temporopolar cortices. AJNR 19: 659-671

Irle E, Markowitsch HJ (1982) Widespread cortical projections of the hippocampal formation in the cat. Neuroscience 7: 2637–2647

Issacson RL, Pribram KH (1975) The hippocampus, 2nd edn. Plenum, New York

Issacson RL (1992) A fuzzy limbic system. Behav Brain Res 52: 129–131

Ishizuka N, Weber J, Amaral DG (1990) Organization of intrahippocampal projections originating from CA3 pyramidal cells in the rat. J Comp Neurol 295: 580–623

Jack CR, Gehring DG, Sharbrough FW, Felmlee JP, Forbes G, Hench VS, Zinsmeister AR (1988) Temporal lobe volume measurement from MR images. Accuracy and left-right asymmetry in normal persons. J Comput Assist Tomogr 12: 21–29

Jack CR, Twomey CK, Zinmeister AR, Sharbrough FW, Petersen RC, Cascino GD (1989) Anterior temporal lobes and hippocampal formations: normative volumetric measurements from MR images in young adults. Radiology 172: 549–554

Klingler J (1948) Die makroskopische anatomie der ammonsformation. Denkschriften der schweizerischen naturforschenden Gesellschaft. Fretz, Zürich, 78:82

Kluver H (1952)

Kluver H, Bucy P (1939) Preliminary analysis of functions of the temporal lobes in monkeys. Arch Neurol Psychiatry 42: 979–1000

Kotter R, Meyer N (1992) The limbic system: a review of its empirical foundation. Behav Brain Res 52: 105–127

Krayniak PF, Siegel A, Meibach RC, Fruchtman D, Scrimenti M (1979) Origin of the fornix system in the squirrel monkey. Brain Res 160: 401–411

Lecaque G, Scialfa G, Salamon G, et al (1978) Les arteres du gyrus para hippocampique. J Neuroradiol 5: 3–12

Lewis FT (1923) The significance of the term hippocampus. J Comp Neurol 35: 213–230

Lilly R, Cummings JL, Benson F, Frankel M (1983) The human Kluver-Bucy syndrome. Neurology 33: 1141–1145

Lorente De No R (1934) Studies on the structure of the cerebral cortex. II. Continuation of the study of the ammonic system. J Psychol 46: 113–177

Ludwig E, Klingler J (1956) Atlas cerebri humani. Karger, Basel

MacLean PD (1952) Some psychiatric implications of physiological studies on frontotemporal portions of limbic system (visceral brain). Electroencephalogr Clin Neurophysiol 4: 407–418

Mark LP, Daniels DL, Naidich TP, Williams AL (1993) Hippocampal anatomy and pathologic alterations on conventional MR images. Am J Neuroradiol 14: 1237–1240

Mark LP, Daniels DL, Naidich TP, Williams AL (1993) The fornix. Am J Neuroradiol 14: 1355–1358

Meibach RC, Siegel A (1977) Efferent connections of the hippocampal formation in the rat. Brain Res 124: 197–224

Mesulam MM (1985) Patterns in behavioral neuroanatomy: association areas, the limbic system and hemispheric specialization. In: Mesulam MM (ed) Principles of behavioral neurology. Davis, Philadelphia

Milner B (1973) Hemispheric specialization: scope and limits. In: Schmitt FO, Worden FG (eds) The neurosciences: third study program. MIT Press, Boston

Nagata S, Rhoton A, Barry M (1988) Microsurgical anatomy of the choroidal fissure. Surg Neurol 30: 3–59

Naidich TP, Daniels DL, Haughton VM, Williams A, Pech P, Pojunas K, Palacios E (1988) The hippocampal formation and related structures of the limbic lobe: anatomic-magnetic resonance correlation. In: Gouaze A, Salamon G (eds) Brain anatomy and magnetic resonance imaging. Springer, Berlin Heidelberg New York, pp 32–64

Narabayashi H (1972) Stereotaxic amygdalatomy. In: Eleftheriou BE (ed) The neurobiology of the amygdala. Plenum, New York, pp 459–483

Narabayashi H, Nagano T, Saito Y, Yoshida M, Nagahata M (1963) Sterotaxic amygdalatomy for behavior disorders. Arch Neurol 9: 1–16

Nauta WJH (1956) An experimental study of the fornix in the rat. J Comp Neurol 104: 247–272

Nieuwenhuys R, Voogd J, van Huijzen CHR (1988) The human central nervous system. A synopsis and atlas, 3rd edn. Springer, Berlin Heidelberg New York

Papez JW (1937) A proposed mechanism of emotion. Arch Neurol Psychiat 38: 725–743

Pearson J, Halliday G, Sakamoto N, Michel JP (1990) Catecholaminergic neurons. In: Paxinos G (ed) The human nervous system. Academic, New York, 1023–1049

Porrino LJ, Crane AM, Goldman Rakic PS (1979) Direct and indirect pathways from the amygdala to the frontal lobe in rhesus monkeys. J Comp Neurol 198: 121–136

Powell TPS, Guillery RW, Cowan WM (1957) A quantitative study of the fornix-mammillo-thalamic system. J Anat 91: 419–432

Ramon y Cajal S (1909, 1911) Histologie du Système Nerveux de l'Homme et des Vertébrés (Azoulay L, translation) Maloine, Paris (Reprinted Consejo Superior De Investigaciones Cientificas, Instituto Ramon y Cajal, Madrid, 1972)

Scott SA, DeKosky ST, Scheff SW (1991) Volumetric atrophy of the amygdala in Alzheimer's disease: quantitative serial reconstruction. Neurology 41: 351–356

Scoville WB, Milner B (1957) Loss of recent memory after bilateral hippocampal lesions. J Neurol Neurosurg Psychiatry 20: 11–21

Squire LR, Zola Morgan S (1991) The medial temporal lobe memory system. Science 253: 1380–1386

Salamon G, Lecaque GL, Strother CM (1978) An angiographic study of the temporal horn. Radiology 128: 387–392

Swanson LW, Cowan WM (1977)An autoradiographic study of the organization of the efferent connections of the hippocampal formation in the rat. J Comp Neurol 172: 49–84

Terzian H (1958) Observations on the clinical symptomatology of bilateral partial or total removal of the temporal lobe in man. In: Baldwin M, Bailey P, (eds) Temporal lobe epilepsy. Thomas, Springfield, pp 510–529

Testut L, Latarjet A (1948) Traité d'anatomie humaine, vol 2. Angiologie, système nerveux central. 9th edn. Doin, Paris

Tilney F (1939) The hippocampus and its relations to the corpus callosum. J Nerv Ment Dis 89: 433–513

Tork I, Hornung JP (1990) Raphe nuclei and the serotonergic system. In: Paxinos G (ed) The human nervous system, Chap. 30. Academic , New York, pp 1001–1022

Williams PL, Warwick R, Dyson M, Bannister LH (1989) Gray's anatomy, 37th edn. Churchill Livingstone, London

Witter MP, Griffioen AW, Jorritsma-Bayham B, Krijnen JOM (1988) Entorhinal projections to the hippocampal CA1 region in the rat: an underestimated pathway. Neurosci Lett 85: 193–198

Witter MP, Van Hoesen GW, Amaral DG (1989) Topographical organisation of the entorhinal projection to the dentate gyrus of the monkey. J Neurosci 9: 216–228

Yazargil MG, Teddy PJ, Roth P (1985) Selective amygdalo-hippocampectomy. Operative anatomy and surgical technique. Adv Tech Stand Neurosurg 12: 93–123

Yeckel MF, Berger TW (1990) Feed-forward excitation of the hippocampus by afferents from the entorhinal cortex: redefinition of the role of the trisynaptic pathway. Proc Natl Acad Sci USA 87: 5832–5836

7 The Basal Forebrain, Diencephalon and Basal Ganglia

I Regional Anatomy and Imaging of the Interbrain

The diencephalon or interbrain is a midline structure with symmetrical right and left portions located on each side of the third ventricle. The topographic limits of this region are, caudally, the plane including the posterior commissure (PC), and the mamillary bodies (MB), and cranially, the plane joining the interventricular foramina to the posterior border of the optic chiasm. Caudally, the diencephalon is continuous with the tegmentum of the mesencephalon, the posterior commissure being located at the midbrain-diencephalic junction. Anteriorly, some portions of the hypothalamus extend at least to the lamina terminalis. Laterally, the diencephalon is bordered by the internal capsule. The diencephalon comprises the thalamus, the subthalamic region and the epithalamus.

Such structures have developmental and phylogenetic significance. It is interesting to add to these main structures, in terms of functional anatomy, other related and regional anatomic structures, such as the basal ganglia consisting of the lenticular and caudate nuclei and the amygdaloid nuclear complex. Moreover, these core brain structures are functionally interrelated but also well displayed together on MR imaging cuts and, particularly, on contiguous coronal cuts oriented parallel to the brainstem long axis, in man and in anthropoids (Fig. 7.1). All these diencephalic and deep telencephalic anatomic structures are located between the coronal plane, tangent to the genu of the corpus callosum and extending posteriorly to the commissural-obex reference plane, the PC-OB (Tamraz et al. 1990, 1991) but excluding, at this level, the pulvinar thalami found behind this plane (see synoptical atlas at end of chapter).

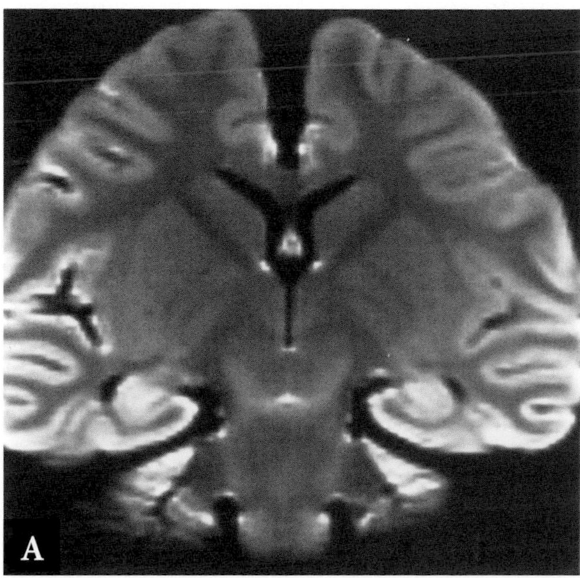

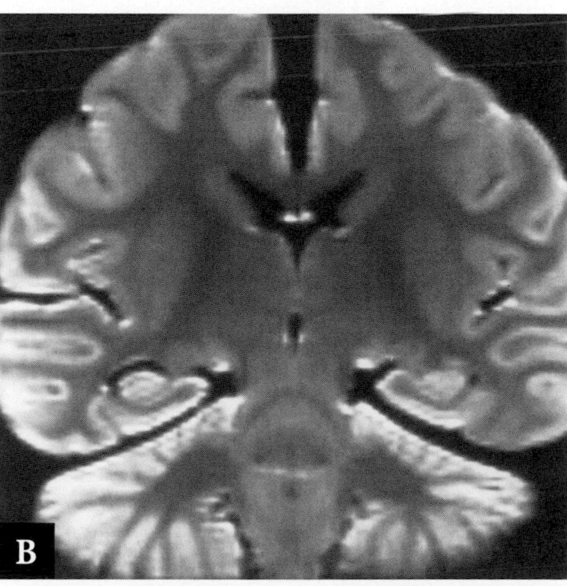

Fig. 7.1A,B. Coronal MR cuts displaying the brainstem and interbrain structures of the chimpanzee brain, using the commissural-obex reference plane (PC-OB). Formalin brain specimen from the collection of the Laboratoire d'Anatomie Comparée, Museum National d'Histoire Naturelle, Paris (R. Saban and J. Repérant)

Anterior to the anterior commissural plane, the cuts involve the paraterminal gyrus and the subcallosal area, together constituting the septal area beneath which are found the septal nuclei functionally linked to the limbic system. Note that the diencephalon corresponds in large measure to the third ventricle and the anatomic gray matter structures which bound it, the thalamus dorsally and the hypothalamus ventrally, separated by the hypothalamic sulcus. The thalamus is contained in the slab extending from the plane of the interventricular-mamillary bodies anteriorly to the plane tangent posteriorly to the quadrigeminal plate and the pineal body.

This functional region is covered by the lateral ventricles, the corpus callosum, the velum interpositum, and the fornix and is limited laterally by the insula on each side.

II The Basal Forebrain and Related Structures

The septal region and the substantia innominata are major components of a heterogeneous group of telencephalic structures which occupy the medial and the ventral aspects of the cerebral hemispheres. This area includes the so-called basal forebrain, which extends from the olfactory tubercles to the hypothalamus overlapping the anterior perforated substance. This ill-defined basal forebrain region includes the septal region and the olfactory tubercle (Figs. 7.2, 7.3), the substantia innominata and a related portion of the amygdala (Figs. 7.4, 7.5). For convenient imaging purposes, this region may be extended to involve anteriorly the related orbitofrontal cortices, already described in Chap. 3. All these basal ana-

A

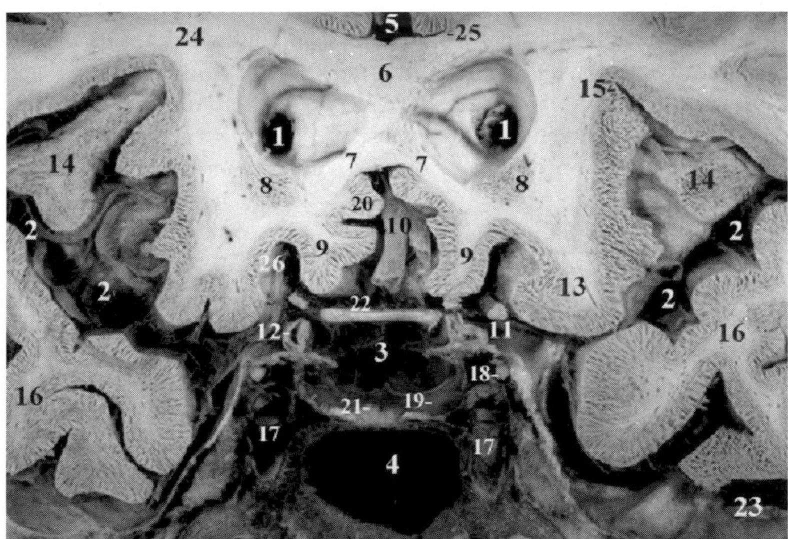

B

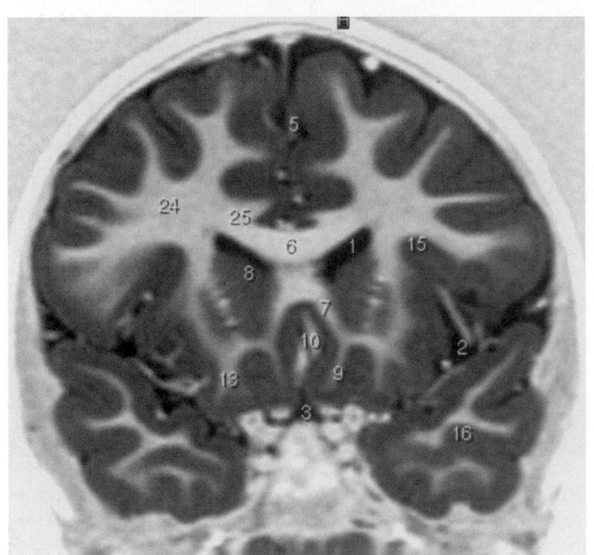

Fig. 7.2A,B. Coronal anatomic cuts through the anterior basal forebrain displayed in a rostrocaudal order (Figs. 7.2–7.5) with MR correlations. Coronal cut through the anterior basal forebrain at the level of the rostrum of corpus callosum. **A** Anatomy, **B** MR IR, T1-w. *1*, Tip of the frontal horn; *2*, lateral fissure; *3*, suprasellar cistern; *4*, sphenoid sinus; *5*, interhemispheric fissure; *6*, genu of corpus callosum; *7*, rostrum of corpus callosum; *8*, head of caudate nucleus; *9*, rectus gyrus; *10*, anterior cerebral artery; *11*, olfactory tract; *12*, supraclinoid internal carotid artery; *13*, orbitofrontal gyri; *14*, insula, anterior pole; *15*, superior border of circular sulcus; *16*, temporal pole; *17*, intracavernous internal carotid artery; *18*, oculomotor nerve (III); *19*, pituitary gland (adenohypophysis); *20*, cingulate gyrus; *21*, pituitary gland (neurohypophysis); *22*, optic chiasm; *23*, middle cranial fossa; *24*, centrum semiovale; *25*, callosal sulcus; *26*, olfactory sulcus

tomic structures are best imaged using the coronal approach perpendicular to the long axis of the temporal ventricular horns and lobes, and will be evaluated according to the PC-OB plane.

A The Septal Region

1 Morphology and Topographical Anatomy and Imaging

The septal region, also named the septum verum or precommissural septum, develops from the telencephalon and is situated anterior and superior to the lamina terminalis and the AC, forming part of the medial wall of the cerebral hemispheres. It consists of nuclear masses of gray matter and important bundles of white fibers. The septal region is bordered dorsally by the corpus callosum and caudally by the AC and the preoptic region. The base of the septal region ventral to the AC is continuous laterally with the substantia innominata (Figs. 7.4, 7.5).

The septal region shows variations in different mammals, being very well developed in lower mammals. In higher primates and in humans, the septal region shows modifications due to the great expansion of the corpus callosum and the neocortex. The upper portion of the septal region is reduced to the thin septum pellucidum constituting the supracommissural part. The precommissural septum verum, corresponding to the lower portion, contains a number of more or less individualized cell groups among which are retained the medial septal nucleus, composed of large cholinergic neurons projecting to the

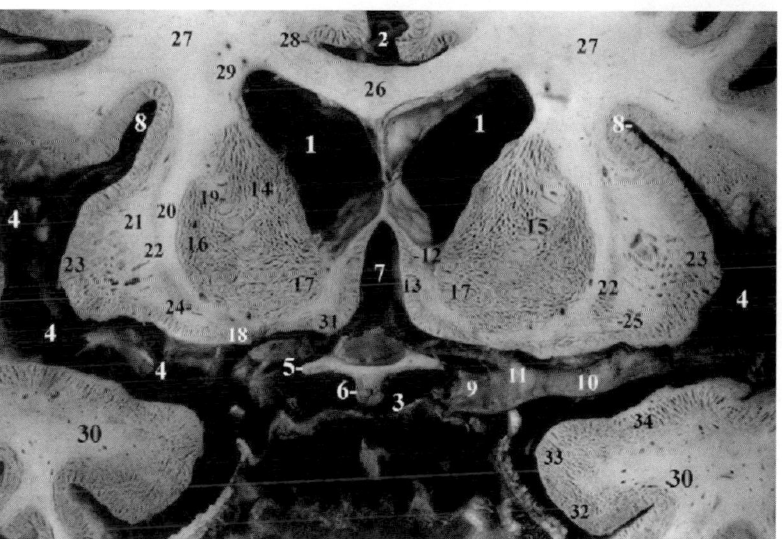

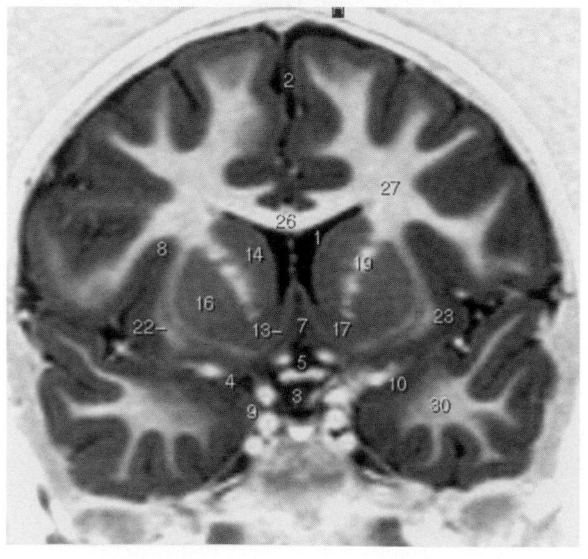

Fig. 7.3A,B. Coronal cuts through the anterior basal forebrain at the level of the subcallosal area, showing the anterior part of the striatum and the ventral striatum comprising the nucleus accumbens septi. **A** Anatomy, **B** MR IR, T1-w. *1*, Frontal horn of lateral ventricle; *2*, interhemispheric fissure; *3*, chiasmal cistern; *4*, lateral fissure; *5*, optic tract; *6*, infundibulum of the third ventricle; *7*, cisterna of lamina terminalis; *8*, circular sulcus of insula; *9*, internal carotid artery; *10*, middle cerebral artery; *11*, anterior cerebral artery; *12*, rostrum and callosal radiation; *13*, paraterminal gyrus (subcallosal area); *14*, head of caudate nucleus; *15*, internal capsule, anterior limb; *16*, putamen; *17*, nucleus accumbens; *18*, olfactory tubercle (olfactory area); *19*, putaminocaudate gray matter bridges; *20*, external capsule; *21*, extreme capsule; *22*, claustrum; *23*, insula; *24*, ventral claustrum; *25*, uncinate fasciculus; *26*, corpus callosum; *27*, centrum semi-ovale; *28*, callosal sulcus; *29*, fronto-occipital bundle; *30*, temporal lobe; *31*, diagonal band; *32*, entorhinal cortex; *33*, gyrus ambiens; *34*, semilunar gyrus

hippocampus, the lateral septal nucleus, consisting of smaller non cholinergic neurons, and the nucleus accumbens septi, located at the base of the septum medial to the junction of the caudate nucleus and the putamen (Fig. 7.3). The ventromedial part of the septum is occupied by the nucleus of the diagonal band of Broca.

More detailed and precise information concerning the septum may be found in the following reviews by Andy and Stephan (1968), Nauta and Haymaker (1969), Stephan (1975), and Mesulam et al. (1983, 1989).

2 Functional and Clinical Considerations

The connections of the septal nuclei have drawn much interest due to the influence of this anatomic region on behavior and autonomic functions. In general, the lateral septal nucleus receives the major afferents and the medial septal complex, comprising the medial septal nucleus and the nucleus of the diagonal band of Broca, giving rise to most of the septal efferents.

The main afferents to the lateral septal nucleus originate from the hippocampal formation, the Ammon's horn and the subiculum, via the precommissural fornix (Swanson and Cowan 1977; Meibach and Siegel 1977). Others arise from the preoptic region and several hypothalamic nuclei, as well as from the locus coeruleus, the raphe nuclei, the parabrachial nuclei and the dorsal tegmental nucleus (Lindvall et al. 1974; Bobillier et al. 1976). The medial septal nuclear complex receives important projections from the lateral septal nucleus, the mamillary nucleus, the lat-

A

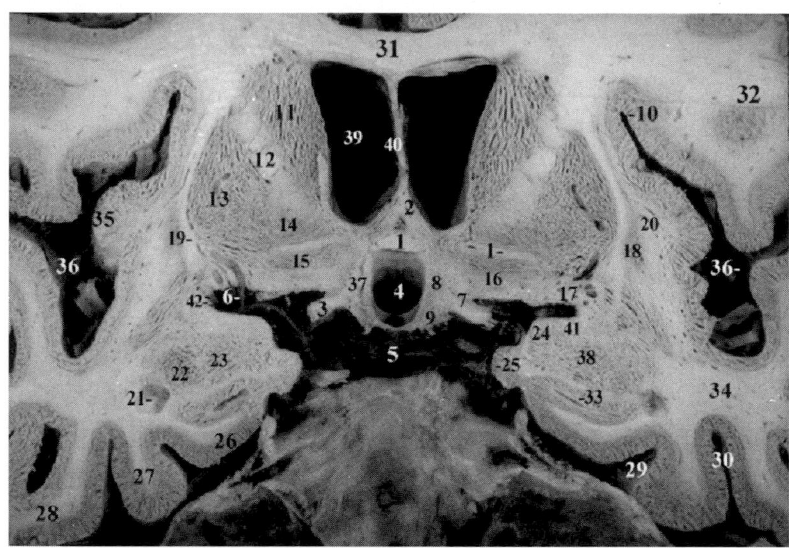

B

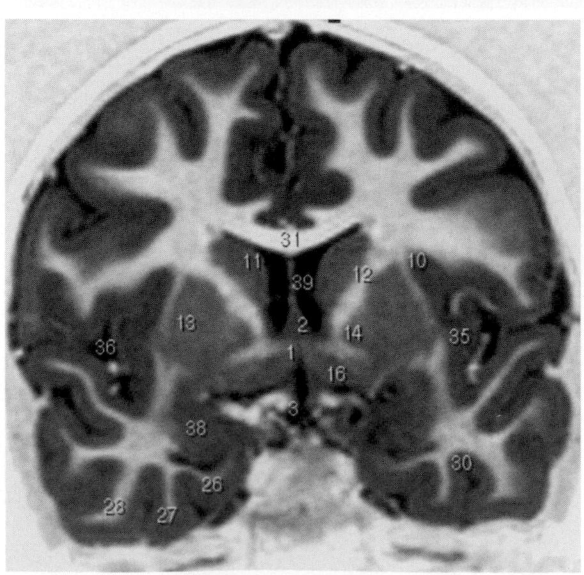

Fig. 7.4A,B. Coronal cuts through the anterior basal forebrain at the level of the anterior commissure passing through the basal ganglia, the substantia innominata, and the amygdala. **A** Anatomy, **B** MR IR, T1-w. *1*, Anterior commissure; *2*, anterior columns of fornix; *3*, optic tract; *4*, third ventricle; *5*, chiasmal cistern; *6*, lenticulostriate artery; *7*, supraoptic nucleus of hypothalamus; *8*, paraventricular nucleus of hypothalamus; *9*, tuber; *10*, circular sulcus of insula; *11*, caudate nucleus; *12*, internal capsule, anterior limb; *13*, putamen; *14*, pallidum, pars lateralis; *15*, ventral pallidum; *16*, substantia innominata; *17*, anterior perforated substance; *18*, claustrum; *19*, external capsule; *20*, extreme capsule; *21*, inferior horn of lateral ventricle; *22*, lateral nucleus of amygdala; *23*, basal nucleus of amygdala; *24*, cortcal nucleus of amygdala (gyrus semilunaris); *25*, gyrus ambiens; *26*, parahippocampal gyrus (entorhinal area); *27*, fusiform gyrus; *28*, inferior temporal gyrus; *29*, collateral/rhinal sulcus; *30*, lateral occipitotemporal sulcus; *31*, corpus callosum; *32*, inferior frontal gyrus; *33*, hippocampus, head; *34*, temporal stem; *35*, insula; *36*, lateral fissure; *37*, hypothalamus; *38*, amygdala; *39*, frontal horn of the lateral ventricle; *40*, septum lucidum; *41*, medial nucleus of amygdala; *42*, endorhinal sulcus

eral preoptico-hypothalamic region, and the dorsal tegmental nucleus.

The main efferents from the lateral septal nucleus project fibers to the medial septal complex, to many hypothalamic nuclei and the midbrain reticular formation via the medial forebrain bundle, and to the habenular nuclei via the stria medullaris thalami (Swanson and Cowan 1979). The efferents originating in the medial septal nuclei and the nuclei of the diagonal band project mostly to the hippocampal formation, the subiculum, and the entorhinal cortex via the fornix. These efferents are reciprocal to the afferents. The septohippocampal fibers appear to be diffusely distributed throughout the hippocampus. Other efferents are distributed to the lateral hypothalamic and preoptic regions, the mamillary nucleus, and the midbrain reticular formation (Swanson and Cowan 1979; Alonso and-Cohler 1984).

Functionally, the septal region appears to be an important region through which major hypothalamic and limbic structures are interconnected, mainly by the hippocampal formation. Contrary to prevailing opinion, the septal nuclei increase in prominence in primates and reach the highest degree of development in humans (Andy and Stephan 1968). Several functions are attributed to the septal region.

The so-called septal syndrome observed after destruction of the septal nuclei is characterized by behavioral overreaction to environmental stimuli. Modifications of behavior occur in feeding and drinking, reproductive functions and rage. A reduction of aggressive behavior is observed following lesions of the septal area. Hormonal modifications are also found in

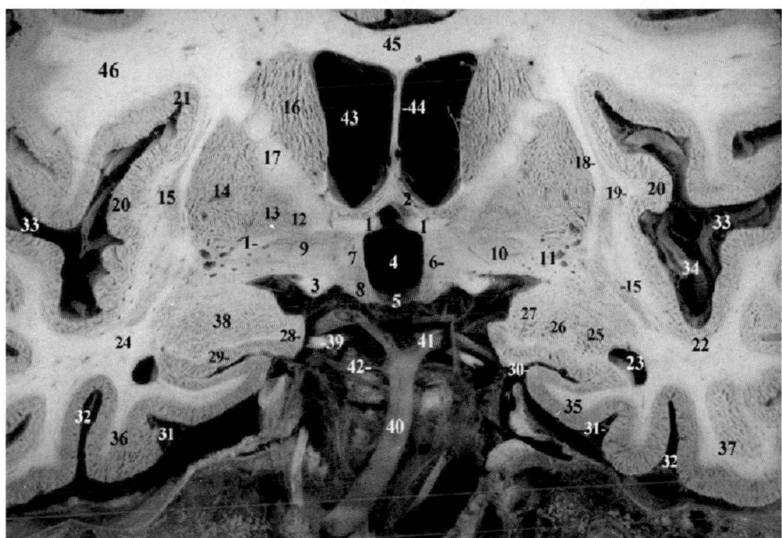

A

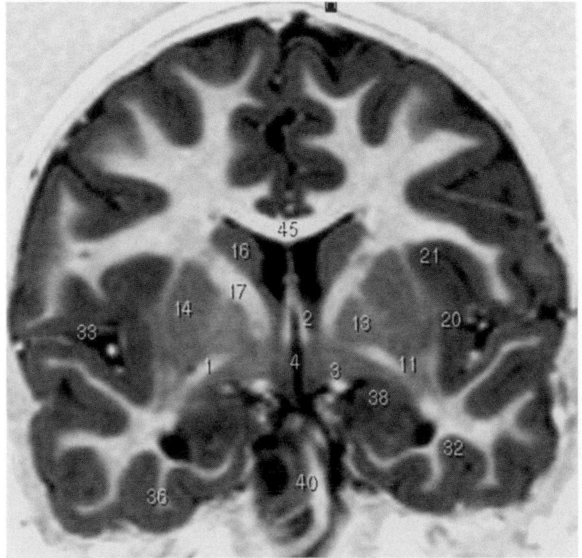

B

Fig. 7.5A,B. Coronal cuts through the anterior basal forebrain at the level of the anterior commissure, passing through the basal ganglia and the amygdala. Note that the substantia innominata lies beneath the globus pallidus. (This cut is almost contiguous to the former.) **A** Anatomy, **B** MR IR, T1-w. *1*, Anterior commissure; *2*, anterior columns of fornix; *3*, optic tract; *4*, third ventricle; *5*, floor of third ventricle; *6*, lateral hypothalamic area; *7*, dorsomedial nucleus of hypothalamus; *8*, ventromedial nucleus of hypothalamus; *9*, substantia innominata; *10*, ventral striatum; *11*, anterior perforated substance; *12*, medial globus pallidus; *13*, lateral globus pallidus; *14*, putamen; *15*, claustrum; *16*, caudate nucleus; *17*, internal capsule, genu; *18*, external capsule; *19*, extreme capsule; *20*, insula; *21*, insular sulcus, superior border; *22*, circular sulcus, inferior border; *23*, inferior horn of lateral ventricle; *24*, temporal stem; *25*, lateral nucleus of amygdala; *26*, basal nucleus of amygdala; *27*, cortical nucleus of amygdala; *28*, gyrus ambiens; *29*, hippocampus; *30*, uncal sulcus; *31*, collateral/rhinal sulcus; *32*, lateral occipitotemporal sulcus; *33*, lateral fissure; *34*, arterial branches of the middle cerebral artery; *35*, parahippocampal gyrus; *36*, fusiform gyrus; *37*, inferior temporal gyrus; *38*, amygdala; *39*, oculomotor nerve (III); *40*, basilar artery; *41*, posterior cerebral artery; *42*, superior cerebellar artery; *43*, lateral ventricle, frontal horn; *44*, septum lucidum; *45*, corpus callosum; *46*, precentral gyrus

association with the behavioral changes, as is also observed with the amygdaloid nuclear complex.

B The Substantia Innominata

1 Morphology and Topographical Anatomy and Imaging

The substantia innominata region is a part of the basal forebrain, located near the surface of the brain and containing telencephalic structures (Fig. 7.6).Located under the pallidum, separating it from the ventral aspect of the anterior forebrain, this heterogeneous region consisting of gray and white matter lacks cortical organization.

Above the substantia innominata is the AC, easily seen on coronal slices tangent to the anterior border of this commissure, which proceeds laterally on each side as the temporal limbs are directed obliquely toward the anterior temporal lobes. The major nuclear cell group found in the substantia innominata is the basal nucleus of Meynert (Viennese neurologist in the nineteenth century). This basal nucleus contains characteristic large cells responsible for the widespread cholinergic innervation of the cerebral cortex. The substantia innominata is bounded medially by the heavily myelinated diagonal band of Broca formed of gray and white matter. These two diagonal bands are followed from the medial part of the septum along the medial aspect of the cerebral hemispheres. There they course downward in front of the AC, diverging to reach the basal aspect of the hemisphere, en route laterally toward the amygdala traversing the substantia innominata. Thus, the diagonal band of Broca morphologically links the preseptal region to the substantia innominata medially. Laterally, the substantia innominata, occupying

A

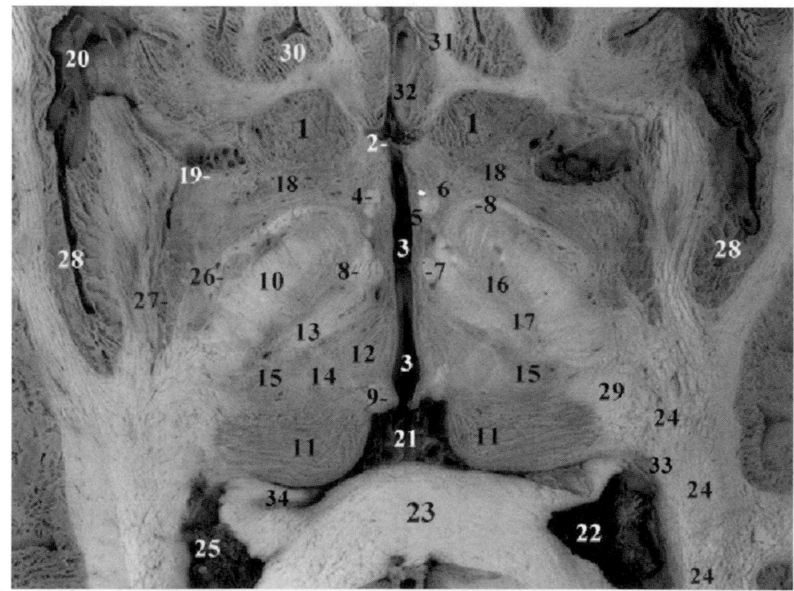

B

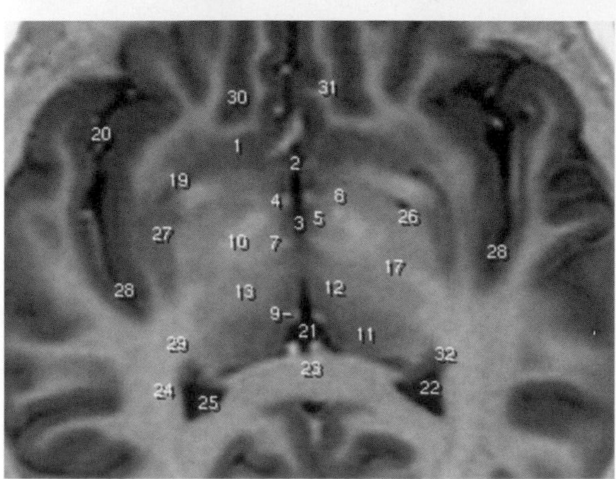

Fig. 7.6A,B. Axial cut through the midbrain-diencephalic junction, including part of the subthalamic nucleus and the innominate substance. Note that the upper midbrain region is bounded laterally and posteriorly by diencephalic structures. **A**, anatomy. **B**, MR IR, T1-w. *1*, Caudate nucleus, head; *2*, lamina terminalis; *3*, third ventricle; *4*, anterior column of fornix; *5*, medial hypothalamus; *6*, lateral hypothalamus; *7*, mamillothalamic tract; *8*, ansa lenticularis; *9*, habenular nuclei; *10*, internal capsule, posterior limb; *11*, pulvinar thalami; *12*, dorsomedian nucleus of thalamus; *13*, thalamic fasciculus; *14*, centromedian nucleus of thalamus; *15*, ventral posterior nuclear group of thalamus; *16*, subthalamic nucleus; *17*, zona incerta; *18*, substantia innominata of Reichert; *19*, anterior perforated substance; *20*, insular branches of middle cerebral artery; *21*, ambient cistern; *22*, lateral ventricle, atrium; *23*, corpus callosum, splenium; *24*, geniculocalcarine tract (optic radiations); *25*, choroid plexus, glomus; *26*, medial pallidum; *27*, putamen; *28*, circular sulcus of insula; *29*, zone of Wernicke (area triangularis); *30*, olfactory sulcus, posterior end; *31*, gyrus rectus, posterior end; *32*, subcallosal area; *33*, tail of caudate nucleus; *34*, crus fornicis

all the subcommissural region, extends toward the dorsal aspect of the amygdaloid nuclear complex from which it is difficult to distinguish on coronal MR slices (Figs. 7.4, 7.5).

The AC constitutes an important frontal central landmark separating, from medial to lateral, the inferior border of the frontal horn and the anterior inferomedial aspect of the head of the caudate nucleus; the internal capsule and the globus pallidus, superiorly; and overlying structures of the basal aspect of the brain, which comprise the diagonal band of Broca and its nucleus anteromedially; the substantia innominata and the olfactory tubercle in the subcommissural region proper; and laterally, the dorsal aspect of the amygdala in its superomedial extension (Fig. 7.5). This region is well displayed on the coronal slices tangent to the anterior border of the AC, and extending to the contiguous slices which pass through the septal region and the anterior striatum-accumbens complex. The region is limited inferiorly by the horizontal reference CH-PC plane, whose projection on the coronal slices appears tangent to the anterior basal forebrain aspect anteriorly and to the dorsal aspects of the optic tracts at the level of the AC (Figs. 7.4, 7.5).

2 Functional and Clinical Considerations

The substantia innominata is characterized by the presence of magnocellular neurons intensely stained for acetylcholinesterase in the normal human brain. These neurons, scattered in the basal forebrain region, extending from the medial to the ventral aspect of the cerebral hemisphere as previously described, are grouped in the subcommissural region to constitute the nucleus basalis of Meynert. The latter gained much interest, recently, with the discovery that this important cell group degenerates specifically in Alzheimer's disease, as well as in senile dementias of the Alzheimer's type (SDAT). Alzheimer's disease, which normally occurs in persons over the age of 50 years, is a progressive dementia associated with the loss of memory, disorientation, apraxia and speech disorders. Pathologically, it is characterized by a diffuse degeneration of the cerebral cortex, and by the presence of amyloid plaques and neurofibrillary tangles. The basal nucleus of Meynert and the nucleus of the diagonal band appear depleted of their magnocellular neurons, which explains the major and diffuse breakdown in cholinergic innervation of the cerebral cortex (Whitehouse et al. 1981, 1982; Coyle et al. 1983). It seems that the basal nucleus and the nucleus of the diagonal band play an essential role in intellectual functions which act through cortical cholinergic innervation. To these major cortical efferents, the substantia innominata receives projections from the amygdaloid nuclei and from portions of the temporal, insular, entorhinal, and piriform cortices.

III The Thalamus

The thalami are the largest, most internal structures of the diencephalon, consisting of two oblique ovoid nuclear masses of gray matter situated at the rostral end of the midbrain on each side of the third ventricle. Each thalamus is about 3–4 cm long, lying between the interventricular foramina-mamillary plane anteriorly, and the posterior PC-OB plane posteriorly; thus, excluding the pulvinar, which extend to the plane tangent to the posterior aspect of the tectal plate, the anterior aspect of the splenium (see synoptical atlas at end of chapter). The thalamus is located dorsally to the hypothalamic sulcus, a shallow groove on the lateral wall of the third ventricle. Note that the coronal slices passing through the cerebral hemispheres, the diencephalon, and the brainstem and oriented according to the PC-OB plane display the thalami and their major subnuclei. They are surrounded, laterally, by the internal capsules, the caudate nuclei, the lentiform nuclei, and the claustrum and inferiorly by the subthalamic and red nuclei, and the substantia nigra in the midbrain-diencephalic region (Figs. 7.7–7.10).

The thalamus has two ends and four surfaces. The anterior end is narrow, located at the level of the interventricular foramen; the posterior end, named the pulvinar, is an expanded portion, which overhangs the superior colliculi and their brachia (Fig. 7.11). The superior surface of the thalamus is slightly convex and covered by the stratum zonale, which is a thin layer of white matter fibers. It is separated laterally from the caudate nucleus by a white band, the stria terminalis, which lies with the terminal vein at the junction of the thalamus and caudate nucleus. The superior surface of the thalamus may be divided into a lateral part, which partially constitutes the floor of the lateral ventricle. The medial part is covered with the tela choroidea of the third ventricle. Near the roof of the third ventricle, a small bundle of white fibers, the stria medullaris thalami, is found at the junction of the superior and medial aspects of the thalamus. The lateral surface of the thalamus is bounded by the posterior limb of the internal capsule, which separates

A

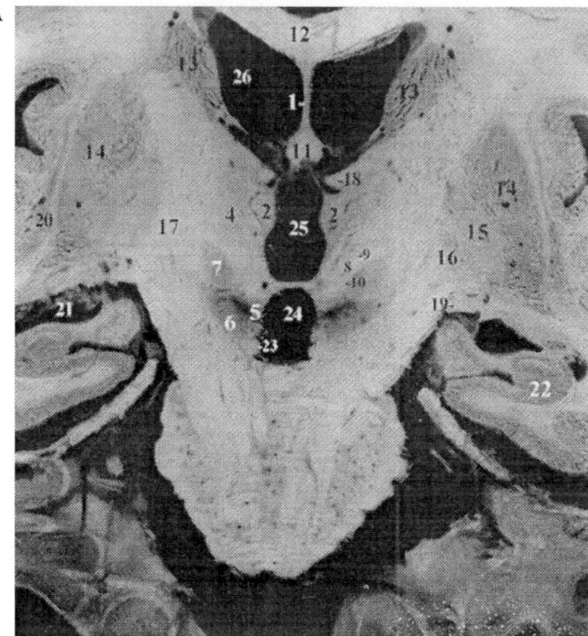

B

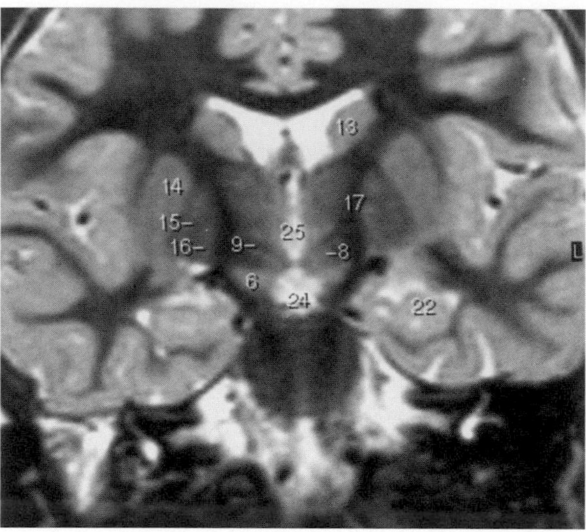

Fig. 7.7A,B. Coronal cuts through the midbrain-diencephalic region at the anterior thalamic level, passing through the Forel's fields, the subthalamic nucleus, and the substantia nigra. **A**, Anatomy. **B**, MR STIR, T2-w. *1*, Septum lucidum; *2*, dorsomedian nucleus of thalamus; *3*, mamillothalamic tract; *4*, ventral lateral nucleus of thalamus; *5*, substantia nigra, pars compacta; *6*, substantia nigra, pars reticulata; *7*, subthalamic nucleus; *8*, zona incerta; *9*, thalamic fasciculus (Forel's field H1); *10*, lenticular fasciculus (Forel's field H2); *11*, fornix; *12*, corpus callosum; *13*, caudate nucleus; *14*, putamen; *15*, globus pallidus, lateral part; *16*, globus pallidus, medial part; *17*, internal capsule; *18*, stria medullaris thalami; *19*, optic tract; *20*, claustrum; *21*, lateral ventricle, temporal horn; *22*, hippocampus; *23*, oculomotor nerve root; *24*, interpeduncular cistern; *25*, third ventricle; *26*, lateral ventricle

A

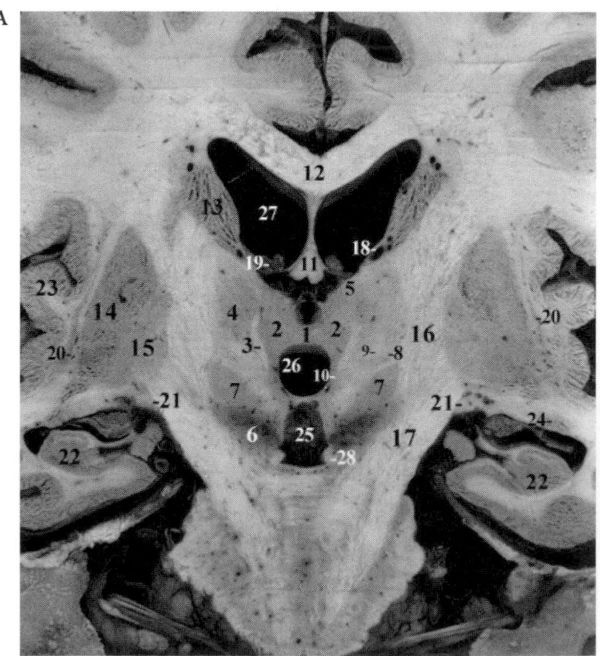

B

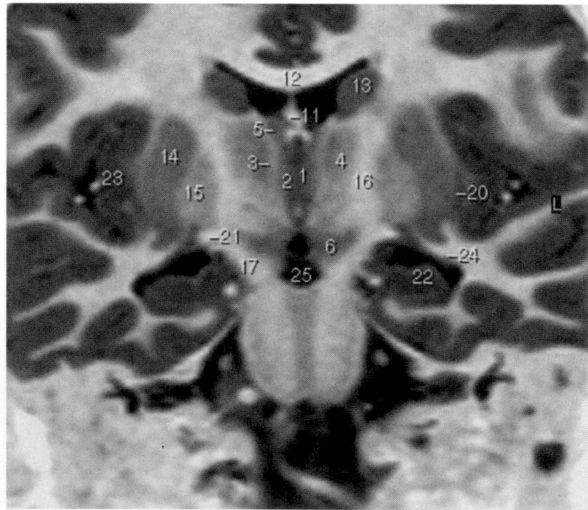

Fig. 7.8A,B. Coronal cuts through the midbrain-diencephalic region at the level of the interpeduncular fossa, passing through the interthalamic adhesion, the mamillothalamic tracts, and the posterior part of the subthalamic nucleus and the substantia nigra. **A**, Anatomy. **B**, MR IR, T1-w. *1*, Interthalamic adhesion and midline thalamic nuclear group; *2*, dorsomedian nucleus of thalamus; *3*, mamillothalamic tract; *4*, ventral lateral nucleus of thalamus; *5*, anterior nucleus of thalamus; *6*, substantia nigra; *7*, subthalamic nucleus; *8*, zona incerta; *9*, thalamic fasciculus; *10*, posterior hypothalamic nucleus; *11*, fornix; *12*, corpus callosum; *13*, caudate nucleus; *14*, putamen; *15*, globus pallidus, lateral segment; *16*, internal capsule; *17*, cerebral peduncle; *18*, thalamostriate vein; *19*, choroid plexus of lateral ventricle; *20*, claustrum; *21*, optic tract; *22*, hippocampus; *23*, insula; *24*, caudate nucleus, tail; *25*, interpeduncular cistern; *26*, third ventricle; *27*, lateral ventricle; *28*, oculomotor nerve root

A

B

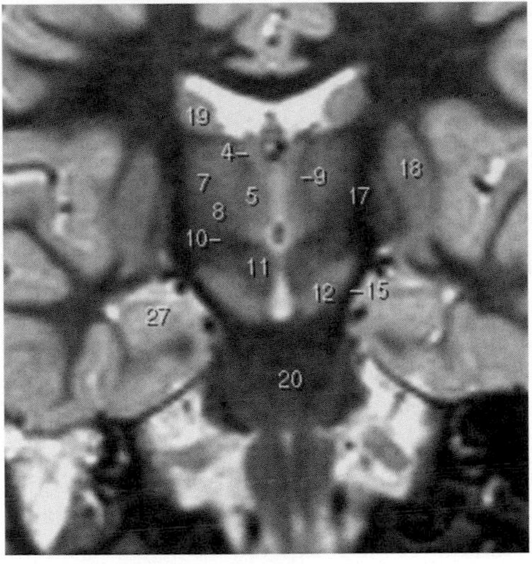

Fig. 7.9A,B. Coronal cuts through the brainstem-diencephalon continuum, displaying the major thalamic nuclear subdivisions at the level of the red nuclei. **A**, Anatomy. **B**, MR STIR, T2-w. *1*, Septum lucidum; *2*, fornix (body); *3*, thalamostriate veins; *4*, lateral dorsal nucleus of thalamus; *5*, dorsomedial nucleus of thalamus; *6*, centromedian nucleus of thalamus; *7*, ventral lateral nucleus of thalamus; *8*, ventral posterolateral nucleus of thalamus; *9*, internal medullary lamina of thalamus; *10*, Forel's fields H; *11*, red nucleus; *12*, substantia nigra; *13*, superior cerebellar peduncle (decussation); *14*, interpeduncular nucleus; *15*, cerebral peduncle (crus cerebri); *16*, lateral geniculate body; *17*, internal capsule, posterior limb; *18*, putamen; *19*, caudate nucleus; *20*, pontine nuclei; *21*, middle cerebellar peduncle; *22*, medial lemniscus; *23*, inferior olivary nuclear complex; *24*, medulla oblongata at medullary-spinal cord junction; *25*, corona radiata; *26*, corpus callosum, body; *27*, hippocampus; *28*, superior edge of tentorium cerebelli at the foramen ovale of Pacchioni

this nuclear mass from the lentiform nucleus of the corpus striatum (Figs. 7.12, 7.13).

The medial surface constitutes the lateral wall of the third ventricle above the hypothalamic sulcus on each side. The medial surfaces are usually connected (in about 80% of human brains they are partially fused) posteriorly to the interventricular foramina. The anteroposterior diameter of this gray commissure, named the interthalamic adhesion or massa intermedia, is about 1 cm (Fig. 7.12).

The inferior surface overlies the midbrain structures and is continuous with the rostral extension of the tegmentum in the subthalamic region.

A Topographical and Nuclear Organization

Most subdivisions of the thalamus are not evident either on anatomical specimens or on high resolution and high contrast MR images. For the identification of the major subnuclear groups on MRI one must rely on different criteria such as the topography with respect to the internal medullary laminae, the knowledge of the relative volume of the nuclear masses, the relative cell density of the subnuclei, and the relative importance of intrinsic myelination as related to the major afferent bundles. Chiefly constituted of gray matter, the dorsal surface of the thalamus is covered by a layer of white matter, named the stratum zonale, and its lateral surface is similarly covered by the external medullary lamina (Fig. 7.13, Table 7.1). The thalamus is incompletely divided internally into anterior, lateral, and medial nuclear groups by a thin layer of myelinated fibers, the internal medullary lamina. This lamina can be seen on coronal cuts of the brain, splitting superiorly in a Y-shaped manner (Fig. 7.12).

The anterior nuclear group, known as the anterior tubercle, forms a rostromedial distinct swelling separated from the other nuclei by a myelinated capsule (Fig. 7.8). It is comprised of the anteroventral, anteromedial, and anterodorsal nuclei. These nuclei are identified in most mammals. The anteromedial and anteroventral nuclei are well developed in apes and humans.

The medial nuclear group is located medial to the internal medullary lamina, containing the dorsomedial nucleus. This nucleus occupies most of the area located between the periventricular gray matter and the internal medullary lamina (Figs. 7.8, 7.12, 7.13).

The dorsomedial nucleus is the second largest nucleus in the human thalamus after the pulvinar.

The lateral part of the thalamic mass is subdivided into ventromedial and dorsolateral parts. The ventral nuclear group occupies the ventromedial moiety of the lateral nuclear mass of the thalamus, containing three separate nuclei which are rostrocaudally: the ventral anterior nucleus, the ventral lateral nucleus, and the ventral posterior nucleus (Fig. 7.14). The latter is subdivided into a ventral-posteromedial nucleus and a ventral posterolateral nucleus. The ventral anterior nucleus is the smallest of these nuclei and the most rostrally located, bounded anteriorly and ventrolaterally by the thalamic reticular nucleus. It occupies the thalamic region lateral to the anterior nuclear group. The mamillothalamic tract of Vicq d'Azyr passes through this nucleus (Figs. 7.8, 7.14). The ventral lateral nucleus is situated caudally to the latter. The ventral posterior nucleus is the largest and most posteriorly located nucleus of the ventral thalamic nuclei. It is subdivided into ventral posteromedial and posterolateral subnuclei, which cannot be separated on MR. The ventral posteromedial nucleus is crescent-shaped and found medially to the ventral posterolateral nucleus and laterally to the centromedian nucleus (Figs. 7.12–7.14).

The lateral nuclear group of this thalamic mass is located dorsal to the ventral nuclear group. It is also subdivided into three separate subnuclei, which are rostrocaudally: the lateral dorsal nucleus, the lateral posterior nucleus, and the pulvinar. This pulvinar forms the most caudal portion of the thalamus, overhanging the geniculate bodies and the posterolateral aspect of the midbrain (Fig. 7.11). The lateral dorsal nucleus is found on the dorsal aspect of the thalamus

A

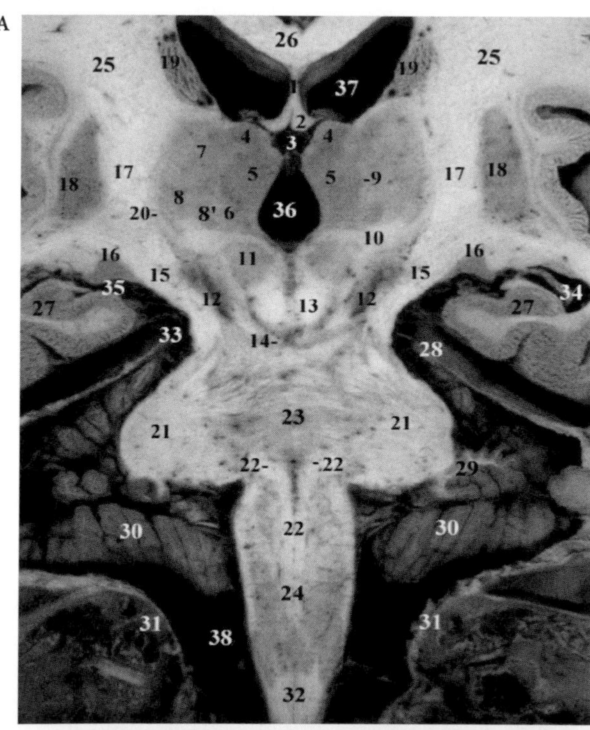

B

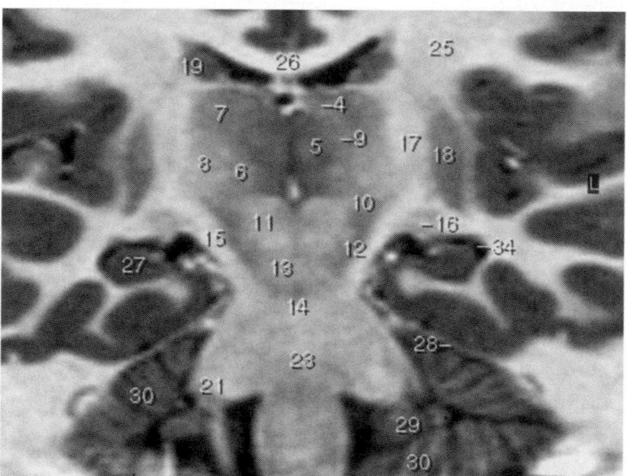

C

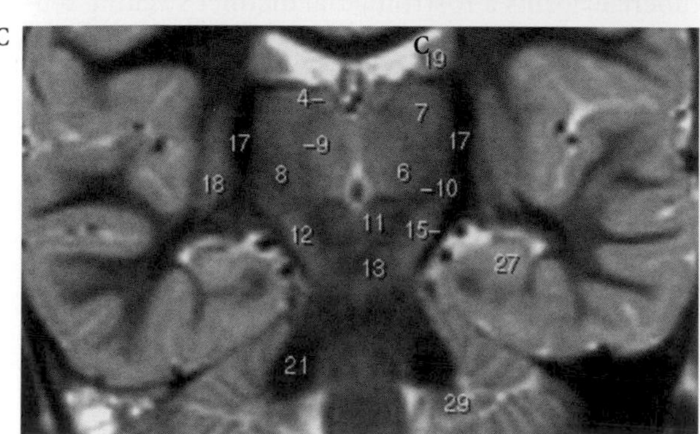

Fig. 7.10A–C. Coronal cuts (contiguous and posterior to Fig. 7.7) through the brainstem-diencephalon continuum, displaying the major thalamic nuclear subdivisions at the level of the decussation of the brachia conjunctiva. **A**, Anatomy. **B**, MR IR-T1-w. **C**, MR STIR T2-w. 1, Septum lucidum; *2*, fornix (body); *3*, internal cerebral veins (under the fornix); *4*, lateral dorsal nucleus of thalamus; *5*, dorsomedial nucleus of thalamus; *6*, centromedian nucleus of thalamus; *7*, ventral lateral nucleus of thalamus; *8*, ventral posterolateral nucleus (and ventral posteromedial); *9*, internal medullary lamina; *10*, Forel's fields H; *11*, red nucleus; *12*, substantia nigra (pars compacta corresponding to pigmented portion); *13*, superior cerebellar peduncle (decussation); *14*, oculomotor nucleus (III); *15*, cerebral peduncle (crus cerebri); *16*, lateral geniculate body; *17*, internal capsule, posterior limb; *18*, putamen; *19*, caudate nucleus body; *20*, reticular nucleus of thalamus; *21*, middle cerebellar peduncle; *22*, medial lemniscus; *23*, pontine nuclei; *24*, medulla oblongata; *25*, corona radiata; *26*, corpus callosum body; *27*, hippocampus; *28*, tentorium cerebelli; *29*, flocculus; *30*, cerebellar hemisphere; *31*, foramen magnum (outer border); *32*, spinal cord; *33*, foramen ovale of Pacchioni; *34*, temporal horn of the lateral ventricle; *35*, choroidal fissure; *36*, third ventricle; *37*, lateral ventricle; *38*, perimedullary cistern

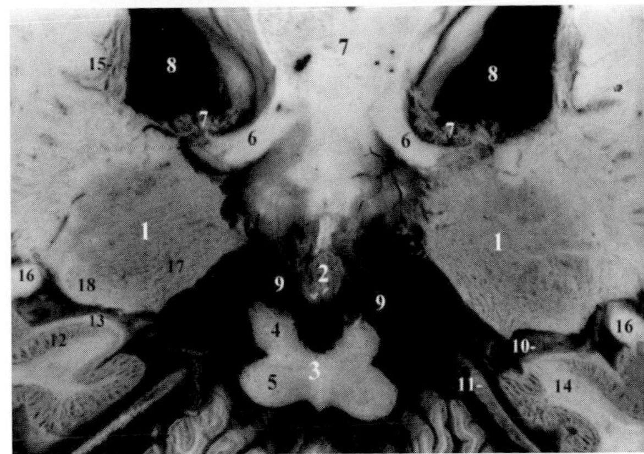

A

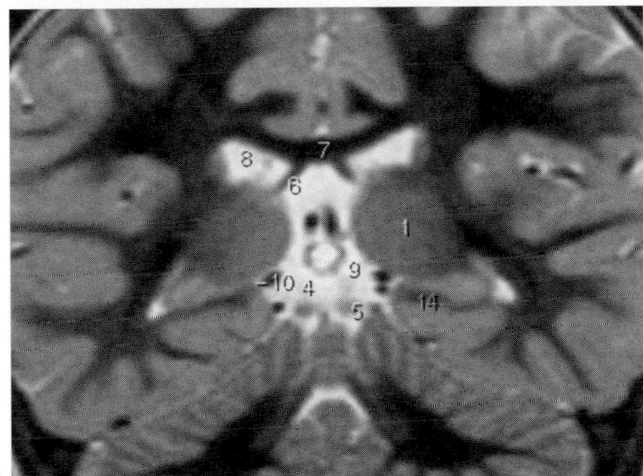

B

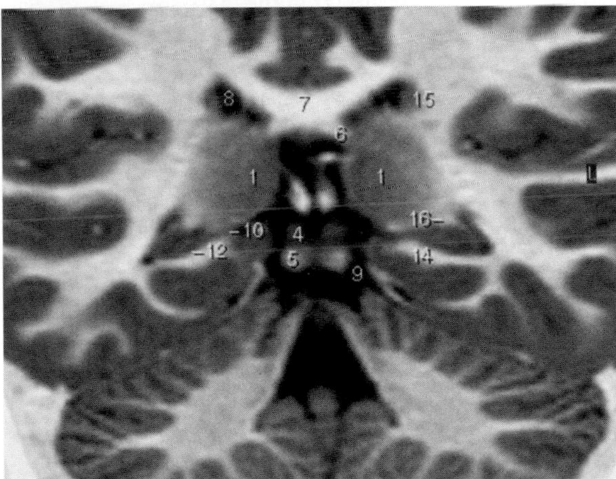

C

Fig. 7.11A–C. Posterior thalamic coronal anatomic cut through the pulvinar nuclei at the level of the pineal body and the ambient cistern. **A**, Anatomy. **B**, MR STIR-T2-w. **C**, MR IR T1-w. *1*, Pulvinar thalami; *2*, pineal body; *3*, quadrigeminal plate; *4*, superior colliculus; *5*, inferior colliculus; *6*, crus of fornix; *7*, splenium of corpus callosum; *8*, lateral ventricle; *9*, quadrigeminal cistern; *10*, wing of ambient cistern; *11*, tentorium cerebelli; *12*, subiculum; *13*, superficial medullary stratum of the subiculum; *14*, parahippocampal gyrus; *15*, body of caudate nucleus; *16*, fimbria of fornix; *17*, nucleus pulvinaris medialis; *18*, nucleus pulvinaris lateralis

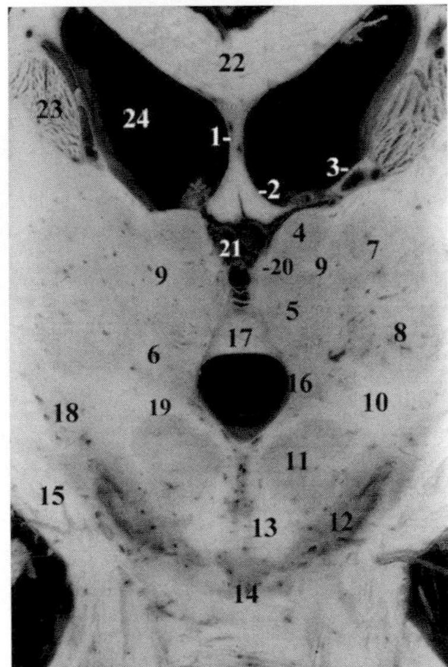

A

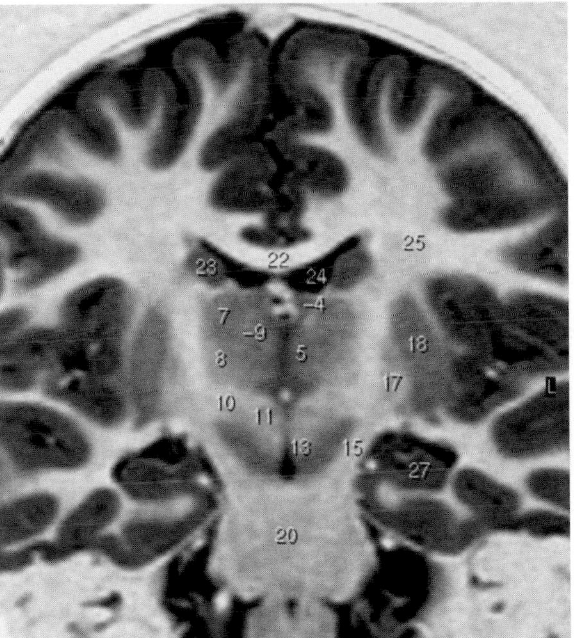

B

Fig. 7.12A,B. Major nuclear groups of the thalamus. Anterior coronal cut through the thalami displaying the internal architecture at the level of the interthalamic adhesion. **A**, Anatomy. **B**, MR IR-T1-w. *1*, Septum lucidum; *2*, fornix; *3*, thalamostriate veins; *4*, lateral dorsal nucleus of thalamus; *5*, dorsomedial nucleus of thalamus; *6*, centromedian nucleus of thalamus; *7*, ventral lateral nucleus of thalamus; *8*, ventral posterolateral nucleus of thalamus; *9*, internal medullary lamina of thalamus; *10*, cerebellorubrothalamic tracts; *11*, red nucleus; *12*, substantia nigra; *13*, superior cerebellar peduncle (decussation); *14*, interpeduncular nucleus; *15*, cerebral peduncle (crus cerebri); *16*, parafascicular nuclei; *17*, interthalamic adhesion; *18*, zona incerta; *19*, prerubral tract and Forel's field H2; *20*, stria medullaris thalami; *21*, internal cerebral veins; *22*, corpus callosum; *23*, caudate nucleus, body; *24*, lateral ventricle

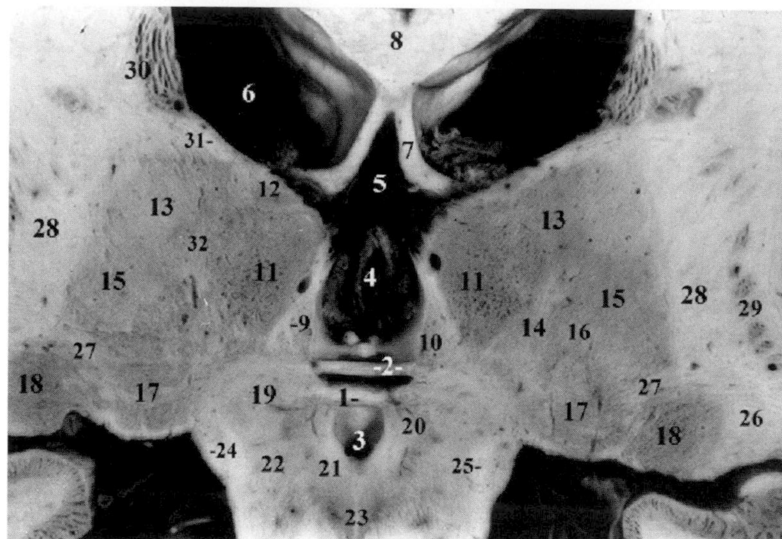

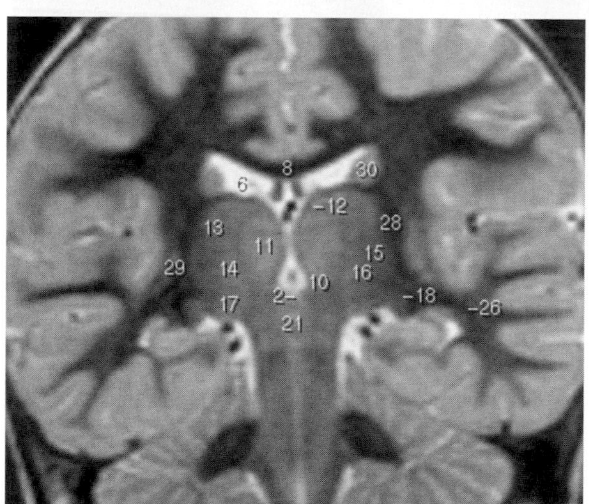

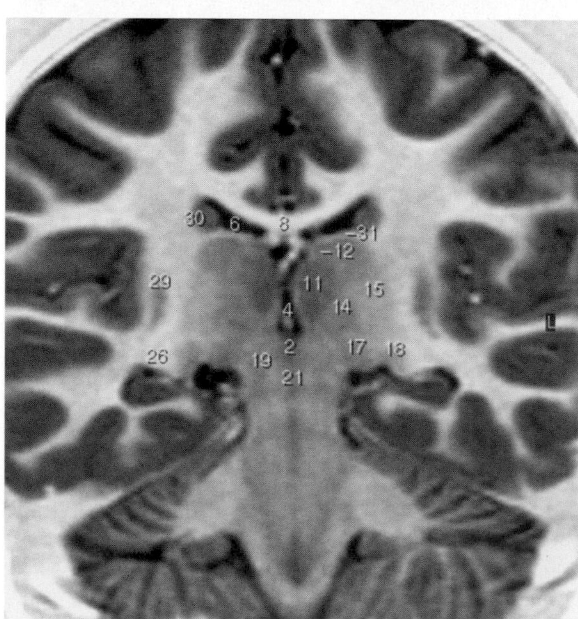

Fig. 7.13A–C. Major nuclear groups of the thalamus. Posterior coronal cut through the thalami displaying their internal architecture at the level of the posterior commissure and the lateral geniculate bodies. **A**, Anatomy. **B**, MR STIR-T2-w. **C**, MR IR T1-w. *1*, Posterior commissure; *2*, habenular commissure; *3*, cerebral aqueduct; *4*, third ventricle; *5*, quadrigeminal cistern; *6*, lateral ventricle; *7*, fornix; *8*, splenium of corpus callosum; *9*, stria medullaris thalami; *10*, habenular nucleus; *11*, dorsomedian nucleus of thalamus; *12*, lateral dorsal nucleus of thalamus; *13*, lateral posterior nucleus of thalamus; *14*, centromedian nucleus of thalamus; *15*, ventral posterolateral nucleus of thalamus; *16*, ventral posteromedial nucleus of thalamus; *17*, medial geniculate body; *18*, lateral geniculate body; *19*, pretectal area; *20*, nucleus of the posterior commissure; *21*, periaqueductal gray mater; *22*, midbrain tegmentum (nucleus tegmenti); *23*, oculomotor nerve root; *24*, brachium of inferior colliculus; *25*, medial lemniscus and spinothalamic tracts; *26*, optic radiation; *27*, auditory radiations; *28*, internal capsule; *29*, putamen (posterior border); *30*, caudate nucleus, body; *31*, external medullary lamina and thalamic reticular nucleus; *32*, internal medullary lamina of thalamus

Table 1. Major nuclear groups of the thalamus

1. Anterior nuclear group
   - Anteroventral nucleus (AV)
   - Anterodorsal nucleus (AD)
   - Anteromedial nucleus (AM)
2. Medial nuclear group
   - Dorsomedial nucleus (DM)
3. Intralaminar nuclear group
   - Centromedian nucleus (CM)
4. Lateral nuclear group
   - Lateral dorsal nucleus (LD)
   - Lateral posterior nucleus (LP)
   - Pulvinar (medial, lateral) (P)
5. Ventral nuclear group
   - Ventral anterior nucleus (VA)
   - Ventral lateral nucleus (VL)
   - Ventral posterolateral nucleus (VPL)
   - Ventral posteromedial nucleus (VPM)
6. Thalamic reticular nucleus (RN)
7. Metathalamus
   - Medial geniculate body (MGB)
   - Lateral geniculate body (LGB)

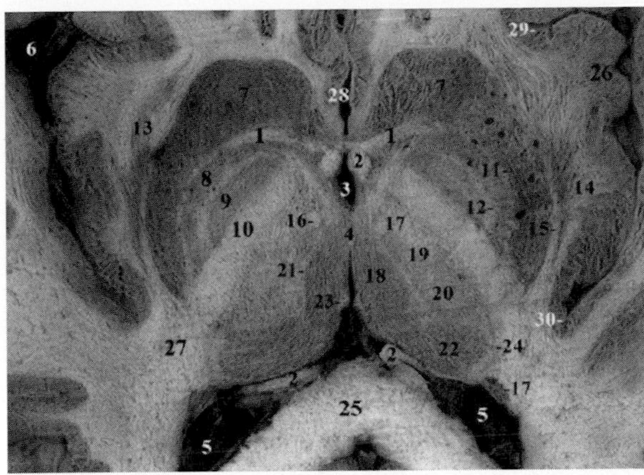

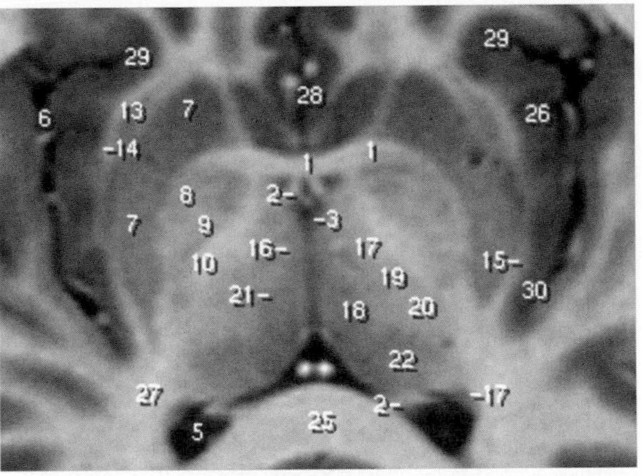

Fig. 7.14A,B. Major nuclear groups of the thalamus. Axial anatomic cut at the level of the anterior commissure and the habenula, displaying the major subdivisions of the lenticular nuclei. **A**, Anatomy. **B**, MR IR-T1-w. *1*, Anterior commissure; *2*, anterior columns of fornix; *3*, third ventricle; *4*, interthalamic adhesion; *5*, lateral ventricle, atrium; *6*, sylvian fissure; *7*, head of caudate nucleus; *8*, globus pallidus, lateral part; *9*, globus pallidus, medial part; *10*, internal capsule; *11*, external medullary lamina; *12*, internal medullary lamina of pallidum; *13*, claustrum; *14*, extreme capsule; *15*, external capsule; *16*, mamillothalamic tract; *17*, ventral anterior nucleus of thalamus; *18*, dorsomedian nucleus of thalamus; *19*, ventral lateral nucleus of thalamus; *20*, ventral posterior lateral and medial nuclei of thalamus; *21*, internal medullary lamina of thalamus; *22*, pulvinar thalami; *23*, habenula; *24*, reticular nucleus of thalamus; *25*, corpus callosum, splenium; *26*, insular cortex; *27*, internal capsule, retrolenticular part; *28*, interhemispheric fissure; *29*, circular sulcus of insula, anterior end; *30*, circular sulcus of insula, posterior end

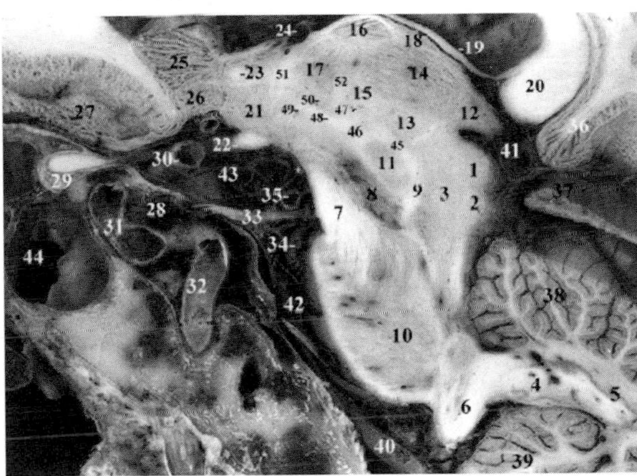

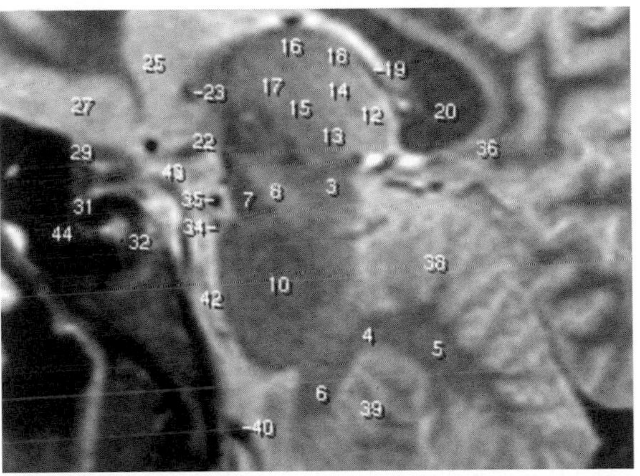

Fig. 7.15A,B. Parasagittal cuts through the thalamus and the midbrain-diencephalic region. **A**, Anatomy. **B**, MR FSE-T2-w. *1*, Superior colliculus; *2*, inferior colliculus; *3*, midbrain tegmentum; *4*, hilus of dentate nucleus; *5*, dentate nucleus; *6*, inferior cerebellar peduncle; *7*, cerebral peduncle; *8*, substantia nigra; *9*, internal carotid artery (anterior genu); *10*, pons (pontine nuclei); *11*, red nucleus; *12*, pulvinar thalami; *13*, centromedian nucleus of thalamus; *14*, dorsomedial nucleus of thalamus; *15*, ventral lateral thalamic nucleus; *16*, anterior nuclear group of thalamus; *17*, ventral anterior thalamic nucleus; *18*, lateral dorsal thalamic nucleus; *19*, fornix; *20*, splenium of corpus callosum; *21*, lateral hypothalamic area; *22*, optic tract; *23*, anterior commissure; *24*, thalamostriate vein; *25*, head of caudate nucleus; *26*, area septalis; *27*, gyrus rectus; *28*, cavernous sinus; *29*, intracanalicular optic nerve; *30*, supraclinoid internal carotid artery; *31*, cavernous internal carotid artery (anterior genu); *32*, cavernous internal carotid artery (ascending segment); *33*, oculomotor nerve (III); *34*, superior cerebellar artery; *35*, posterior cerebral artery; *36*, isthmus cinguli; *37*, tentorium cerebelli; *38*, anterior lobe of cerebellum; *39*, tonsil of cerebellum; *40*, vertebral artery; *41*, ambient cistern; *42*, prepontine cistern; *43*, chiasmal cistern; *44*, sphenoid sinus; *45*, prerubral tract; *46*, Forel's field H (prerubral field); *47*, Forel's field H1 (thalamic fasciculus); *48*, Forel's field H2 (lenticular fasciculus and ansa lenticularis); *49*, ansa lenticularis; *50*, zona incerta; *51*, anterior thalamic peduncle (anterior radiations); *52*, mamillothalamic tract

surrounded by a thin myelin fiber capsule along the upper margin of the internal medullary lamina (Figs. 7.12, 7.13, 7.15). The lateral posterior nucleus is found caudal, ventral, and lateral to the lateral dorsal nucleus, irregularly shaped but unlike the former, this nucleus lacks myelin capsule. It is found dorsal to the ventral posterolateral nucleus, contiguous to the lateral medullary lamina (Figs. 7.13, 7.16, 7.17).

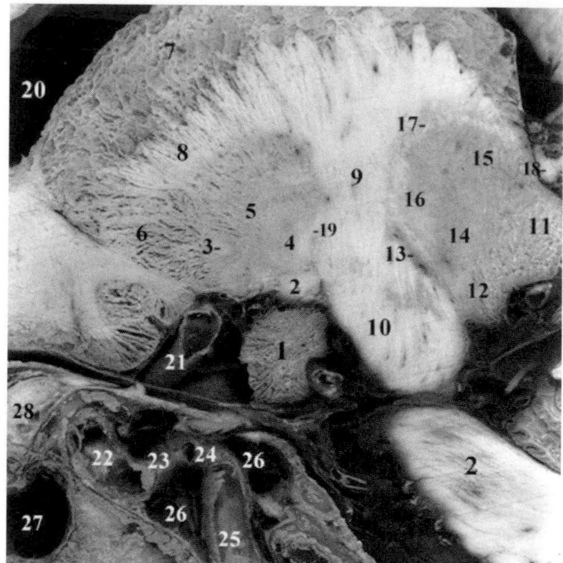

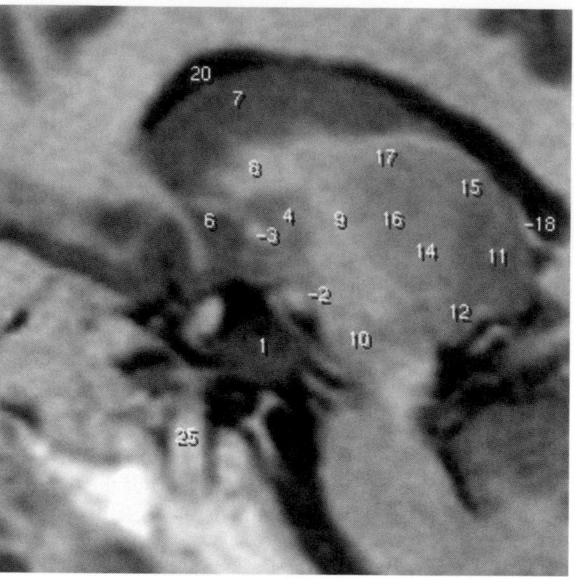

Fig. 7.16A,B. Parasagittal cuts through the basal ganglia at the level of the uncus and the intracanalicular optic nerve. **A**, Anatomy. **B**, MR IR T1-w. *1*, Uncus; *2*, optic tract; *3*, anterior commissure; *4*, medial pallidum; *5*, lateral pallidum; *6*, caudate nucleus, head; *7*, caudate nucleus, body; *8*, internal capsule, anterior limb; *9*, internal capsule; *10*, cerebral peduncle; *11*, pulvinar thalami; *12*, medial geniculate body; *13*, zona incerta (and subthalamic nucleus); *14*, ventral posterolateral nucleus of thalamus; *15*, lateral posterior nucleus of thalamus; *16*, ventral lateral nucleus of thalamus; *17*, external medullary lamina and reticular nucleus; *18*, fornix, crus; *19*, lenticular fasciculus; *20*, lateral ventricle, body; *21*, internal carotid artery, supraclinoid segment; *22*, cavernous internal carotid artery, anterior genu (C2); *23*, cavernous internal carotid artery, horizontal segment (C3); *24*, cavernous internal carotid artery, posterior genu (C4); *25*, cavernous internal carotid artery, ascending segment (C5); *26*, cavernous sinus, venous spaces; *27*, sphenoidal sinus; *28*, intracanalicular optic nerve

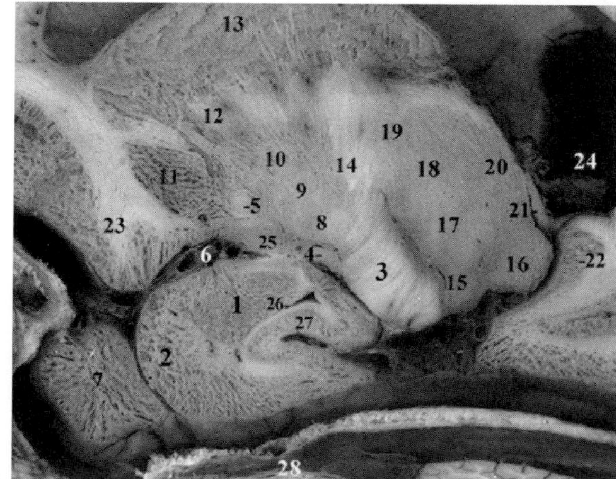

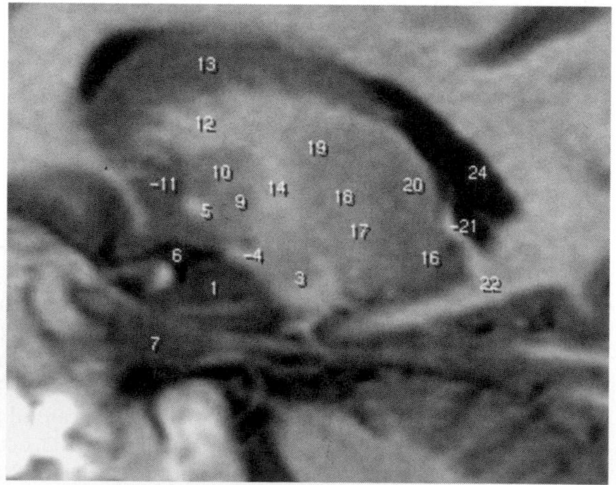

Fig. 7.17A,B. Parasagittal cuts through the core brain structures at the level of the amygdala and the hippocampal head, showing the intimate relationships between the medial border of the pallidum and the optic tract. **A**, Anatomy. **B**, MR IR T1-w. *1*, Amygdaloid body; *2*, uncus; *3*, cerebral peduncle; *4*, optic tract; *5*, anterior commissure; *6*, lateral fissure; *7*, temporal pole; *8*, globus pallidus, medial part; *9*, globus pallidus, lateral part; *10*, lateral globus pallidus; *11*, putamen; *12*, internal capsule, anterior limb; *13*, caudate nucleus, body; *14*, internal capsule; *15*, medial geniculate body; *16*, pulvinar thalami; *17*, ventral posterolateral and intermediate nuclei of thalamus; *18*, ventral lateral nucleus of thalamus; *19*, ventral anterior nucleus of thalamus; *20*, lateral posterior nucleus of thalamus; *21*, fornix; *22*, hippocampal tail; *23*, medial orbital gyrus; *24*, lateral ventricle, atrium; *25*, substantia innominata and anterior perforated space; *26*, temporal horn; *27*, hippocampal head; *28*, trigeminal nerve root

The intralaminar nuclear group consists of small cell groups embedded within the internal medullary lamina, which separates the medial from the lateral thalamic nuclei. The largest nucleus of this group is the centromedian nucleus, which is wedged between the dorsomedial nucleus and the ventral posterior nucleus caudally, and is almost completely surrounded by the white matter of the internal medullary lamina (Figs. 7.12, 7.13, 7.15).

The midline nuclear group lies in the periventricular gray matter of the upper half of the ventricular wall, as well as in the interthalamic adhesion (Figs. 7.8, 7.14). This group is very difficult to delimit in humans. It constitutes part of the periventricular gray matter separating the medial aspect of the thalamus from the ependyma of the third ventricular wall.

The reticular nucleus is a thin lamina of gray matter separating the posterior limb of the internal capsule from the external medullary lamina of the thalamus (Dekaban 1954). It surrounds the lateral, superior and the anteroinferior surface of the thalamus (Figs. 7.13, 7.16). The anterior portion of the reticular nucleus surrounds completely the anterior pole of the thalamus, becoming thinner at the posterior around its lateral aspect. Morphologically, the reticular nucleus is closely related to the zona incerta (Figs. 7.9, 7.10), as well as to the lateral geniculate body. The reticular nucleus is considered a derivative of the ventral thalamus which has migrated dorsally (Kuhlenbeck 1948).

It is, of course, beyond the scope of this work and useless for MR at the present time to give details about microscopic subdivisions of the thalamic nuclei. Major groups and nuclei have been described here in order to help with clinical and pathological correlations that may be obtained to some extent on high resolution, high contrast MR images. The classification used in this chapter is modified from Le Gros Clark (1932), Walker (1938), Van Buren and Borke (1972), Jones (1985), and Parent (1996).

B Functional Aspects and Clinical Considerations

1 The Thalamic Radiations

The thalamus is connected with all parts of the cerebral cortex by well defined fiber bundles designated as the thalamic peduncles. These fibers are reciprocally organized into thalamocortical and corticothalamic fibers, which form a continuous fan contributing to a large portion of the internal capsule and the corona radiata. The thalami are also connected with the main subcortical structures of the central nervous system such as the brainstem, the spinal cord, the cerebellum, the hypothalamus, and the corpus striatum.

The thalamic radiations are grouped into four peduncles or stalks. These peduncles are the following: (1) the anterior or frontal peduncle, which interconnects the anterior and medial thalamic nuclei with the frontal lobe; (2) the superior peduncle, which interconnects the central tier thalamic nuclei with the pre- and postcentral gyri and the adjacent parts of the frontal and parietal lobes; (3) the posterior or occipital peduncle, which connects the posterior parietal gyri and the occipital lobes with the caudal portions of the thalamus, including the pulvinar and the lateral geniculate body, as well as the geniculocalcarine tract projecting to the striate cortex; (4) the inferior or temporal peduncle, smaller than the others, which interconnects the posterior thalamus and the medial geniculate body to restricted areas of the temporal lower cortex and, particularly, to the transverse temporal gyrus of Heschl. These extensive projections appear as a radiating band of fibers named the corona radiata (Fig. 7.16) which converges toward the thalamus. The most abundant of these are the projections to the central gyri, the frontal granular cortex, the transverse gyrus, and the calcarine cortex.

A complete and authoritative review of the morphological and functional aspects of the thalamus may be found in a recent work by Jones (1985). The major function of the thalamus consists of the integration and relay of sensory information, with the exception of olfactory signals, all of which terminate in the thalamus and are then projected to specific regions of the cerebral cortex by the thalamocortical radiations. The thalamus also plays a particular role in the conscious perception and interpretation of pain, the only peripheral sensory stimulus to be interpreted at the thalamic level. Moreover, the thalamus serves as an integrative center for motor functions since it receives major afferent projections from the cerebellum, as well as from the basal ganglia, and also from various limbic structures. On the other hand, specific portions of the thalamus play a major role in maintaining and regulating consciousness, alertness and attention state, via nonspecific thalamic diffuse projections. Based on physiologic data, the EEG arousal response seems largely mediated by the nonspecific intralaminar and midline thalamic nuclei.

C The Vascular Supply to the Thalamus

The arterial supply of the thalamus is derived from branches of the posterior cerebral artery. The medial and anterior regions of the thalamus receive their major blood supply from the thalamoperforating branches. These arteries arise from the most internal segment of the posterior cerebral artery, as well as from the terminal portion of the basilar artery (Foix and Hillemand 1925; Salamon and Lazorthes 1971; Hara and Fujino 1966). The posteromedial arteries, which course dorsally into the diencephalon, vascularize the medial regions of the thalamus and the paraventricular region of the hypothalamus. The thalamogeniculate branches, consisting of posterolateral arteries, nourish the lateral nuclei of the thalamus and the pulvinar. These branches arise from the lateromesencephalic segment of the posterior cerebral artery, as well as from the choroidal arteries (Lazorthes and Salamon 1971). The inferior thalamic arteries are branches of the posterior communicating artery, but may also arise from the bifurcation of the basilar artery. These arteries penetrate the inferior portions of the thalamus to vascularize the region rostral to the vascular territory of the thalamoperforating branches. The superior and medial portions of the thalamus are supplied by the inferior thalamic arteries, branches of the posterior communicating artery, which also perfuse the choroid plexus of the third ventricle. The pineal body, or epiphysis, and the habenula receive their blood supply from branches of the medial posterior choroidal artery.

IV The Epithalamus

The epithalamus occupies the caudal roof of the diencephalon. It consists of the pineal body, or epiphysis, the right and left habenular nuclei, each receiving the stria medullaris thalami, the taenia thalami, the habenular and posterior commissures, which cross the midline, and the cranial and caudal laminae of the epiphyseal stalk.

A The Pineal Gland

The epiphysis is a small cone-shaped body attached to the roof of the third ventricle above the PC. It consists of a vascular connective tissue, containing glial cells and pinealocytes (Figs. 7.6, 7.11). The epiphysis is a rudimentary gland and regarded in mammals as a photosensitive neuroendocrine organ. The main pineal secretions are serotonin, norepinephrine, and melatonin, synthesized from serotonin. The pineal gland shows rhythmic modifications in neuroendocrine activity, suggesting that this gland functions as a biologic clock. The circadian rhythms have a periodicity of 24 h. Tumors such as pinealomas cause depression of gonadal function and delayed pubescence, while tumors destroying the gland are generally associated with precocious puberty (Relkin 1976). Calcareous bodies are frequently observed in the pineal gland of young adults, visible in skull radiography, and help to identify indirectly, if needed, the topography of the pineal body.

B The Habenula

The habenular nucleus, consisting of a smaller medial and a larger lateral nucleus in humans, is deeply situated beneath the floor of the habenular trigone. Each nuclei receives the terminal of the stria medullaris and gives rise to either the habenulo-interpeduncular tract or the fasciculus retroflexus (Figs. 7.6, 7.13, 7.14). The stria medullares are complex bundles arising from the septal nuclei, the lateral preoptico-hypothalamic area, and the anterior thalamic nuclei. Some of the fibers cross to the opposite side through the habenular commissure in the cranial leaflet of the pineal stalk. The main outflow pathways from the habenular nucleus consisting of the fasciculus retroflexus of Meynert pass to the interpeduncular nucleus. This tract passes to the rostromedial part of the red nucleus to reach the interpeduncular nucleus, the latter projecting to the midbrain reticular formation. Functionally, the habenular nuclei may be considered as a site of conversion of limbic forebrain pathways which transmit impulses to the upper midbrain.

C The Posterior Commissure

The PC is a complex fiber bundle which crosses the midline in the caudal lamina of the pineal stalk (Fig. 7.13). Dorsally, it marks the junction between midbrain and diencephalon, as previously reported. Its size is relatively reduced in primates. Located dorsal to the periaqueductal gray matter and rostral to the superior colliculi at the upper aperture of the cerebral aqueduct, the PC lies near the rostral end of the oculomotor nucleus and is closely linked with the medial longitudinal fasciculus. The PC acquires its

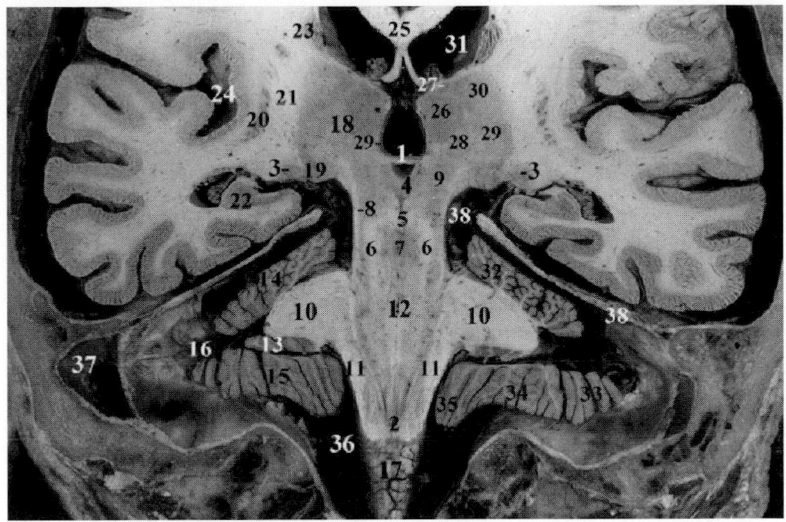

Fig. 7.18. Referential PC-OB coronal anatomic cut, including the posterior commissure on the midline, the inferior end of the calamus scriptorius and, laterally, the lateral geniculate bodies. The cut, oriented according to the brainstem long axis, passes through the major posterior extent of the thalami. *1*, Posterior commissure; *2*, calamus scriptorius, inferior extremity; *3*, lateral geniculate body; *4*, cerebral aqueduct (superior aperture); *5*, decussation of brachium conjunctivum; *6*, superior cerebellar peduncle (brachium conjunctivum); *7*, midbrain tegmentum; *8*, lateral lemniscus; *9*, midbrain-thalamic region; *10*, middle cerebellar peduncle; *11*, inferior cerebellar peduncle; *12*, pontine tegmentum; *13*, flocculus and paraflocculus; *14*, superior aspect of cerebellar hemisphere; *15*, inferior aspect of cerebellar hemisphere; *16*, horizontal fissure of Vicq d'Azyr; *17*, medulla oblongata; *18*, thalamus; *19*, medial geniculate body; *20*, putamen (posterior limit); *21*, internal capsule; *22*, hippocampus; *23*, caudate nucleus; *24*, insula; *25*, corpus callosum (posterior columns of fornix beneath); *26*, dorsomedian nucleus of thalamus; *27*, lateral dorsal nucleus of thalamus; *28*, centromedian nucleus of thalamus; *29*, ventral posterior nuclei of thalamus; *30*, ventral lateral nucleus of thalamus; *31*, lateral ventricle; *32*, anterior lobe of cerebellar hemisphere; *33*, inferior semilunar lobule; *34*, biventer lobule; *35*, cerebellar tonsil; *36*, cerebellomedullary cistern; *37*, lateral (transverse) sinus; *38*, tentorium cerebelli

myelin sheaths very early. The fibers of the PC are surrounded laterally by small groups of various nuclei called the interstitial nuclei (Figs. 7.13, 7.18). These small nuclei contributing fibers to the commissure include the nuclei of the PC, the pretectal nuclei, the nucleus of Darkshewitsch, and the interstitial nucleus of Cajal. Note that the lesions in the PC reduce the consensual pupillary right reflex (Magoun et al. 1935). Lesions destroying the fibers from the nuclei of Cajal produce impairment of vertical eye movements and bilateral eyelid traction (Carpenter et al. 1970). Other centers also contribute fibers to the commissure.

Caudal and ventral to the PC, in the roof of the cerebral aqueduct, is a modified ependymal area called the subcommissural organ which shows secretary function. The function of this circumventricular organ is unknown in human, but it is probably concerned with thirst and water intake (Gilbert 1960). Note that the commissural organ is one of the brain structures not included in the blood brain barrier and may show enhancement on MR.

V The Hypothalamus

An important portion of the diencephalon, the hypothalamus lies ventral to the hypothalamic sulcus, extending from the lamina terminalis at the chiasmal notch in the region of the optic chiasm through a vertical plane caudal to the MB (Figs. 7.6, 7.19), and including the structures forming the lateral walls and the floor of the third ventricle.

The hypothalamus is divided mediolaterally into medial and lateral groups of nuclei separated by a paramedian plane, which includes the fibers of the fornix ending in the MB (Fig. 7.20), as well as the mamillothalamic tracts and the fasciculus retroflexus (Fig. 7.6, 7.8). The anterior columns of the fornix may be used as a landmark to separate the medial and lateral zones.

Three rostrocaudal areas may be distinguished: (1) an anterior area between the lamina terminalis and the posterior edge of the chiasm, including the preoptic and the supraoptic regions dorsal to the chiasm (Fig. 7.3); (2) a tuberal or tubero-infundibular

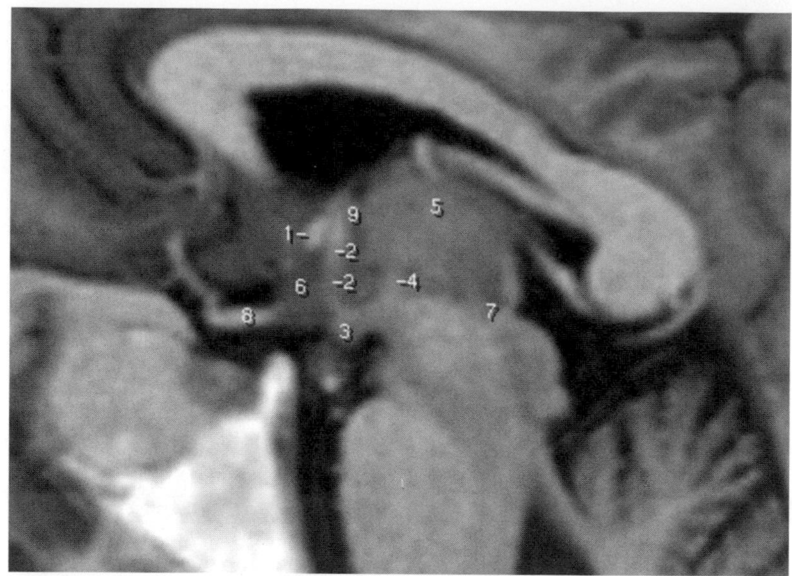

Fig. 7.19. Sagittal MR cut showing the fornix and the mamillo-Thalamic track. *1*, Anterior commissure; *2*, anterior columns of fornix; *3*, mamillary body; *4*, mamillo-thalamic tract; *5*, thalamus; *6*, third ventricle and lamina terminalis in front; *7*, posterior commissure; *8*, optic chiasm; *9*, interventricular foramen

A

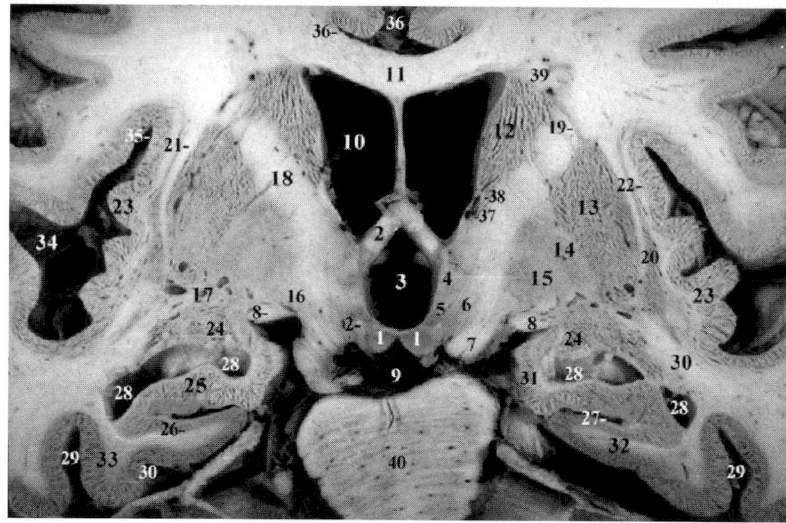

B

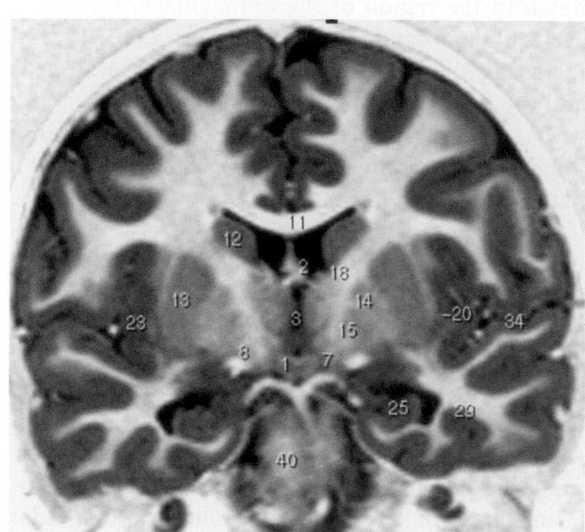

Fig. 7.20A,B. The hypothalamus: coronal anatomic cut through the anterior columns of the fornix and the mamillary bodies. **A**, Anatomy. **B**, MR IR T1-w. *1*, Mamillary bodies; *2*, anterior columns of fornix; *3*, third ventricle; *4*, dorsomedial hypothalamic nucleus; *5*, ventromedial hypothalamic nucleus; *6*, lateral hypothalamic area; *7*, crus cerebri; *8*, optic tract, pericrural portion; *9*, interpeduncular cistern; 10, lateral ventricle, frontal horn; *11*, corpus callosum; *12*, caudate nucleus; *13*, putamen; *14*, globus pallidus, lateral part; *15*, globus pallidus, medial part; *16*, globus pallidus, tip of the medial part; *17*, anterior perforated substance; *18*, internal capsule, genu; *19*, gray striatal bridges (caudate-lenticular); *20*, claustrum; *21*, external capsule; *22*, extreme capsule; *23*, insula; *24*, amygdala; *25*, hippocampus; *26*, subiculum; *27*, uncal sulcus; *28*, inferior horn of lateral ventricle; *29*, lateral occipitotemporal sulcus; *30*, collateral sulcus; *31*, uncinate gyrus; *32*, parahippocampal gyrus; *33*, fusiform gyrus; *34*, lateral fissure; *35*, circular sulcus of insula; *36*, callosal sulcus; *37*, thalamostriate vein; *38*, stria terminalis; *39*, superior longitudinal fasciculus; *40*, pons

region centrally, where the hypothalamus reaches its widest extent (Figs. 7.4, 7.5); and (3) a posterior region referred to as the mamillary region (Fig. 7.20).

The hypothalamus is continuous rostrally and laterally with the basal olfactory region which corresponds to the gray mass area located beneath the rostral portion of the lenticular nucleus and the head of the caudate nucleus (Figs. 7.3, 7.6). In the midsagittal area, the hypothalamus extends rostral to the AC to become the septal region (Figs. 7.3, 7.6). The latter is comprised of medial and lateral septal nuclei and the nucleus accumbens septi lying medially at the junction of the putamen and the caudate nucleus (Fig. 7.3). The gray mass of the basal olfactory region also extends more laterally beneath the lentiform nucleus toward the amygdaloid nuclear complex, called the substantia innominata, which contains the basal nucleus of Meynert (Figs. 7.4, 7.5).

Considering its relationships, the hypothalamus, which corresponds to the central portion of the diencephalon, is bounded rostrally by the optic chiasm, posteriorly by the MB, and laterally by the optic tracts (Fig. 7.21). The thalamus lies caudodorsally and the subthalamic region is lateral and caudal to the hypothalamus. A ventral protrusion of the hypothalamus, along with the third ventricular recess, is the infundibulum, the most distal portion of which constitutes the neurohypophysis (Fig. 7.22).

The anterior to posterior length of the hypothalamus is about 10 mm. Despite its small size, the hypothalamus contains the neural systems critical for the survival of the organism and for the regulation of hormones from the pituitary gland. The importance of the hypothalamus in maintaining the "milieu intérieur" has been emphasized by the French physiologist C. Bernard at the end of the nineteenth century (1878). This condition was later called "homeostasis" by Cannon and Britton (1925).

A Cytoarchitecture of the Hypothalamus

The cytoarchitecture of the human hypothalamus is similar to that observed in other primates but the nuclear masses are not as well delineated as in the other species. Detailed and comprehensive reviews can be found in Le Gros Clark et al. (1938), Haymaker et al. (1969), and Saper (1990). MRI, therefore, cannot presently identify the hypothalamic subnuclei. Only topographical delimitation of rostrocaudal regions may be obtained if needed. A detailed description of the architectonics of these nuclei will not, therefore, be detailed due to the present impossibility, with the exception of the mamillary bodies (Fig. 7.20), to discriminate most subnuclei on MR slices (Miller et al. 1994; Naidich et al. 1986), even if most of them are sharply circumscribed but embedded in a continuous cellular matrix.

1 The Medial Hypothalamic Zone

Located medially to the fornix and the mamillothalamic tract of Vicq d'Azyr, the medial hypothalamic zone borders the wall of the third ventricle. It is divided rostrocaudally into a preoptic region, which constitutes the periventricular gray matter of the most rostral portion of the third ventricle, a supraoptic region containing two well delimited hypothalamic nuclei, the supraoptic nucleus and the paraventricular nucleus, the tubero-infundibular region in which a large roughly oval ventromedial nucleus and a smaller less distinct dorsomedial nucleus, as well as an arcuate nucleus located near the entrance of the infundibular recess with an arcuate shape, are found on frontal cuts, and finally, the mamillary region which consists, in humans, mainly of a spherical medial mamillary nucleus surrounded by a capsule of myelinated fibers (Fig. 7.20). Dorsal to the MB is the posterior hypothalamic nucleus.

2 The Lateral Hypothalamic Region

The lateral hypothalamic area is located lateral to the anterior column of the fornix and the mamillothalamic tracts (Fig. 7.6). Its lateral boundary is formed by the internal capsule and the subthalamic region. Its rostral and caudal portions are narrow, being

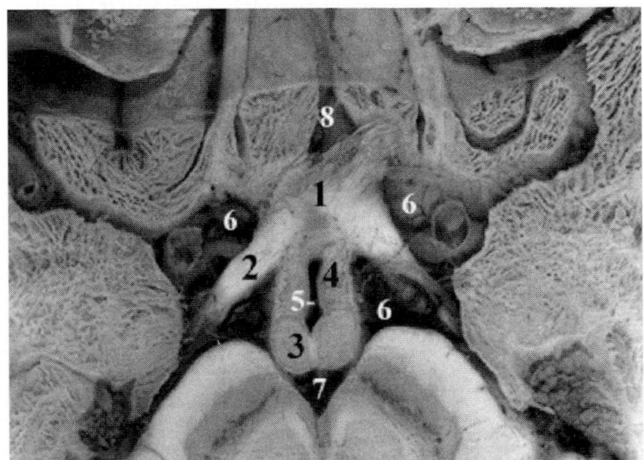

Fig. 7.21. The hypothalamus: axial anatomic cut through the chiasmal cistern. *1*, Optic chiasm; *2*, cisternal optic tract; *3*, mamillary body; *4*, hypothalamus; *5*, infundibular recess of third ventricle; *6*, chiasmal cistern; *7*, interpeduncular cistern

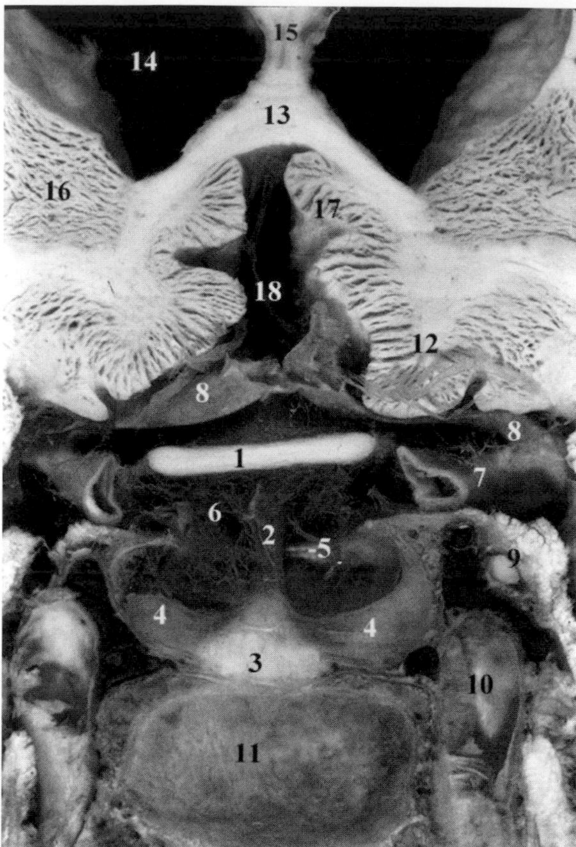

Fig. 7.22. The preoptic and tubero-infundibular regions. Coronal anatomic cut at the level of the rostrum of corpus callosum, passing through the chiasm and the pituitary, and including the infundibulum. *1*, Optic chiasm; *2*, pituitary stalk; *3*, neurohypophysis (posterior pituitary gland); *4*, adenohypophysis (anterior pituitary gland); *5*, diaphragma sellae; *6*, suprasellar cistern; *7*, supraclinoid internal carotid artery; *8*, proximal segment of anterior cerebral artery; *9*, oculomotor nerve (III); *10*, intracavernous internal carotid artery; *11*, sphenoid sinus; *12*, gyrus rectus; *13*, rostrum of corpus callosum; *14*, frontal horn of lateral ventricle; *15*, septum lucidum; *16*, head of caudate nucleus; *17*, subcallosal area; *18*, cistern of lamina terminalis

developed in the tuberal region. Caudally, this region is continuous with the ventral tegmental area of the midbrain and rostrally it merges with the lateral preoptic area. This region contains well delineated nuclear masses which are the lateral preoptic nucleus, the nuclei tuberales, and the largest tuberomamillary nucleus.

B Connections of the Hypothalamus

The hypothalamus shows extensive fiber connections, some of which are well defined, forming compact bundles, while the remaining are more diffuse. Some may be identified using MRI as shown. The major fiber systems converging on the hypothalamus are related to all types of visceral activities, the hypothalamus being the major subcortical center for the regulation of the peripheral autonomic sympathetic and parasympathetic nervous system. Other pathways such as the olfactory pathways and various tracts coming from the midbrain, the diencephalon, the limbic structures, as well as from the neocortex, terminate in the hypothalamus.

The major connections are: (1) the medial forebrain bundle, which is a very well developed tract in nonmammalian vertebrates but relatively small in humans, and contains ascending serotoninergic, noradrenergic and dopaminergic fiber systems; (2)the amygdalo-hypothalamic tracts, which are the stria terminalis arising from the corticomedial nuclei of the amygdala, and the ventral amygdalo-fugal tract arising from the basolateral amygdaloid nuclei and the pyriform cortex; (3) the hippocampal-hypothalamic fibers, which constitute the heavily myelinated fibers of the fornix. The latter divides in the septal region dorsal to the AC into precommissural fibers and postcommissural fibers that terminate in the MB. Note that a large number of the fibers constituting the columns of the fornix lose their myelination along their route within the hypothalamus. (4) The retinohypothalamic fibers project bilaterally to the suprachiasmatic nucleus, considered to be the pacemaker for circadian rhythms (Moore 1973, 1992); (5) the brainstem reticular formation sends two major efferent pathways, the mamillary peduncle and the dorsal longitudinal fasciculus of Schutz, the former projecting to the lateral mamillary nucleus originating from the midbrain, which is not well differentiated in humans; the other constituting a fiber system originating from the midbrain and the tegmentum, and running longitudinally through the periaqueductal gray matter; (6) the corticohypothalamic fibers project to the hypothalamus from wide areas of the prefrontal, the parietal and the occipital cortices. The major forebrain afferents arise from the two phylogenetically oldest cortical regions: the hippocampal formation and the pyriform cortex.

The efferent connections seem to be, in part, reciprocal to the afferent. The hypothalamus is connected to the hippocampal formation via the medial forebrain bundle, to the amygdaloid nuclear complex via the stria terminalis and the ventral pathway, and to the midbrain tegmentum mainly via the dorsal longitudinal fasciculus, which is a major pathway of communication between the hypothalamus and the brainstem that contains very poorly myelinated fibers. This bundle, together with the medial forebrain bundle, constitutes the major path connecting the hypothalamus and the brainstem. The hypothalamic fibers descending to the brainstem, as well as to the spinal cord, transmit the regulatory influences of the hypothalamus to the central autonomic neurons. Several efferent hypothalamic pathways have no counterpart among the afferent systems. The mamillary nuclei, and the medial nucleus of the MB, give rise to a large ascending fiber bundle, the fasciculus mamillaris princeps, which diverges into a mamillothalamic tract of Vicq d'Azyr, projecting to the ipsilateral anterior thalamic nuclei, and a mamillotegmental tract, which arches caudally to enter the midbrain tegmentum towards the tegmental nuclei of the reticular formation, ventral to the medial longitudinal fasciculus.

Other major efferent hypothalamic pathways are represented by the connections of the hypothalamus with the hypophysis by means of a supraopticohypophyseal tract and a tubero-infundibular tract. The former arises from the supraoptic and paraventricular nuclei of the hypothalamus, and projects to the posterior lobe of the hypophysis. Cells of these nuclei are neurosecretory neurons. Neurosecretions are synthesized within the cell bodies, and transported by axonal flow to be liberated by the axon terminals near the capillaries in the posterior lobe of the pituitary gland, the neurohypophysis (Fig. 7.22). This process of neurosecretion is responsible for the synthesis and release of the posterior lobe hormones, oxytocin and vasopressin. The other system originating from the infundibular nucleus is also called the arcuate nucleus. It is located in the tuberal region and ends in the infundibulum on the capillary loops near the sinusoids of the hypophyseal portal system. It is responsible for conveying releasing-inhibiting hormones which are transmitted by the portal vessels to the adenohypophysis. These releasing factors modulate the synthesis and release of the pituitary hormones, and constitute a neurohumoral link between the hypothalamus and the anterior pituitary gland.

C Functional Aspects and Clinical Considerations

The hypothalamus acts as the "head ganglion" of the autonomic nervous system (Sherrington 1906). It is, in fact, related to all types of visceral activities, and is considered the major subcortical center for the regulation and coordination of the autonomic nervous system. An enormous literature has accumulated with the development of the science of neuroendocrinology concerning the functional roles of the hypothalamus. Stimulation or destruction of the different hypothalamic areas causes various disturbances of autonomic functions. The major functions of the hypothalamus are concerned with endocrine control and neurosecretion as described, regulation of body temperature, maintenance of water balance and food intake, control of sexual behavior and reproductive functions, and control of growth and behavior and emotional reactions such as fear, pleasure, aversion or rage. Interestingly, the hypothalamus is concerned with circadian rhythms, the suprachiasmatic nucleus being in many animals considered an endogenous neural pacemaker which acts as a biological clock and is found in all vertebrates. Finally, studies by Jouvet (1964, 1965, 1972) show that the hypothalamus may be involved in the sleep-waking cycle, suggesting that the posterior hypothalamus, including the tuberomamillary nucleus, plays an important role in the arousal mechanisms. These periodic conditions of sleep and wakefulness are a major example of the circadian rhythm.

D Vascular Supply to the Hypothalamus

The vascularization of the hypothalamus and the pituitary gland has been studied by Haymaker (1969). Characterized by a rich anastomotic network, the hypothalamic region is vascularized by small arteries arising from the circle of Willis. The anterior hypothalamus and preoptic region are supplied by branches of the anterior cerebral artery, the anterior communicating artery, and the internal carotid artery (Marinkovic et al. 1986). The posterior part of the hypothalamus is vascularized by the posterior communicating artery and the posterior cerebral artery. Both arteries supply the mamillary region. The internal carotid artery, from which arises the superior hypophyseal artery (Haymaker 1969), and the posterior communicating artery together give rise to the tubero-infundibular arterial branches.

VI The Subthalamic Region, Subthalamus, or Ventral Thalamus

The subthalamic region is a portion of the diencephalon which constitutes the transitional zone bounded laterally by the internal capsule, medially by the hypothalamus, and dorsally by the thalami. Ventrolaterally, the subthalamic region is in contact with the junctional zone where the cerebral peduncles merge into the internal capsules, these latter separating the subthalamus from the pallidum. This area contains important nuclei and is traversed by many important fiber bundles on their route toward the thalamus. These nuclei include the nucleus subthalamicus, the zona incerta, the nuclei of the tegmental fields of Forel (Forel's field H) extending to the midbrain-thalamic junction, the red nuclei, and the substantia nigra. The main tracts passing through this region are the lenticular fasciculus (Forel's field H2), the ansa lenticularis, the thalamic fasciculus (Forel's field H1), and the subthalamic fasciculus. The rostral ends of the medial and the trigeminal lemnisci and the dentatothalamic tract originating from the opposite superior cerebellar peduncle, as well as the ipsilateral rubrothalamic fibers, pass through this region as they reach their terminations in the thalamus (Figs. 7.6, 7.10, 7.15).

The topographical anatomy of the subthalamic area is best evaluated on the coronal cuts obtained with MR using the PC-OB orientation. Successive cross-sectional views in the coronal plane (Figs. 7.7, 7.8, 7.10, 7.12) show most of the anatomic structures contained in this rather complex upper midbrain-thalamic region. The anatomic imaging correlations are also well displayed on contiguous sagittal slices (Figs. 7.15–7.17). For imaging purposes, and better understanding, the complex organization of this region with its rostrocaudal relationships and the major structures of the upper midbrain are included in this part of the chapter.

A The Subthalamic Nucleus (Corpus Luysi)

1 Morphology and Topographical Anatomy

Included in the "région mésencéphalo-sous-optique", as denominated by Foix and Nicolesco (1925), the subthalamic nuclear mass is a lens-shaped structure found on the inner aspect of the internal capsule. Well delineated, it is prominent in primates and humans, but it is small in most mammalian groups and absent in the submammalian species. On the coronal cuts, this nucleus is biconvex, lying in the caudal subthalamic region, and even extends into the subthalamus-midbrain tegmentum junctional zone. Its caudal portion lies dorsolateral to the rostral end of the substantia nigra and lateral to the upper border of the red nucleus. It is separated from the globus pallidus of the lenticular nucleus by the medial aspect of the internal capsule. Medially, the subthalamic nucleus abuts upon the thalamus and dorsally it is separated from the ventral tier of the thalamic nuclei by the zona incerta (Figs. 7.7, 7.8).

2 Functional and Clinical Considerations

The major afferent projections originate from: the precentral motor cortex and regions of the frontal lobe, the globus pallidus, and the pedunculopontine nucleus. The corticosubthalamic projections are topographically organized. The subthalamic nucleus may in fact be divided into a large dorsolateral part corresponding to the sensory-motor cortex and a smaller ventromedial portion corresponding to the associative cortical areas. The external segment of the globus pallidus projects the largest number of subcortical fibers to the subthalamic nucleus. The fibers traverse the internal segment of the pallidum and the internal capsule. A massive cholinergic projection to the subthalamic nucleus has been identified in monkeys by Lavoie and Parent (1994) and Mesulam et al. (1992).

Concerning the efferent projections, the subthalamic nucleus gives rise to subthalamopallidal, subthalamonigral, and subthalamostriatal projections. The subthalamopallidal efferent fibers traverse the internal capsule and radiate into all parts of the pallidum in a manner parallel to the medullary laminae of the globus pallidus.

The subthalamic nucleus is believed to modulate the activities of the neurons making up the output system of the basal ganglia based on the presence of efferents to both the pallidum and the substantia nigra. Small lesions of the human subthalamic nucleus, usually hemorrhagic, result in the clinical condition of hemiballismus, which is characterized by uncontrollable violent and involuntary torsional movements of the choreiform type, occurring on the contralateral side of the body. These abnormal movements affect primarily the axial and proximal musculature of the upper and lower limbs. The facial musculature may also be involved (Martin 1927; Whittier 1947).

B The Zona Incerta

The zona incerta is a small area of gray matter located ventral to the thalamus, from which it is separated by the thalamic fasciculus, and laterally continuous with the reticular nucleus of the thalamus (Figs. 7.7, 7.8). These diffuse cell groups receive corticofugal projections from the precentral cortex.

C The Prerubral Field

Also called the Forel's field H (Figs. 7.7, 7.12), this area is functionally associated with the zona incerta. It contains scattered groups of neurons situated caudomedially to the latter, which constitute the nucleus of the prerubral field.

D Vascular Supply to the Subthalamic Region

The subthalamic region is supplied by posteromedian arteries derived from the posterior communicating and the posterior cerebral arteries. More specifically, blood supply to the subthalamic nucleus is derived from branches of the posterior cerebral artery, premamillary branches of the posterior communicating artery, and from peduncular branches of the anterior choroidal artery as well (Foix and Hillemand 1925). The substantia nigra is supplied in its rostral part by the premamillary branches of the posterior communicating artery and by the peduncular branches of the anterior choroidal artery. Its caudal portion receives blood supply from peduncular branches of the posterior cerebral artery, the medial posterior choroidal artery, and the superior cerebellar arteries (Duvernoy 1978; Rhoton et al. 1979).

VII The Basal Ganglia

A Morphology and Imaging

The basal ganglia are large subcortical nuclear masses of gray matter which are in close relationship to the diencephalic structures but are separated from it by the fibers of the internal capsule (Fig. 7.23). These basal nuclei derive largely from the telencephalon.

The anatomic structures included under this general terminology vary between authors, leading to confusion. The anatomists generally refer to the subcortical nuclei located in the basal forebrain, including the corpus striatum, which comprises the caudate nucleus, and the putamen, the pallidum or globus pallidus, which forms with the putamen, the lentiform nucleus, and finally, the amygdala and the claustrum.

From a functional and clinical point of view, the basal ganglia may be restricted to the striatum and

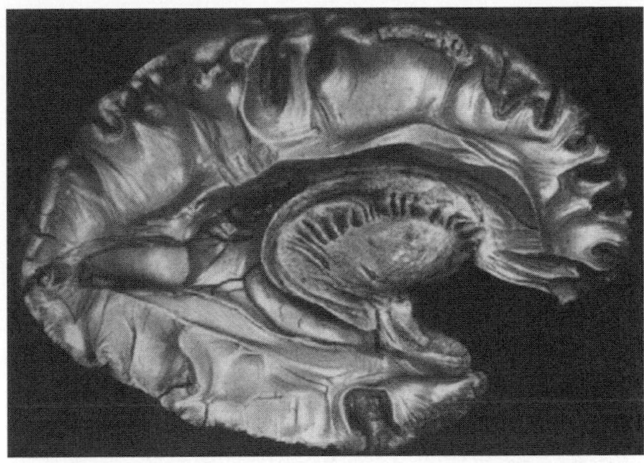

Fig. 7.23. Topographical anatomy of the basal ganglia; dissection from Klingler. (In Ludwig and Klingler 1956, Tabula 18)

the pallidum while excluding the claustrum and amygdala, as the former show no major connections with the basal nuclear structures and the latter are generally considered as part of the limbic system previously described in Chap. 6 on the mesial temporal region.

Imaging may be completed most efficiently using coronal cuts through the basal forebrain which display these core structures in a way that benefits from such sectional orientation. The anatomic structures studied are the diencephalic structures as previously described, to which the lenticular nuclei as well as the caudate nuclei, and the related ventral striatopallidal area obviously should be added. These core structures of the brain benefit from the coronal approach parallel to the PC-OB reference plane and are displayed extending from the level of the rostrum of corpus callosum to the PC-OB plane (Figs. 7.3–7.5, 7.7–7.10, 7.20). The MR coronal cuts include the plane roughly parallel to the CA-CM plane of Guiot (1958), which shows a strict relationship with the medial border of the medial pallidum (see Chap. 2). The axial cuts performed according to the "Flechsig" classical orientation, as represented in the anatomic cuts shown and oriented in the neuro-ocular plane, close to the Frankfurt-Virchow plane (Figs. 7.14, 7.24–7.26), display the basal ganglia between the level of the AC to the roof of the lateral ventricles, bounded laterally by the claustrum and the insula on each side. The MR horizontal cuts are performed parallel to the CH-CP plane, very close to a sylvian plane orientation, and differ largely from the bicommissural orientation of the stereotactic neurosurgery (AC-PC is angled 24° with respect to the CH-PC plane).

The ventral striatopallidal region (Figs. 7.3–7.5) comprises an ill-defined anatomic region corre-

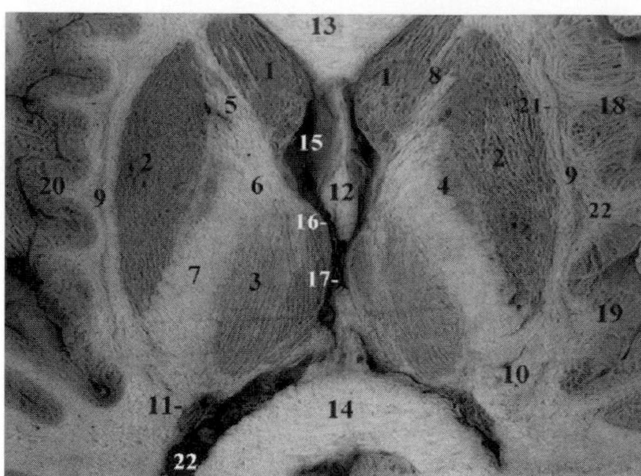

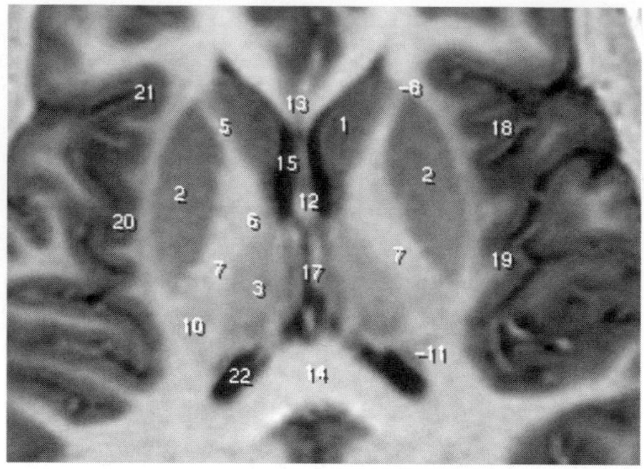

A B

Fig. 7.24A,B. The basal ganglia: axial anatomic cut at the level of the insular and frontal horns, displaying the caudate and lenticular nuclei, and including the thalami and the internal capsules. *1*, Caudate nucleus, head; *2*, putamen; *3*, thalamus; *4*, pallidum, lateral segment; *5*, internal capsule, anterior limb; *6*, internal capsule, genu; *7*, internal capsule, posterior limb; *8*, putaminocaudate gray matter bridges; *9*, claustrum; *10*, internal capsule, retrolenticular part; *11*, caudate nucleus, tail; *12*, fornix; *13*, corpus callosum, genu; *14*, corpus callosum, splenium; *15*, lateral ventricle, frontal horn; *16*, interventricular foramen (Monro); *17*, third ventricle; *18*, insular cortex, short gyri; *19*, insular cortex, long gyri; *20*, insula; *21*, circular sulcus of insula; *22*, lateral ventricle, atrium

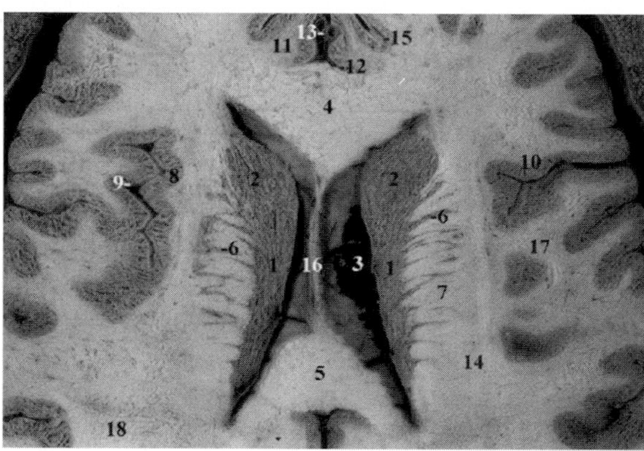

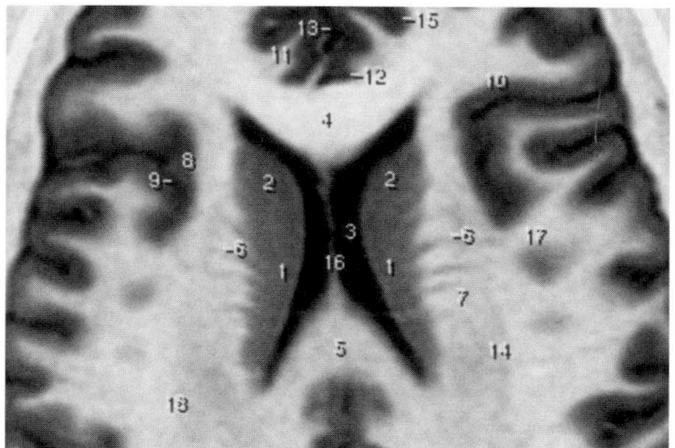

A B

Fig. 7.25A,B. The basal ganglia: axial anatomic cut through the bodies of the lateral ventricles, displaying the rostrocaudal extent of the caudate nuclei, superior to the level of lenticular nuclei. *1*, Caudate nucleus, body; *2*, caudate nucleus, head; *3*, lateral ventricle, body; *4*, corpus callosum, genu; *5*, corpus callosum, splenium; *6*, putaminocaudate gray matter bridges; *7*, corona radiata; *8*, insular cortex; *9*, interlocking gyral surfaces; *10*, lateral fissure, ascending ramus; *11*, cingulate gyrus; *12*, callosal sulcus; *13*, pericallosal arteries; *14*, centrum semiovale; *15*, cingulate sulcus; *16*, septum lucidum; *17*, frontal operculum; *18*, parietal lobe

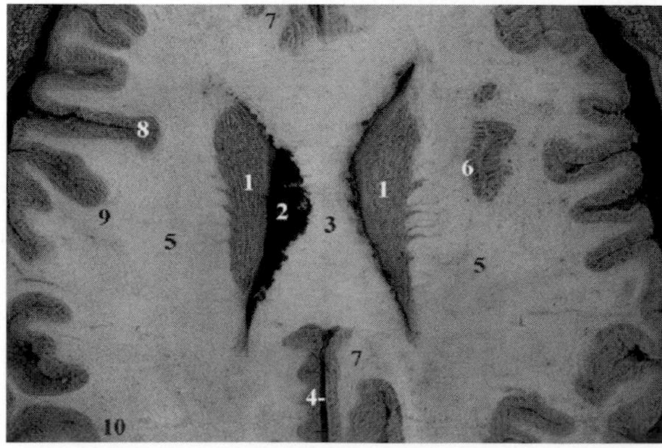

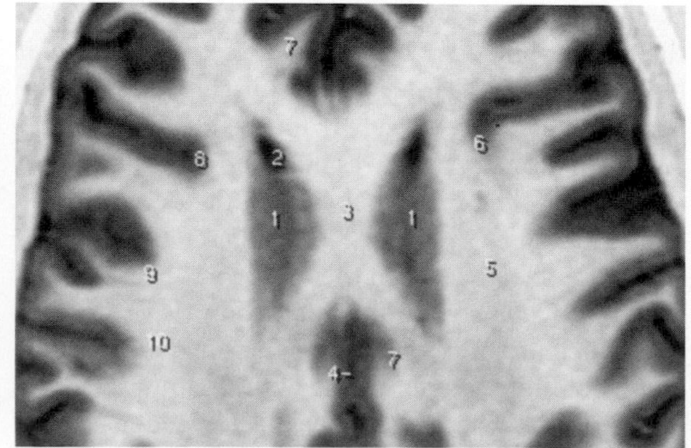

A B

Fig. 7.26A,B. The basal ganglia: axial anatomic cut through the roof of the lateral ventricles and the body of the corpus callosum, displaying the corona radiata lateral to the caudate nuclei. *1*, Caudate nucleus, body; *2*, lateral ventricle, body; *3*, corpus callosum; *4*, interhemispheric fissure; *5*, centrum semiovale; *6*, superior insular cortex; *7*, cingulate gyrus; *8*, lateral fissure, ascending ramus; *9*, frontal operculum; *10*, parietal lobe

sponding to a ventral extension of both the striatum and the pallidum to the inferior basal surface of the brain (Heimer et al. 1982). The ventral striatum includes the nucleus accumbens septi and the anterior perforated substance and the ventral pallidum corresponds partly to the substantia innominata.

B Topographical Anatomy of the Lenticular Nucleus

The lentiform or lenticular nucleus refers to the putamen and pallidum. It is shaped like a biconvex lens completely buried in the hemispheric white matter, and covered laterally by the external capsule and limited medially by the internal capsule.

In transverse sections, the lenticular nucleus takes the form of a wedge with the apex directed medially and the base laterally. This nucleus is divided into two portions: a larger outer portion, the putamen, and a smaller medial portion lighter in color, named the pallidum or globus pallidus (Figs. 7.7, 7.14). The anterior-posterior and superior margins of the lentiform nucleus are related to the corona radiata (Figs. 7.7, 7.8) and its inferior aspect is grooved by the AC (Fig. 7.14) en route laterally towards the temporal lobes, as shown on the coronal (Figs. 7.4, 7.5, 7.20) and parasagittal cuts (Figs. 7.15 7.17). The rostral portion of the putamen is continuous with the head of the caudate nucleus (Figs. 7.3, 7.6). In front of the groove of the AC, the gray matter of the striatum is continuous with the anterior perforated substance (Figs. 7.4–7.6). The lateral striate arteries penetrating the brain at this level are clearly seen on the coronal slices (Fig. 7.4). The inferior aspect of the lenticular nucleus lies above the temporal horn of the lateral ventricle from which it is separated by the fibers of the external capsule.

The globus pallidus, which forms the medial portion of the lenticular nucleus, is subdivided into two segments separated by the internal medullary lamina. It is traversed by numerous heavily myelinated fibers which explains its pale color as compared with the putamen or the caudate nuclei on anatomic as well as on MR cuts. The pallidum is separated from the putamen by the external medullary lamina (Figs. 7.14, 7.20).

C Topographical Anatomy of the Caudate Nucleus

This nucleus is an elongated arcuate mass of gray matter related throughout its extent to the lateral ventricle, occupying the floor of the anterior or frontal horn and the roof of the temporal horn. Its anteriorly enlarged portion is termed the head and protrudes into the frontal horn of the lateral ventricle (Figs. 7.2–7.4). At the interventricular foramen, the nucleus narrows to constitute the body of the nucleus, which lies dorsolateral to the thalamus and contiguous to the lateral wall of the lateral ventricle (Figs. 7.20, 7.25, 7.26). The remaining portion, called the tail of the caudate, follows the curvature of the temporal horn of the lateral ventricle, penetrates into the temporal lobe, and ends in the region of the amygdaloid body. In all portions of the lateral ventricle, the caudate nucleus is covered by the ependyma. At its anterior extremity, the head of the caudate nucleus is fused with the putamen above the anterior perforated substance (Figs. 7.3, 7.6). Above this inferior fusion, the putamen and the head of the caudate are connected by strands of gray matter traversing the anterior limb of the internal capsule (Figs. 7.4, 7.5, 7.16, 7.25).

This striped appearance of these gray matter bridges suggested the term corpus striatum. Along the anterior horn and the central portion of the lateral ventricle, the caudate nucleus is related to the corpus callosum but separated from it by the fronto-occipital bundle. Its lateral flat surface is related to the internal capsule. In the temporal lobe, the tail of the caudate nucleus is separated from the inferior aspect of the globus pallidus by the sublentiform portion of the internal capsule and by the fibers from the external capsule.

The intrinsic architecture of the caudate nucleus and the putamen is similar; both are highly cellular and richly vascularized, as shown on FLAIR (Fig. 7.27) and particularly on SE-T1 weighted coronal cuts performed with magnetization transfer after Gd contrast infusion (Fig. 7.28). Morphometric data has shown that the putamen is around 13% larger than the caudate nucleus in humans and the external globus pallidus constitutes 70% of the volume of the pallidum (Parent 1996).

D Functional Aspects and Clinical Considerations

Afferent connections to the striatum derive mainly from the cerebral cortex, the intralaminar thalamic nuclei, and the substantia nigra. These afferent systems are topographically organized.

1. The corticostriatal projections arise from large areas of the cerebral cortex and project to the cau-

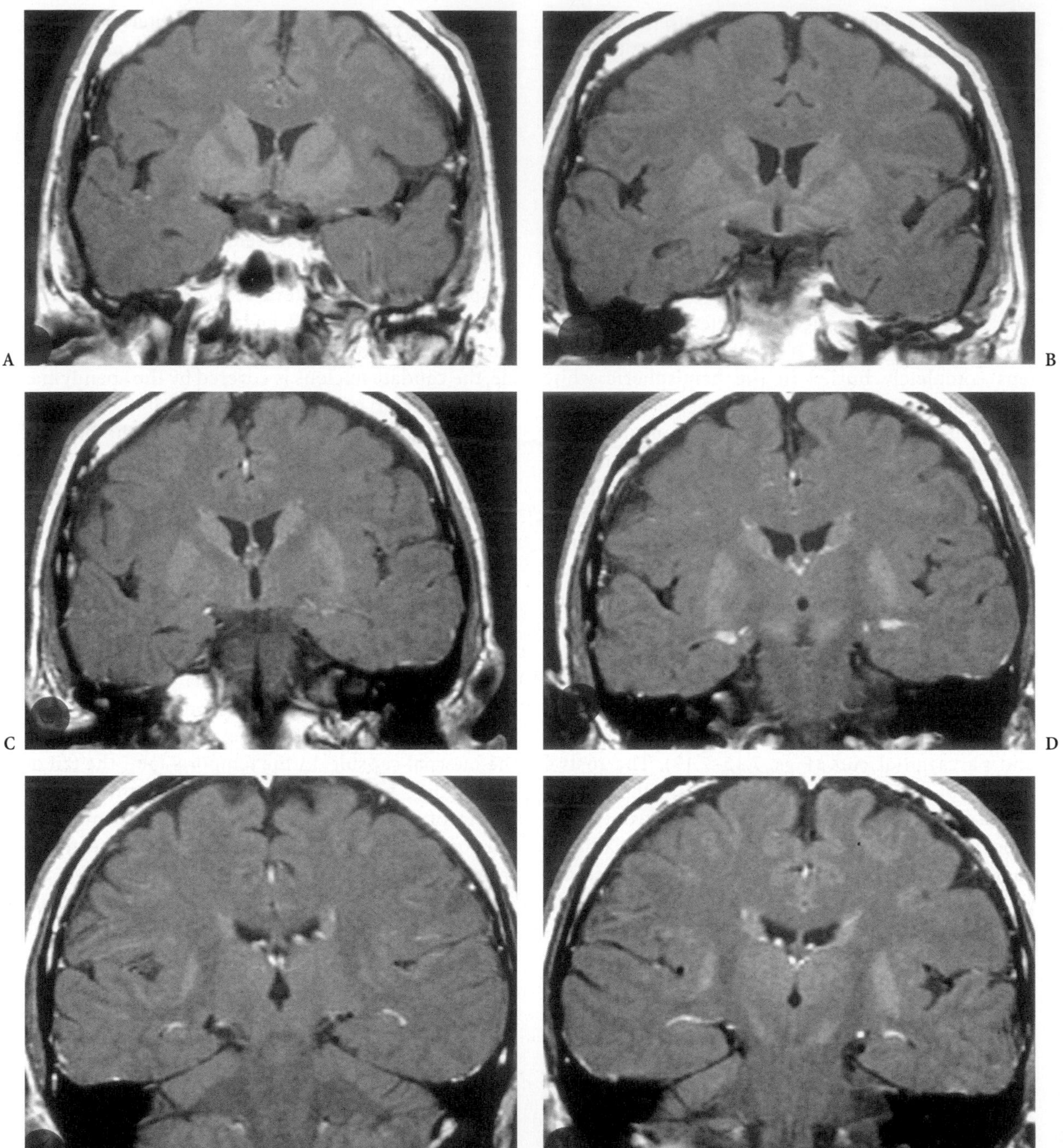

Fig. 7.27A–F. The interbrain structures: MR correlations in the coronal (PC-OB) plane, using FLAIR sequence (note the relative increase in signal intensity of the striatum, the substantia innominata and the substantia nigra as compared to the cortex and the remaining deep nuclei) **A** Anterior striatum and accumbens; **B** striatum and innominate substance; **C** caudate and putamen; **D** substantia nigra; **E** putamen and substantia nigra; **F** posterior border of putamen at PC-OB level

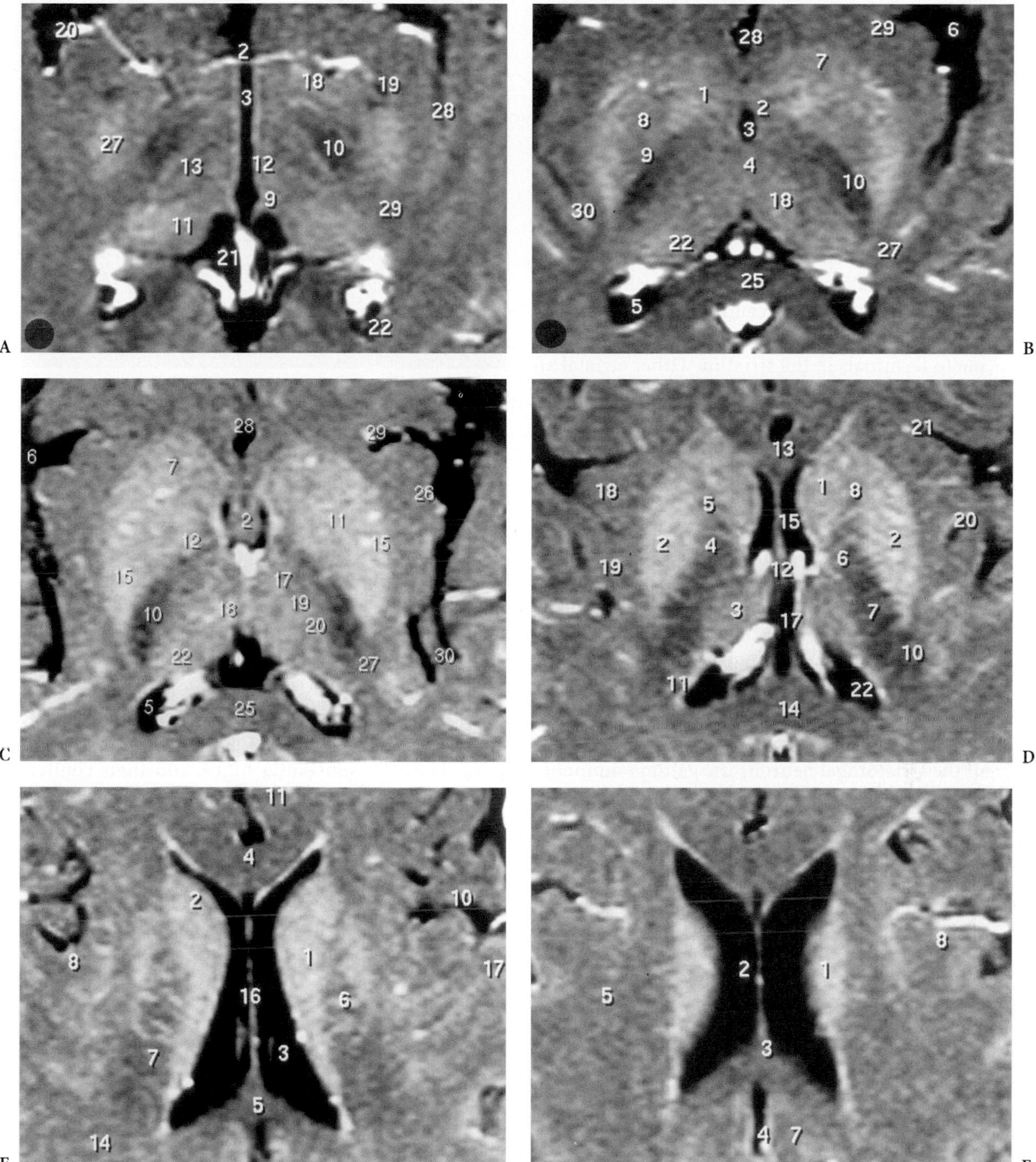

Fig. 7.28A–F. The interbrain structures including the basal ganglia: MR correlations in the axial (CH-PC) plane, using SE-T1 weighted pulse sequence with magnetization transfer and contrast (Gd) infusion. Note the high contrast resolution due partly to the relatively rich vascularization of most of the basal ganglionic structures, mainly, the ventral striatum-accumbens complex, the striatum, the pulvinar and dorsomedian thalamic nuclei. **A** The ventral striatum-accumbens and pulvinar level; **B** the striatum, inferior level; **C** the striatum, mid-level; **D** the striatum, upper level; **E,F** the body of the caudate nucleus. **A** (see fig. 7.6B), **B** (see fig. 7.14A), **C** (see fig. 7.14A), **D** (see fig. 7.22A), **E** (see fig. 7.25A), **F** (see fig. 7.26A),

date nucleus and the putamen. The cortical striatal fibers arising from area 4 project bilaterally and somatotopically to the putamen and use glutamate as a neurotransmitter.
2. The thalamostriatal projections constitute another profuse afferent system, arising mainly from the centromedian, but also other intralaminar and midline nuclei.
3. The nigrostriatal fibers originate from the cells of the pars compacta of the substantia nigra, ascend to the subthalamic region to reach the internal capsule, and end in the caudate and the putamen nuclei. These nigrostriatal fibers convey dopamine to terminals in the striatum. Other striatal afferents reach the striatum, such as those originating from serotoninergic cell groups located in the dorsal raphe nucleus of the midbrain.

The efferents are more limited. The majority of the striatofugal fibers terminate in the pallidum and the substantia nigra. The striatopallidal fibers are topographically organized; the lateral portion of the putamen projects to the external segment of the pallidum while the medial portion of the putamen and the caudate nucleus projects to both segments of the pallidum.

Topographically organized fibers arising from the subthalamic nucleus project to both segments of the globus pallidus. From a neurochemical aspect, nearly all the striatofugal neurons use gamma-aminobutyric acid (GABA) as an inhibitory neurotransmitter. The most important outflow from the striatum is represented by the pallidofugal system which is comprised of thick and heavily myelinated fibers topographically organized in a series of pathways including: the ansa lenticularis, the lenticular fasciculus, the thalamic fasciculus, the subthalamic fasciculus, and between other pallido-tegmental, pallido-nigral, and pallidohabenular projections (Fig. 7.29).

The ansa lenticularis, the lenticular fasciculus and pallido-tegmental fibers originate exclusively from the internal segment of the globus pallidus with the exception of the pallidosubthalamic fibers that arise from the external segment of the pallidum. The pallidofugal system is arranged in a rostrocaudal sequence with the ansa lenticularis situated most rostrally, the pallidosubthalamic fibers caudally, and the lenticular fasciculus in the intermediate position (Fig. 7.29). The main destination of the pallidothalamic crossed and uncrossed fibers is to the ventral anterior and ventral lateral thalamic nuclei, which in turn project to the cerebral cortex. Thalamostriatal fibers arising from the centromedian nucleus also

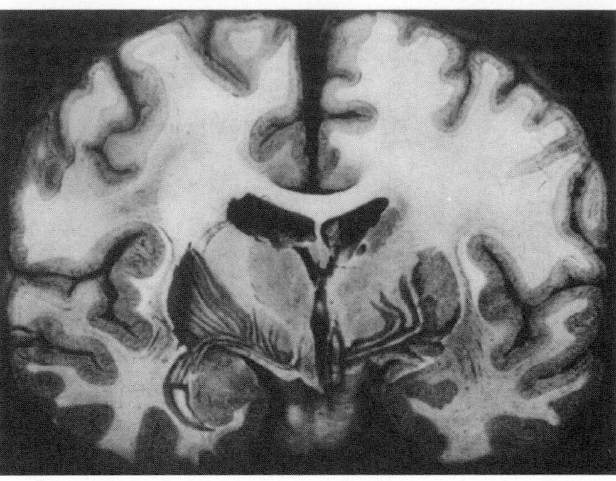

Fig. 7.29. Dissection of the major fiber bundles in the basal ganglia. (From Klingler, in Ludwig and Klingler 1956, Tabula 65)

project to the putamen as part of a feed-back system. The topographical route of the main pallidofugal fiber systems may be seen on coronal MR cuts and helps with clinical and anatomic correlations to some extent.

The basal ganglia functionally include the putamen, the globus pallidus, the caudate nucleus, the ventral anterior nucleus of thalamus, the subthalamic nucleus, the substantia nigra, and their connections, which exert influences on the motor activities by way of projections to the frontal cortex. The frontal cortex, in turn, exerts motor control, mainly contralaterally, at all levels of the central nervous system. Note that the basal ganglia do not project fibers directly to the level of the spinal cord. The basal ganglia control system is organized in circuits and acts as a modulating system, inhibiting or facilitating motor activities. Physiologic data suggest that this inhibition is the basic mechanism subjacent to the expression of striatal function (Chevalier and Deniau 1990). The output systems of the basal ganglia are in fact GABAergic. Pallidothalamic and nigrothalamic projections may result in inhibition of the thalamic neurons projecting on the cerebral cortex. In turn, the striatum, which is the receptive component of the basal ganglia, receives major inputs from the cerebral cortex and from subcortical nuclei such as the substantia nigra, and the intralaminar thalamic nuclei and the raphe nuclei of the midbrain, all of which are projections mediated by different neurotransmitters.

Pathologic conditions are observed when the balance in this complex, modulating and interrelated system is disrupted. Movement disorders consecutive to the basal dysfunction comprise a wide spectrum of abnormalities, ranging from hypokinesia to hyperkinesia or dyskinesia. The pathophysiologic basis of the associated disease processes is often the consequence of a deficiency in one or more involved neurotransmitters.

Parkinson's disease is the best representative of hypokinetic disorders. It is characterized by a reduction or loss of movement with reduction of initiation, implementation and facility of execution of movements, as well as in the velocity of voluntary movements known as bradykinesia. Hypokinesia is usually associated with muscular rigidity and tremor at rest.

On the other hand, the negative symptoms characterizing parkinsonism are thought to reflect primary functional deficits due to destruction of the related anatomical structures. In Parkinson's disease, the pathologic changes affect mainly the substantia nigra and are characterized by a reduced dopaminergic input from the cells of the pars compacta to the striatum. The clinical picture of this syndrome includes akinesia and bradykinesia with little facial expression and slowness of movements, flexed posture and immobility, muscular rigidity, and static or postural tremor. An experimental model of parkinsonism is available since the discovery of the meperidine analogue, MPTP (1-Methyl-4-Phenyl-4–1-2–5-6-Tetrahydropyridine), a neurotoxin, which produces a chronic form of parkinsonism in monkeys, the signs of which are identical to human Parkinson's disease (Langston et al. 1983; Bédard et al. 1992; Agid 1991).

Hyperkinetic disorders, such as Huntington's and Sydenham's choreas or ballism, are characterized by the presence of involuntary movements including tremor, choreiform or athetoid movements, or hemiballismus. This excessive motor activity is due to the release of pallidal and thalamic activities following the degeneration of striatal neurons which normally modulate the pallidum. The cerebral cortex plays an important role in the neural mechanisms, causing dyskinesias.

Most of the abnormal involuntary movements and dyskinetic states are abolished with interruption of the corticospinal pathway or surgical ablation of the motor cortex (Bucy 1958; Carpenter et al. 1960). Stereotaxic surgery has focused mainly on the ventral lateral nucleus of the thalamus and on the pallidum. Localized lesions focused to these nuclear structures have significantly reduced, and even abolished, some forms of dyskinesia (Cooper 1956; Cooper and Bravo 1958; Hassler 1959, 1982; Martin and McCaul 1959; Talairach et al. 1950). Such surgical attempts to alleviate various forms of involuntary movements are based on the hypothesis that dyskinesias are the physiologic expression of release phenomena, the involuntary movements observed being the result of excessive neural activity.

Experimental models clarified part of the pathophysiology of hypokinetic disorders, which seem to be due to increased thalamic inhibition caused by increased excitatory effects acting on the internal globus pallidus and the substantia nigra reticulata and originating from the subthalamic nucleus. Clinical results obtained from selective lesioning of the subthalamic nucleus produce, in fact, dramatic improvement of hypokinesia, rigidity and tremor in the contralateral limbs (DeLong 1990; Guridi et al. 1993; Wichmann and DeLong 1993; Gerfen 1992; Aziz et al. 1991; Bergman et al. 1990). The positive role of the subthalamic nucleus in the genesis of akinesia as postulated is also supported by experimental high frequency stimulation of this nucleus (Benazouz et al. 1993).

E Functional Neurosurgery

Imaging of the thalamus and the basal ganglia has its application in the surgical treatment of movement disorders. This treatment modality has recently received much attention and consists of lesional surgery directed to specific targets or neuro-augmentative procedures using high frequency stimulation.

The localization of these targets has classically relied on the identification, under stereotaxic conditions, of the AC and PC by means of a ventriculogram.

With high resolution MRI performed in a coronal and axial plane, the AC and PC coordinates can be determined easily and accurately. Using the standard brain atlases, which are incorporated frequently in the stereotaxy software, the approximate location of specific targets can be derived. The precise location of the target is selected, based on stimulation studies and single-cell electrode recordings. At present, most units performing functional neurosurgery supplement the coordinates derived by neuroimaging with intraoperative physiological testing to determine the exact target location.

The treatment of Parkinson's disease has evolved. Previously, lateral thalamic lesions were the most accepted surgical treatment modalities. More recently, the treatment is individualized based on the most disabling symptoms. In addition, high frequency stimulation has been found to produce the same effects as lesional surgery with fewer complications.

For intractable tumor associated with Parkinson's disease, a lesional or high frequency stimulation is applied to the ventral intermedius (VIM) nucleus of the thalamus. Although VIM does not receive any input from the ansa lenticularis fibers, it appears to play a fundamental role in tremor genesis. VIM can be localized by reference to a standard atlas such as that of Schaltenbrand and Bailey, or more easily by using the Guiot parallelogram. This method consists in determination of the AC-PC coordinates and thalamic height. The mid AC-PC thalamic height line is constructed and a parallel to the AC-PC line is drawn from the midthalamic height line. The AC-PC and midthalamic height lines are divided into 12 segments. The specific thalamic nuclei are located in the parallelogram drawn between these two lines and correspond to Hassler's terminology (Figs. 7.30–7.32; Taren et al. 1968).

As predicted from animal experiments, the subthalamic nucleus (Fig. 7.33) appears to play a cardinal role in the pathogenesis of motor disturbances associated with Parkinson's disease. Consequently, recent work has demonstrated that high frequency stimulation of this nucleus is exceedingly effective in a kinetic-rigid parkinsonism. Moreover, it can be performed bilaterally in the same setting. Visualization of the subthalamic nucleus is performed under stereotactic conditions, using a protocol developed by Benebid et al. (1987, 1991).

High-resolution imaging has contributed to the resurgence of interest in pallidotomy in Parkinson's disease. This technique, reported in 1962, was rarely used until recently. Localization of internal globus pallidus relies heavily on thin cut, using T1 and T2 weighted pulse sequences, performed parallel to the AC-PC line. Again, the AC-PC coordinates are derived from a stereotactic atlas. Since the internal segment of the globus pallidus (Gpi) lies in close approximation with the optic tract and the internal capsule, stimulation is used to avoid these structures and locate induced neuronal activity within Gpi movement. A lesion is then created while patient vision and movement are tested (Guiot et al. 1958).

F Arterial Supply to the Basal Ganglia

The lateral striate arteries, branches of the middle cerebral artery, vascularize the striatum. Most of the putamen is nourished by these lateral striate branches except the medial part, which is supplied by the recurrent artery of Heubner, and the caudal part, by branches of the anterior choroidal artery (Gillilan 1968; Dunker and Harris 1976). The rostromedial portion of the head of the caudate nucleus is nourished by Heubner's artery which originates from the A1 segment of the anterior cerebral artery, according to Perlmutter and Rhoton (1976). The dorsolateral portion of the head and the body of the caudate nucleus are supplied by the lateral striate branches of the middle cerebral artery. Note that the head of the caudate may be supplied entirely by the lateral striate perforators of the middle cerebral artery or the Heubner artery. The tail of the caudate nucleus is supplied by branches of the anterior choroidal artery and the lateral posterior choroidal artery.

The lateral segment of the globus pallidus is supplied by the lateral striate branches of the middle cerebral artery, and also from medial striate branches of the anterior cerebral artery and even the anterior choroidal artery. The medial pallidal segment receives branches from the anterior choroidal artery vascularizing its lateral part, while its medial part receives major blood flow from branches of the posterior communicating artery.

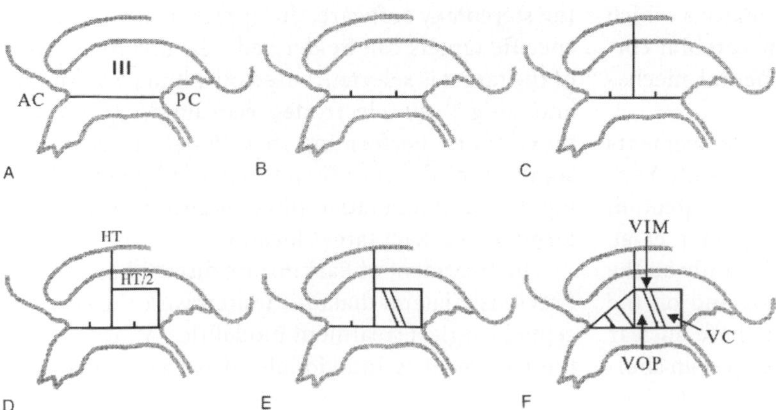

Fig. 7.30. Methodology of Guiot for the localization of the ventral intermedius (VIM) thalamic subnucleus, using ventriculography, and based on the intercommissural (CA-CP) reference line. *AC*, anterior commissure; *PC*, posterior commissure; *HT*, thalamic height; *VOp*, nucleus ventralis oralis posterior; *VC*, nucleus ventralis caudalis (Taren et al, 1968)

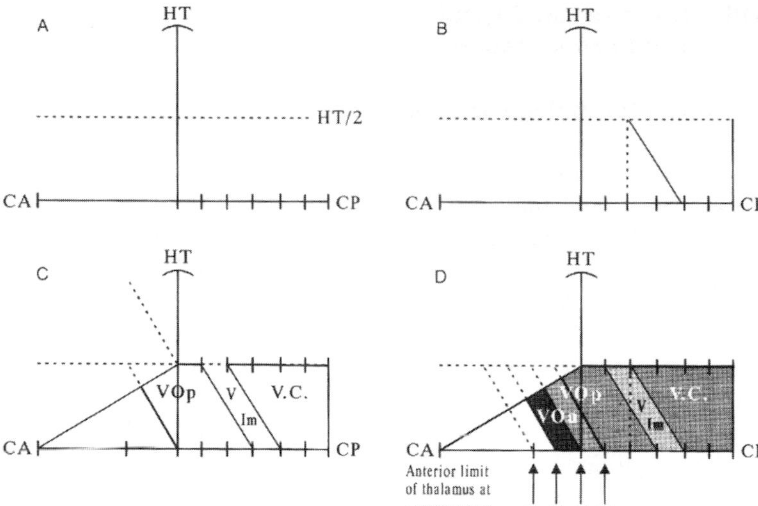

Fig. 7.31. Methodology of Guiot for the localization of the ventral intermedius (VIM) thalamic subnucleus, using ventriculography, and based on the intercommissural (CA-CP) reference. *CA*, commissura anterior; *CP*, commissura posterior commissure (Taren et al, 1968)

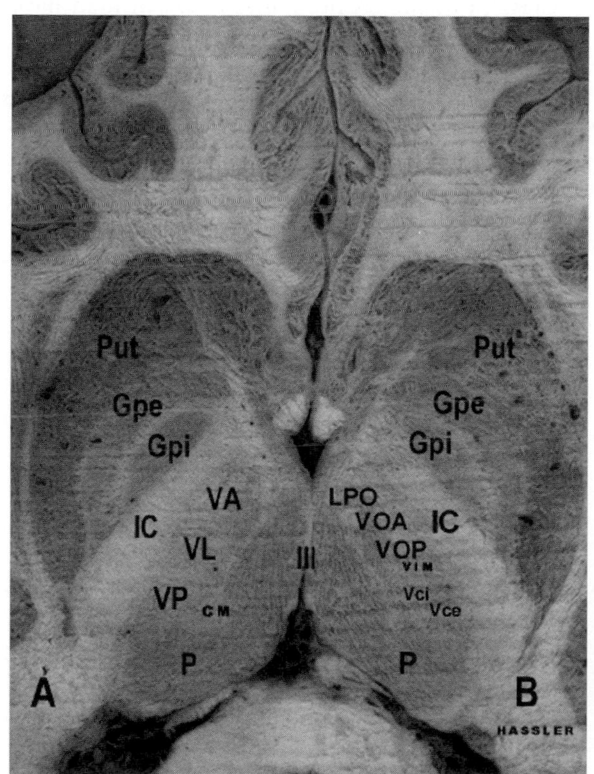

Fig. 7.32. Thalamic subnuclei terminology. *A*, Anglo-Saxon: *VA*, ventral anterior; *VL*, ventral lateral; *VP*, ventral posterior; *Gpi*, internal segment of globus pallidus; *Gpe*, external segment of globus pallidus; *Put*, putamen. *B*, Hassler's: *LPO*, lateralis polaris; *VOa*, ventralis oralis anterior; *VOp*, ventralis oralis posterior; *Vim*, ventralis intermedius; *Vci*, ventralis caudalis internus; *Vce*, ventralis caudalis externus; *CM*, centrum medianum

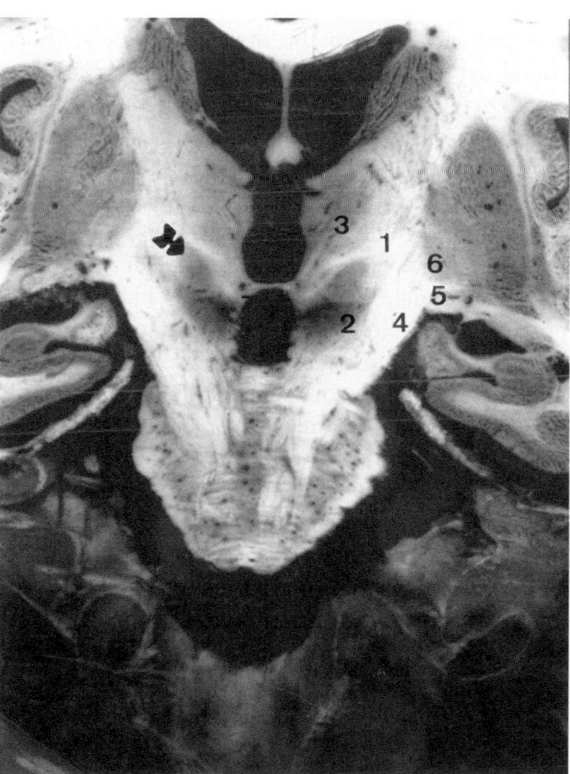

Fig. 7.33. The subthalamic nucleus (*arrow*): topographical anatomy and relationships. *1*, Internal capsule; *2*, substantia nigra; *3*, thalamus; *4*, cerebral peduncle; *5*, optic tract; *6*, internal pallidum

VIII The Internal Capsule and Corona Radiata

A Gross Morphology and Imaging

The cerebral cortex is connected with the thalamus, the brainstem and the spinal cord by an extensive projection fiber system which penetrates the white matter of the centrum semiovale of Vieussens and converges as the corona radiata toward the thalamus (Figs. 7.26, 7.10, 7.16). At this level, these radiating fibers constitute a compact band interposed between the thalamus and the caudate on the medial side, and the lentiform nucleus on the lateral aspect. This mass of fibers is designated as the internal capsule (Fig. 7.24). Afferent fibers constituting the thalamic radiations, described previously, and the corticofugal fiber systems, compose a large amount of the fibers of the internal capsule. The denomination of internal capsule is widely used since Burdach.

The morphological aspect and the relationship of the internal capsule are best visualized on horizontal cuts passing through the optostriate nuclei (horizontal cut superiorly to the sylvian fissure as proposed by Flechsig). In such orientation, the internal capsule presents a "boomerang" shape composed of a short anterior limb, meeting at an obtuse angle open laterally, and a longer posterior limb. The genu constitutes the junction between the anterior and posterior limbs (Fig. 7.24). The anterior limb separates the caudate from the lentiform nuclei and the posterior limb lies between the thalamus medially and the lentiform nucleus laterally. The posterior limb extends posteriorly behind the posterior border of the lentiform nucleus, constituting the retrolenticular portion of the internal capsule. Some of the fibers pass beneath the lentiform nucleus toward the temporal lobe, constituting the sublenticular portion of the internal capsule (Figs. 7.9, 7.10). Morphometric data has shown that the anterior limb is around 2 cm long, with the posterior limb measuring 3–4 cm. The retrolenticular portion extends caudally behind the lentiform nucleus to an extent of 10–12 mm (Fig. 7.13).

B Topographical and Functional Anatomy

Considering the fiber systems contained in the internal capsule, the anterior limb contains the anterior thalamic peduncle and the prefrontal corticopontine tracts; the genu contains the corticobulbar and corticoreticular tracts; and in the posterior limb are found the superior thalamic peduncle, the corticospinal and frontopontine tracts, and the smaller bundles representing the corticotectal, corticorubral and corticoreticular fibers. The retrolenticular portion of Déjerine contain the posterior thalamic peduncle including the parieto-occipital, corticopontine fibers, the optic radiations and projections from the occipital cortex to the superior colliculi, and the pretectal region. The sublenticular portion contains the inferior thalamic peduncle including the auditory radiations and the temporal corticopontine fiber bundle, as well as parieto-occipital projections (Fig. 7.6).

The localization of the corticospinal fibers of the pyramidal tract in their route through the corona radiata, the internal capsule, the basis pontis and the cerebral peduncles to reach the pyramids at the anterior aspect of the medulla, has been disputed by several authors in the last 30 years (Hardy et al. 1979; Ross 1980; Englander et al. 1975; Déjerine 1901; Kretschmann 1988; Yagishita et al. 1994).

Classically, the corticospinal fibers in man have been considered to lie in the anterior half of the posterior limb near the genu (Déjerine 1901; Crosby et al. 1962) or in the anterior two third portion of the posterior limb (Testut and Latarjet 1948). This traditional localization has been disputed by several authors in view of their results from electrical stimulations and careful neuropathological studies (Hirayama et al. 1962; Brion and Guiot 1964; Bertrand et al. 1965; Hanaway and Young 1977). The data provided by these authors suggest that the corticospinal tract is largely confined to a region in the posterior half of the posterior limb of the internal capsule. Ross and Elliot (1980) demonstrated that the controversy which exists concerning the different anatomic topographical data reported is explained by a failure to take into account the modification in the rostrocaudal and anterior posterior topography of the pyramidal tract in its descending route through the posterior limb of the internal capsule. The authors showed that the pyramidal tract is located in the anterior half of the posterior limb at the upper level of the internal capsule, but shifts to the posterior half of the posterior limb in the lower aspect of the internal capsule as seen on the horizontal cuts passing through the upper portion, the mid-portion and the lower portion of the optostriate nuclei (Figs. 7.14, 7.24, 7.25, 4.22, 4.28).

The explanation is that the pyramidal tract shifts posteriorly in order to accommodate the fibers contained in the anterior limb. These fibers are displaced to the posterior limb at the lower thalamic level contiguous to the crus cerebri. This posterior shift of the corticospinal tract is also apparent and obvious at the level of the corona radiata, and the centrum semiovale due to the anterior-posterior displacement of the central sulcus according to the brain reference line used in performing the horizontal cuts. The pyramidal tract is located more posteriorly in the CH-PC plane or sylvian plane orientation than in the AC-PC plane, as may be observed on MR using FLAIR sequences or SE-T2 weighted sequences in degenerative or toxic diseases of white matter tracts (see Chap. 4). On the other hand, the fibers contained in the corticospinal tract are somatotopically arranged in the posterior limb of the internal capsule with a rostrocaudal sequence, cervicothoracic fibers being found anterior to the lumbosacral fibers. Lesions involving the internal capsule produce a more extended disability than similar insults involving another region of the brain.

C Arterial Supply to the Internal Capsule

The internal capsule may be subdivided into an anterior limb, a genu, a posterior limb, and a retrolenticular part. The anterior limb is supplied by branches of the Heubner medial striate artery, which vascularize its rostromedial portion, while the dorsolateral portion is supplied from lateral striate branches of the middle cerebral artery. The genu is vascularized by the lateral striate branches of the middle cerebral artery supplying its dorsal portion and by branches from the internal carotid artery, as well as the anterior cerebral and the anterior communicating arteries. The dorsal aspect of the posterior limb of the internal capsule is supplied primarily by the lateral striate branches of the middle cerebral artery, while its ventral part is supplied by branches of the anterior choroidal artery (Salamon and Lazorthes 1971). Thalamogeniculate branches of the posterior cerebral artery may also supply the posterior limb (Schlesinger 1976). The retrolenticular portion of the internal capsule is vascularized by branches of the anterior choroidal artery.

References

Agid Y (1991) Parkinson's disease: pathophysiology. Lancet 337:1321–1324

Alonso A, Kohler C (1984) A study of the reciprocal connections between the septum and the entorhinal area using anterograde and retrograde axonal transport methods in the rat brain. J Comp Neurol 225:327–343

Andy OJ, Stephan H (1968) The septum in the human brain. J Comp Neurol 133:383–410

Aziz TZ, Peggs D, Sambrook MA, Crossman AR (1991) Lesion of the subthalamic nucleus for the alleviation of 1-methyl-4-phenyl1-1,2,3,6-tetrahydropyridine (MPTP) – induced Parkinsonism in the primate. Mov Disord 6:288–293

Bédard PJ, Boucher R, Gomez Mancilla B, Blanchette P (1992) Animal models of Parkinson's disease. In: Boultol A, Baker G, Butterworth R (eds) Animal models of neurological disease. Humana, Totowa, pp 159–173

Benazzouz A, Gross CH, Féger J, Boraud T, Bioulac B (1993) Reveral of rigidity and improvement in motor performance by subthalamic high frequency stimulation in MPTP treated monkeys. Eur J Neurosci 5:382–389

Benebid AL, Pollak P, Louveau A et al (1987) Combined (thalamotomy and stimulation) stereotactic surgery of the Vim thalamic nucleus for bilateral Parkinson'sdisease. Appl Neurophysiol 50:344–346

Benebid AL, Pollak P, Gervason C et al (1991) Long term suppression tremor by chronic stimulation of the ventral intermediate thalamic nucleus. Lancet 377:403–406

Bergman H, Wichmann T, Delong MR (1990) Reversal of experimental Parkinsonism by lesion of the subthalamic nucleus. Science 249:1436–1438

Bernard C (1878) Leçons sur les phénomènes de la vie commune aux animaux et aux végétaux. Baillière, Paris

Bertrand GL, Blundelle J, Musella R (1965) Electrical exploration of the internal capsule and neighboring structures during stereotaxic procedures. J Neurosurg 22:333–343

Bobillier P, Seguin S, Petitjean F, Salvert D, Touret M, Jouvet M (1976) The raphe nuclei of the cat brain stem: a topographical atlas of their efferent projections as revealed by autoradiography Brain Res 113:449–486

Braak H, Braak E (1991) Alzheimer's disease affects limbic nuclei of the thalamus. Acta Neuropathol (Berl) 81:261–268

Brion S, Guiot G (1964) Topographie des faisceaux de projection du cortex dans la capsule interne et dans le pédoncule cérébral. Revue Neurologique Paris 110:123–144

Brodal A (1981) Neurological anatomy in relation to clinical medicine, 3rd edn, vol 9. Oxford University Press, New York

Bucy PC (1958) The cortico-spinal tract. In: Fields WS (ed) Pathogenesis and treatment of parkinsonism, chap 11. Thomas, Springfield, pp 271–293

Burdach KF (1819–1824) Vom Bau und Leben des Gehirns. Dyksche Buchhandlung, Leipzig

Cannon WB, Britton SW (1925) Studies on the conditions of activity in endocrine glands. XV. Pseudoaffective medulliadrenal secretion. Am J Physiol 72:283–294

Carpenter MB (1981) Anatomy of the corpus striatum and brainstem integrating systems, vol 197. In: Brooks V (ed) Handbook of physiology, vol II, sect 1. Motor control, chap 19. Americal Physiological Society, Washington DC, pp 579–603

Carpenter MB, Harbison JW, Peter P (1970) Accessory oculomotor nuclei in the monkey. Projections and effects of discrete lesions. J Comp Neurol 140:131–154

Chevalier G, Deniau JM (1990) Disinhibition as a basic process in the expression of striatal functions. Trends Neurosci 13:277–280

Cooper IS (1956) Neurosurgical alleviation of Parkinsonism. Thomas, Springfield

Copper IS, Bravo GJ (1958) Anterior choroidal artery occlusion, chemopallidectomy and chemothalamectomy in parkinsonism: a consecutive series of 700 operations. In: Fields WS (ed) Pathogenesis and treatment of parkinsonism, chap 15. Thomas, Springfield, pp 325–352

Coyle JT, Price DL, DeLong MR (1983) Alzheimer's disease: a disorder of cortical cholinergic innervation. Science 219:484-490

Crosby EC, Humphrey T, Lauer EW (1962) Correlative anatomy of the nervous system. Macmillan, New York, p 731

Déjerine J (1901) Anatomie des centres nerveux, vol 2. Rueff, Paris

Dekaban A (1954) Human thalamus. An anatomical developmental and pathological study. II. Development of the human thalamic nuclei. J Comp Neurol 100:63–97

DeLong MR (1990) Primate models of movement disorders of the basal ganglia. Trends Neurosci 13:281–285

Dunker RO, Harris AB (1976) Surgical anatomy of the proximal anterior cerebral artery. J Neurosurg 44:359–367

Duvernoy HM (1978) Human brainstem vessels. Springer, Berlin Heidelberg New York

Englander RN, Netsky MG, Adelman LS (1975) Location of human pyramidal tract in the internal capsule: anatomical evidence. Neurology 25:823–826

Flechsig P (1905) Einige Bemerkungen über die Untersuchungsmethoden der Grosshirnrinden insbesondere des Menschen. Arch Anat Entwickl-Gesch 337–444

Foix C, Hillemand J (1925) Irrigation de la couche optique. CR Soc Biol (Paris) 92:52–54

Foix C, Nicolesco J (1925) Les noyaux gris centraux et la région mésencéphalo-sous-optique. Masson, Paris

Gerfen CR (1992) The neostriatal mosaic: multiple levels of compartmental organization in the basal ganglia. Annu Rev Neurosci 15:285–320

Gilbert GJ (1960) The subcommissural organ. Neurology 10:138–142

Gillilan LA (1968) The arterial and venous supplies to the forebrain of primates. Neurology 18:653–670

Guiot G, Brion S (1958) La destruction stéréotaxique du pallidum interne dans les syndromes parkinsonniens. Ann Chir 17/18

Guridi J, Luquin MR, Herrero MT, Obeso JA (1993) The subthalamic nucleus: a possible target for stereotaxic surgery in Parkinson's disease. Mov Disord 8:421–429

Hanaway J, Young RR (1977) Localization of the pyramidal tract in the internal capsule of man. J Neurol Sci 34:63–70

Hara K, Fujino Y (1966) The thalamoperforate artery. Acta Radiol 5:192–200

Hardy TL, Bertrand G, Thompson CJ (1979) The position and organization of motor fibers in the internal capsule found during stereotactic surgery. Appl Neurophysiol 42:160–170

Hassler R (1959) Anatomy of the thalamus. In: Schaltenbrand G, Bailey P (eds) Introduction to stereotaxis with an atlas of human brain, vol I. Thieme, Stuttgart, pp 230–290

Hassler R (1982) Architectonic organization of the thalamic nuclei. In: Schaltenbrand G, Walker AE (eds) Stereotaxy of the human brain – anatomical, physiological, and clinical applications, 2nd edn. Thieme, Stuttgart, pp 140–180

Hassler R, Mundinger F, Riechert T (1979) Stereotaxis in Parkinson's syndrome. Springer, Berlin Heidelberg New York

Haymaker W (1969) Hypothalamo-pituitary neural pathways and the circulatory system of the pituitary. In: Haymaker W et al. (eds), The hypothalamus, chap 6. Thomas, Springfield, Ill., pp 219–250

Haymaker W, Anderson E, Nauta W (1969) The hypothalamus. Thomas, Springfield

Heimer L, Switzer RC III, van Hoesen GW (1982) Ventral striatum and ventral pallidum: components of the motor system? Trends Neurosci 5:83–87

Hirayama K, Tsubaki T, Toyokura Y, Okinaka S (1962) The representation of the pyramidal tract in the internal capsule and basis pedunculi. Neurology 12:337–342

Jones EG (1985) The thalamus. Plenum, New York

Jouvet M (1972) The role of monoamines and acetylcholine containing neurons in the regulation of sleep-waking cycle. Rev Physiol Biochem Exp Pharmacol 64:166–307

Jouvet M (1964) Etude neurophysiologique clinique des troubles de la conscience. Acta Neurochir Wien 12:258–269

Jouvet M (1965) Paradoxical sleep. A study of its nature and mechanisms. Prog Brain Res 18:20–62

Kretschmann HJ (1988) Localization of the corticospinal fibres in the internal capsule in man. J Anat 160:219–225

Kuhlenbeck H (1948) The derivatives of the thalamus ventralis in the human brain and their relation to the so-colled subthalamus. Milit Surg 102:433–447

Langston JW, Ballard P, Tetrud JW, Irwin I (1983) Chronic parkinsonism in humans due to a product meperidine-analog synthesis. Science 249:979–980

Lavoie B, Parent A (1994) The pedunculopontine nucleus in the squirrel monkey. Cholinergic and glutamatergic projections to the substantia nigra. J Comp Neurol 344: 232–241

Lewy FH (1942) Historical introduction. In: The basal ganglia and their diseases. Res Publ Ass Nerv Ment Dis 21:1–20

Le Gros Clark WE (1932) The structure and connections of the thalamus. Brain 55:406–470

Le Gros Clark WE, Beattie J, Riddoch G, Dott NM (eds) (1938) The hypothalamus. Oliver and Boyd, Edinburgh

Lindvall O, Bjorklund A, Moore RY, Stenevi U (1974) Mesencephalic dopamine neurons projecting to neocortex. Brain Res 81:325–331

Ludwig E, Klingler J (1956) Atlas cerebri humani. Karger, Basel

Magoun HW, Ranson SW, Mayer LL (1935) The pupillary light reflex after lesions of the posterior commissure in the cat. Am J Ophthal 18:624–630

Marinkovic SV, Milisavljejic MM, Kovacevic MS (1986) Anatomical bases for surgical approach to the initial segment of the anterior cerebral artery. Surg Radiol Anat 8:7–18

Martin JP (1927) Hemichorea resulting from a local lesion of the brain (the syndrome of body of Luys). Brain 50:637–651

Martin JP, McCaul IR (1959) Acute hemiballismus treated by ventrolateral thalamolysis. Brain 82:104–108

Meibach RC, Siegel A (1977) Efferent connections of the septal area in the rat: an analysis utilizing retrograde and anterograde transport methods. Brain Res 119:1–20

Mesulam MM, Mufson EJ, Levey AI, Wainer BH (1983) Cholinergic nnervation of cortex connections of the septal area, diagonal band nuclei, nucleus basalis (substantia innominata) and hypothalamus in the rhesus monkey. J Comp Neurol 214:170–197

Mesulam MM, Geula C, Bothwell MA, Hersh LB (1989) Human reticular formation: cholinergic neurons of pedunculopontine and laterodorsal tegmental nuclei and some cytochemical comparisons to forebrain cholinergic neurons. J Comp Neurol 283:611–633

Mesulam MM, Mash D, Hersh L, Bothwell M, Geula C (1992) Cholinergic innervation of the human striatum, globus pallidus, subthalamic nucleus, substantia nigra, and red nucleus. J Comp Neurol 323:252–268

Miller MJ, Mark L. P, Yetkin F. Z, Khang-Cheng Ho, Haughton VM, Estkowski L, Wong E (1994) Imaging white matter tracts and nuclei of the hypothalamus: an MR anatomic comparative study. Am J Neuroradiol 15:117–121

Moore RY (1973) Retinohypothalamic projection in mammals: a comparative study. Brain Res 49:403–409

Moore RY (1992) The organization of the human circadian timing system. Prog Brain Res 93:99–105

Naidich TP, Daniels DL, Pech P, Haughton VM, Williams A, Pojunas K (1986) Anterior commissure: anatomic-MR correlation and use as a landmark in three orthogonal planes. Radiology 158:421–429

Nauta WJH, Haymaker W (1969) Hypothalamic nuclei and fiber connections. In: Haymaker W, Anderson E, Nauta WJH (eds) The hypothalamus, chap 4. Thomas, Springfield, pp 136–209

Parent A (1996) Carpenter's human neuroanatomy, 9th edn. Williams and Wilkins, Baltimore

Perlmutter D, Rhoton AL (1976) Microsurgical anatomy of the anterior cerebral anterior communicating-recurrent artery complex. J Neurosurg 45:259–272

Relkin R (1976) The pineal. Eden, Montreal

Rhoton AL, Fujii K, Saeki N (1979) Microsurgical anatomy of the anterior choroidal artery. Surg Neurol 12:171–187

Ross ED, Elliot D (1980) Localization of the pyramidal tract in the internal capsule by whole brain dissection. Neurology 30:59–64

Salamon G, Lazorthes G (1971) Atlas of the arteries of the human brain. Sandoz, Paris

Saper CB (1990) Hypothalamus. In: Paxinos G (ed) The human nervous system, chap 15. Academic, New York, pp 389–413

Schlesinger B (1976) The upper brainstemin the human. Its nuclear configuration and vascular supply. Springer, Berlin Heidelberg New York

Sherrington CS (1906) The integrative action of the nervous system. Scribner, New York (Reprinted 1947, Yale University Press, New Haven)

Stephan H (1975) Handbuch der mikroskopischen Anatomie des Menschen, vol. 4, part 9: Allocortex. Springer, Berlin Heidelberg New York

Swanson LW, Cowan WM (1977) An autoradiographic study of the organization of the efferent connections of the hippocampal formation in the rat. J Comp Neurol 172:49–84

Swanson LW, Cowan WM (1979) The connections of the septal region in the rat. J Comp Neurol 186:621–655

Talairach J, Paillas JE, David M (1950) Dykinésie de type hémiballique traitée par cortectomie frontale limitée, puis par coagulation de l'anse lenticulaire de la portion interne du globus pallidus. Rev Neurol (Paris) 83:440–451

Tamraz J (1983) Atlas d'anatomie céphalique dans le plan neuro-oculaire (PNO), Md thesis. Schering, Paris (1986)

Tamraz J, Iba-Zizen MT, Cabanis EA (1984) Atlas d'anatomie céphalique dans le plan neuro-oculaire (PNO). J Fr Ophtalmol 7(5):371–379

Tamraz J, Iba-Zizen MT, Atiyeh M, Cabanis EA (1985) Atlas d'anatomie céphalique dans le plan neuro-oculaire (PNO). Bull Soc Fr Ophtalmol 8/9(85):853–857

Tamraz J et al (1989) The chiasmato-commissural plane. Scientific session (poster), Joint meeting of the European society of neuroradiology (ESNR) and the International congress of radiology (ICR), July 6, Paris

Tamraz J, Saban R, Reperant J, Cabanis EA (1990) Définition d'un plan de référence céphalique en imagerie par résonance magnétique: le plan chiasmato-commissural. CR Acad Sci Paris 311(III):115–121

Tamraz J, Saban R, Reperant J, Cabanis EA (1991) A new cephalic reference plane for use with magnetic resonance imaging: the chiasmato-commissural plane. Surg Radiol Anat 13:197–201

Taren J, Guiot G, Derome P, Trigo JC (1968) Hazards of stereotaxic thalamectomy. Added safety factor in corroborating x-ray target localization with neurophysiological methods. J Neurosurg 29:173–182

Testut L, Latarjet A (1948) Traité d'anatomie humaine. Tome 2: angiologie, système nerveux central, 9th edn. Doin, Paris

Van Buren JM, Borke RC (1972) Variations and connections of the human thalamus. Springer, Berlin Heidelberg New York

Walker AE (1938) The primate thalamus. University of Chicago Press, Chicago

Whitehouse PJ, Price DL, Clark AW, Coyle JT, Delong MR (1981) Alzheimer's disease: evidence for selective loss of cholinergic neurons in the nucleus basalis. Ann Neurol 10:122–126

Whitehouse PJ, Price DL, Struble RG, Clark AW, Coyle JT, Delong MR (1982) Alzheimer's disease and senile dementia: loss of neurons in the basal forebrain. Science 215:1237–1239

Whittier JR (1947) Ballism and the subthalamic nucleus (nucleus hypothalamicus; corpus Luysi) Arch Neuro Psychiatry 58:672–692

Wichmann T, DeLong MR (1993) Pathophysiology of parkinsonian motor abnormalities. In: Narabayashi H, Nagatsu T, Yanagisawa N, Mizuno Y, (eds) Advances in neurology, vol 60. Raven, New York, pp 53–61

Williams PL, Warwick R, Dyson M, Bannister LH (1989) Gray's anatomy, 37th edn. Churchill Livingstone, London

Willis T (1664) Cerebri anatome, cui accessit nervorum descriptio et usus. Martyn and Allestry, London

Yagishita A, Nakano I, Oda M, Hirano A (1994) Location of the corticospinal tract in the internal capsule at MR imaging. Radiology 191:455–460

Synoptical Atlas of Cross-Sectional Anatomy of the Interbrain Using the Commissural-Obex (PC-OB) Reference Plane

The aim of this synoptical atlas of cross sections of the human brain is to display those successive anatomic landmarks routinely observed on MR. These successive cuts are performed according to the long axis of the brainstem, as obtained using the PC-OB reference line (Tamraz 1983; Tamraz et al. 1984, 1985, 1989, 1990, 1991)

These successive coronal cuts are performed using a high field system, at 3 mm slice thickness and 1 mm gap, in an inversion recovery T1 weighted pulse sequence, in order to achieve the best contrast resolution and discriminate gray from white matter, mainly for interbrain structures (Fig. A1). Correlations with major structures are emphasized to assist the imaging specialist in determining the exact topography and extent of the slab in reference to the anatomic structure under investigation (Figs. A2--A19). From front to back, five major anatomical regions are defined, separated by constant anatomic cuts passing through easily identified and topometrically reliable anatomic landmarks. This coronal approach to brain anatomy is in routine use in our department.

A

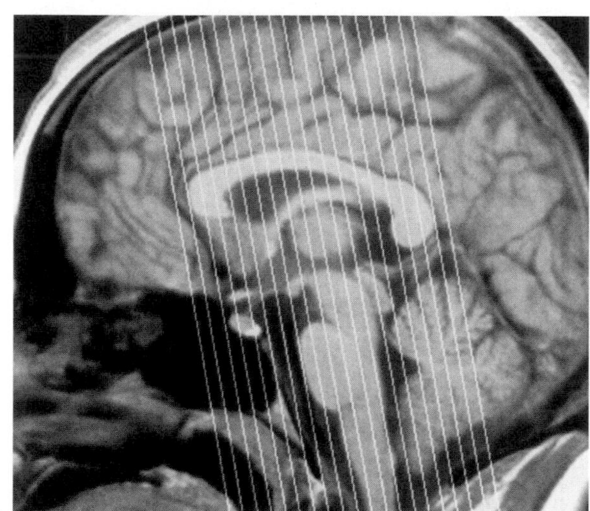

B

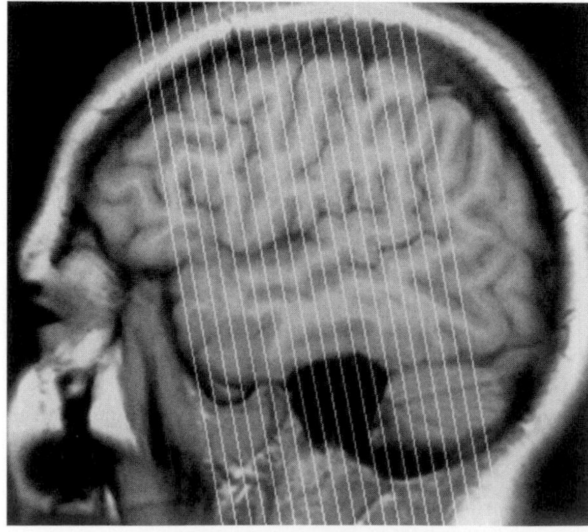

Fig. A1. Successive coronal cuts made using the commissural-obex reference line and a high field system, with 3 mm slice thickness and 1 mm gap, in an inversion recovery T1 weighted, pulse sequence

From the Genu of Corpus Callosum to the Anterior Commissure

(Figs. A2–A7)

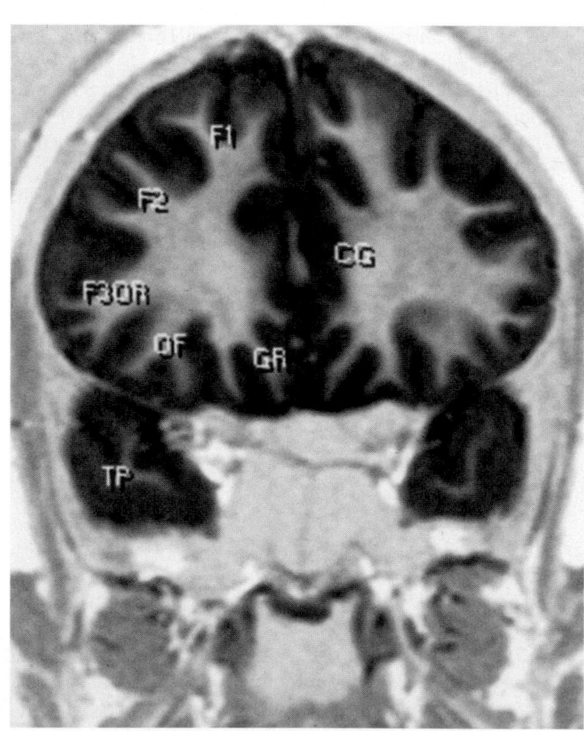

Fig. A2. Cut through the temporal poles

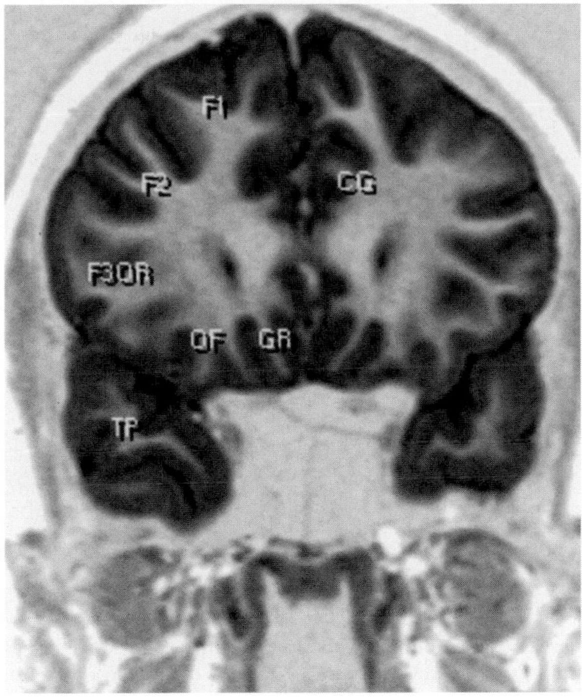

Fig. A3. Cut through the tip of the frontal horns

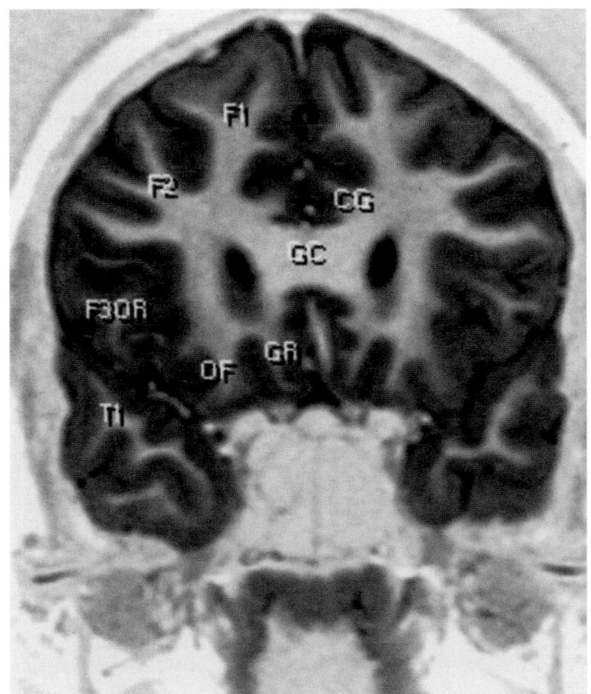

Fig. A4. Cut through the heads of the caudate nuclei

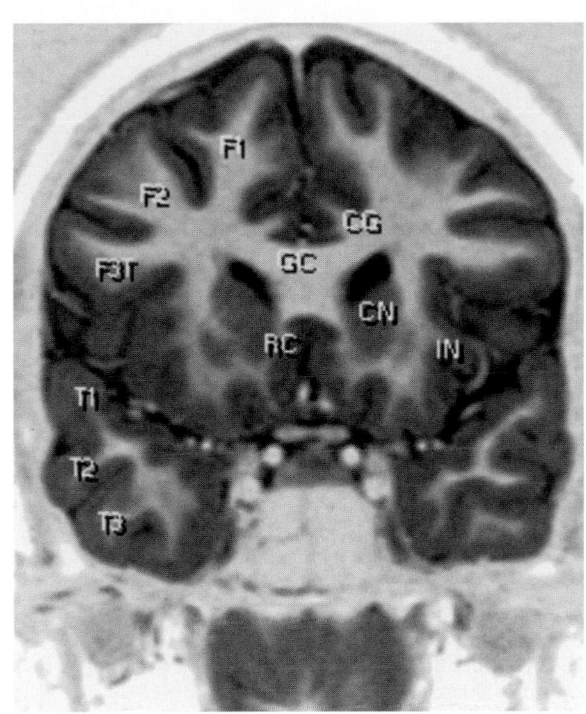

Fig. A5. Cut through the rostrum of corpus callosum

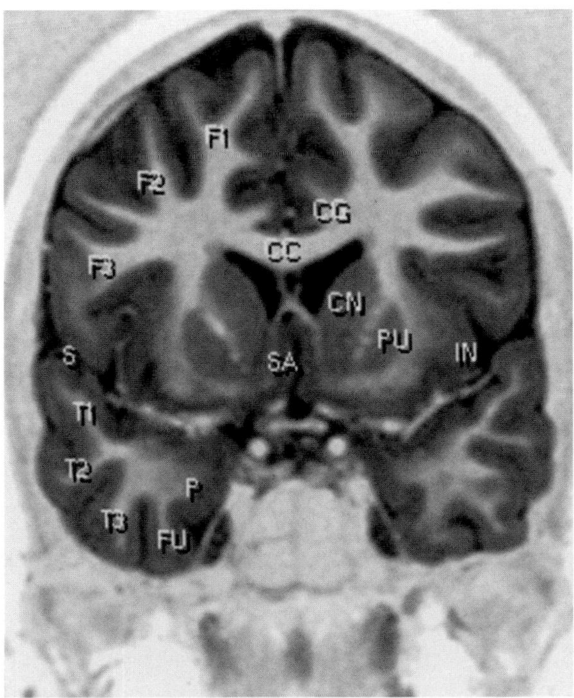

Fig. A6. Cut through the limen insulae and septal region

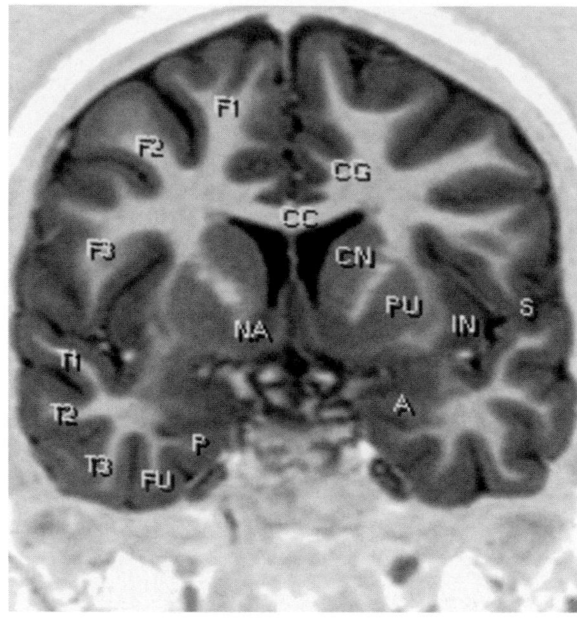

Fig. A7. Cut through the temporal stem, accumbens and amygdaloid nuclei

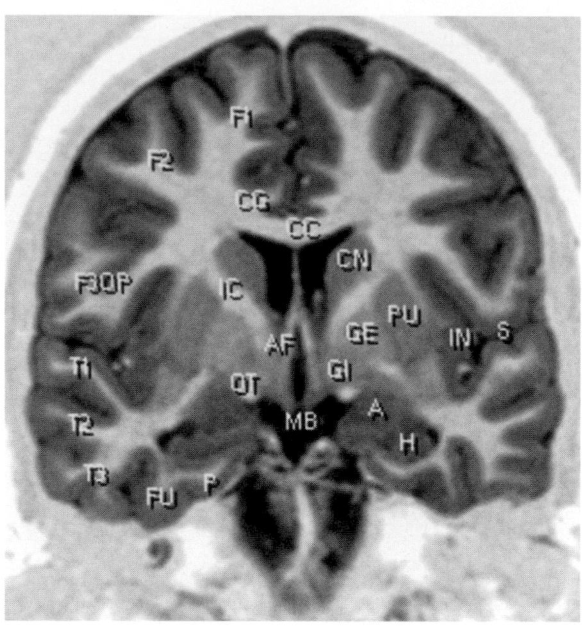

Fig. A9. Cut through the anterior columns of fornix

From the Anterior Commissure to the PC-OB Reference Plane

(Figs. A8–A13)

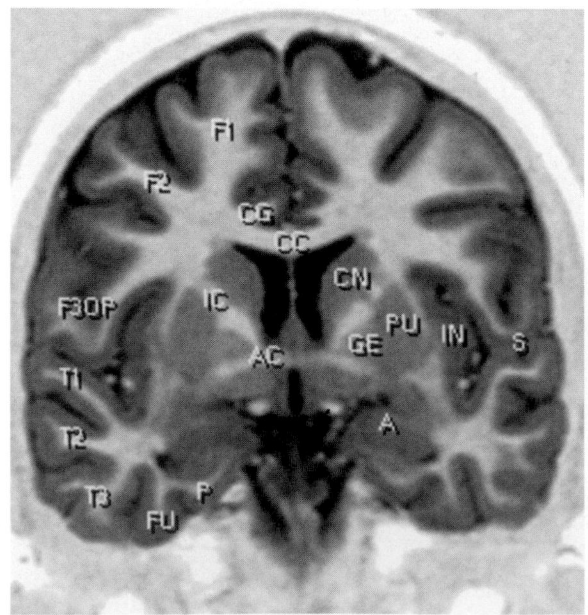

Fig. A8. Cut through the anterior commissure

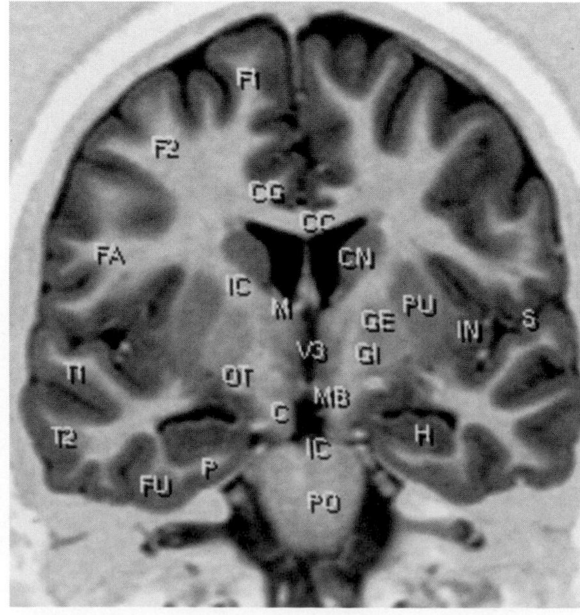

Fig. A10. Cut through the interventricular foramen and the mamillary bodies

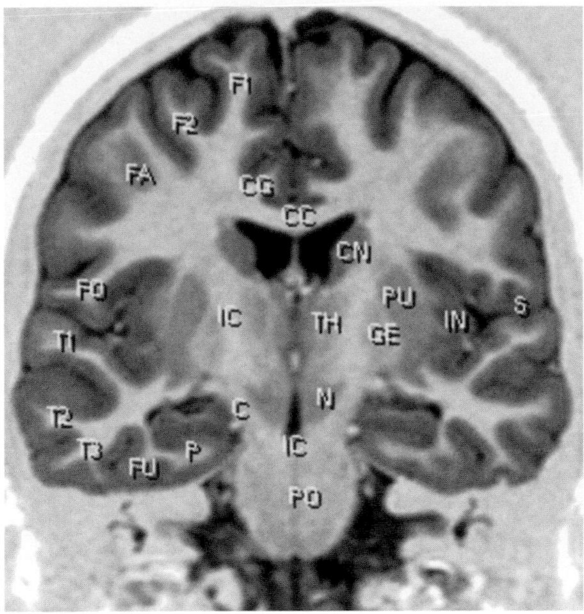

Fig. A11. Cut through the thalamus and the interpeduncular space

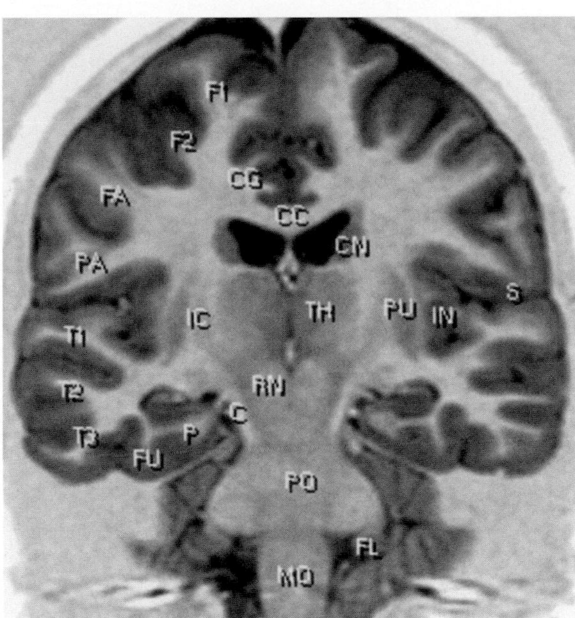

Fig. A13. Cut through the advent of the cerebellum

From the PC-OB Plane to the Splenium of Corpus Callosum

(Figs. A14–A19)

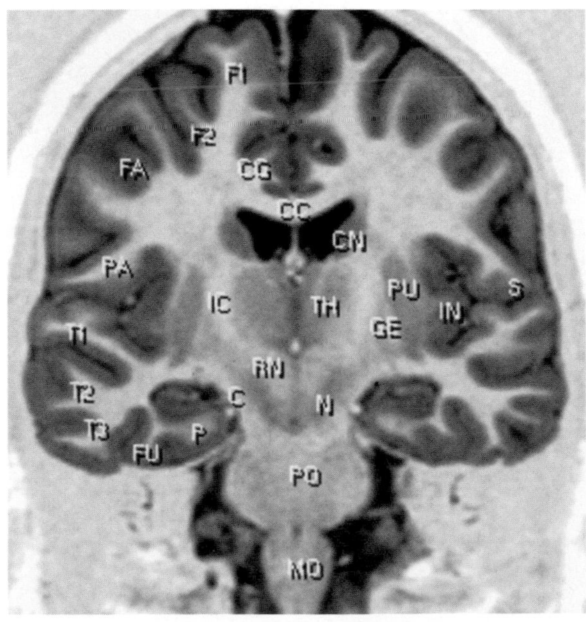

Fig. A12. Cut through the whole brainstem

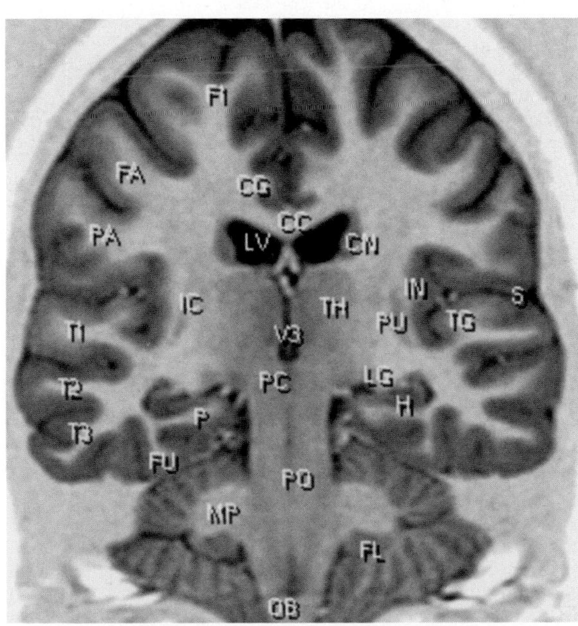

Fig. A14. Cut through PC-OB, lateral geniculate bodies and midthalamus

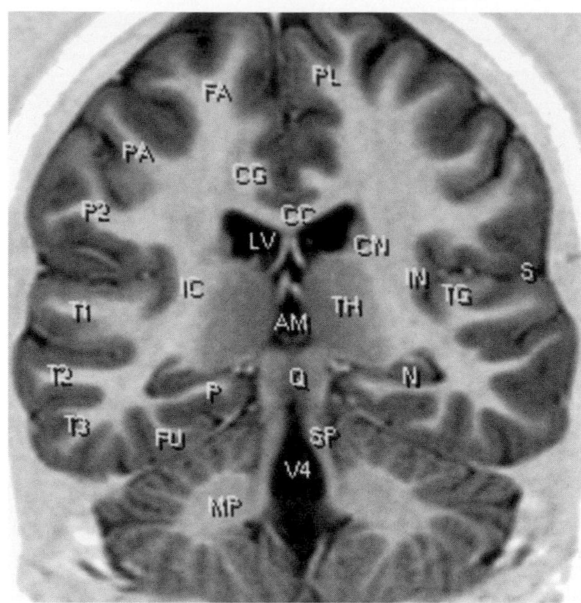

Fig. A15. Cut through the tectal plate

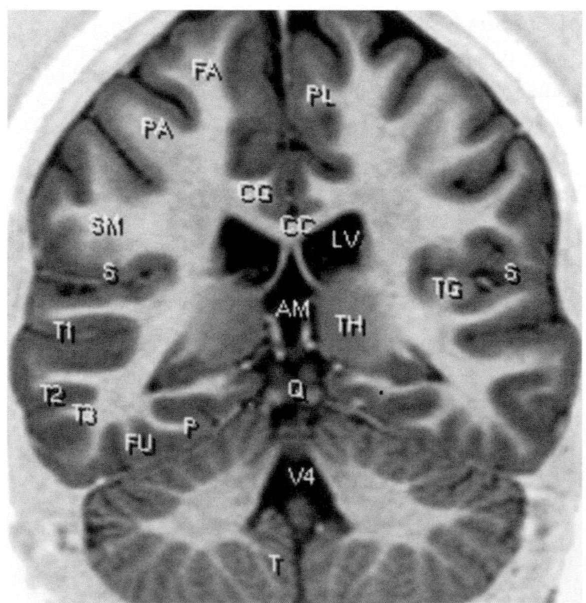

Fig. A16. Cut through the pulvinar

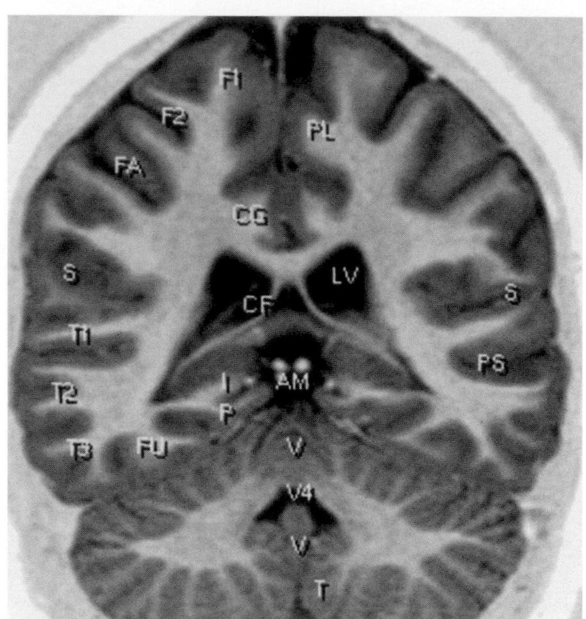

Fig. A17. Cut through the crus fornicis

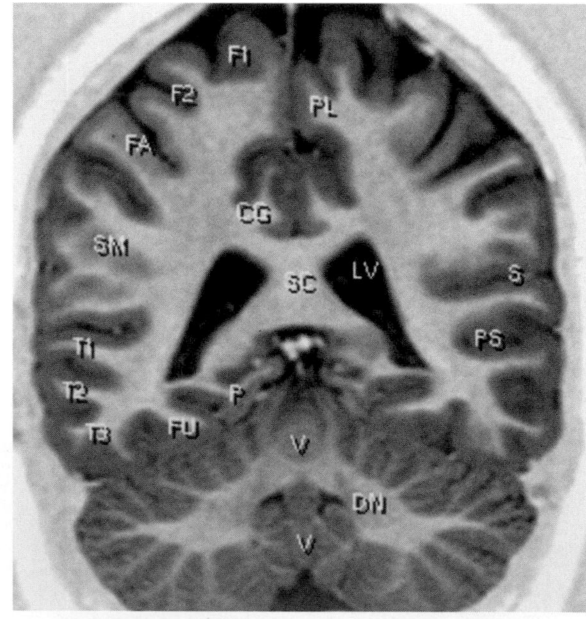

Fig. A18. Cut through the atrium of lateral ventricles

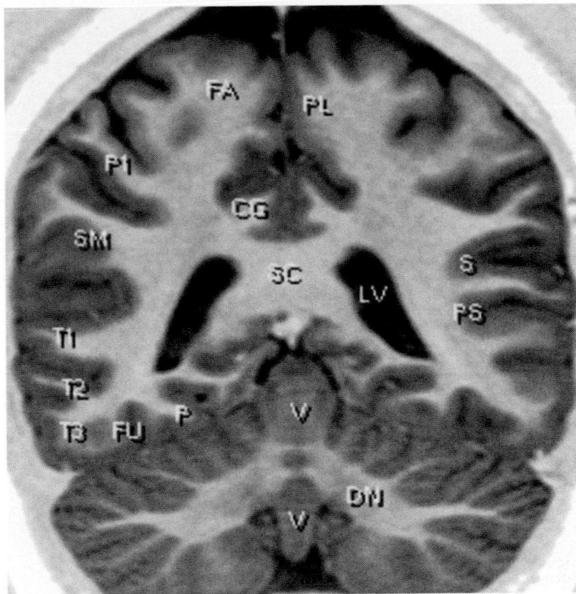

Fig. A19. Cut through the isthmus cinguli and culmen vermis

Abbreviations

A	Amygdala
AC	Anterior commissure
AF	Fornix, anterior column
AG	Angular gyrus
AN	Accumbens nucleus
C	Crus cerebri
CA	Cisterna ambiens
CC	Corpus callosum
CF	Fornix, crus
CG	Cingulate gyrus *or* Corpus callosum, genu
CN	Caudate nucleus
CR	Corpus callosum, rostrum
CS	Calcarine sulcus
D	Decussation of brachia conjunctiva
DN	Dentate nucleus of cerebellum
F1	Superior frontal gyrus
F2	Middle frontal gyrus
F3	Inferior frontal gyrus
F3Op	Inferior frontal gyrus, pars opercularis
F3Or	Inferior frontal gyrus, pars orbitalis
F3Tr	Inferior frontal gyrus, pars triangularis
FA	Precentral gyrus
FL	Flocculus
FU	Fusiform gyrus or lateral occipital gyrus
GE	Globus pallidus, lateral segment
GI	Globus pallidus, medial segment
GR	Gyrus rectus
H	Hippocampus
I	Isthmus of cingulate gyrus
IC	Internal capsule *or* Interpeduncular cistern
IN	Insula
LG	Lateral geniculate body
M	Interventricular foramen of Monro
MB	Mamillary body
MP	Middle cerebellar peduncle
OB	Obex
OF	Orbitofrontal gyri
OL	Occipital lobe
OT	Optic tract
P1	Superior parietal gyrus
PA	Postcentral gyrus
PC	Posterior commissure
PH	Parahippocampal gyrus
PL	Paracentral lobule
PO	Pons
PS	Superior temporal sulcus, parallel
PU	Putamen
Q	Tectal or quadrigeminal plate
R	Central sulcus of Rolando
RN	Red nucleus
S	Lateral fissure of Sylvius
Sa	Septal area
SC	Splenium of corpus callosum
SI	Substantia innominata
SM	Supramarginal gyrus
SN	Substantia nigra
SP	Superior cerebellar peduncle
T	Tonsil of cerebellum
T1	Superior temporal gyrus
T2	Middle temporal gyrus
T3	Inferior temporal gyrus
TG	Transverse temporal gyrus of Heschl
TH	Thalamus
TP	Temporal pole
V	Vermis of cerebellum
V3	Third ventricle
V4	Fourth ventricle

8 The Brainstem and Cerebellum

I Introduction

Magnetic resonance (MR) has dramatically improved visualization of structures of the posterior fossa. This is due to MR's high contrast resolution, direct multiplanar capabilities and absence of beam hardening artifacts of the petrous bone such as usually observed with computed tomography. The functional anatomy of the brainstem and cerebellum, necessary for accurate clinical and anatomic correlations, is reviewed in this chapter.

The structures contained in the posterior fossa are the hindbrain and the midbrain. The hindbrain comprises the pons, the medulla oblongata, and the cerebellum, the latter forming the roof of the fourth ventricle which is the cavity of the rhombencephalon. The last portion of the brainstem, the midbrain, corresponds to the upper portion connecting the pons and cerebellum with the forebrain. The relationships of the brainstem to the cerebellum posteriorly and laterally and to the diencephalon superiorly are best appreciated on midsagittal (Fig. 8.1) and coronal cuts oriented parallel to the PC-OB reference plane which limits anteriorly the fourth ventricular cavity and the mass of the cerebellar hemispheres (Fig. 8.2).

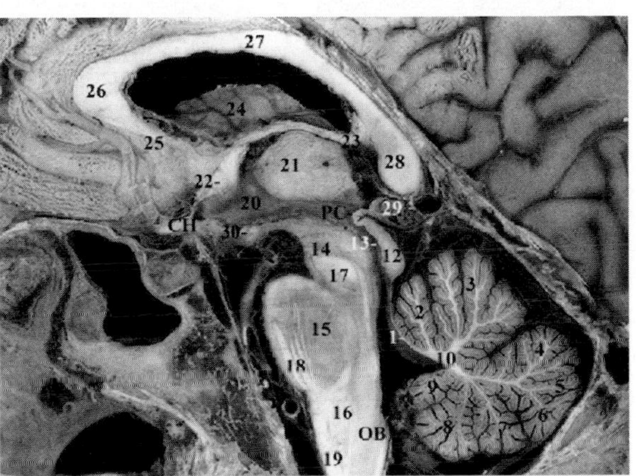

A

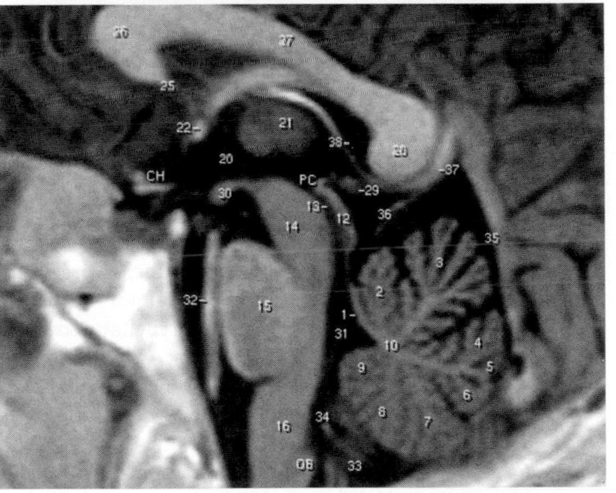

B

Fig. 8.1. A,B *1*, Lingula, vermis; *2*, central lobule, vermis; *3*, culmen, vermis; *4*, declive, vermis; *5*, folium, vermis; *6*, tuber, vermis; *7*, pyramis, vermis; *8*, uvula, vermis; *9*, nodulus, vermis; *10*, central white matter; *11*, superior medullary velum; *12*, tectal plate; *13*, cerebral aqueduct; *14*, midbrain; *15*, pons; *16*, medulla oblongata; *17*, decussation of superior cerebellar peduncles; *18*, corticospinal (pyramidal tract); *19*, pyramid (pyramidal tract); *20*, third ventricle; *21*, thalamus; *22*, anterior commissure; *23*, fornix; *24*, caudate nucleus; *25*, rostrum of corpus callosum; *26*, genu of corpus callosum; *27*, body of corpus callosum; *28*, splenium of corpus callosum; *29*, epiphysis (pineal body); *30*, mamillary bodies

II The Brainstem

The brainstem, or truncus cerebri, comprises the midbrain or mesencephalon, the pons and the medulla oblongata which is continuous below with the spinal cord. The definition of the term "brainstem" is variable and for some authors may include the diencephalon. In the following, we will exclude the diencephalon, considered as part of the deep core structures of the brain and discussed in Chap. 7.

The CH-PC plane separates the diencephalic structures from the brainstem and cerebellum and passes through the midbrain diencephalic junction. This corresponds to a supratentorial part and infratentorial posterior fossa structures. Such a distinction seems

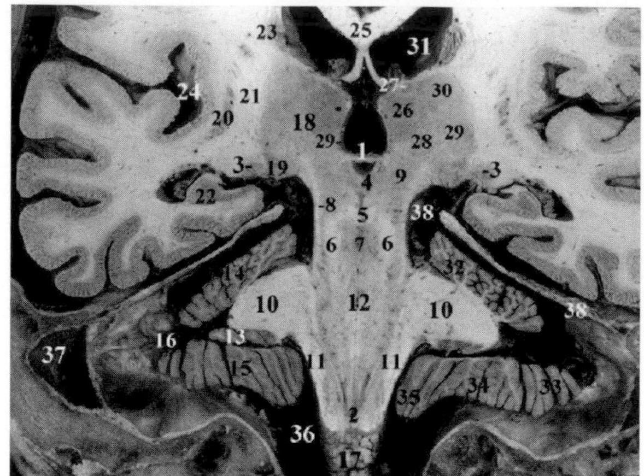

A

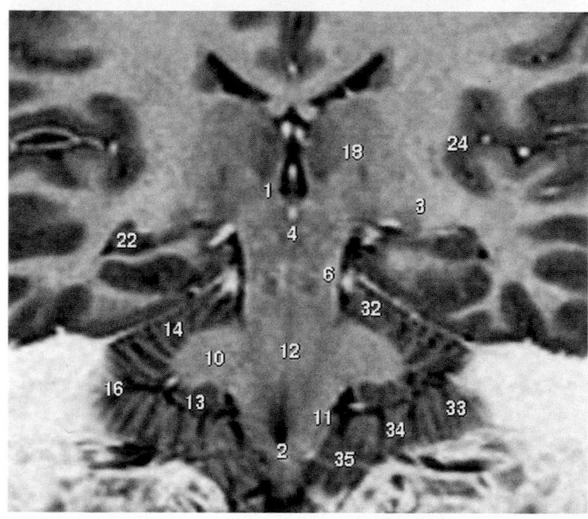

B

Fig. 8.2. A,B *1*, Posterior commissure; *2*, calamus scriptorius, inferior extremity; *3*, lateral geniculate body; *4*, cerebral aqueduct (superior aperture); *5*, decussation of brachium conjunctivum; *6*, superior cerebellar peduncle (brachium conjunctivum); *7*, midbrain tegmentum; *8*, lateral lemniscus; *9*, midbrain-thalamic region; *10*, middle cerebellar peduncle; *11*, inferior cerebellar peduncle; *12*, pontine tegmentum; *13*, flocculus and paraflocculus; *14*, superior aspect of cerebellar hemisphere; *15*, inferior aspect of cerebellar hemisphere; *16*, horizontal fissure of Vicq d'Azyr; *17*, medulla oblongata; *18*, thalamus; *19*, medial geniculate body; *20*, putamen (posterior limit); *21*, internal capsule; *22*, hippocampus; *23*, caudate nucleus; *24*, insula; *25*, corpus callosum (posterior columns of fornix beneath); *26*, dorsomedian nucleus of thalamus; *27*, lateral dorsal nucleus of thalamus; *28*, centromedian nucleus of thalamus; *29*, ventral posterior nuclei of thalamus; *30*, ventral lateral nucleus of thalamus; *31*, lateral ventricle; *32*, anterior lobe of cerebellar hemisphere; *33*, inferior semilunar lobule; *34*, biventer lobule; *35*, cerebellar tonsil; *36*, cerebellomedullary cistern; *37*, lateral (transverse) sinus; *38*, tentorium cerebelli

more practical from an imaging point of view, because axial or horizontal cuts performed perpendicular to the long axis of the brainstem contribute more to anatomic imaging correlations and structural analysis. Such cuts are best obtained parallel to the CH-PC plane (Fig. 6.13, 2.41). The coronal approach parallel to the PC-OB plane and oriented along the vertical long axis of the brainstem efficiently displays the diencephalon-brainstem continuum, corresponding morphologically to the part of the brain remaining after removal of the cerebral hemisphere and the cerebellum (Fig. 8.4), and the cerebellum posterior to the referential plane.

In the following, we will develop the gross morphology and the structural and functional anatomy of the mesencephalon, or midbrain, with special emphasis on the functional aspects of the colliculi, the mesencephalon, composed of both the pons and the cerebellum, and the myelencephalon or medulla oblongata.

A The Midbrain

The midbrain is the smallest of the three major subdivisions of the brainstem, situated between the pons caudally and the diencephalon dorsally. Its upper boundary passes through the PC dorsally and the MB ventrally, excluding the hypothalamic nuclei located in the floor of the third ventricle. This boundary is ontogenetically and phylogenetically situated at the junction between the telencephalon and the mesencephalon as obtained in the CH-PC reference plane orientation. The midbrain connects the pons and the cerebellum caudally with the diencephalon rostrally. It is the shortest segment of the brainstem, measuring 2 cm in length. Its long axis inclines ventrally from its caudal to its rostral aspect. This explains why the cuts parallel to the rhombencephalic floor of the fourth ventricle are less accurate for the study of midbrain than the coronal cuts performed parallel to the PC-OB line or the axial cuts perpendicular to the brainstem vertical axis (Tamraz et al. 1990, 1991).

The midbrain may be divided into right and left cerebral peduncles, each of which includes a ventral part, the crus cerebri, and a dorsal portion, the tegmentum, located ventral to the cerebral aqueduct and separated from the crura cerebri by the substantia nigra. The tegmentum is traversed by the cerebral aqueduct connecting the fourth ventricle to the third. Dorsal to the cerebral aqueduct is the tectum, represented by the superior and inferior colliculi

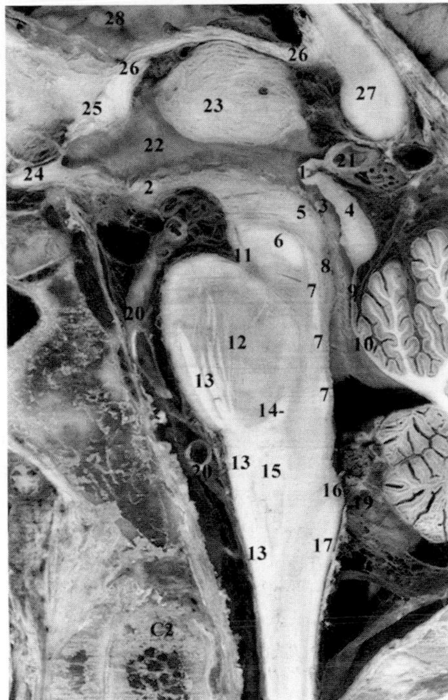

A

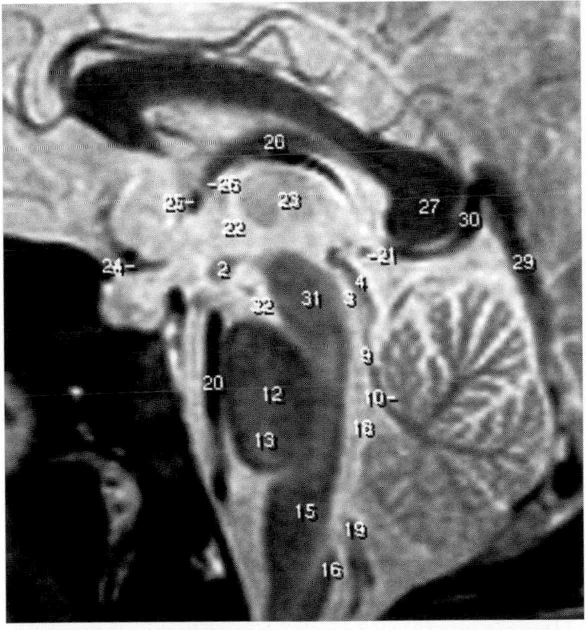

B

Fig. 8.3. A,B *1*, Posterior commissure; *2*, mamillary body; *3*, cerebral aqueduct; *4*, tectal plate; *5*, oculomotor nucleus (III); *6*, decussation of superior cerebellar peduncle; *7*, medial longitudinal fasciculus; *8*, dorsal nucleus of raphe; *9*, superior medullary velum; *10*, lingula vermis; *11*, interpeduncular nucleus; *12*, basis pontis; *13*, pyramidal corticospinal tract; *14*, trapezoid body; *15*, medial lemniscus; *16*, gracile nucleus (obex); *17*, gracile fasciculus; *18*, fourth ventricle; *19*, foramen of Magendie; *20*, basilar artery; *21*, epiphysis; *22*, third ventricle; *23*, thalamus; *24*, optic chiasm; *25*, anterior commissure; *26*, fornix; *27*, splenium of corpus callosum; *28*, caudate nucleus

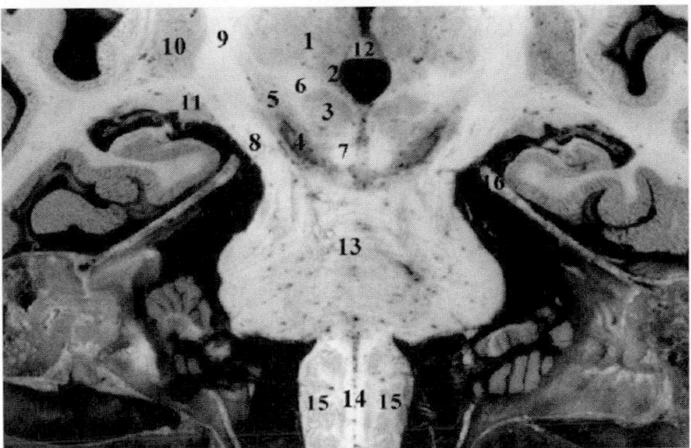

Fig. 8.4. *1*, Thalamus; *2*, hypothalamus; *3*, red nucleus; *4*, substantia nigra; *5*, subthalamic nucleus; *6*, Forel's fields; *7*, superior cerebellar peduncle (decussation); *8*, crus cerebri (cerebral peduncle); *9*, internal capsule; *10*, putamen; *11*, lateral geniculate body; *12*, interthalamic adhesion; *13*, pons; *14*, medulla oblongata; *15*, inferior olivary nuclear complex; *16*, tentorium cerebelli (upper border of foramen ovale of Pacchioni)

and consisting of four rounded elevations arranged in superior and inferior symmetrical pairs. The crura cerebri are massive bundles of white fibers constituting the ventral surface of the midbrain and emerging from the cerebral hemispheres on each side of the median plane. As they descend, they converge to meet at the entry into the pons. The peduncles form the posterior and lateral boundaries of the interpeduncular fossa, the posterior portion of which corresponds to the posterior perforated substance, through which pass the central branches of the posterior cerebral arteries. The crura cerebri consist almost entirely of descending fibers, the corticospinal tract projecting to the spinal cord, the corticopontine tracts terminating in the pontine nuclei and the corticobulbar tract projecting into specific regions of the lower brainstem and mainly to the brainstem reticular formation. From the medial surface of each crus emerge the roots of the oculomotor nerves (III cranial nerve). The ventral surface of each crus is crossed from medial to lateral by the proximal segments of the posterior cerebral and superior cerebellar arteries. Superiorly, as they emerge from the cerebral hemispheres, the crura cerebri are surrounded by the optic tracts.

Two transverse sections, the first at the level of the superior colliculus and the second at the level of the inferior colliculus, reveal the internal structures of the midbrain. The main anatomic structures found are the cerebral aqueduct, surrounded by the central gray matter (periaqueductal gray) separating the tectum, represented by the quadrigeminal plate, from the tegmentum. The latter is separated by the darkly pigmented substantia nigra from the cerebral peduncles or crura cerebri most ventrally. Particularly prominent are the red nuclei and the substantia nigra as well as the cerebral peduncles, which are also well depicted on routine MR imaging.

1 The Rostral Midbrain: Superior Collicular Level

Major structures are identified at this level: (1) the superior colliculi at the rostral part of the tectal plate, (2) the periaqueductal gray matter and the V-shaped oculomotor nuclear complex, (3) the tegmentum, occupied centrally by the red nuclei surrounded by the white fiber bundles of the superior cerebellar peduncles, (4) lateral to the red nuclei, curved white matter bundles corresponding dorsally to the spinothalamic tract and ventromedially to the medial lemniscus, (5) the substantia nigra, ventral to the tegmental region and dorsal to the crus cerebri or cerebral peduncle, (6) the cerebral peduncles, with its concavity directed towards the substantia nigra and the tegmentum, corresponding to massive white matter tracts.

The Superior Colliculi: Morphology and Functional Anatomy

The superior colliculi are large and flattened swellings constituting the rostral half of the tectal plate, primarily associated with the optic system. Unlike the inferior colliculi, they are simplified in higher vertebrates, becoming reduced in size in primates and in humans. Each colliculus consists of alternate gray and white layers. In human, the superior colliculus presents a complex laminar organization, as observed in the optic tectum of nonmammalian vertebrates. Seven variously named (Cajal 1909; Crosby et al. 1962; Carpenter 1983) laminae are described and the pattern of organization resembles that of the cerebral cortex. From the outer aspect inward are the stratum zonale, the stratum cinereum, the stratum opticum, and the stratum lemnisci, consisting of four layers.

The superficial layers of the superior colliculus receive most of the afferents from the retina and the visual cortex, concerned mainly with the detection of movement of objects in the visual field. The retinotectal fibers contained in the optic tracts project to the superior colliculus via its brachium conjunctivum before they terminate in the lateral geniculate body. This projection is topographically organized. The contralateral peripheral visual field is represented in the caudal two thirds of the superior colliculus, the rostral portion receiving the fibers concerned with central vision. The corticotectal projections, mainly from the visual cortex, are also highly organized, reaching the superior colliculus via its brachium. A correspondence exists between terminations of both retinotectal and corticotectal fibers in the superior colliculus. Other corticotectal fibers arise from the frontal lobe, and particularly the frontal eye field, from the temporal lobe, such as the auditory cortex, and from the parietal lobe. The deep layers of the superior colliculus receive afferent fibers from the spinal cord via the spinotectal tract and from the brainstem, mainly the inferior colliculus and the auditory relay nuclei.

Considering the efferent pathways arising from the superior colliculus, these may be divided into ascending tectothalamic fibers originating from the superficial layers and projecting ipsilaterally to the lateral geniculate body, the pulvinar and the pretectum. The descending fibers originating from the deep layers project to the brainstem and the spinal cord as tectoreticular, tectopontine, tectobulbar and tectospinal tracts.

The superior colliculi may be considered as reflex centers influencing the position of the head and eyes in response to external stimuli, visual, auditory or somatic (Gordon 1972; Sterling and Wickelgren 1969; Kunzle and Akert 1977). Experimental unilateral lesions of the superior colliculus in animals show no disturbance of eye movements (Sprague 1972). However, if the visual cortex in animals is removed, the superior colliculus loses its functional ability to detect movements in the visual field (Wickelgren and Sterling 1969).

2 The Caudal Midbrain: Inferior Collicular Level

This transverse section passing through the inferior colliculi at the caudal aspect of the midbrain at a level superior to the isthmus of the pons is characterized by the presence of: (1) the inferior colliculi, which present as ovoid eminences more prominent than the superior colliculi and occupy the caudal part of the quadrigeminal plate, covered by the lateral lemniscus; (2) the cerebral aqueduct and the periaqueductal central gray matter. Ventral to the gray matter and close to the midline are the nuclei of the trochlear nerves, bordered anteriorly by the fibers of the medial longitudinal fasciculi whose dorsal surfaces are somehow invaginated by these nuclei; (3) the decussation of the fibers of the superior cerebellar peduncles occupying the central portion of the central tegmentum which at this level is reduced in size compared to the rostral midbrain. Its ventrolateral border is occupied by fibers of the medial lemniscus; (4) the inferior portion of the substantia nigra, separatings the central tegmental area from the massive white fiber tracts constituting the crus cerebri.

The Inferior Colliculi: Morphology and Functional Anatomy

The inferior colliculus consists mainly of a central ovoid mass (the central nucleus) associated with a pericentral nucleus dorsally and an external nucleus laterally. The inferior colliculus is surrounded by a laminar zone of myelinated nerve fibers, most of which correspond to the lateral lemniscus and end in the central nucleus. The nuclear and neuronal organization of the inferior colliculi have been described extensively (Rockel and Jones 1973; Meininger and Baudrimont 1977).

The inferior colliculus is the major brainstem auditory relay nucleus to which auditory impulses are transmitted via the lateral lemniscus, its chief afferent pathway. Auditory information is further projected to the medial geniculate body and then to the primary auditory cortex. Most cells of the inferior colliculus respond to bineural stimulation and may encode information about sound localization. The inferior collicular nuclei show a definite tonotopic localization (Aitkin et al. 1975). Fibers from the auditory cortex project back to some of the subnuclei of the inferior colliculus.

3 The Midbrain-Diencephalic Junction

The PC is found rostral to the superior collicular level and dorsal to the periaqueductal gray matter, overhanging the superior aperture of the cerebral aqueduct. It marks the transitional zone between the midbrain and the diencephalon. The PC is the small commissure well displayed on the midsagittal cuts, constituting an important landmark used in various cephalic reference lines. At the level of the PC and rostral to the superior colliculi are found the nuclei of the pretectal area, the midbrain center involved in pupillary light reflex (Magoun and Ranson 1935A–C). In fact, the pretectal nuclei receive afferent fibers from the optic tracts, the lateral geniculate bodies and regions of the cerebral cortex. Lesions involving the PC do not impair the pupillary light reflex but reduce only the consensual pupillary light reflex.

4 The Red Nuclei and Substantia Nigra

The midbrain tegmentum covers the area situated ventral to the cerebral aqueduct and dorsal to the substantia nigra, containing the red nuclei, the mesencephalic reticular formation and the oculomotor and trochlear nuclei, as shown on the axial cuts passing through the superior (Figs. 8.5, 8.6) and inferior colliculi (Figs. 8.7, 8.8). Due to their topographical, clinical importance and accurate visibility on MR imaging, the morphological and functional aspects concerning the red nucleus and the substantia nigra will be further discussed below.

a The Red Nucleus: Morphology and Functional Anatomy

Situated dorsomedially to the substantia nigra, the red nucleus is an ovoid mass of gray matter presenting an elliptical shape, as shown on the parasagittal cuts (Figs. 8.9, 8.10), and roughly round on the transverse cuts (Figs. 8.5, 8.6) and the coronal cuts (Figs. 8.11, 8.12). This nucleus extends from the subthalamic region to the decussation of the superior cerebellar peduncle and measures around 5 mm in diameter. The red nucleus is very richly vascularized and contains iron in many of its pigmented cells. It is traversed in its upper part by fibers of the fasciculus retroflexus, well shown medially on the axial cut. Its caudal and lateral aspects are traversed by fibers of the superior cerebellar peduncle. The rootlets of the

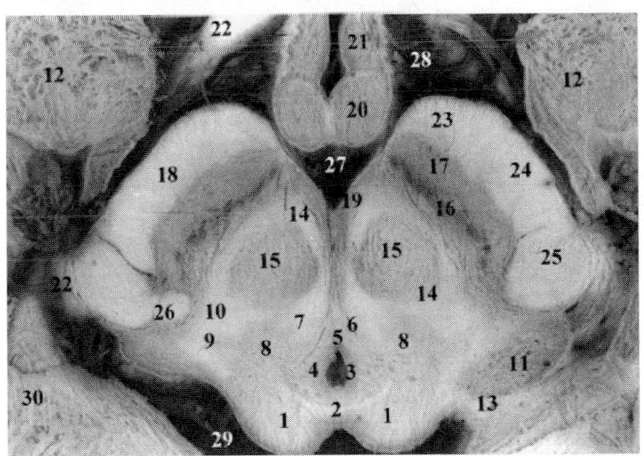

Fig. 8.5. *1*, Superior colliculus; *2*, commissure of superior colliculus; *3*, cerebral aqueduct (Sylvius); *4*, periaqueductal gray matter; *5*, oculomotor nucleus (III); *6*, medial longitudinal fasciculus; *7*, central tegmental tract; *8*, midbrain reticular formation; *9*, spinothalamic tracts; *10*, medial lemniscus; *11*, medial geniculate body; *12*, uncus (amygdala); *13*, brachium of superior colliculus; *14*, cerebellorubrothalamic tract; *15*, red nucleus; *16*, substantia nigra, pars compacta; *17*, substantia nigra, pars reticulata; *18*, crus cerebri (cerebral peduncle); *19*, ventral tegmental area; *20*, mamillary body; *21*, hypothalamus; *22*, optic tract; *23*, frontopontine tract; *24*, pyramidal tract (corticospinal and corticobulbar); *25*, occipitotemporopontine tract; *26*, pallidonigral and corticonigral tracts; *27*, interpeduncular cistern; *28*, chiasmal cistern; *29*, ambient cistern; *30*, mesial temporal region

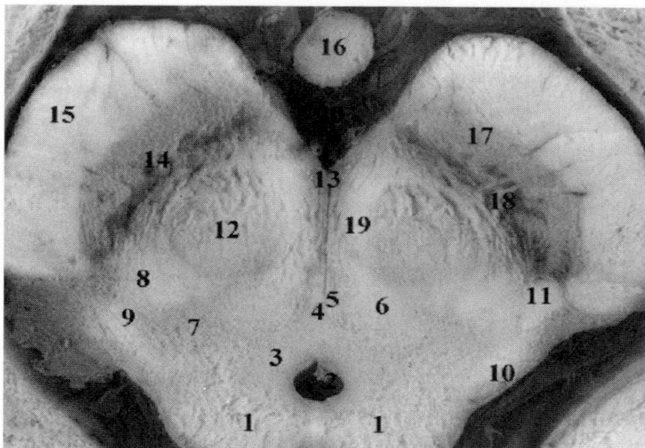

Fig. 8.6. *1*, Superior colliculus; *2*, cerebral aqueduct; *3*, periaqueductal gray matter; *4*, oculomotor nucleus (III); *5*, medial longitudinal fasciculus; *6*, central tegmental tract; *7*, midbrain reticular formation; *8*, medial lemniscus; *9*, spinothalamic tracts; *10*, brachium of inferior colliculus; *11*, pallidonigral and corticonigral tracts; *12*, red nucleus; *13*, ventral tegmental area; *14*, substantia nigra; *15*, crus cerebri (cerebral peduncle); *16*, mamillary body; *17*, substantia nigra, pars reticulata; *18*, substantia nigra, pars compacta; *19*, cerebellorubrothalamic tract; *20*, interpeduncular cistern

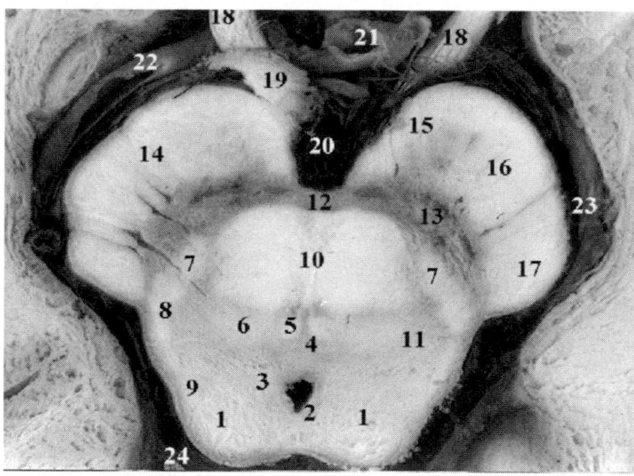

Fig. 8.7. *1*, Inferior colliculus; *2*, cerebral aqueduct; *3*, periaqueductal gray matter; *4*, trochlear nucleus; *5*, medial longitudinal fasciculus; *6*, central tegmental tract; *7*, medial lemniscus; *8*, spinothalamic tracts; *9*, lateral lemniscus; *10*, decussation of superior cerebellar peduncle (brachium conjunctivum); *11*, midbrain reticular formation; *12*, interpeduncular nucleus; *13*, substantia nigra; *14*, cerebral peduncle; *15*, frontopontine tract; *16*, pyramidal tract; *17*, occipitotemporopontine tract; *18*, oculomotor nerve; *19*, brachium pontis; *20*, interpeduncular cistern; *21*, basilar artery; *22*, posterior cerebral artery; *23*, lateromesencephalic cistern; *24*, ambient cistern

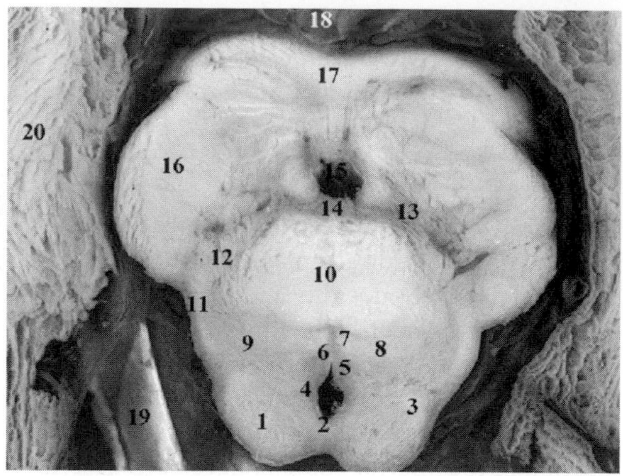

Fig. 8.8. 1, Inferior colliculus; *2*, cerebral aqueduct; *3*, lateral lemniscus; *4*, periaqueductal gray matter; *5*, dorsal tegmental nucleus; *6*, trochlear nucleus (IV); *7*, medial longitudinal fasciculus; *8*, central tegmental tract; *9*, midbrain reticular formation; *10*, decussation of superior cerebellar peduncle (brachium conjunctivum); *11*, spinothalamic tracts; *12*, medial lemniscus; *13*, substantia nigra; *14*, interpeduncular nucleus; *15*, interpeduncular fossa; *16*, crus cerebri; *17*, middle cerebellar peduncle; *18*, basilar artery; *19*, edge of tentorium cerebelli; *20*, mesial temporal region

oculomotor nerve (III) dorsoventrally traverse its central portion on their route toward the interpeduncular fossa (Fig. 8.7).

b Functional and Clinical Considerations

Functionally, the red nucleus receives afferent fibers from the deep cerebellar nuclei and the cerebral cortex. The corticorubral projections originate from the precentral and the premotor cortex and project somatotopically onto the red nucleus. Projections from the precentral motor cortex are ipsilateral and correspond somatotopically to the origin of the rubrospinal fibers. Fibers originating from the deep cerebellar nuclei decussate in the caudal midbrain before traversing and surrounding the contralateral red nucleus. Those originating in the dentate nucleus terminate in the rostral third of the contralateral red nucleus while those from the globose and emboliform nuclei terminate somatotopically in the caudal two thirds. Cells of the caudal portion give rise to the crossed rubrospinal tract, which influences flexor motor tone. Stimulation of the red nucleus in animals produces flexion of the ipsilateral limb due to the fact that both systems, the superior cerebellar peduncle as well as the rubrospinal tract, are crossed. Clinically, lesions involving the red nucleus are responsible for an ipsilateral oculomotor disturbance associated with contralateral involuntary move-

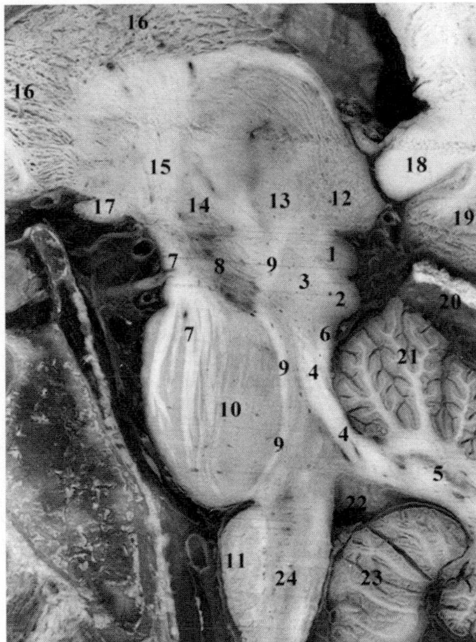

Fig. 8.9. *1*, Superior colliculus; *2*, inferior colliculus; *3*, central gray matter; *4*, superior cerebellar peduncle; *5*, dentate nucleus; *6*, red nucleus; *7*, corticospinal tract; *8*, substantia nigra; *9*, medial lemniscus; *10*, basis pontis; *11*, inferior olivary nucleus; *12*, pulvinar thalami; *13*, centromedian nucleus of thalamus; *14*, Forel's fields H; *15*, internal capsule; *16*, caudate nucleus; *17*, optic tract; *18*, cisternal optic nerve; *19*, splenium of corpus callosum; *20*, isthmus; *21*, culmen cerebelli; *22*, fourth ventricle; *23*, tonsil of cerebellum; *24*, medulla oblongata

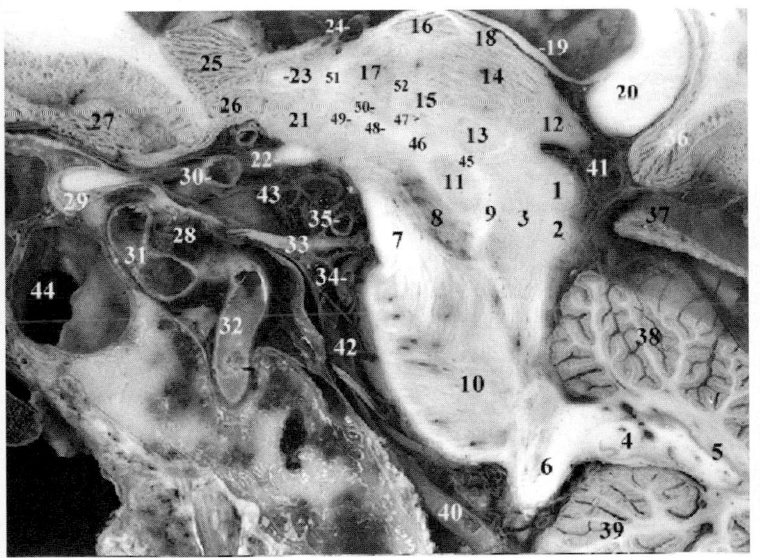

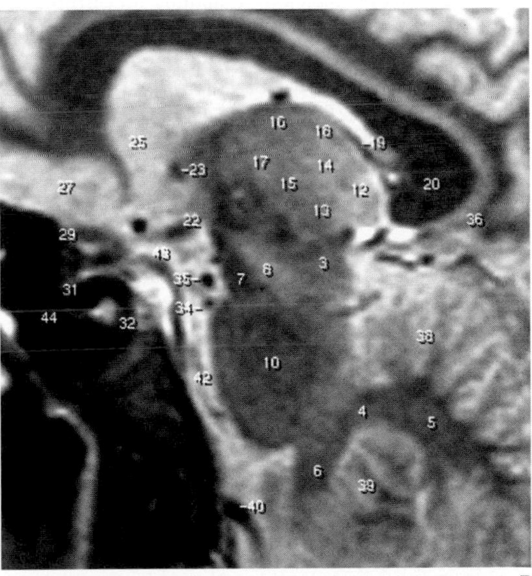

Fig. 8.10. A,B *1*, Superior colliculus; *2*, inferior colliculus; *3*, midbrain tegmentum; *4*, hilus of dentate nucleus; *5*, dentate nucleus; *6*, inferior cerebellar peduncle; *7*, cerebral peduncle; *8*, substantia nigra; *9*, cerebellothalamic tract; *10*, pons (pontine nuclei); *11*, red nucleus; *12*, pulvinar thalami; *13*, centromedian nucleus of thalamus; *14*, dorsomedial nucleus of thalamus; *15*, ventral lateral thalamic nucleus; *16*, anterior nuclear group of thalamus; *17*, ventral anterior thalamic nucleus; *18*, lateral dorsal thalamic nucleus; *19*, fornix; *20*, splenium of corpus callosum; *21*, lateral hypothalamic area; *22*, optic tract; *23*, anterior commissure; *24*, thalamostriate vein; *25*, head of caudate nucleus; *26*, area septalis; *27*, gyrus rectus; *28*, cavernous sinus; *29*, intracanalicular optic nerve; *30*, supraclinoid internal carotid artery; *31*, cavernous internal carotid artery (anterior genu); *32*, cavernous internal carotid artery (ascending segment); *33*, oculomotor nerve (III); *34*, superior cerebellar artery; *35*, posterior cerebral artery; *36*, isthmus cinguli; *37*, tentorium cerebelli; *38*, anterior lobe of cerebellum; *39*, tonsil of cerebellum; *40*, vertebral artery; *41*, ambient cistern; *42*, prepontine cistern; *43*, chiasmal cistern; *44*, sphenoid sinus; *45*, prerubral tract; *46*, Forel's field H (prerubral field); *47*, Forel's field H1 (thalamic fasciculus); *48*, Forel's field H2 (lenticular fasciculus and ansa lenticularis); *49*, ansa lenticularis; *50*, zona incerta; *51*, anterior thalamic peduncle (anterior radiations); *52*, mamillothalamic tract

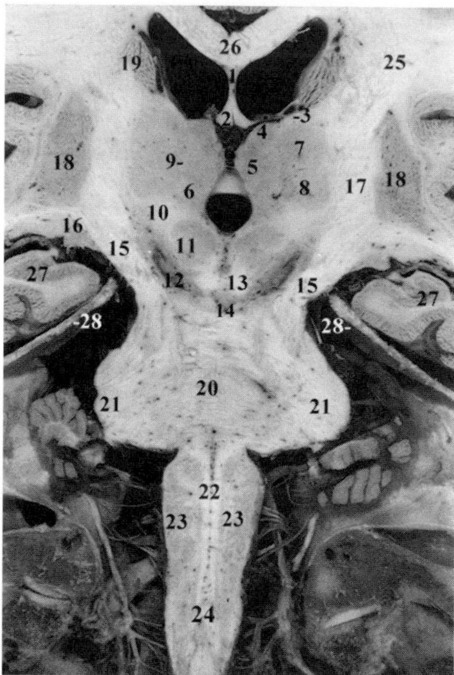

Fig. 8.11. *1*, Septum lucidum; *2*, fornix (body); *3*, thalamostriate veins; *4*, lateral dorsal nucleus of thalamus; *5*, dorsomedial nucleus of thalamus; *6*, centromedian nucleus of thalamus; *7*, ventral lateral nucleus of thalamus; *8*, ventral posterolateral nucleus of thalamus; *9*, internal medullary lamina of thalamus; *10*, Forel's fields H; *11*, red nucleus; *12*, substantia nigra; *13*, superior cerebellar peduncle (decussation); *14*, interpeduncular nucleus; *15*, cerebral peduncle (crus cerebri); *16*, lateral geniculate body; *17*, internal capsule, posterior limb; *18*, putamen; *19*, caudate nucleus; *20*, pontine nuclei; *21*, middle cerebellar peduncle; *22*, medial lemniscus; *23*, inferior olivary nuclear complex; *24*, medulla oblongata at medullary-spinal cord junction; *25*, corona radiata; *26*, corpus callosum, body; *27*, hippocampus; *28*, superior edge of tentorium cerebelli at the foramen ovale of Pacchioni

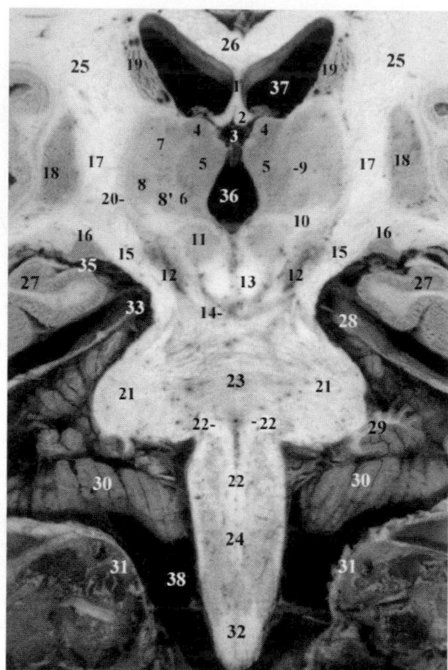

Fig. 8.12. *1*, Septum lucidum; *2*, fornix (body); *3*, internal cerebral veins (under the fornix); *4*, lateral dorsal nucleus of thalamus; *5*, dorsomedial nucleus of thalamus; *6*, centromedian nucleus of thalamus; *7*, ventral lateral nucleus of thalamus; *8*, ventral posterolateral nucleus (and ventral posteromedial); *9*, internal medullary lamina; *10*, Forel's fields H; *11*, red nucleus; *12*, substantia nigra (pars compacta corresponding to pigmented portion); *13*, superior cerebellar peduncle (decussation); *14*, oculomotor nerve (III); *15*, cerebral peduncle (crus cerebri); *16*, lateral geniculate body; *17*, internal capsule, posterior limb; *18*, putamen; *19*, caudate nucleus body; *20*, corpus callosum body; *21*, middle cerebellar peduncle; *22*, medial lemniscus; *23*, pontine nuclei; *24*, medulla oblongata; *25*, corona radiata; *26*, corpus callosum body; *27*, hippocampus; *28*, tentorium cerebelli; *29*, flocculus; *30*, cerebellar hemisphere; *31*, foramen magnum (outer border); *32*, spinal cord; *33*, foramen ovale of Pacchioni; *34*, temporal horn of the lateral ventricle; *35*, choroidal fissure; *36*, third ventricle; *37*, lateral ventricle; *38*, perimedullary cistern

ments such as ataxia, tremor or choreiform movements. This is known as the syndrome of Benedikt.

c The Substantia Nigra: Morphology and Functional Anatomy

The substantia nigra, also called the locus niger, is located in the midbrain between the crus cerebri and the tegmentum, as shown on the parasagittal (Figs. 8.10, 8.13) and coronal (Figs. 8.11, 8.12) cuts, lateral to the red nuclei and medial to the crus cerebri. It has a characteristic V-shape on MR imaging and is present in mammals, and reaches its highest level of development in primates. The substantia nigra is divided into a pars compacta, richly cellular and containing melanin pigments, and a pars reticulata, characterized by the presence of the dense striatonigral fibers. The pars compacta may also be subdivided into ventral and dorsal tiers, the former containing most of the pigmented cells. This pigmentation is maximum in humans, appearing after the fourth or fifth year of life and increasing in melanin content with age. The neurons of the pars compacta contain high concentrations of dopamine whereas the cells in the pars reticulata show the presence of GABA. Other neurotransmitters are also found in the substantia nigra.

d Functional and Clinical Considerations

The major afferents of the substantia nigra originate from the striatum as the striatonigral fibers that are topographically organized and terminate on

GABAergic neurons of the pars reticulata of the substantia nigra. Other afferents originate from the lateral segment of the globus pallidus and end in the pars reticulata as pallidonigral fibers, considered to be GABAergic, from the subthalamic nucleus constituting subthalamonigral projections to the pars reticulata and mediating a glutamate excitatory influence, and, finally, from the raphe nucleus dorsalis as the raphe nigral serotoninergic fibers. Other fiber projections end in the pars compacta of the substantia nigra, represented by the pedunculonigral fibers originating from the pedunculopontine nucleus and the corticonigral fibers originating from the prefrontal cortex.

A

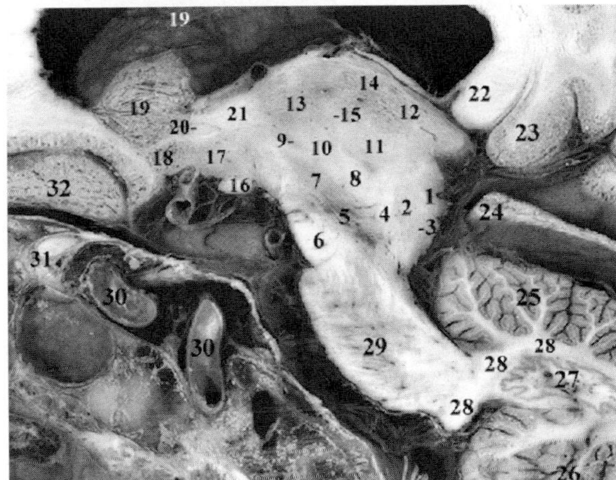

B

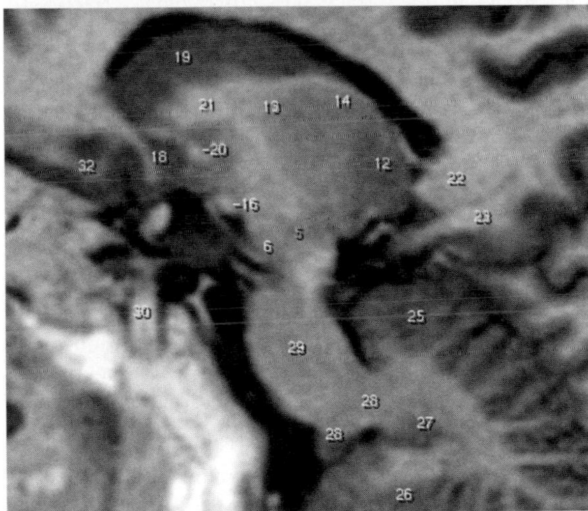

Fig. 8.13. A,B *1*, Quadrigeminal plate; *2*, central gray matter; *3*, lateral lemniscus; *4*, medial lemniscus; *5*, substantia nigra; *6*, cerebral peduncle (crus cerebri); *7*, subthalamic nucleus; *8*, thalamic fasciculus; *9*, zona incerta; *10*, Forel's fields H; *11*, centromedian nucleus of thalamus; *12*, pulvinar thalami; *13*, ventral anterior and lateral nuclei of thalamus; *14*, lateral posterior thalamic nucleus; *15*, internal medullary lamina; *16*, optic tract; *17*, globus pallidus; *18*, putamen; *19*, caudate nucleus; *20*, anterior commissure; *21*, genu of internal capsule; *22*, splenium of corpus callosum; *23*, isthmus; *24*, tentorium cerebelli; *25*, superior surface of the cerebellar hemisphere; *26*, inferior surface of cerebellar hemisphere; *27*, dentate nucleus; *28*, inferior cerebellar peduncle; *29*, pontine nuclei; *30*, intracavernous carotid artery; *31*, intracanalicular optic nerve; *32*, gyrus rectus

Efferent connections of the substantia nigra are represented by the nigrostriatal dopaminergic fibers arising from the pars compacta and projecting to the striatum, the rostral two thirds of the substantia nigra terminating in the head of the caudate nucleus and the caudal part in the putamen. A reciprocal arrangement characterizes the striatonigral and the nigrostriatal fibers constituting a closed feed-back loop. Other efferent projection systems arising from GABAergic neurons in the pars reticulata of the substantia nigra, comprising the nigrothalamic, nigrotectal and nigrotegmental fibers, constitute a major part of the output system of the basal ganglia. In primates, the nigrothalamic fibers terminate in those thalamic motor nuclei lacking input from the cerebellum or the basal ganglia. The nigrotectal fibers end in the superior colliculus and play an important role in the initiation of saccadic eye movements (Hikosaka and Wurtz 1983a–d). The nigrotegmental fibers terminate in the pedunculopontine nucleus, the latter projecting fibers back to the pars compacta of the substantia nigra, constituting a nigrotegmentonigral feed-back loop.

The importance of the substantia nigra is due to its involvement in many diseases of the basal ganglia, such as Parkinson's disease and other parkinsonian syndromes of different etiologies. Most of these diseases are characterized by involuntary movements such as tremor, dystonia, chorea, athetosis, or ballism. Other cardinal signs include akinesia and bradykinesia and disorders of muscle tone and posture. The most common of these diseases is Parkinson's disease, or paralysis agitans. The neuropathologic basis of this idiopathic disease is a massive loss of the pigmented cells in the substantia nigra and the ventral tegmental area. The nigral cell loss ranging from 50% to 90% and is associated with reactive gliosis and the presence of Lewy bodies. Degeneration of the nigral neurons is responsible for the marked decrease in dopamine concentration in the striatum, the dopaminergic depletion being more significant in the putamen than in the caudate nucleus and the nigrostriatal system being more severely affected than the mesolimbicocortical system. The decrease in striatal dopamine is directly proportional to the neuronal degeneration in the substantia nigra.

5 The Cerebral Peduncles or Crus Cerebri

The cerebral peduncles are massive white matter tracts occupying the most ventral portion of the midbrain, separated posteriorly from the tegmental area by the deeply pigmented substantia nigra. Semilunar in shape on transverse sections (Figs. 8.5–8.8), the crus cerebri consist of corticofugal fibers – mainly corticospinal, corticobulbar and corticopontine. On coronal cuts, the crus cerebri constitute the medial boundary of the lateral wings of the transverse cerebral fissure (Figs. 8.11, 8.12) encircled by the superior border of the tentorium cerebelli.

The exact topography of these corticofugal fibers in the crus cerebri differs to some extent according to different authors. Déjerine (1901) places the corticospinal and the corticobulbar fibers in the medial three fifths of the cerebral peduncle and considers that they are somatotopically arranged. Flechsig (1905) and Von Monakow (1905) concluded that these tracts occupy a smaller portion of the central segment of the cerebral peduncle. Classically, the corticospinal and corticobulbar fibers occupy the middle two thirds of the crus cerebri, that is, its extreme medial and lateral portions, containing corticopontine fibers, the frontopontine fibers located medially and the temporopontine, parietopontine and occipitopontine fibers located laterally. The corticospinal fibers are topographically arranged, the fibers concerned with the upper extremity being disposed more laterally than the most medial fibers innervating the facial musculature. The medial and lateral portions correspond each to a sixth of the crus cerebri.

B The Pons

The pons derives from the mesencephalic vesicle constituting the anterior portion of the hindbrain. It may be subdivided into a dorsal portion, the tegmentum, and a ventral portion, the pons proper, which is particularly developed in humans. As completed for the midbrain, and in order to facilitate imaging-clinical correlations, the morphological aspect and the internal architecture of the pons will be analyzed with reference to representative axial anatomical cuts, involving specifically and rostrocaudally the isthmus of the hindbrain, the midportion of the pons at the level of the trigeminal nerve roots and the caudal portion at the level of the abducens nuclei and the massive middle cerebellar peduncles.

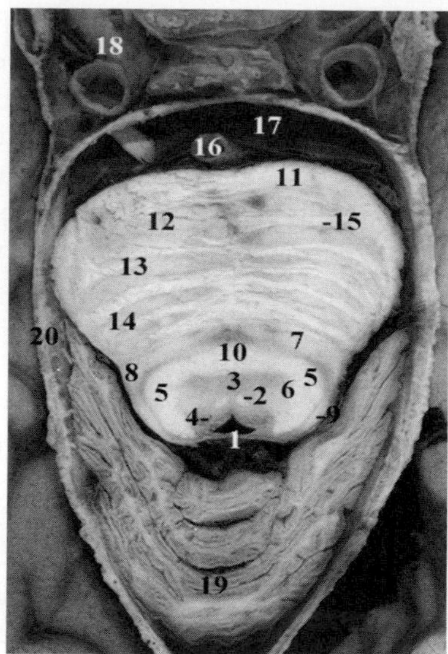

Fig. 8.14. *1*, Superior extremity of the fourth ventricle and superior medullary velum; *2*, medial longitudinal fasciculus; *3*, reticular formation; *4*, locus coeruleus; *5*, brachium conjunctivum; *6*, central tegmental tract; *7*, medial lemniscus and ventral trigeminothalamic tract; *8*, lateral and ventral spinothalamic and spinotectal tracts; *9*, lateral lemniscus; *10*, decussation of brachium conjunctivum; *11*, brachium pontis; *12*, frontopontine tract; *13*, pyramidal tract; *14*, occipitotemporopontine tract; *15*, pontocerebellar fiber bundle; *16*, basilar artery; *17*, prepontine cistern; *18*, intracavernous and internal carotid artery; *19*, culmen cerebelli; *20*, superior edge of tentorium cerebelli (delimiting foramen ovale of Pacchioni)

1 Isthmus Rhombencephali: Upper Pons Level

This transverse cut orthogonal to the brainstem long axis and passing through the upper portion of the pons is well shown at the level of the foramen ovale of Pacchioni, involving posteriorly the upper border of the superior vermis of the cerebellum, mainly the culmen (Fig. 8.14). This cut, rostral to the cerebellum and immediately caudal to the mesencephalon, is bordered laterally by the inferior medial aspects of the temporal lobes in a horizontal orientation of the cuts. As in the midbrain, this brainstem segment may be divided into a posterior or roof portion, a tegmental portion anterior to the latter and a ventral portion.

The roof of the isthmus is represented by the upper extremity of the superior medullary velum, shown as the thin membrane limiting posteriorly the most rostral portion of the fourth ventricle. Ventral to the fourth ventricle is the tegmental region, formed by the central gray matter bounded laterally by the white fibers of the superior cerebellar peduncles and shifting ventromedially in order to decussate at the inferior mesencephalic level above. The lateral border of the central gray matter contains the nucleus and tract of the trigeminal nerve. In the midline, anterior to the rostral fourth ventricle, are the medial longitudinal fasciculi on each side of the midsagittal plane, bordered anteriorly by the gray matter substance of the reticular formation. Laterally are found the central tegmental tracts. The locus coeruleus and posterolaterally the mesencephalic nucleus of the trigeminal nerve occupy the posterolateral margins of the periventricular gray matter at the lateral border of the upper fourth ventricle on each side. The locus coeruleus is also called the locus pigmentosus pontis and is easily depicted on gross specimens due to its characteristic pigmentation, which is caused by melanin-containing pigment granules. The major importance of this nucleus is due to the fact that it provides a widespread noradrenergic innervation of the entire neuraxis. Lateral to the superior cerebellar peduncle, at the external surface of the tegmentum, the lateral lemniscus is found on each side; it projects rostrally at the level of the inferior colliculus. Ventral to the anteromedial portion of the superior cerebellar peduncle is the ascending medial lemniscus, merging laterally between the medial and the lateral lemnisci, with the spinothalamic and spinotectal tracts. The fibers of the medial lemnisci also include the secondary trigeminal fibers.

It is interesting to note the characteristic disposition of the superior cerebellar peduncles lateral and ventral to the gray matter of the tegmentum, surrounded more laterally and ventrally by the major ascending sensory tracts on each side. Finally, the ventral portion of the isthmus, which is much more expanded than the tegmental portion, is constituted by the corticospinal and corticopontine tracts surrounded by the pontine nuclei. These are separated by the transverse pontine fiber bundles which join the middle cerebellar peduncle or brachium pontis laterally and inferiorly.

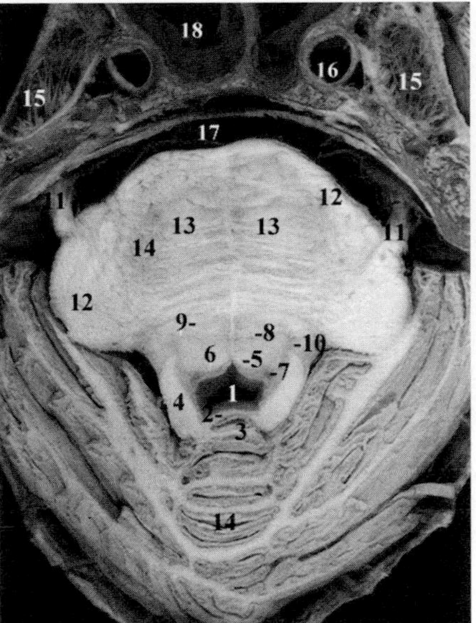

Fig. 8.15. *1*, Fourth ventricle; *2*, superior (anterior) medullary velum; *3*, lingula of cerebellum; *4*, superior cerebellar peduncle; *5*, medial longitudinal fasciculus and tectospinal tracts anteriorly; *6*, pontine (oral) reticular formation; *7*, locus coeruleus; *8*, central tegmental tract; *9*, medial lemniscus; *10*, trigeminal main sensory and motor nuclei; *11*, trigeminal nerve root; *12*, middle cerebellar peduncle (brachium pontis); *13*, pyramidal tract (corticospinal and corticobulbar); *14*, pontine nuclei and culmen cerebelli (posteriorly); *15*, trigeminal (Meckel) cave; *16*, internal carotid artery (carotid canal); *17*, prepontine cistern; *18*, sphenoid sinus

2 The Pons at the Level of the Trigeminal Nerve Root

At this level, the fourth ventricle is wider, with its roof formed by the superior medullary velum covered posteriorly by the upper vermis (Fig. 8.15). Its lateral walls are formed by the superior cerebellar peduncles. The pontine tegmentum is reduced as compared to the large ventral portion, which appears even larger than at the upper or lower levels. The medial longitudinal fasciculi are still visible beneath the floor of the fourth ventricle in their paramedian position. The central part of the pontine tegmentum is formed by the pontine reticular formation. Fibers composing the central tegmental tract are situated dorsal to the external part of the medial lemniscus. In the more ventral part of the tegmentum, immediately dorsal to the basilar portion of the pons, are the medial lemnisci, which appear flattened into two fiber bundles cut transversely. The spinothalamic tracts are situated lateral to the medial lemnisci. Anteriorly, the ventral portion of the pons shows transverse and longitudinal fibers bundles. The corticospinal and corticopontine tracts are more or less arranged in compact bundles in the anterior half of this ventral portion of the pons. At the lateral aspects of the pons, dorsolateral to the entry zone of the trigeminal roots, the upper aspect of the middle cerebellar peduncles is shown.

3 The Pons at the Level of the Advent of the Cerebellum

This axial cut, situated at the advent of the cerebellum, passes through the caudal pons, showing later-

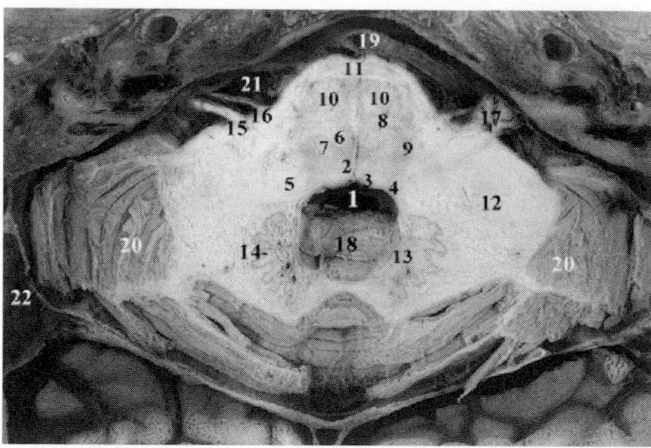

Fig. 8.16. *1*, Fourth ventricle; *2*, medial longitudinal fasciculus; *3*, nucleus prepositus hypoglossi; *4*, vestibular nuclei; *5*, restiform body (inferior cerebellar peduncle); *6*, medial lemniscus; *7*, central tegmental tract; *8*, trapezoid body; *9*, facial nucleus and dorsally the spinal trigeminal nucleus; *10*, pyramidal tract; *11*, transverse pontine bundles; *12*, brachium pontis (middle cerebellar peduncle); *13*, brachium conjunctivum (superior cerebellar peduncle); *14*, dentate nucleus; *15*, vestibular nerve; *16*, facial nerve; *17*, flocculus; *18*, nodulus; *19*, basilar artery; *20*, cerebellar hemisphere; *21*, cerebellopontine angle; *22*, transverse sinus; *23*, tonsil of cerebellum; *24*, cochlea; *25*, semicircular canals; *26*, internal auditory canal; *27*, cochlear nerve; *28*, inferior vestibular nerve; *29*, middle cerebellar peduncle; *30*, pons.

ally the massive middle cerebellar peduncles (Fig. 8.16). The cavity of the fourth ventricle is enlarged at this level as compared to the upper level, the nodule of the inferior vermis occupying its roof, bordered laterally in the cerebellar white matter by the dentate nuclei. The ventral portion shows anteriorly the massive bundles of the corticofugal, corticospinal, and corticobulbar fibers and, in the anterior portion, the transverse pontine fibers which contribute to form the middle cerebellar peduncles. Posterior to the longitudinal corticospinal tracts are the crossing fibers bundles of the trapezoid body, traversing horizontally the ventral portion of the medial lemnisci which occupy a paramedian topography. Laterally are found the lateral and ventral spinothalamic tracts and dorsolaterally the central tegmental tracts. Dorsolateral to the latter is a nuclear mass corresponding at least partly to the facial motor nucleus. The reticular formation occupying the pontine tegmentum is mainly represented by the nucleus reticularis pontis caudalis, which posterolateral to the medial lemniscus contains the large bundle representing the central tegmental tract. This tract consists mainly of descending fibers from the mesencephalic nuclei which project to the inferior olivary complex in the medulla and ascending fibers originating from the lower brainstem reticular formation projecting to the thalamus. Most anteriorly and laterally in the cerebellopontine cisterns emerge the root fibers of the cochleovestibular and facial nerves. Note the proximity of the flocculus.

C The Medulla Oblongata

This section passes through the inferior part of the floor of the fourth ventricle. The medulla oblongata is cut in its full development showing in the periventricular gray matter, from the midline to the dorsolateral aspect on each side, the medial longitudinal fasciculus, the vestibular nuclei, and laterally the bulky inferior cerebellar peduncle. Anterior to the restiform body on the midlateral aspect of the medulla, the most characteristic structure of the cut is represented by the large inferior olivary nuclear complex, which is a convoluted band of gray matter appearing as a folded bag with a hilus opening medially. Anterior to this olivary nucleus and its surrounding myelinated fibers forming the amiculum are found anteromedially the pyramids, containing the corticospinal or pyramidal descending tract. Dorsal to the pyramids are the medial lemnisci, occupying the paramedian areas on each side of the median raphe, medial to the inferior olivary nuclei. Immediately dorsolateral to the inferior olive on the lateral aspect of the medulla are situated the anterior and lateral spinothalamic tracts, which are separated from the medial lemnisci (Figs. 8.17, 8.18).

The central gray matter spreads out over the floor of the fourth ventricle cutting and containing ventrolaterally the hypoglossal nucleus, the dorsal nucleus of the vagus and the nucleus of the tractus solitarius. At the mid-olivary level, the medullary reticular formation occupies the area ventral to the periventricular gray matter and dorsal to the inferior olivary complex. The central region at mid-olivary level is mainly represented by the gigantocellular reticular nucleus, in the area medial and dorsal to the inferior olive. The medulla is surrounded anteriorly and laterally by the perimedullary cistern, containing anteriorly the vertebral arteries and laterally, in the cerebellobulbar cistern, the glossopharyngeal nerve, which emerges from the posterolateral sulcus dorsal to the olive and courses caudally to leave the posterior cranial fossa through the jugular foramen.

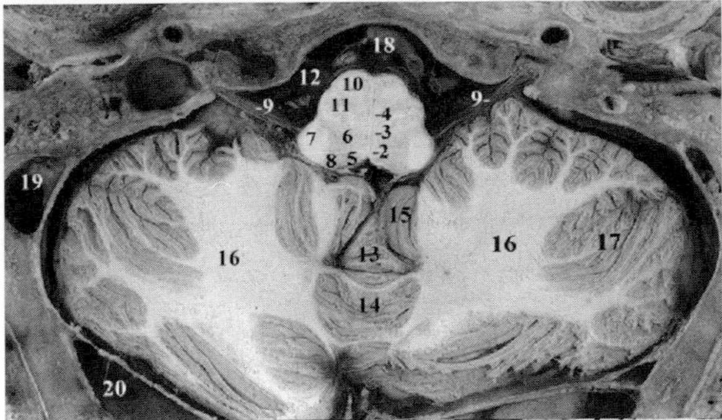

Fig. 8.17. *1*, Inferior portion of the fourth ventricle; *2*, medial longitudinal fasciculus; *3*, tectospinal tract; *4*, medial lemniscus; *5*, hypoglossal nucleus; *6*, bulbar reticular formation (nucleus gigantocellularis); *7*, restiform body (inferior cerebellar peduncle); *8*, vestibular nuclei; *9*, glossopharyngeal nerve (IX); *10*, pyramid (pyramidal tract); *11*, inferior olivary nucleus and amiculum; *12*, cerebellobulbar cistern; *13*, urula vermis; *14*, pyramis vermis; *15*, tonsil of cerebellum; *16*, album cerebelli; *17*, cortex of cerebellar hemisphere; *18*, vertebral artery; *19*, sigmoid sinus; *20*, lateral or transverse sinus

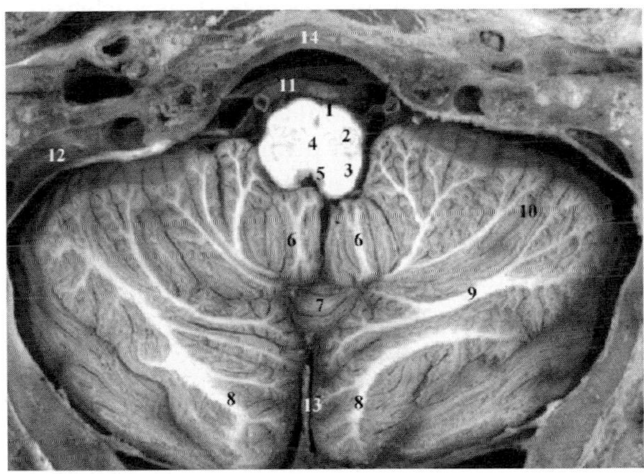

Fig. 8.18. *1*, Pyramid of the medulla oblongata; *2*, inferior olivary nucleus and accessory nuclei; *3*, inferior cerebellar peduncle; *4*, medial lemniscus; *5*, hypoglossal nucleus; *6*, tonsil cerebelli; *7*, pyramis, vermis; *8*, inferior semilunar lobule; *9*, lamina alba cerebelli; *10*, cerebellar cortex (inferior aspect of cerebellar hemisphere); *11*, vertebral artery; *12*, sigmoid sinus; *13*, cerebellar falx; *14*, clivus

D The Brainstem Reticular Formation

The reticular formation is a phylogenetically old portion of the brain, occupying the central region of the brainstem throughout most of its extent and consisting of intermingled gray and white matter. The term reticular formation refers to the fact that the cytoarchitecture of this region is composed of loosely arranged cells and diffusely organized related fibers arranged in a complex network. The reticular formation of the brainstem is continuous rostrally with the intralaminar nuclear group of the thalamus and some of the subthalamic region, and caudally with the intermediate gray matter of the spinal cord. In the brainstem, the reticular formation is bound by the long ascending and descending tracts as well as the nuclei of the origin of the cranial nerves, occupying a large area of the brainstem tegmentum. The reticular formation plays an important role in the regulation of autonomic functions, muscle reflexes, pain sensation, and behavioral arousal.

1 Morphology and Topographical Anatomy

The reticular formation of the brainstem may be divided into three longitudinal zones (Nieuwenhuys et al. 1988): (1) the median zone corresponding to the raphe nuclei, (2) the medial zone in which large cells are found, (3) the lateral parvocellular zone. These longitudinal zones show distinctive cytoarchitectural organization as well as fiber connections (Brodal 1957, 1981; Martin et al 1990; Olszewsky and Baxter 1954). In addition, the longitudinal subdivisions are not independent entities, but are largely interconnected. In fact, almost all neurons of the reticular formation project axonal fibers in both rostral and caudal directions with collaterals oriented in all directions. Many of these establish connections with the cranial nerve nuclei (Ramon-Moliner and Nauta 1966). It is often impossible, in fact, to define anatomically definite conduction paths in the reticular formation due to the diffused patterns of connections. Physiological data indicate that the impulses are conducted through polysynaptic systems. The reticular nuclei are often very poorly delineated, consisting mainly of groups of aggregated neurons embedded in complex fiber networks, even if obvious architectonic differences exist between some areas of the reticular formation. It is not surprising that within this structure MR imaging does not even separate any of the more aggregated subnuclei. Thus, currently, only topographical data may help in localizing some of the major nuclear formations described below.

2 Functional and Clinical Considerations

a The Raphe Nuclei or Median Zone

The median zone contains the raphe nuclei, which include the dorsal raphe nucleus in the midbrain, the superior central nucleus, the pontine raphe nucleus, and the nucleus raphes magnus in the pons, and the nuclei raphes obscurus and raphes pallidus in the medulla oblongata. Topographically, the large dorsal raphe nucleus is located in and ventral to the periaqueductal gray matter. The nucleus raphes magnus is located in the caudal pons. The pontine raphe nucleus is located between the nucleus raphe magnus and the central superior nucleus, which is situated in the rostral pontomesencephalic tegmentum. The nucleus raphes pallidus is found in the ventral medulla oblongata, and the nucleus raphes obscurus is found more dorsally to the latter at the same level. Histofluorescence and immunohistochemical techniques have shown that many cell groups lying in this median zone are serotoninergic neurons expressing indolamine serotonin. Other neurons display immunoreactivity through neuropeptides and amino acids. The fibers originating from serotoninergic neurons in the brainstem are extensively distributed to almost the entire central nervous system.

b The Medial Reticular Zone

The medial reticular zone includes: in the midbrain, the mesencephalic cuneiform and subcuneiform nuclei, in the pons the nuclei reticulares pontis caudalis and oralis and the reticulotegmental nucleus, and in the medulla, at mid-olivary levels, the gigantocellular reticular nucleus. The latter is situated medial and dorsal to the rostral half of the inferior olivary nuclear complex, containing characteristically large cells and extending rostrally to the medullary pontine junction. Descending fibers from the gigantocellular reticular nucleus constitute the medullary reticulospinal tract. The reticular nuclei pontis caudalis and oralis constitute the major portion of the pontine reticular formation, the nucleus reticularis pontis oralis extending rostrally into the caudal midbrain. Uncrossed reticulospinal fibers arise from cells of the pontine reticular formation. These ascend in the central tegmental tract, projecting to intralaminar thalamic nuclei and influencing the electrical activity of the cerebral cortex. The reticulotegmental nucleus, located dorsal to the medial lemniscus, constitutes a nuclear relay in the corticocerebellar motor circuits. The midbrain cuneiform and subcuneiform nuclei are situated ventral to the tectum, the former extending throughout the rostrocaudal extent of the mesencephalon. The nucleus subcuneiformis is ventral to the latter. The connections of the medial zone, largely confined to the reticular formation even though some of the projections ascend to the diencephalon or descend to the spinal cord, suggest that it is linked to both the motor and sensory pathways.

c The Lateral Reticular Zone

The lateral reticular formation is limited to the pons and the medulla oblongata. This lateral group includes the pedunculopontine nucleus, the medial and the lateral parabrachial nuclei in the pons, and the lateral reticular nucleus in the medulla. The pedunculopontine nucleus is found in the lateral tegmentum, ventral to the inferior colliculus. At the pontine level, surrounding the medial and lateral regions of the superior cerebellar peduncle, are found the medial and lateral parabrachial nuclei. The medial nucleus receives inputs from the gustatory nucleus of the nucleus solitarius, and the lateral nucleus receives general visceral afferents from the caudal portion of the nucleus solitarius. These nuclei project efferents to the hypothalamus and the amygdaloid body. The cellular population of the parabrachial nuclei contain a great variety of neuromodulators. The lateral reticular nucleus of the medulla occupies the anterolateral region of the medulla, beginning caudal to the inferior olive and extending to the mid-olivary level. This nucleus is a cerebellar relay nucleus receiving afferents from the spinal cord as the spinoreticular tract, collaterals from the spinothalamic tracts and projecting fibers via the inferior cerebellar peduncle that end bilaterally in the anterior lobe as mossy fibers. The lateral pontine reticular formation, constituting the enlarged rostral portion of the lateral reticular zone, is primarily involved in the regulation of cardiovascular, respiratory and gastrointestinal activities.

E Vascular Supply to the Brainstem

According to Duvernoy (1978), the midbrain, pons and medulla receive their blood supply from anteromedial, anterolateral, lateral, and dorsal arteries.

1 At the Midbrain Level

At the midbrain level, the anteromedial or paramedian arteries give rise to medial pedicles which vascularize the red nucleus, the periaqueductal gray matter, and the oculomotor and trochlear nuclei. The lateral pedicles supply the medial lemniscus, the medial portion of the substantia nigra, and the decussation of the superior cerebellar peduncles. The anterolateral arteries, also called the short circumferential arteries, arise from different vessels and vascularize the cerebral peduncle, the substantia nigra, and the medial lemniscus. These peduncular branches arise from the posterior cerebral artery, the posterior communicating artery, the superior cerebellar artery, and the anterior and posterior choroidal arteries (Zeal and Rhoton 1978; Duvernoy 1978). The lateral arteries vascularize the lateral tegmentum including the lateral lemniscus, the reticular formation, and the central tegmental tract. They are represented by the superior cerebellar artery, the collicular artery, and the medial posterior choroidal artery, all of which perforate the midbrain at the level of the mesencephalic sulcus. The posterior arteries are branches of the superior cerebellar artery and the collicular artery, which penetrates the tectal region to supply the superior and inferior colliculi and the periaqueductal gray matter (Fig. 8.19).

2 At the Pontine Level

The anteromedial or paramedian arteries are branches of the basilar artery and the adjacent segment of the vertebral artery which supply the paramedian region of the tegmentum, including the pyramidal tract, the medial lemniscus, the reticular formation, the medial longitudinal fasciculus, and the abducens nucleus. The lateral pontine region is vascularized by arterial perforators originating from the superior cerebellar artery supplying the rostrolateral portion of the pons, mainly the superior cerebellar peduncle, the central tegmental tract and pontine reticular formation, the lateral lemniscus, and the locus coeruleus. The caudal and lateral portion of the pons is supplied by the anterior inferior cerebellar artery, which vascularizes the facial nucleus, the middle cerebellar peduncle, the principal sensory nucleus of the trigeminal nerve, the abducens nucleus, the lateral lemniscus, and the superior olivary nucleus. The long pontine arteries supply the pontine nuclei, the lateral lemniscus, the central tegmental tract, and the lateral portion of the pyramidal tract. The terminal segment of the superior cerebellar artery supplies the superior cerebellar peduncle, the locus coeruleus, and the mesencephalic trigeminal nucleus (Fig. 8.20).

3 At the Medullary Level

The anteromedial, or paramedian medullary, arteries arise from the vertebral artery and the anterior spinal artery and supply the pyramid and the medial lemniscus, as well as the medial portion of the inferior olive and the central reticular formation. The anterolateral arteries also supply the inferior olive and the pyramidal tract. The lateral pedicles arise from the posterior inferior cerebellar artery, the anterior inferior cerebellar artery, and the basilar and vertebral arteries. Branches from these arteries vascularize the inferior olive and lateral medullary fossa, comprising the inferior cerebellar peduncle, the spinothalamic and spinocerebellar tracts, the dorsal motor nucleus of the vagus, the nucleus and tractus solitarius, the spinal trigeminal nucleus, the vestibular nuclei, and the ambiguous nucleus. The posterior inferior cerebellar artery vascularizes the posterior medullary region including the cuneate and gracile nuclei and the vagal, vestibular and solitary nuclei (Fig. 8.21).

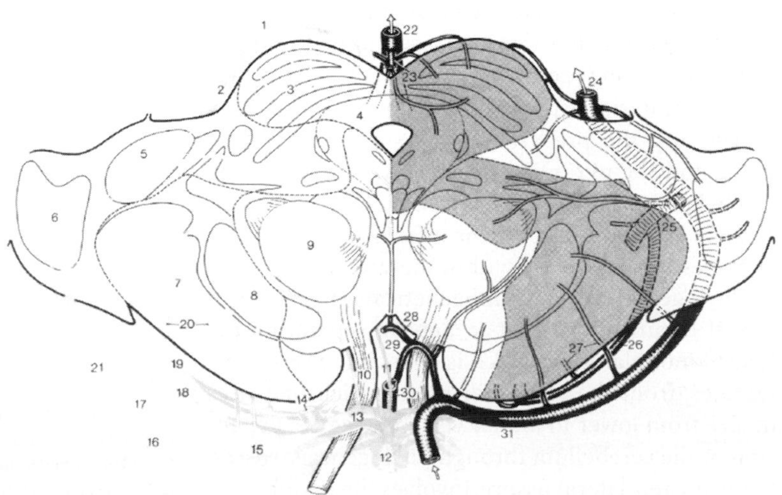

Fig. 8.19. Vascular supply to the brainstem: midbrain level. Vascular territories (arterial on the *right* and venous on the *left*). (According to Duvernoy 1978)

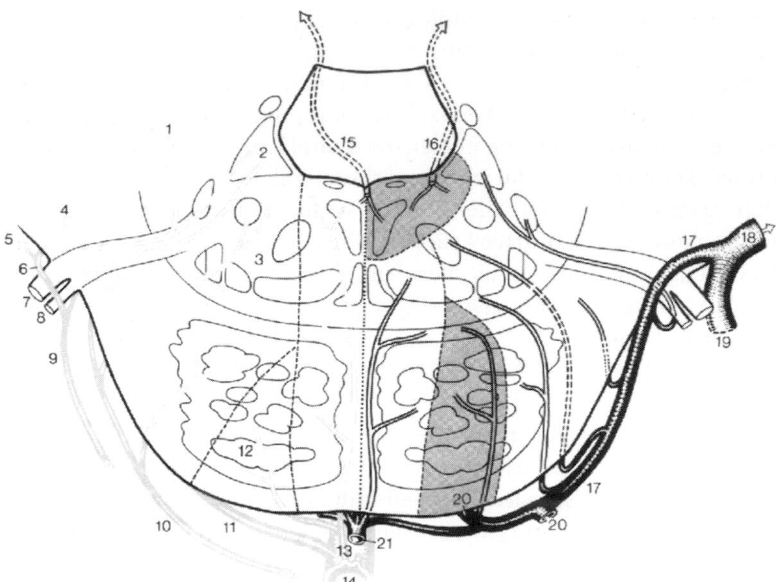

Fig. 8.20. Vascular supply to the brainstem: pontine level. Vascular territories (arterial on the *right* and venous on the *left*). (According to Duvernoy 1978)

II The Cerebellum

A Developmental Anatomy and Phylogenesis

In order to better understand cerebellar functioning, some developmental and comparative data are required. The cerebellar rudiment develops from the cranial portion of the rhombencephalic vesicle as early as the beginning of the third month. The rudiment consists of a bilobar mass corresponding to the cerebellar hemispheres and separated by a median region which will form the vermis. The first fissure to appear is the posterolateral, separating the caudal portion of the mass from the cerebellar rudiment and demarcating the flocculonodular lobe. At the end of the third month, the primary fissure appears and deepens to separate the most cranial portion of the rostral cerebellar slope corresponding to the anterior lobe. At the same time, two other fissures deepen on the inferior aspect of the vermis, the secondary fissure and the prepyramidal fissure, limiting the uvula and the pyramid respectively. Meanwhile the cerebellar mass, especially the cerebellar hemispheres, develops to cover the inferior vermis, which becomes buried deeply within the vallecula.

Phylogenetically and ontogenetically, the posterolateral fissure is the first to appear, separating the flocculonodular lobe, which is constant in most vertebrates, from the cerebellar mass, which increases in size from lower to higher vertebrates. The expansion of the cerebellum through phylogenesis, rostral to the posterolateral fissure, involves the middle portion of the corpus cerebelli, the anterior lobe demarcated posteriorly by the primary fissure as well as the pyramid and the uvula. This expansion is present in most vertebrates and undergoes moderate modifications. The major development of the middle portion, mainly in mammals, including human and nonhuman primates, involves the neocerebellum, corresponding roughly to the cerebellar hemispheres. The flocculonodular lobe is also named the archicerebellum, and the paleocerebellum includes portions of the vermis located in the anterior lobe as well as the

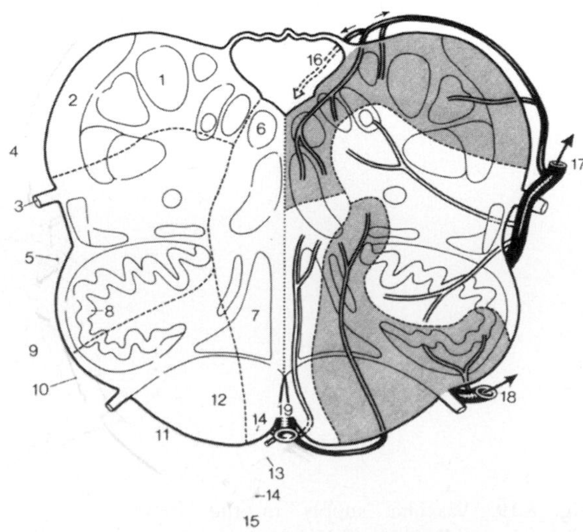

Fig. 8.21. Vascular supply to the brainstem: level of medulla. Vascular territories (arterial on the *right* and venous on the *left*). (According to Duvernoy 1978)

pyramid, the uvula and the paraflocculus. The paraflocculus of mammals is the homologue of the human tonsil and the biventer lobule of the human cerebellum.

The subdivision of the human cerebellum, based on comparative studies in mammals, corresponds to the subdivision reached on the basis of the cerebellar afferents. In fact, the archicerebellum is also named the vestibulocerebellum, the paleocerebellum corresponds to the spinocerebellum, and the neocerebellum corresponds to the pontocerebellum. These anatomic regions are connected with other parts of the central nervous system, respectively, the spinal cord and the cerebral cortex. To this lobular organization of the cerebellum a longitudinal zonal subdivision, based on the corticonuclear projections of the cerebellum, was proposed by Jansen and Brodal (1940, 1942, 1958). These authors subdivided the cerebellar cortex into three longitudinal zones of functional importance: the medial zone corresponds to the vermis and projects to the fastigial nucleus, the intermediate zone projects to the nuclei interpositi and corresponds to a paramedian region, and the lateral zone is related to the dentate nucleus. This latter subdivision, based on anatomical and physiological data, seems more precise. A further longitudinal subdivision of these functional areas of the cerebellar cortex has been mapped by Voogd (1969).

1 Morphology and Topographical Anatomy

The cerebellum, or little brain, lies in the posterior cranial fossa covered by the tentorium cerebelli. In humans, the size ratio of cerebellum to cerebrum is about 1:8 in the adult and 1:20 in the infant. The cerebellum is the largest portion of the hindbrain overlying the posterior aspect of the pons and the medulla oblongata. Morphologically it consists of two cerebellar hemispheres joined by a midline portion, the vermis. The vermis is a wedge-shaped structure presenting a superior and an inferior surface separated by the horizontal fissure of Vicq d'Azyr, the most conspicuous of the cerebellar fissures. The superior surface of the cerebellum is flattened, showing no deep grooves in the paramedian regions as the superior vermis is directly continuous with the cerebellar hemispheres on each side. Anteriorly, the superior vermis continues beyond the free margin of the tentorium cerebelli. Superiorly, it is bound by a wide, shallow, anterior cerebellar incisure. The posterior inferior surface of the cerebellum is convex and lies in the occipital region. The inferior vermis is separated from the paramedian region of the cerebellar hemisphere by deep sulci. Posteriorly and inferiorly a narrow median fossa, the vallecula cerebelli, separates the hemispheres and contains the falx cerebelli (Fig. 8.1). The anterior-posterior coronal cuts through the cerebellum oriented parallel to the PC-OB plane display the morphological and topographical anatomy of the cerebellum and disclose its internal structure (Figs. 8.25–8.28).

a *Structural Organization*

Structurally, the cerebellum differs from the medulla oblongata and the pons, consisting of a superficial gray cortical mantle, the cerebellar cortex, and an internal white matter core containing four pairs of intrinsic nuclei. The cortical gray matter covers the total surface of the cerebellum, folding into the fissures. The white matter forms the medullary core and is thicker laterally than medially. Thus, the cerebellum is structurally similar to the cerebrum. The internal structure of the cerebellum is best appreciated on a midsagittal section, passing through the cerebellar vermis and showing the characteristic branched organization of the laminae (the arbor vitae cerebelli) (Fig. 8.1).

The cerebellum is connected with the three rostrocaudal portions of the brainstem by three paired cerebellar peduncles, superior, middle and inferior. The middle cerebellar peduncles are shown on the axial cuts at the pontine level (Fig. 8.16), on the most anterior coronal cuts at the PC-OB level (Fig. 8.2), and on the parasagittal cuts passing through the trigeminal root (Fig. 8.29). The superior cerebellar peduncles, constituting the lateral walls of the roof of the fourth ventricle, are well displayed on both the coronal cuts (Fig. 8.25) and the parasagittal cuts (Fig. 8.29), proceeding from the hilum of the dentate cerebellar nuclei to their decussation at the inferior collicular level, well shown on the axial cut passing through the inferior midbrain (Figs. 8.7, 8.8). The inferior cerebellar peduncles are visualized on the parasagittal cuts (Figs. 8.10, 8.13).

The cerebellar cortex is actually composed of numerous primary laminae oriented transversally and cut at right angles, containing secondary and tertiary folia disposed more or less at right angles to the primary laminae and well shown on midsagittal (Fig. 8.1) and parasagittal (Fig. 8.30) cuts. Five deep fissures are identified on median sagittal sections and on the external aspect of the cerebellum. These are: the primary, the posterior superior, the horizontal, the prepyramidal, and the posterolateral fissures. The fissures divide the cerebellum into several lobes and lobules (Figs. 8.30, 8.1) and con-

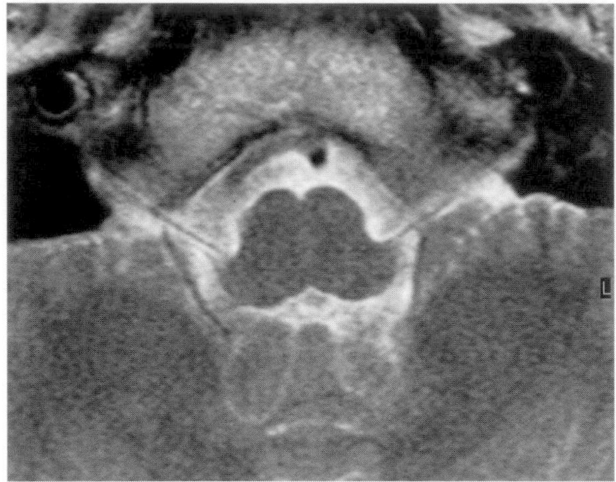

A

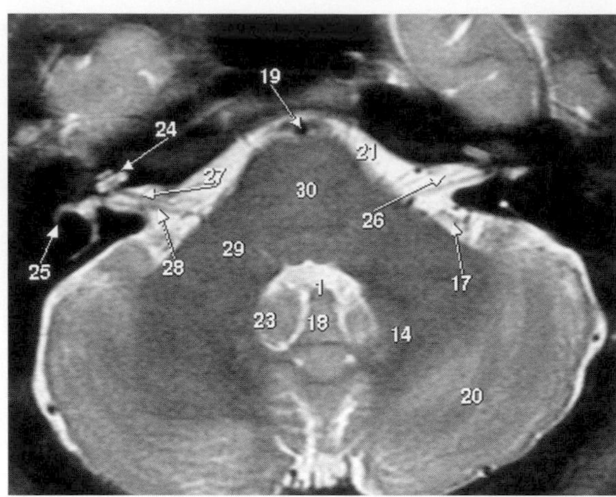

B

A: At the medullary level showing the glossopharyngeal nerves (see anatomical correlation fig 8.17)

B: At the caudal pontine level, showing the emergence of the facial and the vestibulocochlear nerves (see anatomical correlation fig. 8.16)

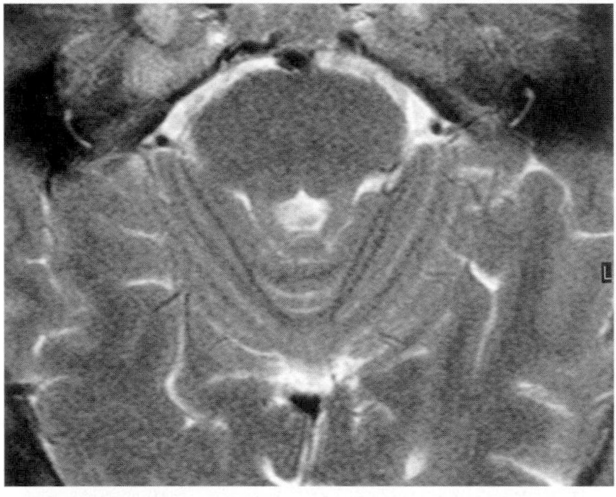

C

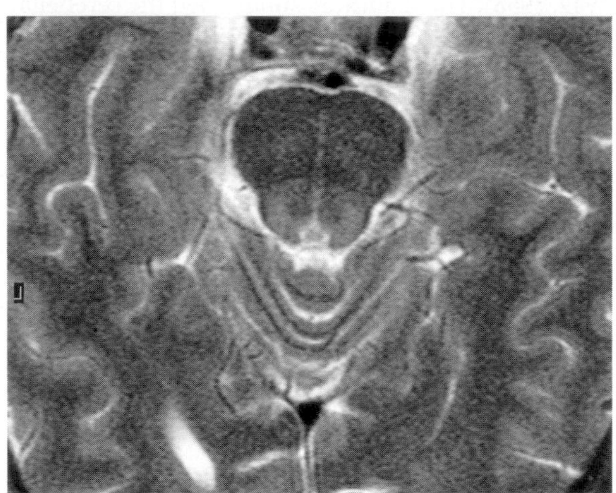

D

C: At the level of entrance of the trigeminal roots in the pons (see anatomical correlation fig 8.15)

D: At the isthmus level and the exit of the cochlear nerves (see anatomical correlation fig 8.14)

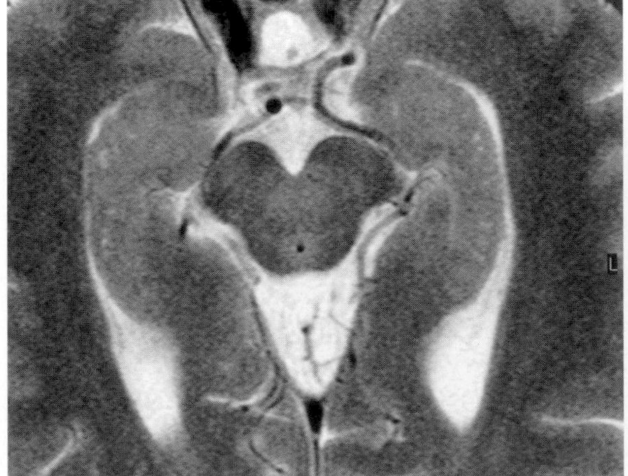

E

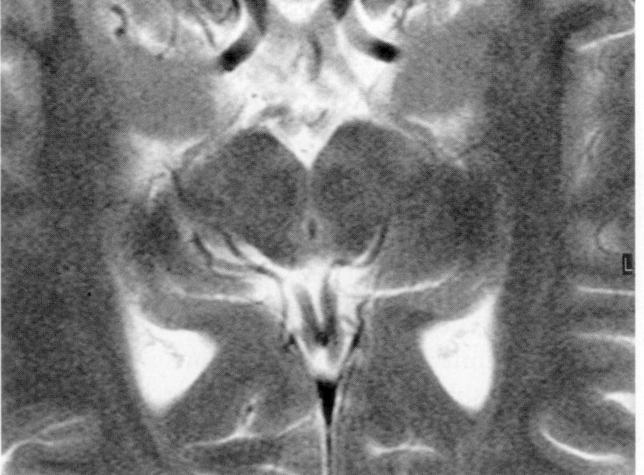

F

E: At the inferior collicular level in the caudal midbrain showing the emergence of the oculomotor nerves from the interpeduncular cistern (see anatomical correlation fig 8.7)

F: At the superior collicular level in the rostral midbrain showing the "X" shape of the cisternal optic nerves and tracts, in the CH-PC plane.

Fig. 8.22. Horizontal chiasmato-commissural (CH-PC) MR cuts, 4 mm thick, through the brainstem using FSE-T2 weighted pulse sequence and showing the general external morphology and the cisternal portions of some of the cranial nerves

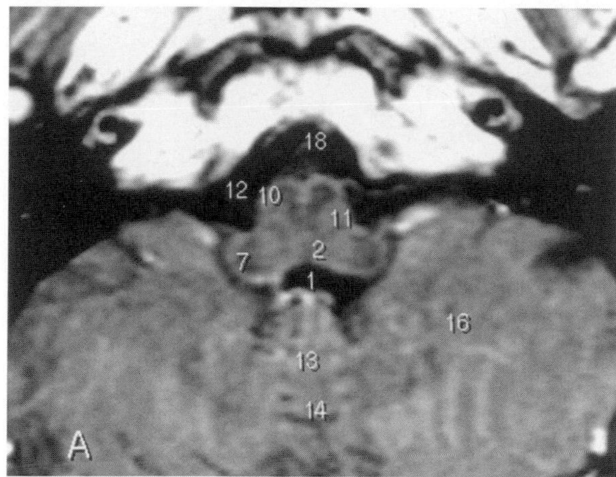

A: At the medullary level (see anatomical correlation fig 8.17)

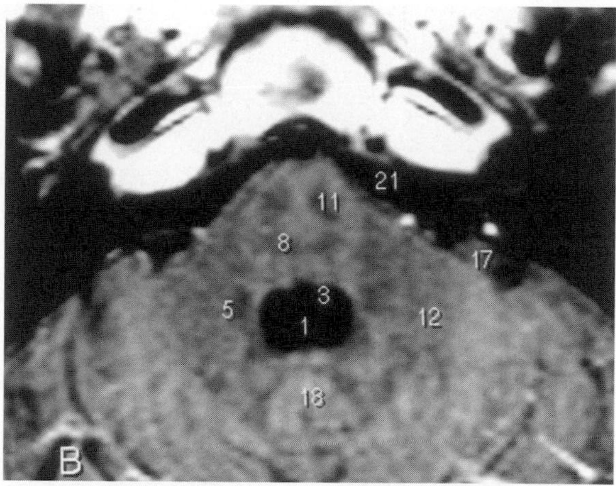

B: At the caudal pontine and middle cerebellar peduncular level (see anatomical correlation fig. 8.16)

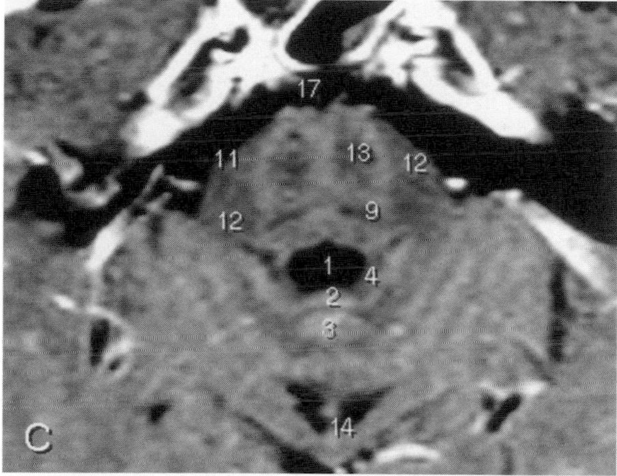

C: At the level of the trigeminal roots in the pons (see anatomical correlation fig 8.15)

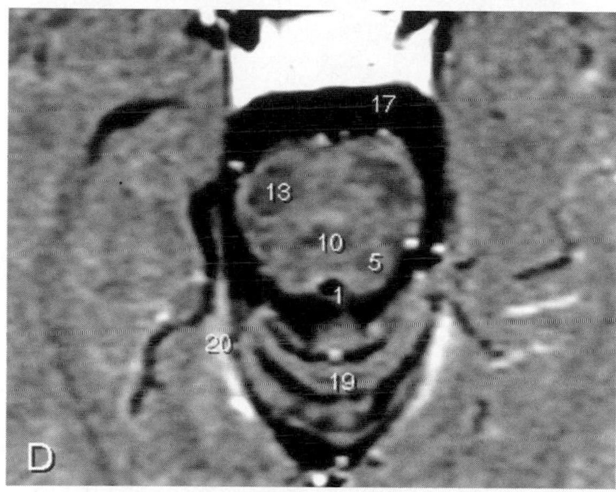

D: At the isthmus level (see anatomical correlation fig 8.14)

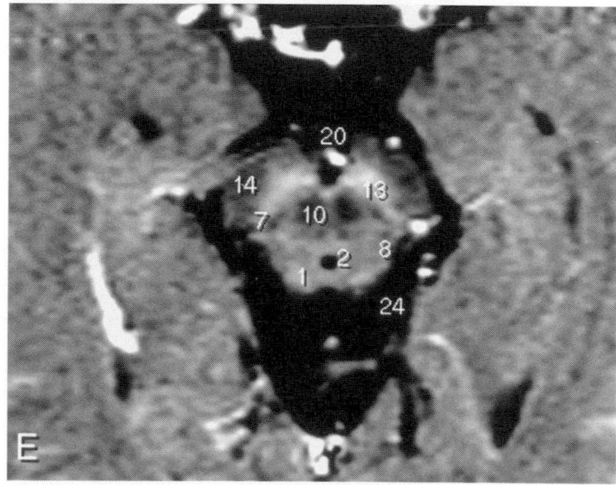

E: At the caudal midbrain and inferior collicular level (see anatomical correlation fig 8.7)

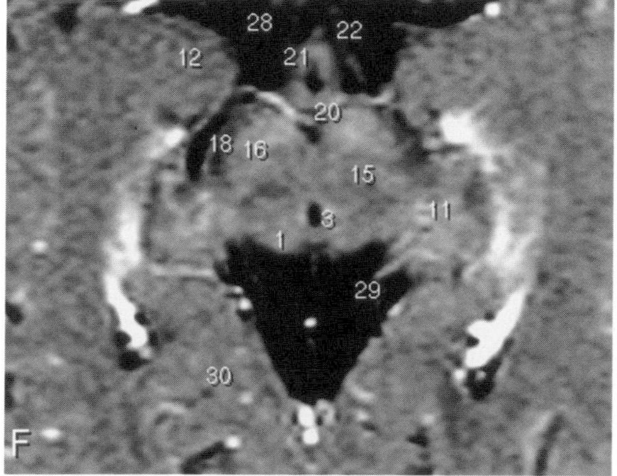

F: At the midbrain-diencephalic junction level and the superior colliculi in the CH-PC plane. (see anatomical correlation, Fig. 8.5)

Fig. 8.23. Horizontal chiasmato-commissural (CH-PC) MR cuts, 4 mm thick, through the brainstem using SE-T_1w. with magnetization transfer and Gd infusion sequence and showing the internal structure of the brainstem, particularly the white matter tracts

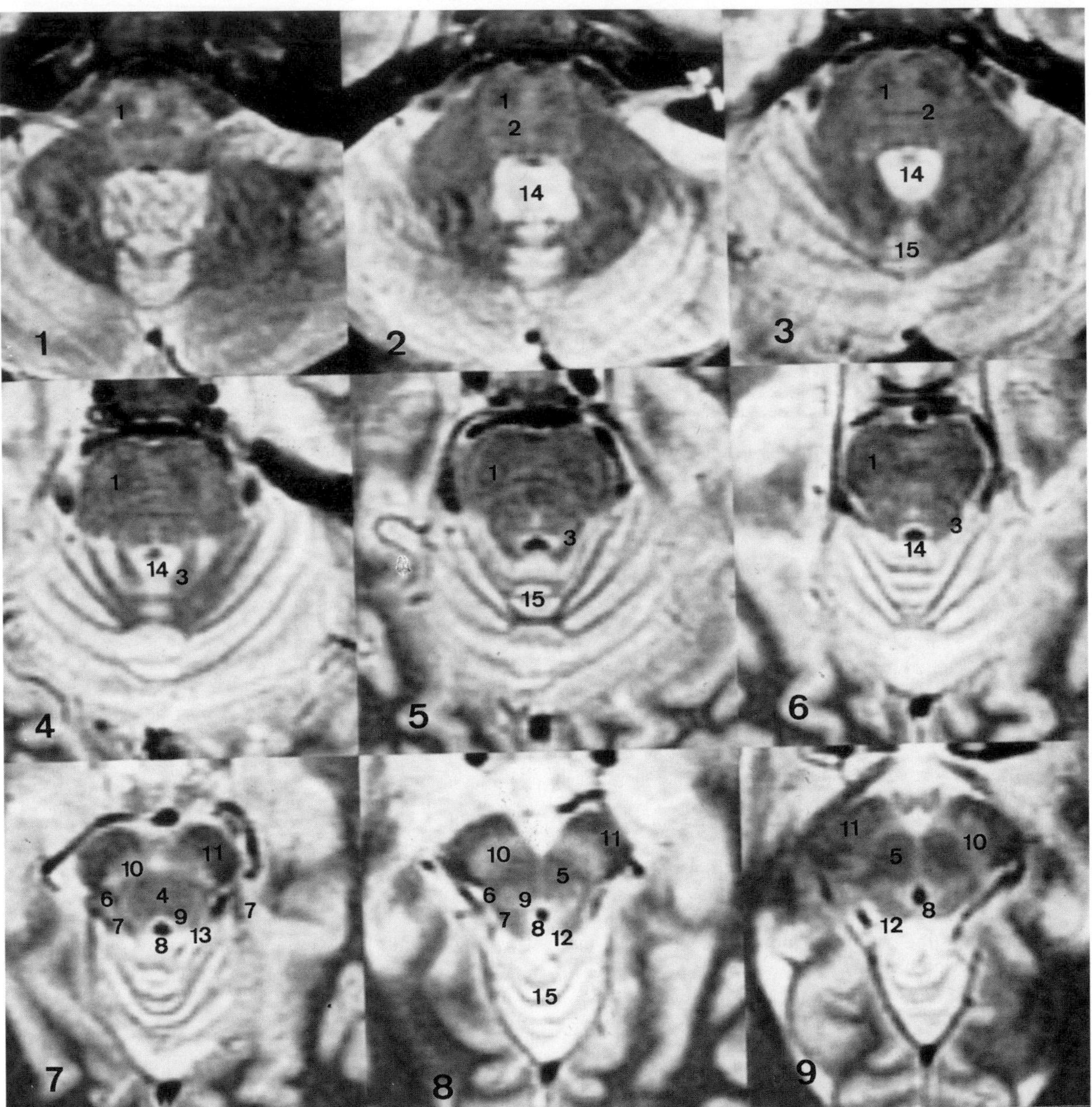

Fig. 8.24. Horizontal chiasmato-commissural (CH-PC) MR cuts, 3 mm thick, through the brainstem using FSE-PD weighted pulse sequence and showing the internal structure of the brainstem. *1*, Corticospinal tract; *2*, medial lemniscus; *3*, superior cerebellar peduncle; *4*, decussation of superior cerebellar peduncle; *5*, red nucleus; *6*, spinothalamic tract; *7*, lateral lemniscus; *8*, cerebral aqueduct; *9*, medial lemniscus; *10*, substantia nigra; *11*, crus cerebri; *12*, superior colliculus; *13*, inferior colliculus; *14*, fourth ventricle; *15*, vermis of cerebellum

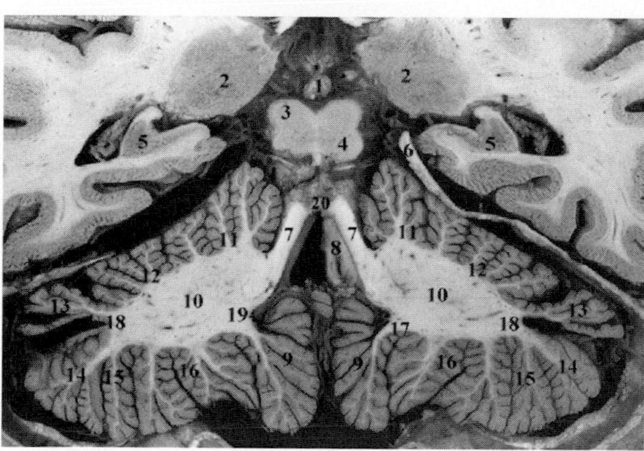

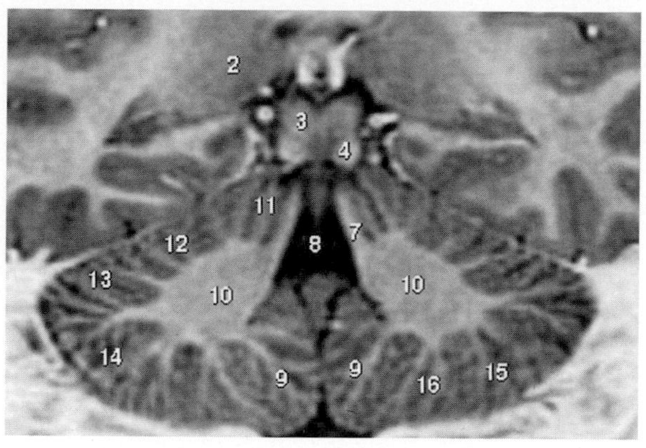

Fig. 8.25. A,B *1*, Pineal body; *2*, pulvinar thalami; *3*, superior colliculus; *4*, inferior colliculus; *5*, hippocampus; *6*, tentorium cerebelli; *7*, superior cerebellar peduncle; *8*, fourth ventricle (floor); *9*, tonsil of cerebellum (and medially the vallecula); *10*, album cerebelli (cerebellar white matter); *11*, anterior quadrangular lobule; *12*, posterior quadrangular lobule; *13*, superior semilunar lobule; *14*, inferior semilunar lobule; *15*, gracilis lobule; *16*, biventer lobule; *17*, secondary fissure; *18*, horizontal fissure of Vicq d'Azyr; *19*, lateral recess of the fourth ventricle; *20*, superior medullary velum (frenulum veli)

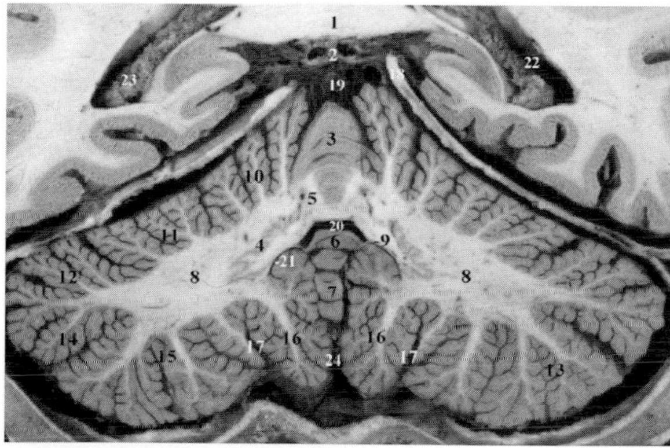

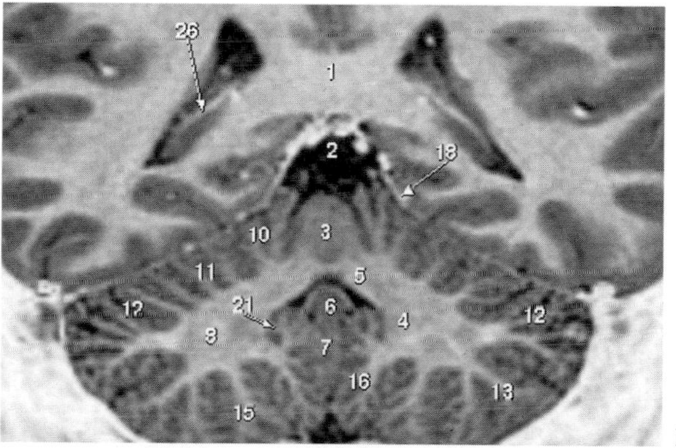

Fig. 8.26. A,B *1*, Splenium of corpus callosum; *2*, internal cerebral vein; *3*, culmen, vermis; *4*, dentate nucleus; *5*, fastigial nucleus; *6*, nodulus, vermis; *7*, uvula, vermis; *8*, cerebellar white matter; *9*, inferior medullary velum; *10*, anterior quadrangular lobule; *11*, posterior quadrangular lobule; *12*, superior semilunar lobule; *13*, inferior semilunar lobule; *14*, gracile lobule; *15*, biventer lobule; *16*, cerebellar tonsil; *17*, secondary fissure; *18*, tentorium cerebelli; *19*, ambient cistern; *20*, fourth ventricle; *21*, lateral recess of fourth ventricle; *22*, atrium of lateral ventricle; *23*, choroid plexus of lateral ventricle; *24*, vallecula cerebelli

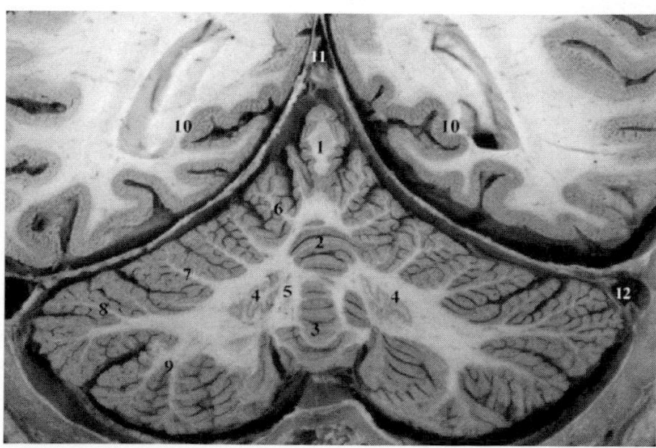

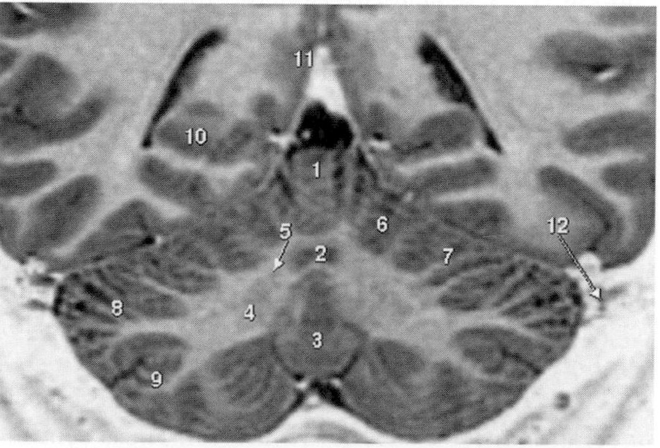

Fig. 8.27. A,B *1*, Culmen, vermis; *2*, declive, vermis; *3*, pyramis, vermis; *4*, dentate nucleus; *5*, globose nuclei; *6*, anterior quadrangular lobule; *7*, posterior quadrangular lobule; *8*, superior semilunar lobule; *9*, inferior semilunar lobule; *10*, calcarine sulcus; *11*, rectus sinus; *12*, transverse lateral sinus

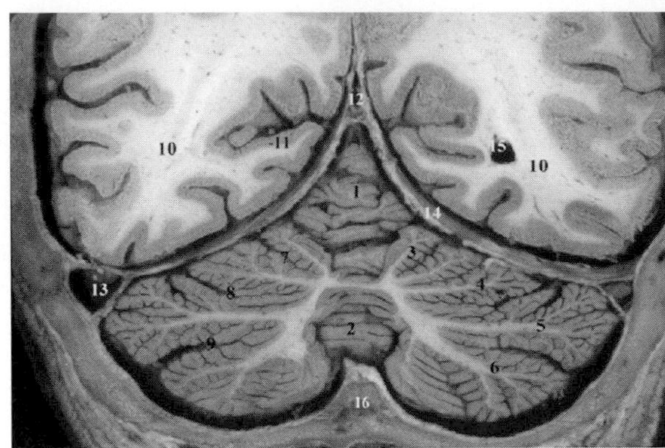

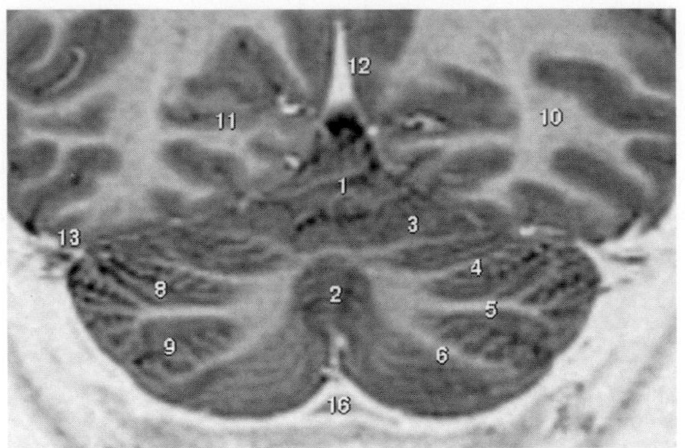

Fig. 8.28. A,B *1*, Declive, vermis; *2*, tuber, vermis; *3*, anterior quadrangular lobule; *4*, posterior quadrangular lobule; *5*, superior semilunar lobule; *6*, inferior semilunar lobule; *7*, primary fissure; *8*, superior posterior fissure; *9*, horizontal fissure; *10*, occipital lobe; *11*, calcarine sulcus; *12*, sinus rectus; *13*, lateral sinus; *14*, tentorium cerebelli; *15*, occipital horn of the lateral ventricle; *16*, internal occipital protuberance

stitute the basics for the morphological and functional subdivisions of the cerebellum (Larsell 1951). Two fissures can be identified on the superior surface of the cerebellum, the primary and the anterior superior fissures. The portion of the vermis and the cerebellar hemispheres situated rostral to the primary fissure constitute the anterior lobe (paleocerebellum or spinocerebellum). The primary fissure indents the superior surface of the vermis between the culmen and the declive. The vermis and the cerebellar hemispheres located between the primary and the posterolateral fissures represent the posterior lobe of the cerebellum (neocerebellum or cerebrocerebellum), which is separated from the flocculonodular lobe (archicerebellum or vestibulocerebellum) by the posterolateral fissure.

The anterior lobe consists of the vermis, the lingula, the central lobule and the culmen (Fig. 8.1). The central lobule corresponds to the central lobule, and the anterior quadrangular lobule corresponds to the culmen (Figs. 8.30, 8.26). Considering the posterior lobe, the largest portion of the cerebellum, it is positioned between the anterior lobe and the flocculonodular lobe, constituting the main bulk of the cerebellar hemispheres. The vermal subdivisions of the posterior lobe are the declive, the folium, the tuber, the pyramis, and the uvula (Fig. 8.1). The posterior quadrangular lobule, or lobulus simplex, corresponds to the declive, the superior semilunar lobule (crus I) corresponds to the folium, and the inferior semilunar nodule corresponds to the tuber (crus II). Note that the horizontal fissure separates the superior semilunar lobule from the inferior. These semilunar lobules form the ansiform lobule, located between the posterior superior fissure and the gracile lobule. Between the prepyramidal fissure and the pos-

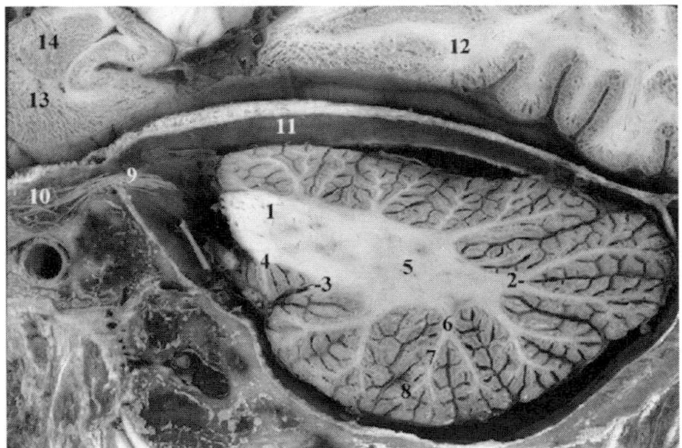

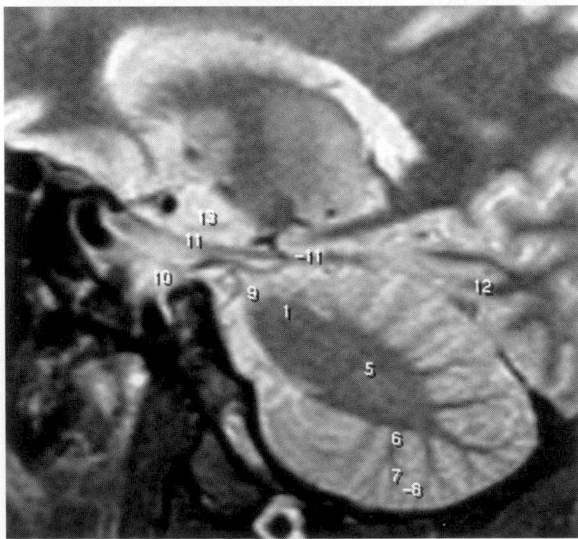

Fig. 8.29. *1*, Middle cerebellar peduncle; *2*, horizontal fissure of Vicq d'Azyr; *3*, posterolateral fissure; *4*, flocculus; *5*, cerebellar white matter (album cerebelli); *6*, lamina alba cerebelli (lobular); *7*, lamina alba cerebelli (sublobular); *8*, lamina alba cerebelli (subcortical); *9*, trigeminal root nerve; *10*, cavum of Meckel; *11*, tentorium cerebelli; *12*, lingual gyrus (occipital lobe); *13*, uncus of temporal lobe; *14*, amygdala

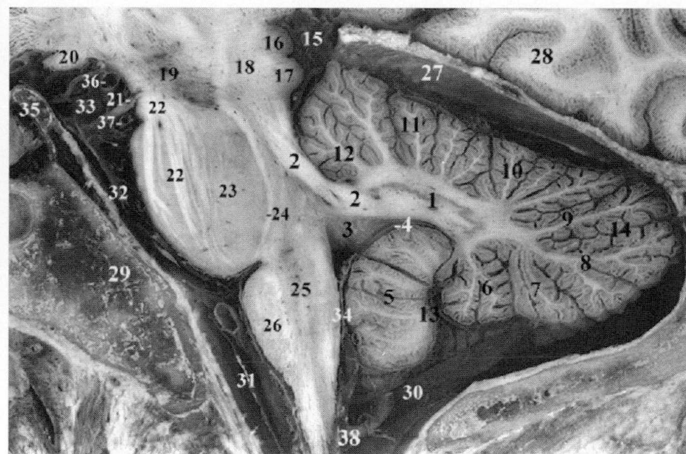

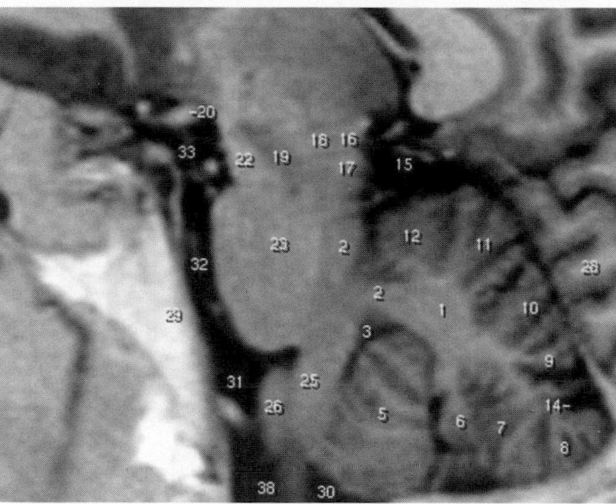

A B

Fig. 8.30A,B. *1*, Dentate nucleus; 2, superior cerebellar peduncle; *3*, superior medullary velum of the fourth ventricle; *4*, inferior medullary velum of the fourth ventricle; *5*, tonsil of cerebellum; *6*, biventer lobule; *7*, gracile lobule; *8*, inferior semilunar lobule; *9*, superior semilunar lobule; *10*, posterior quadrangular lobule; *11*, anterior quadrangular lobule; *12*, central lobule; *13*, secondary fissure; *14*, horizontal fissure; *15*, ambient and midbrain cerebellar cisterns (inferiorly); *16*, superior colliculus; *17*, inferior colliculus; *18*, tegmentum of midbrain; *19*, substantia nigra; *20*, optic tract; *21*, oculomotor nerve (III); *22*, cerebral peduncle and corticospinal bundles; *23*, pons (pontine nuclei); *24*, medial lemniscus; *25*, medulla oblongata; *26*, inferior olivary nucleus (olive); *27*, tentorium cerebelli; *28*, occipital lobe; *29*, clivus; *30*, cisterna magna; *31*, prebulbar cistern; *32*, prepontine cistern; *33*, interpeduncular cistern; *34*, forum of Magendie; *35*, dorsum sellae; *36*, posterior cerebral artery; *37*, superior cerebellar artery; *38*, foramen magnum

terolateral fissure, the inferior vermal segments, the pyramis and the uvula are related to the biventer lobule and the cerebellar tonsil of the cerebellar hemisphere, respectively (Figs. 8.30, 8.27). Finally, in the vermis, the nodule found immediately caudal to the inferior medullary velum is separated from the uvula by the posterolateral fissure (Fig. 8.31). The nodule is part of the flocculonodular lobe consisting of both flocculi and their related peduncles. The flocculi (Fig. 8.2) are small cerebellar portions partially detached and lying immediately below the vestibulocochlear nerves, in the cerebellopontine angle, crossed anteriorly by the glossopharyngeal and vagus nerves in their route toward the jugular foramen (Fig. 8.16).

b The Deep Cerebellar Nuclei

Coronal and parasagittal sections through the white medullary core of the cerebellum (Fig. 8.16, 8.30–8.32) and the parasagittal sections of the cerebellum show the deep cerebellar nuclei, positioned dorsally and dorsolaterally to the fourth ventricle. These nuclei are the dentate, the emboliform, the globose, and the fastigial.

The dentate nuclei are the most laterally placed and the largest, resembling a folded bag with its opening directed medially, as clearly demonstrated on the anatomic dissection by Klingler (Fig. 8.33). These are well displayed when cut in the coronal (Figs. 8.31, 8.32) and in the horizontal plane (Fig. 8.16). Their shape is similar to that of the inferior olivary nucleus (Fig. 8.18). Afferent fibers originating from the Purkinje cells form a dense fiber plexus around the nucleus, named the amiculum. The emboliform nucleus lies just medial to the dentate, close to the hilus and is often difficult to separate from the dentate (Figs. 8.32, 8.31). The globose nucleus consists of two or more small, ovoid, nuclear masses lying medial to the emboliform nucleus and lateral to the fastigial nucleus (Fig. 8.32). Despite its name, this nucleus is elongated anteroposteriorly. The emboliform and globose nuclei correspond in nonprimate mammals to the nucleus interpositus (Jansen and Brodal 1954; Courville and Cooper 1970). The fastigial nucleus, phylogenetically the oldest, is the most medial of the subcortical cerebellar nuclei, located just lateral to the fastigium of the roof of the fourth ventricle, close to the median plane in the anterior part of the superior vermis (Figs. 8.31, 8.26). It is the second largest in size, after the dentate nucleus, in humans.

2 Functional and Clinical Considerations

The cerebellar nuclei receive projections mainly from the ipsilateral Purkinje cells, the corticonuclear afferent fibers which are inhibitory and use GABA as their neurotransmitter. All areas of the cerebellar cortex project upon the subcortical cerebellar nuclei.

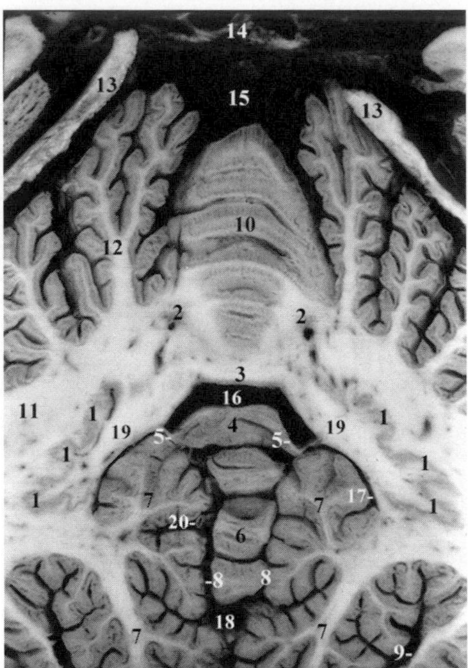

Fig. 8.31. *1*, Dentate nucleus; *2*, fastigial nucleus; *3*, superior medullary velum; *4*, nodule of vermis; *5*, inferior medullary velum (on each side of the nodule); *6*, uvula of inferior vermis; *7*, tonsil of cerebellar hemisphere; *8*, postero-lateral fissure (between the uvula-nodulus complex and the cerebellar hemispheres); *9*, secondary fissure (between the tonsil and the biventer lobule on the cerebellar hemisphere); *10*, culmen of the superior vermis; *11*, album cerebelli (white matter of cerebellar hemisphere); *12*, anterior quadrangular lobule; *13*, tentorium cerebelli; *14*, internal cerebral veins; *15*, median portion of the ambient cistern; *16*, fourth ventricle; *17*, lateral recess of fourth ventricle; *18*, vallecula of cerebellum; *19*, superior cerebellar peduncle (at the level of the hilum of the dentate nucleus); *20*, posterior inferior cerebellar artery

These projections originate from three rostrocaudal longitudinal zones. The median, or vermal, zone projects to the fastigial nucleus ipsilaterally, the paramedian or paravermal zone projects to the emboliform nucleus, and the lateral or hemispheric zone projects to the dentate nucleus (Eager 1963; Jansen and Brodal 1940; Voogd 1964). The tonic inhibitory output from the cerebellar cortex with respect to neurons of the subcortical cerebellar nuclei is overcome by excitatory input originating from extracerebellar sources, mainly the inferior olivary nucleus via the olivocerebellar fibers, the pontine nuclei via the pontocerebellar fibers, and the reticulotegmental nucleus via reticulocerebellar fibers.

The olivocerebellar fibers arise from the contralateral inferior olivary nuclear complex, constitute the largest component of the inferior cerebellar peduncle and project to all parts of the cerebellar cortex as well as to the cerebellar nuclei. The olivocerebellar fibers are distributed in an orderly pattern, each portion of the olive projecting to a specific cerebellar area. The fibers which terminate in the cerebellar nuclei are believed to be collaterals of those projecting to the cerebellar cortex (Brodal 1976). The inferior olivary complex is the major source of climbing excitatory fibers, terminating on Purkinje cell dendrites (Courville and Faraco-Cantin 1978).

The pontocerebellar afferents originating in the pontine nuclei project via the medial cerebellar peduncle mainly to the contralateral cerebellar hemisphere and bilaterally to the vermis, constituting the most important relay and receiving inputs from all of the four cerebral lobes to the cerebellar cortex specifically (Mihailoff 1993). The most important cortical projection arises from the sensory motor cortex and projects somatotopically to the pontine nuclei. Concerning the reticulocerebellar fibers, these arise from the reticulotegmental nucleus and the paramedian and lateral reticular nuclei of the medulla. The reticulotegmental fibers participate in a cerebellar reticular feed-back system. The reticulotegmental nucleus, receiving afferents mainly from both the ipsilateral frontoparietal cortex and the dentate as the crossed descending division of the superior cerebellar peduncle, projects via the middle

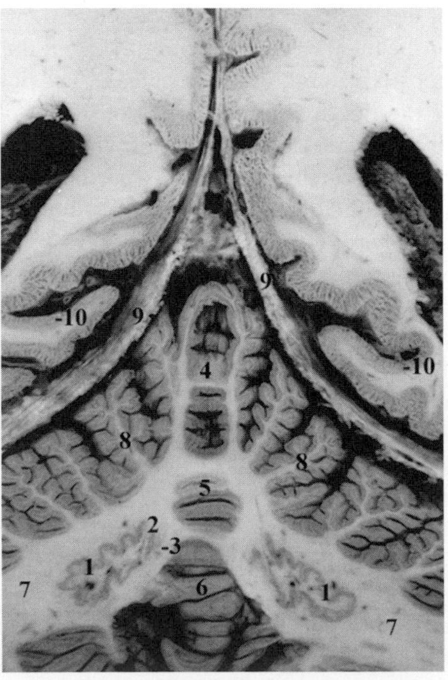

Fig. 8.32. *1*, Dentate nucleus; *2*, emboliform nucleus; *3*, globose nuclei; *4*, culmen, vermis; *5*, declive, vermis; *6*, pyramis, vermis; *7*, album cerebelli; *8*, anterior quadrangular lobule; *9*, tentorium cerebelli; *10*, calcarine sulcus

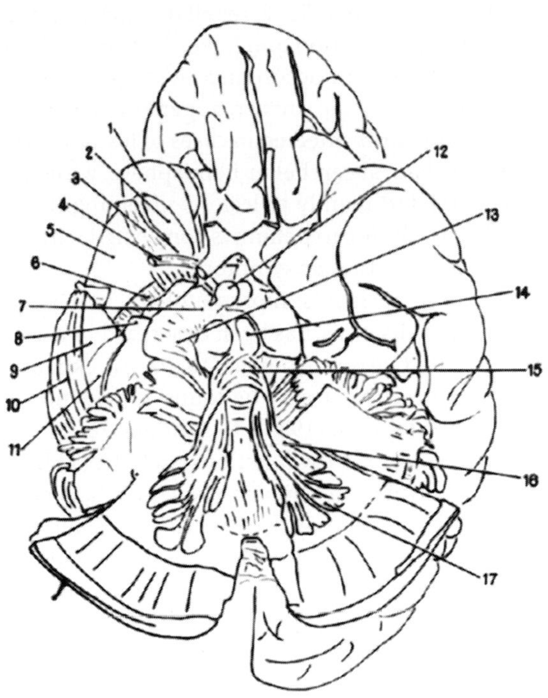

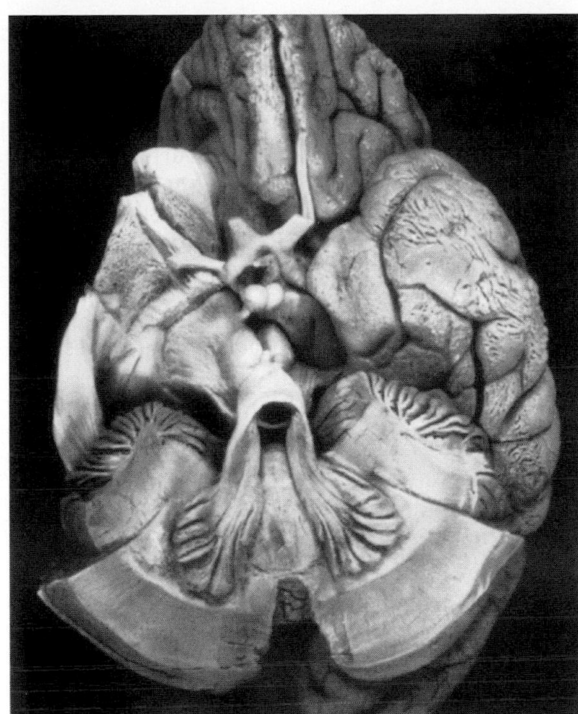

Fig. 8.33. Dissection of the cerebellum disclosing the dentate nuclei (17) and the superior cerebellar peduncles (16) and their decussation (15). (From Klingler 1956)

cerebellar peduncle to the vermis. The reticulotegmental projections end bilaterally as mossy fibers in the granular layer of the cerebellar cortex. The lateral and the paramedian reticular nuclei of the medulla seem to transmit exteroceptive information coming from the spinal cord and the cerebral cortex to the cerebellar cortex.

The vestibulocerebellar fibers are conveyed by the juxtarestiform body and divided into primary and secondary afferents. The primary vestibulocerebellar fibers arise in the semicircular canals and in otoliths, whereas the secondary vestibular fibers arise mainly from the inferior vestibular nucleus. The vestibulocerebellar fibers show a similar pattern of distribution within the entire vermis.

The spinocerebellar path includes the anterior, posterior, and rostral spinocerebellar tracts, arising from cells within the spinal cord and the cuneocerebellar fibers, arising from the lower medulla. These tracts project to the cerebellum, the inferior cerebellar peduncle conveying the fibers of the posterior spinocerebellar and the cuneocerebellar fibers, whereas the superior cerebellar peduncle conveys the anterior spinocerebellar tract. The rostral spinocerebellar tract enters the cerebellum via both the superior and the inferior cerebellar peduncles. Functionally, the fibers of the anterior spinocerebellar tract, which are crossed, are activated by impulses originating from Golgi tendon organs. The fibers of the posterior spinocerebellar tract are uncrossed and are activated by impulses from Golgi organs and muscle spindles. The cuneocerebellar tract, which is uncrossed, may be considered as the upper limb equivalent of the posterior spinocerebellar tract. The rostral spinocerebellar tract in the cat is considered as the upper limb equivalent of the anterior spinocerebellar tract. The information conveyed by the anterior and the posterior spinocerebellar tracts do not reach conscious levels.

The cerebellar efferent fibers originate from the cerebellar nuclei and the flocculonodular cortex (vestibulocerebellum) and make up three major efferent systems: the superior cerebellar peduncle, the fastigial efferent fibers, and the cerebellovestibular fibers. The superior cerebellar peduncle conveys primarily efferent fibers arising from the dentate, emboliform, and globose nuclei. The entire outflow forms a compact bundle which decussates completely in the lower midbrain, constituting the decussation of the brachium conjunctivum (Figs. 8.7, 8.8). Most of the ascending efferent fibers enter and surround the contralateral red nucleus, some terminating in its rostral third, before projecting and ending in the ventral lateral and ventral posterolateral thalamic nuclei. Fibers from the dentate nucleus terminate somatotopically in these nuclei which project in a topical manner upon the primary motor cortex (area 4). The dentate nucleus can therefore monitor the activity of the motor cerebral cortex. The cerebellar nuclei may also send projection fibers to the mediodorsal nucleus of the thalamus, which projects to the prefrontal cortex (Yamamoto et al. 1992). The fastigial efferent bundle consists of uncrossed efferent fibers, conveyed in the juxtarestiform body and projecting mainly to the lateral and inferior vestibular nuclei, and crossed fastigioreticular fibers, projecting to reticular nuclei of the pons and medulla. The cerebellovestibular fibers are ipsilateral projections originating from the flocculonodular lobe and projecting to the vestibular nuclei. The vestibulocerebellum therefore plays a role in equilibrium and contributes in controlling eye movement in coordination with movements of the head.

A great number of studies have been performed in order to elucidate the functional role of the cerebellum. In the preceding sections of this chapter, findings concerning the main cerebellar circuitry were reported. Excellent reviews are available and should be consulted (Holmes 1939; Brown 1949; Dow and Moruzzi 1958; Dow 1969; Eccles et al. 1967). In view of its major cerebellar connections, the cerebellum plays an important role in the integration of inputs originating from various cutaneous receptors, proprioceptors, eyes and ears, as well as from the brainstem reticular formation and the cerebral cortex, before discharging to the motor centers in the brainstem and the cerebrum.

Actually, the cerebellum has been divided into three sagittal cortical zones and their connecting subcortical nuclei, referred to as vermal, paravermal, and lateral zones. The vermal zone, related to fastigial nuclei, is responsible for the motor control of posture and locomotion, muscle tone, and equilibrium. The intermediate paravermal zone is related to the emboliform and globose nuclei and is concerned with motor control of the distal musculature. The lateral zone is related to the dentate nucleus and is concerned with initiation, planning, and timing as well as coordination of ipsilateral motor activity. It is clear that the different parasagittal zones of the cerebellum differ functionally with regard to their connections.

The important question, whether particular signs and symptoms can be related to dysfunction of specific portions of the cerebellum, remains poorly settled. Most cerebellar lesions are usually not restricted to a discrete anatomic region and the results of destruction of specific cerebellar nuclei are not known. Yet, localization and lateralization of clinical signs are usually in accordance with the anatomic cerebellar connection. In fact, upper and lower limbs are clinically more affected in cases of lesions involving the ipsilateral cerebellar hemisphere, while axial ataxia is related mainly to lesions involving the vermis. The vestibulocerebellum is concerned with oculomotor and vestibular symptoms.

The characteristic symptomatology, as observed in cerebellar diseases, has been described in a classical paper by Gordon Holmes (1939). An exhaustive review of the subject may be found in the more recent work of Gilman (1985). To summarize, the main effects of cerebellar dysfunctions include: (1) loss of motor coordination, known as cerebellar ataxia, manifested in disturbance of posture and gait, asynergia with dysmetria or dysdiadochokinesis, decomposition of movement, intention tremor, cerebellar dysarthria with scanning and slurring of speech, and ocular nystagmus, (2) changes in muscle tone usually manifested as hypotonia, (3) asthenia and increased fatiguability of the muscles, (4) a proposed effect on the learning of motor skills (Marr 1969) and in motor adaptation (McCormick 1984; Ito 1989; Tach et al.1992), (5) still controversial, monitoring of the prefrontal regions and thus cerebellar involvement in higher cognitive functions (Leiner et al. 1989; Schmahmann 1991; Lalonde and Botez 1990; Wallesch and Horm 1990).

3 Vascular Supply to the Cerebellum

The cerebellum receives its blood supply through three paired arteries which course from the brainstem anteriorly towards the posterior aspect of the cerebellum:

1. The superior cerebellar artery originates from the basilar artery just before its superior terminal division into posterior cerebral arteries. It courses around the lateral aspect of the crus cerebri in the lateral wing of the ambient cistern. At its origin it is situated beneath the oculomotor nerve. It ends with two branches at the level of the inferior colliculi posteriorly. These arteries vascularize the superior aspect of the cerebellar hemispheres as well as the deep cerebellar nuclei.
2. The anterior inferior cerebellar artery (AICA) originates from the basilar artery and projects laterally in the cerebellopontine cistern, usually giving rise to a labyrinthine branch, and ends at the flocculus. In its route through the cerebellopontine

cistern, the artery courses along the cochleovestibular and facial nerve roots, frequently visualized on high resolution, T2 weighted, MR axial cuts.

3. The posterior inferior cerebellar artery (PICA) originates from the vertebral artery about 2 cm before its union with the basilar artery. It courses around the lateral aspect of the medulla oblongata to reach its posterior aspect, where it supplies the choroid plexus. The artery then loops as the retrotonsillar segment around the cerebellar tonsil to end at and vascularize the inferior aspect of the cerebellum.

References

Adams RD, Victor M, Ropper AH (1997) Principles of neurology. McGraw-Hill, New York

Angevine JB Jr, Mancall EL, Yakovlev PI (1961) The human cerebellum. An atlas of gross topography in serial sections. Little, Brown, Boston

Afshar F, Watkins ES, Yap JC (1978) Stereotaxic atlas of the human brainstem and cerebellar nuclei. A variability study. Raven, New York

Aitkin LM, Webster WR, Veale JL, Crosby DC (1975) Inferior colliculus. I. Comparison of response properties of neurons in central, pericentral and external nuclei of adult cat. J Neurophysiol 38:1196–1207

Aitkin L M (1989) The auditory system. In: Björklund A, Hökfelt T, Swanson LW (eds) Handbook of chemical neuroanatomy, vol 7: Integrated systems of the CNS, part II. Elsevier, Amsterdam, pp 165–218

Braitenberg V, Atwood RP (1958) Morphological observations on the cerebellar cortex. J Comp Neurol 109:1–27

Bobillier R, Seguin S, Petitjean F, Salvert D, Touret M, Jouvet M (1976) The raphe nuclei of the cat brain stem:a topographical atlas of their efferent projections as revealed by autoradiography. Brain Res 113:449–486

Brodal A (1957) The reticular formation of the brain stem. Anatomical aspects and functional correlations. The Henderson Trust Lectures, vol XVIII. Olivier and Boyd, Edinburgh, VII

Brodal A (1976) The olivocerebellar projection in the cat as studied with the method of retrograde axonal transport of horseradish peroxidase. II. The projection of the uvula. J Comp Neurol 166:417–426

Brodal A (1981) Neurological anatomy in relation to clinical medicine, 3rd edn. Oxford University Press, New York

Braitenberg V, Atwood RP (1958) Morphological observations on the cerebellar cortex. J Comp Neurol 109:1–27

<reference>Brown JR (1949) Localising cerebellar syndromes. J Am Med Assoc 141:518–21

Courville J, Cooper CW (1970) The cerebellar nuclei of *Macaca mulatta*, a morphological study. J Comp Neurol 140:241–254

Courville J, Faraco-Cantin F (1978) On the origin of the climbing fibers of the cerebellum: an experimental study in the cat with an autoradiographic tracing method. Neuroscience 3:797–809

De Coene B, Hajnal J V, Pennock J M, Bydder G M (1993) MRI of the brain stem using fluid attenuated inversion recovery pulse sequences. Neuroradiology 35:327–331

Déjerine J (1901, 1986) Anatomie des centres nerveux, vol 2. Rueff, Paris

Dow RS, Moruzzi G (1958) The physiology and pathology of the cerebellum. University of Minnesota Press, Minneapolis

Duvernoy HM (1978) Human brainstem vessels. Springer, Berlin Heidelberg New York

Duvernoy HM (1991) The human brain stem and cerebellum. Springer, Vienna New York

Eager RP (1963) Efferent cortico-nuclear pathways in the cerebellum of the cat. J Comp Neurol 120:81–83

Eccles JC, Ito M, Szentagothai J (1967) The cerebellum as a neuronal machine. Springer, New York Berlin Heidelberg

Flechsig P (1905) Einige Bemerkungen über die Untersuchungsmethoden der Grosshirnrinde, insbesondere des Menschen. Arch Anat Entwickl Gesch:337–444

Ghez C (1991) The cerebellum. In: Kandel ER, Scwartz JH, Jessel TM (eds) Principles of neural science, 3rd edn. Elsevier, New York, pp 626–646

Gilbert GJ (1960) The subcommissural organ. Neurology 10:138–142

Gilman S, Bloedel JR, Lechtenberg (1981) Disorders of the cerebellum. Contemp Neurol Ser, vol 210. Davis, Philadelphia

Gilman S (1985) The cerebellum: its role in posture and movement. In: Swasch M, Kennard C (eds) Scientific basis of clinical neurology. Churchill Livingstone, New York

Gordon B (1972) The superior colliculus of the brain. Sci Am 227:72–82

Henry JM (1982) Anatomy of the brainstem. In: Schaltenbrand G, Walker AE (eds) Stereotaxy of the human brain – anatomical, physiological, and clinical applications, 2nd edn. Thieme, Stuttgart, pp 37–59

Hikosaka O, Wurtz RH (1983a) Visual and oculomotor functions of monkey substantia nigra pars reticulata. I. Relation of visual and auditory responses to saccades. J Neurophysiol 49:1230–1252

Hikosaka O, Wurtz RH (1983b) Visual and oculomotor functions of monkey substantia nigra pars reticulata. II. Visual responses related to fixation of gaze. J Neurophysiol 49:1254–1267

Hikosaka O, Wurtz RH (1983c) Visual and oculomotor functions of monkey substantia nigra pars reticulata. III. Memory-contingent visual and saccade responses. J Neurophysiol 49:1268–1284

Hikosaka O, Wurtz RH (1983d) Visual and oculomotor functions of monkey substantia nigra pars reticulata. IV. Relation of substantia nigra to superior colliculus. J Neurophysiol 49:1285–1301

Holmes G (1922) The Croonian lectures of the clinical symptoms of cerebellar disease and their interpretation. Lancet i:1177–1182

Holmes G (1939) The cerebellum of man. Brain 62:1–30

Ito M (1989) Long-term depression. Annu Rev Neurosci 12:85–102

Jansen J, Brodal A (1940) Experimental studies on the intrinsic fibers of the cerebellum. II. The corticonuclear projection. J Comp Neurol 73: 267–321

Jansen J, Brodal A (eds) (1954) Aspect of cerebellar anatomy. Tanum, Oslo

Joseph JP (1980) Communications: Le rôle fonctionnel du cortex auditif: comparaison homme-animal. Rev Laryngol 101:327–334

Keene MFL, Hewer EE (1935) The subcommissural organ and the mesocoelic recess in human brain, with a note on Reissner's fibre. J Anat 69:501–7

Korneliussen HK (1972) The comparative anatomy and histology of the cerebellum: the human cerebellum, cerebellar connections and cerebellar cortex. University of Minnesota Press, Minneapolis, pp 164–174

Kunzle H, Akert K (1977) Efferent connections of cortical area 8 (frontal eye field) in *Macaca fascicularis:* a reinvestigation using the autoradiographic technique. J.Comp Neurol 173:147–164

Kunzle H, Akert K, Wurtz RH (1976) Projections of area 8 (frontal eye field) to superior colliculus in monkey: an autoradiographic study . Brain Res 117:487–492

Kuypers HGJM (1958) Corticobulbar connections to the pons and lower brainstem in man. Brain 81:364–388

Kuypers HGJM (1981) Anatomy of the descending pathways. In: Brooks VB (ed): Handbook of physiology, sect 1 The nervous system, vol 2: Motor control, part 2 (American Physiological Society Series) Williams and Wilkins, Baltimore, pp 597–666

Lalonde R, Boetz MI (1990) The cerebellum and learning process in animals. Brain Res Rev 15:325–332

Larsell O (1951) Anatomy of the nervous system, 2d edn. Appleton-Century-Crofts, New York

Larsell O, Jansen J (1972) (eds) The comparative anatomy and histology of the cerebellum: the human cerebellum, cerebellar connections and cerebellar cortex. University of Minnesota Press, Minneapolis

Lassek AM (1954) The pyramidal tract. Thomas, Springfield, Ill

Leblanc A (1995) The cranial nerves. Anatomy, imaging, vascularisation. Springer, Berlin Heidelberg New York

Leiner HC, Leiner AL, Dow RS (1989) Reappraising the cerebellum: What does the hindbrain contribute to the forebrain? Behav Neurosci 103:998–1008

Ludwig E, Klingler J (1956) Atlas cerebri humani. Karger, Basel

Magoun HW, Ranson SW (1935a) The central path of the light reflex: a study of the effect of lesions. Arch Ophthalmol 13:791–811

Magoun HW, Ranson SW (1935b) The afferent path of the light reflex: a review of literature. Arch Ophthalmol 13: 862–874

Magoun HW, Ranson SW, Mayer LL (1935c) The pupillary light reflex after lesions of the posterior commissure in the cat. Am J Ophthalmol 18:624–630

Martin GF, Holstege G, Mehler WR (1990) Reticular formation of the pons and medulla. In: Paxinos G (ed) The human nervous system. Academic Press, New York

Marr D (1969) A theory of cerebellar cortex. J Physiol (Lond) 202:437–470

McCormick DA, Thompson RF (1984) Cerebellum: Essential involvment in the classicaly conditioned eyelid response. Science 223:296–299

Mihailoff GA (1993) Cerebellar nuclear projections from the basilar pontine nuclei and nucleus reticularis tegmenti pontis as demonstrated with PHA-L tracing in the rat. J Comp Neurol 330:130–146

Moore JK (1987) The human auditory brain stem: a comparison view. Hearing Res 29:1–32

Nauta WJH, Kuypers HGJM (1958) Some ascending pathways in the brain stem reticular formation. In: Jasper HH et al. (eds) Reticular formation of the brain. Little Brown, Toronto, vol 99, pp 3–31

Nieuwenhuys R (1985) Chemoarchitecture of the brain. Springer, Berlin Heidelberg New York

Nieuwenhuys R, Voogd J, Van Huijzen Chr (1988) The human central nervous system. A synopsis and atlas, 3rd edn. Springer, Berlin Heidelberg New York

Olszeweski J, Baxter C (1954) Cytoarchitecture of the human brain stem. Lippincott, Philadelphia

Parent A (1986) . Comparative neurobiology of the basal ganglia. Wiley, New York

Parent A (1996) Carpenter's human neuroanatomy, 9th edn. Williams and Wilkins, Baltimore

Paturet G (1964) Traité d'anatomie humaine, vol 4: Système nerveux. Masson, Paris

Phillips DP (1988) Introduction to anatomy and physiology of the central auditory nervous system. In: Jahn AF, Santos-Sacchi J (eds) Physiology of the ear. Raven Press, New York, pp 407–427

Ramon-Moliner E, Nauta WJH (1966) The isodendritic core of the brain stem. J Comp Neurol 126:311–335

Riley HA (1943) An atlas of the basal ganglia, brain stem and spinal cord. Williams and Wilkins, Baltimore

Schlesinger B (1976) The upper brainstem in the human. Its nuclear configuration and vascular supply. Springer, Berlin Heidelberg New York

Schmahmann JD (1991) An emerging concept. The cerebellar contribution to higher function. Arch Neurol 48:1178–1187

Seeger W (1978) Atlas of topographical anatomy of the brain and surrounding structures. Springer, Vienna New York

Sherrington CS (1906) The integrative action of the nervous system. Scribner, New York (reprinted by Yale University Press in 1947)

Sprague JM (1972) The superior colliculus and pretectum in visual behaviour. Invest Ophthalmol 11:473–482

Sprague JM, Meikle T Jr (1965) The role of the superior colliculus in visually guided behaviour. Exp Neurol 11:115–146

Sterling P, Wickelgren BG (1969) Visual receptive fields in the superior colliculus of the cat. J Neurophysiol 32:1–15

Tamraz J (1983) Atlas d'anatomie céphalique dans le plan neuro-oculaire (PNO) MD Thesis. Schering, Paris

Tamraz J, Iba-Zizen MT, Cabanis EA (1984) Atlas d'anatomie céphalique dans le plan neuro-oculaire (PNO) . J Fr Ophtalmol 7:371–379

Tamraz J, Iba-Zizen MT, Atiyeh M, Cabanis EA (1985) Atlas d'anatomie céphalique dans le plan neuro-oculaire (PNO) Bull Soc Fr Ophtalmol, 8–9, 85: 853–857

Tamraz J, Saban R, Reperant J, Cabanis EA (1990) Définition d'un plan de référence céphalique en imagerie par résonance magnétique: le plan chiasmato-commissural. CR Acad Sciences, Paris, 311, III:115–121

Tamraz J, Saban R, Reperant J, Cabanis EA (1991) A new cephalic reference plane for use with magnetic resonance imaging: the chiasmato-commissural plane. Surg Radiol Anat 13:197–201

Testut L, Latarjet A (1948) Traité d'anatomie humaine, vol 2: Angiologie, système nerveux central, 9th edn. Doin, Paris

Tomasch J (1969) The numerical capacity of the human cortico-ponto-cerebellar system. Brain Res 13:476–484

Thach WT, Goodkin HP, Keating JG (1992) The cerebellum and the adaptive coordination of movement. Annu Rev Neurosci 15:403–442

Von Monakov C (1905) Gehirnpathologie, 2d edn. Holde, Vienna

Voogd J (1964) The morphology of the cerebellum the last 25 years. Eur J Morphol 3:81–96

Voogd J, Feirabend HKP, Schoen JHR (1990) The cerebellum and precerebellar nuclei. In: Paxinos G (ed) The human nervous system. Academic Press, New York, pp 321–386

Wallesch CW, Horn A (1990) A long-term effect of cerebellar pathology on cognitive functions. Brain Cogn 14:19–25

Wickelgren BG, Sterling P (1969) Influence of visual cortex on receptive fields in the superior colliculus of the cat. J Neurophysiol 32:16–32

Williams PL, Warwick R, Dyson M, Bannister LH (1989) Gray's anatomy, 37th edition. Churchill Livingstone, London

Wyke BD (1947) Clinical physiology of the cerebellum, Med J Aust 2:533–40

Yamamoto T, Yoshida K, Yoshikawa H, Kishimoto Y, Oka H (1992) The medial dorsal nucleus is one of the thalamic relays of the cerebellocerebral responses to the frontal association cortex in the monkey: horseradish peroxidase and fluorescent dye double staining study. Brain Res 579:315–320

9 Optic Pathway and Striate Cortex

I Introduction

The visual pathways extend from anterior to posterior as the optic nerves, chiasm, optic tracts and optic radiations, terminating in the striate or visual cortex on the medial aspect of the occipital lobes. Along this orbitocranial route, the visual paths maintain a roughly axial and horizontal orientation from the eyes to the calcarine fissure.

We will proceed in this chapter, after a short history of the anatomy of the visual pathways, to a step-by-step investigation of the anatomy of these very long sensory tracts, focusing on the MR images which best depict the anatomic details and disease processes. This aim is essential because of the great sensitivity of the visual and the oculomotor systems to injury and to small mass lesions.

Anatomical correlations using MR imaging and routine thin slices (2, 3 or 5 mm) at high field strength (Signa 1.5 Tesla and Gyroscan 1.0 Tesla) are shown. Images are obtained using mainly T1 weighted inversion recovery (IR) or 3D gradient echo (SPGR) pulse sequences for studying the anterior optic pathways, and long TR FSE-T2 weighted or STIR sequences more specifically for exploration of the optic radiations. The objective is to achieve maximal contrast between the optic pathways and the various adjacent structures. Diagnostic algorithms applicable to specific regional pathology are proposed with the respective clinical correlations.

II Short History of the Anatomy of the Visual Pathways

During the second century, Galen (131–201), whose experiments on the nervous system of animals marked him as the first physiologist, described the optic nerves as pneumatic canals carrying sensation from the eyes to the brain. These canals connected each eye to the corresponding cerebral ventricle without any possibility of crossing over between right and left side. However, Galen thought that the canals joined each other at the midline, taking the aspect of an "X" before they separated immediately afterwards. He believed that this kind of exchange at the level of the chiasm allowed the pneuma to go to the opposite eyeball and double its strength if the other eye was destroyed. Furthermore, Galen attempted to justify the arrangement of the optic nerves and chiasm by an explanation of the binocular visual fields based on the geometry of converging cones whose apices were located at the pupils.

During the eighth century, medicine was reaching its apogee in Baghdad under the guidance of the Calif Al Ma'mun, who initiated an important work of translation of the scientific and philosophic heritage of antiquity. He asked the physician Abu Zayd Hunayn Ibn Ishaq Al'Ibadi (808–873), who belonged to a Christian tribe from Hiza and who was fluent in Arabic, Persian, Greek and Syrian, to take charge of this mission. Hunayn translated Galen and was particularly interested in the anatomical description of the eye, which he presented as the first figure. He was the author of the first Arabic textbook of ophthalmology, *Kitab al-ashr maqalat fi al'ayn*, a series of ten books. These were preserved thanks to different medieval Latin translations (*liber de oculis translatus a Demetrio et liber de oculis Constantini africani*).

The first representation of the chiasm showing a total crossing over of the optic nerves was in 1266, in an Arabic book of ophthalmology by the Syrian Khalifah Ibn Abi Al-Mahasin Al-Halabi from Alep (Hirschberg 1905). The figure (reproduced in Fig. 9.1) shows the brain and its ventricles. These were considered to be the sites of the five senses, as reported by Abou el Ala Hossein Ibn Sina in his *Al-Kanun*, a three-volume textbook written around the year 1000. The figure also shows the hollow nerves, in which the visual spirit emanates from the brain. Moreover, the optic nerve is represented with its two sheaths which penetrate the eye. The structure of the eye is also detailed.

The contribution of Arabian authors to the field of the anatomy of the visual system is generally

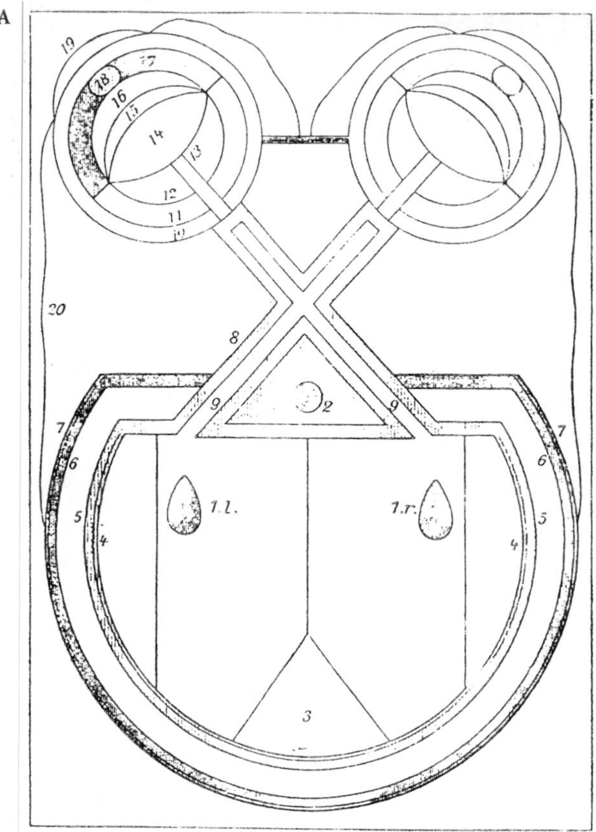

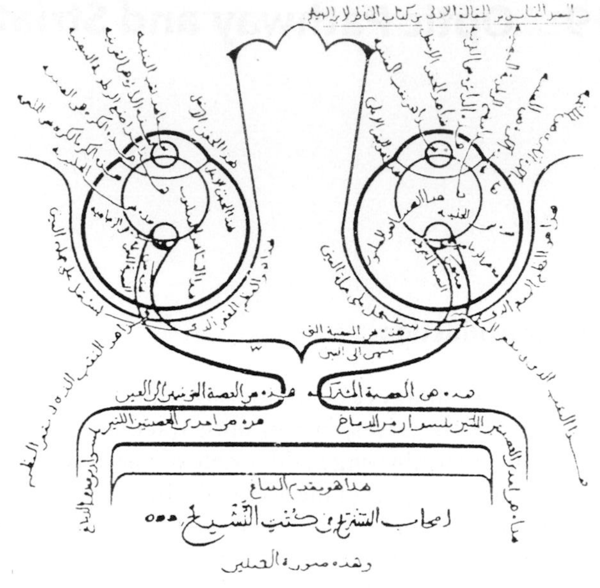

Fig. 9.1. First representation of the chiasm showing a complete crossing-over of the optic nerve fibers, attributed to Khalifah (1266), and first realistic representation of the eyes and the anterior optic pathways, annotated in Arabic and including the chiasma that could be attributed to Ibn Al. Haysem (965–1039)

grossly underestimated. Thus, it should be emphasized that Arabic manuscripts of ophthalmology books contain the oldest representations of the eye, the chiasm and the brain. It is of course true that they followed Galen's work, but they also tried to correct some of his mistakes.

Moreover, the first attempt at a comparative anatomy of animal eyes is found in Al-Shadhili's book of ophthalmology. Nonetheless, Arabic anatomy was not free of the traditional mistakes, such as the unusually deep posterior chamber of the eye, the location of the lens lying in the center of the eyeball or the canal within the optic nerves.

In the Renaissance era, the discovery of printing with moveable type greatly advanced the diffusion of knowledge. In 1543, Vesali, (1514–1664) in Belgium, in the *Fabrica,* his first textbook of modern anatomy,, revealed Galen's mistakes and showed the first exact reproduction of the inferior surface of the brain and the chiasm (Fig. 9.2). He also suggested the existence of a cavity inside the optic nerves, except possibly for the chiasm. However, he persisted in believing that there is no real crossing-over of the nerves, but rather a simple juxtaposition at the chiasmatic level. A half a century before, Da Vinci, following the concept of total decussation of the optic nerves elaborated by the Arabs, was the first to describe in his anatomical drawings the true crossing. Unfortunately the drawings remained confidential until his "cahiers" were discovered at the end of the nineteenth century.

In 1573, Varoli (1543–1575), in Italy, published the first book devoted to the optic nerve and demonstrated its thalamic origin from the lateral aspect of the third ventricle (Fig. 9.3). This had been already reported by Eustache, in 1551, but had not been shown. Being very poor, Eustache was unable to print the plates of his anatomical atlas, which were edited in 1617 by the physician Lancisi. Lancisi, after a very long search, found this work 50 years after the author's death.

The concepts of Galen were still very widely accepted by the middle of the seventeenth century. Descartes (1596–1650), in France, still believed in this mechanistic representation of vision, i.e., that optic nerves do not decussate at the level of the chiasm. Each nerve was thought to originate from a precise region of the lateral ventricle and follow a paral-

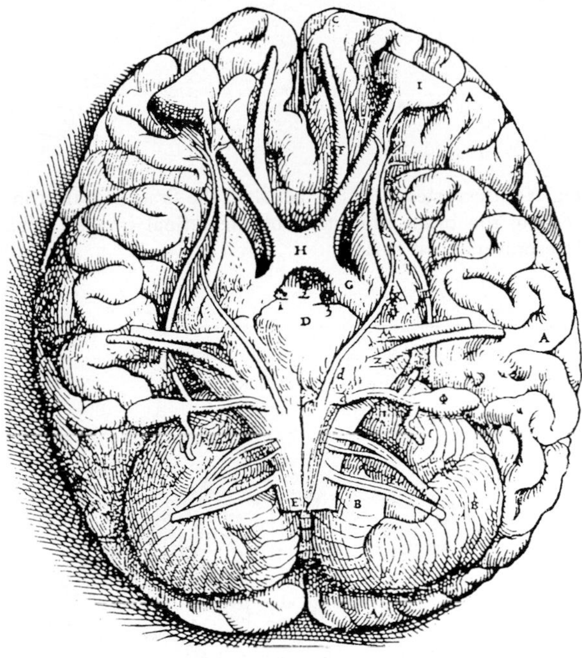

Fig. 9.2. Vesali (1543) shows the first exact reproduction of the inferior surface of the brain and the chiasm (Bibl. Museum National d'Histoire Naturelle, Paris)

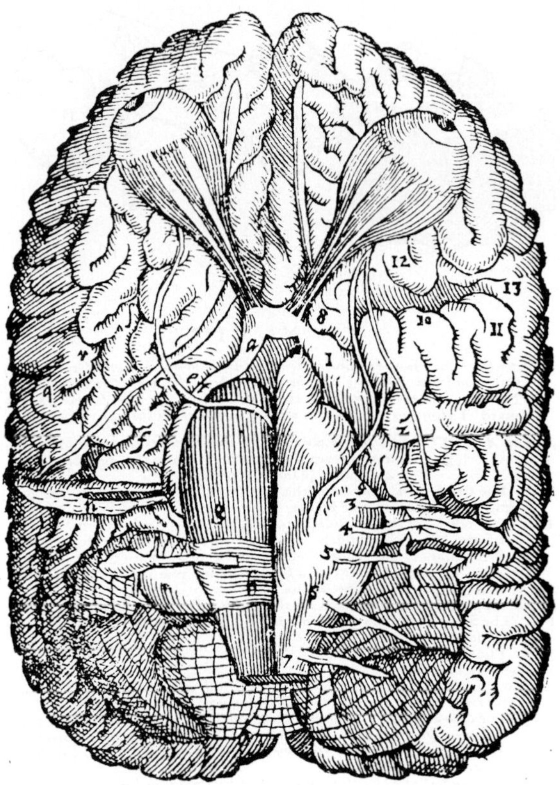

Fig. 9.3. Varoli (1573) shows the optic nerves and the chiasm as well as a dissection of the optic radiations (Bibl. Museum National d'Histoire Naturelle, Paris)

lel chiasmatic route before terminating in the retina in a precisely defined manner. Images were thus thought to be transmitted to the pineal gland, separately for each eye, before they were memorized inside the brain (Fig. 9.4). These speculations may be considered as the preliminary steps in understanding regionalization of the retinal projections.

In 1644, Willis (1622–1675); in Great Britain, published the first textbook on brain anatomy. He demonstrated that the optic nerve is composed of fascicles of nervous fibers, instead of a hollow tube, originating from the thalamus. Willis also discovered the tracts connecting the internal structures to the cortex and recognized the existence of higher centers responsible for voluntary motility. The superior and inferior colliculi were described as glands. Collins, in 1685, showed a very good representation of the optic tracts and their connections to the thalami; he also dissected the temporal horns of the lateral ventricle (Fig. 9.5).

A century later in France, Vicq d'Azyr (1775–1794), demonstrated, in 1786, the diversity of cortical structures inside the occipital lobe. He defined the tracts connecting the structures observed by Willis and Vieussens (1641–1715) and showed, in his *Traité d'Anatomie et de Physiologie*, devoted to the brain, a cut of the cerebral hemisphere passing through the optic pathways. This cut (Fig. 9.6), similar to what is obtained presently on magnetic resonance imaging, shows the optic nerve junction, the optic tract, the enlargement of the posterior tubercle of the optic tectum and the implantation of the brain "legs."

From that time, anatomical knowledge of the visual pathways progressed quickly and continued during the nineteenth century. Burdach, in 1819, and later Gratiolet, in 1854, described the continuity of the fibers of the visual tract projecting as terminal fibers to the vicinity of the calcarine fissure. In 1869 Meynert demonstrated the role of the lateral geniculate body in vision and its connections with the temporal and occipital lobes via the optic radiations. Finally, Flechsig (1896 1900) was the first to elaborate the time course of myelination in the fetus and showed that, just before birth, myelination commences in the optic nerve and the geniculocalcarine tract.

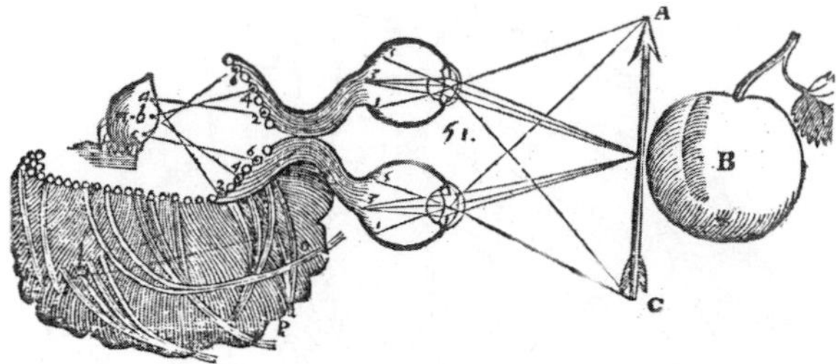

Fig. 9.4. Descartes (1664) established the first diagram concerning the brain projection of the retinal images (Bibl. Interuniversitaire, Paris)

Tab. XLVIII.

Repreſents an Humane Brain, with its Baſis upward, and diveſted of the Dura *and* Pia Mater ; *the better to ſhew the true Origination of the Nerves, and the running of the Fibres, laid open by Learned* Dr. Edward Tyſon, *in the* Theater *of the Colledge of Phyſicians in* London.

A A A A. THE four Lobes of the Brain, wherein the diviſion of the Anterior from the Poſterior, as alſo the *Anfractus* in each, are more plainly repreſented

B B. The *Cerebellum*, and here the Circles which compoſe it, are plainer and truer than in any Figure yet.

C C. The edges of the Medullary part of the Brain, which lines the inſides of the Ventricles which were here opened, only by ſeparating the Membranes, and Blood-veſſels, and gently dilating it with my Fingers, only at (*c c c c.*) a ſmall Inciſion was made with the knife.

D D. The Ventricles of the Brain.

e e e e. Four large Blood-veſſels on the inſide of the Ventricles.

F F. The *Tunica*, or *Plexus Coroides* in its natural ſituation, but a little expanded.

g g g. The Carotide Arteries.

h. The *Infundibulum.*

i i. Two round protuberant Bodies which Dr. *Willis* calls Glands, but are of the ſame ſubſtance with the Medullary part of the Brain.

K K. The *Crura Medullæ oblongatæ*, compoſed of ſeveral *Faſciculi* of nervous Fibres, which continued, makes the *Striæ* in the *Corpora Striata* ; between theſe *Faſciculi*, run ſeveral Blood-veſſels, which pierce them quite through.

L L. The *Caudex Medullæ oblongatæ*, whereby the *Cerebellum* is joyned to the *Cerebrum*, and is covered with ſeveral *Faſciculi* of Fibres, which make the *Protuberantia annularis* of Dr. *Willis*.

M. The *Medulla oblongata, ſeu Medullæ Spinalis principium.* This, as likewiſe the former body (*L L*) by Dr. *Willis*, are both called *Medulla oblongata* ; but I think there is great reaſon to diſtinguiſh them, ſince Nature has ſo remarkably done it to our hands ; for the Surface of one is ſtriated, the other plain ; the former is common to the *Cerebrum* and *Cerebellum* ; the latter is conjoyned to neither of them, but immediately to the *Caudex*.

N N. The Olfactory, or firſt pair of Nerves, where it is obſervable

o o o o. Its double Origination, not before remarked.

P P. The Optic, or Second pair of Nerves.

Q Q. Of the *Thalami nervorum Opticorum.*

r r. The Motory, or Third pair of Nerves.

s s. The Pathetic, or Fourth pair of Nerves.

t t. The Fifth pair of Nerves

v v. The Sixth pair of Nerves.

w w. The Auditory, or Seventh pair of Nerves, which are double.

x x. The *Par vagum*, or Eighth pair of Nerves.

y y. The acceſſary Nerve, that runs to the *Par vagum*, or Eighth pair.

z z. The Ninth pair of Nerves.

« «. The Tenth pair of Nerves.

Tab. XLIX

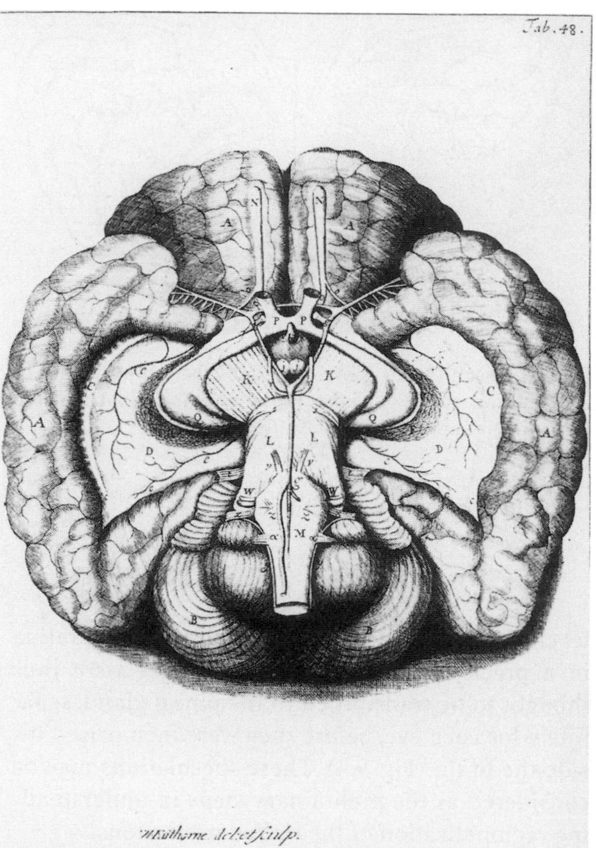

Fig. 9.5. Collins (1685) shows an excellent representation of the optic tracts and their connections to the optic thalami, as well as a dissection of the temporal horns of the lateral ventricles (Bibl. Museum National d'Histoire Naturelle, Paris)

III Elements of Ontogenesis, Phylogenesis and Teratology

A Ontogenesis of the Visual System

The visual pathways develop from the rostral portion of the neural tube which contribute to form the prosencephalon and the posterior optic pathways in higher mammals, and the mesencephalon, related to the visual sense in lower vertebrates and to the visuomotor systems in higher vertebrates including human (Polyak 1957; Hamilton et al. 1962; Duke-Elder 1973).

Before complete closure of the anterior end of the neural tube, the spherical optic vesicles grow on either side, connected to the prosencephalon by the optic stalks. This pattern of development is visible in a 4 mm human embryo at the 3 weeks stage. The optic stalks contain a circular lumen which is continuous with both cavities, the optic vesicles distally and the prosencephalon proximally. A simultaneous invagination of the lower aspect of the optic vesicles and stalks forms the fetal, or choroidal, fissure, which will allow penetration of the vascular mesoderm. A progressive narrowing, until closure of the choroidal fissure and leaving a small opening to the hyaloid artery, is completed at the 6 weeks stage. At this time the general structure of the eyeball is determined (Mann 1964).

Soon after, at the 17 mm stage, the nerve fibers begin to grow from the ganglion cells of the retina and reach the optic stalk. Penetrating the stalk, the nerve fibers proceed proximally toward the brain, forming the future optic nerves. At the 25 mm stage, the stalk is invaded and the optic nerves are already formed by 7 weeks. The optic vesicles and stalks no longer communicate with the prosencephalic cavity.

By the fifth month, the dura mater is noticeable and formation of the arachnoid sheath takes place 1 or 2 months later. During this period, the optic nerves increase in length and diameter, reaching 7–8 mm. At birth, the optic nerves measure about 24 mm and lengthen progressively to adapt to orbital growth until puberty, averaging at this time 40 mm in length and 3 or 4 mm in diameter.

Between the fourth and sixth weeks of development, an intermixing of the optic nerve fibers takes place, forming the optic chiasm at the seventh week. The chiasm occupies the third ventricular floor at the junction of the telencephalon and diencephalon. Note that uncrossed fibers do not appear until the eleventh week, a partial decussation similar to the adult being present at the thirteenth week. The chiasm attains its shape about 2 weeks later, at the 100 mm stage.

Myelination of the optic fibers, dependent on glial oligodendrocytes, becomes evident about the fifth month and develops in the opposite direction to fiber growth, beginning in the lateral geniculate body. The optic tracts and the chiasm become myelinated by the sixth month, and at the eighth month the myelination process involves the optic nerves, progressing distally to reach at birth and some weeks after the level of the lamina cribrosa (Bembridge 1956; Magoon and Robb 1981). At this period the posterior visual pathways undergo their myelination process, which proceeds from the occipital poles centrifugally and ends around 5 months after birth.

B Phylogenesis of the Anterior Optic Pathways

Observation of vertebrates shows that the human brain resembles the brains of other animals, specifically primates, more than it differs from them. The divergent characteristics of the vertebrate central nervous system are explained by the fact that its components have failed to evolve consistently. Hence, the study of comparable anatomic structures in different species can be carried out. Evolution of the visual system best illustrates this fact (Crescitelli 1977). The main observations concerning evolution of the eyes and the optic pathways of vertebrates are discussed below.

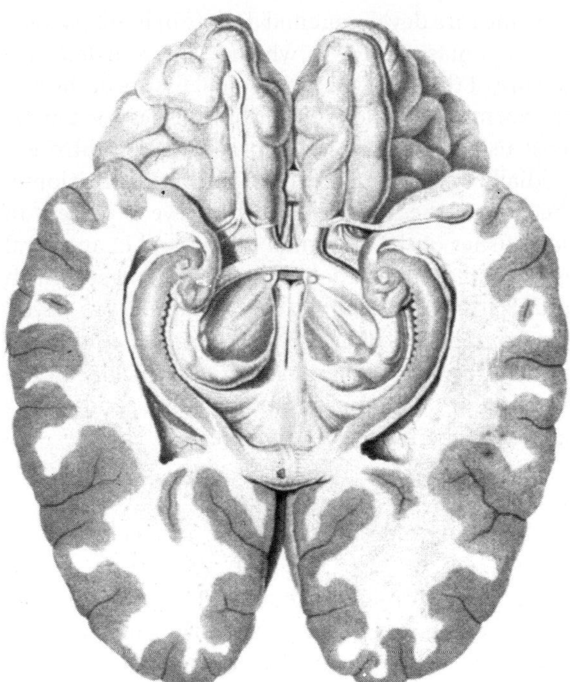

Fig. 9.6. Vicq d'Azyr (1786) shows a realistic anatomical cut passing through the retro-chiasmal optic pathways, including the chiasm and the pericrural optic tracts surrounded laterally by the hippocampal formations, nicely displayed in relation to the temporal horns. The cut is strictly temporal, showing the basal aspect of the orbitofrontal cortex, as observed in a MR cut oriented according to a chiasmato-commissural (CH-PC) orientation (Bibl. Museum National d'Histoire Naturelle, Paris)

1 The Eyes

Eyes are fundamentally similar in all vertebrates but function in a specialized manner in each class. Comparative anatomy of the eyes has been exhaustively reviewed by several authors, including Rochon-Duvigneaud (1943) and Polyak (1957). Paired eyes occur in almost all vertebrates, even though very small in some species, and the diameter of the optic nerve depends on the size of the eyeball. In primates, the size of the eye is about 30 mm, more exactly 24 mm in humans. In blind animals, e.g., the golden mole, eyes become very filiform.

Some rare developmental defects in humans, such as colobomas of the eyes, which result from defective closure of the embryonic choroidal fissure of the eye, are normal conditions in certain species such as teleost fish. Some lower vertebrates show a third eye medially situated on the forehead, in a depression in the roof of the skull. This median eye is present in bony fishes of the Devonian period and in ancestral amphibians and reptiles. It is still found in some fish and lizards. Embryologically, the parietal eye develops from the pineal organ. This parietal eye of lower vertebrates is not homologous to the cyclopean eye found in human monsters which is the result of fusion of the paired eyes of humans.

2 The Optic Nerves

Optic nerves are found in all vertebrates with eyes and are composed of axons of retinal ganglion cells. The fibers terminate in the optic tectum of lower animals and in the lateral geniculate body in mammals. In lower vertebrates the fibers are thought to be collateral ramifications of the opticotectal fibers. Fibers projecting to the lateral geniculate body predominate in mammals. In humans and other mammals, and probably in all vertebrates, optic nerve fibers are arranged in a precise retinotopic manner.

Myelination of these fibers is sparse in lower vertebrates and becomes very extensive in terrestrial vertebrates (Fig. 9.7). Recent research using electronic microscopy (Repérant and Saban 1986) and performed in mammals has permitted evaluation of the number of fibers contained in the optic nerves of different species,. For example, in marsupials, there are 230,000 fibers, 98% of which are myelinated; in carnivores the number is reduced to 145,000 fibers. In rodents there are 130,000 fibers and in cetaceans 155,000 fibers.

3 The Chiasm

Optic nerves form the chiasm by decussating in the floor of the third ventricle. In primates, when comparing prosimians, such as the lemur, and catarrhinians , such as the gibbon, the chiasm appears increasingly embedded between the temporal lobes which undergo an anterior displacement due to the significant development of the occipital lobes. Considering the size of the chiasm, it is relatively more voluminous in primates whose activity is mainly crepuscular, such as the lemur, than in, e.g., the gibbon (Fig. 9.8).

The need for decussation of optic nerves to compensate for image reversal in all vertebrates eyes was well demonstrated by Cajal. In humans and older primates, optic tracts contains an almost equal number of fibers originating from each eye. In other mammals, contralateral eye fibers predominate in each tract. In nonmammalian vertebrates, optic nerve axons do not decussate completely. Thus, the presence of at least a small uncrossed component of fibers in the optic nerves is phylogenetically very old (Fig. 9.9).

4 The Lateral Geniculate Body

The lateral geniculate body, the major relay structure transmitting optic impulses to the visual cortex in humans and other mammals, is found also in many lower vertebrates – even if in some species it is not entirely homologous to the structure found in humans (Le Gros Clark 1941) (Fig. 9.10). The lateral geniculate body is very large in reptiles and in lower mammals. In most vertebrates, it consists of ventral and dorsal nuclei.

5 The Visual Cortex

It is commonly accepted, even if not entirely correct, that the optic tectum is the principal visual center in submammalian vertebrates and that its function shifts to the cerebral cortex in mammals. This concept of cephalization of visual function in phylogeny is suggested by the relative volume of the optic tectum in comparison with the very small forebrain in lower vertebrates, and the extensive development of the cortical mantle in mammals. In the latter, the neocortical region for vision is clearly differentiated in the occipital lobe.

The primary visual cortex is relatively isolated in placental mammals, lying along the calcarine fissure in the medial aspect of the cerebral hemisphere. In reptiles and especially in birds, a laminated structure similar to the primary visual cortex of mammals is demonstrated in the hyperstriatum. This means that the highest visual center in birds is similarly located in the telencephalon and suggests that vision is a telencephalic function that evolved early in both lower vertebrates and in mammals (Repérant and Saban 1986; Repérant et al. 1989).

Perhaps the most interesting characteristic of the occipital lobe in primates is represented by the evolution of its gyral pattern, mainly of the striate area. Actually, the calcarine fissure is composed on the mesial aspect of the cerebral hemispheres in lemuri-

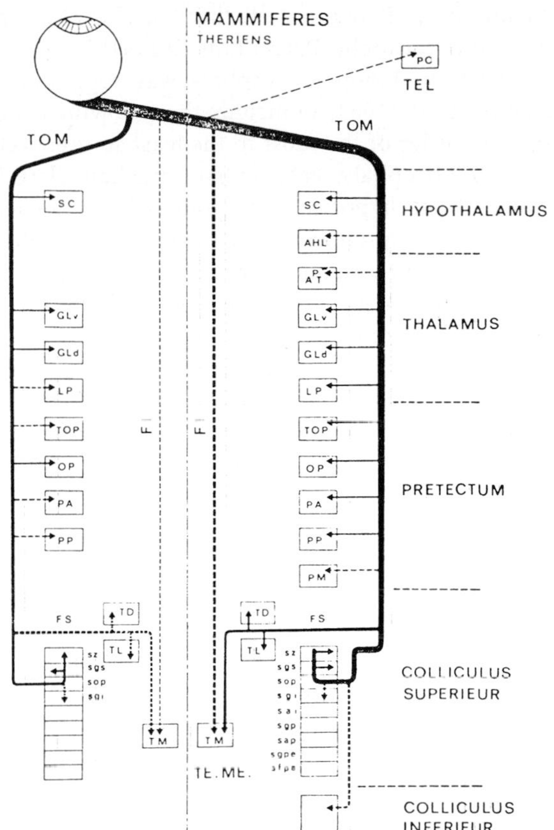

Fig. 9.7. Diagram of the primary visual system in mammals. (According to Repérant and Saban 1986)

ans as in humans of a complex combining a short sulcus somehow vertically oriented and a long posterior extension, the retrocalcarine sulcus. The short sulcus is hidden by the lips of retrocalcarine sulcus beginning with the simians (Fig. 9.11). The retrocalcarine fissure is the only one usually visible on the mesial aspect of the cerebral hemisphere. This fissure is exteriorized on the lateral aspect of the brain in platyrrhinians and certain catarrhinian cynomorphs (*Papio* and *Cercocebus*) as the lateral calcarine fissure (Osman Hill 1974).

6 Approach to Evolution Using Magnetic Resonance Imaging

Modern imaging modalities have given us the opportunity to approach the comparative anatomy of the head based on MR imaging of formalin specimens taken from the very large collection (500 specimens) of the Laboratoire d'Anatomie Comparée (R. Saban and J. Repérant) of the Museum National d'Histoire Naturelle in Paris (Tamraz 1991).

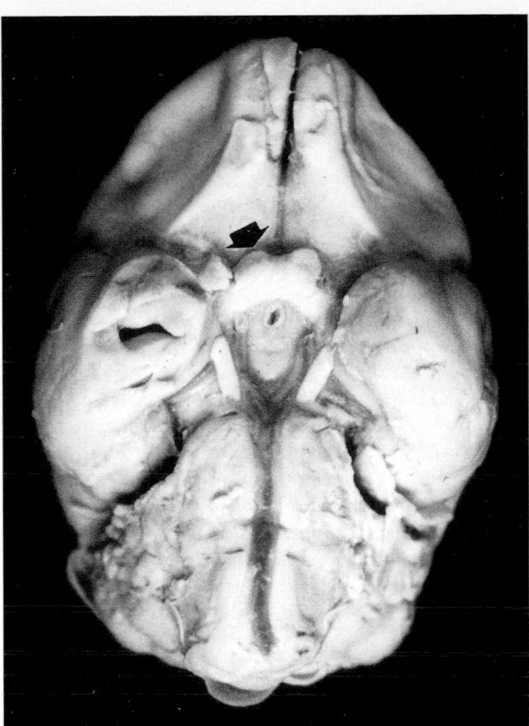

A

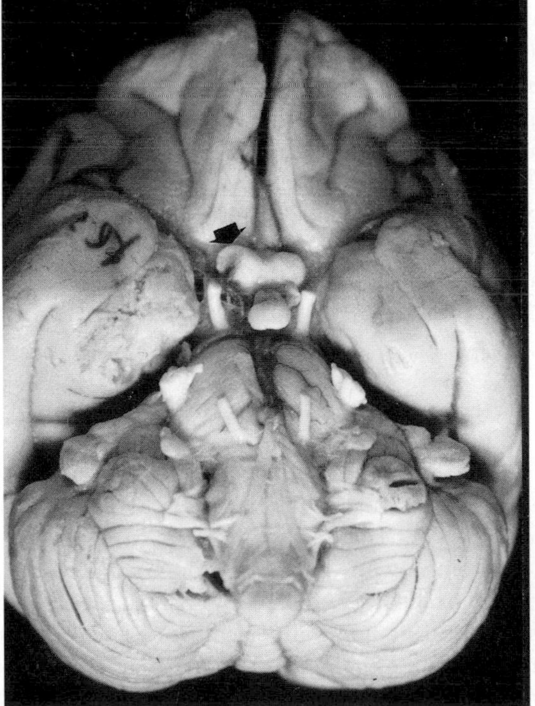

B

Fig. 9.8. A, B. Inferior view of the brain of a lemur (**A**) as compared to a gibbon (**B**), showing the chiasm (*arrow*) the size of which is relatively more voluminous in primates with crepuscular activity, e.g. lemurians (**A**). (Formalin specimen from the Museum National d'Histoire Naturelle, Laboratoire d'Anatomie Comparée, Paris; courtesy of R. Saban and J. Repérant)

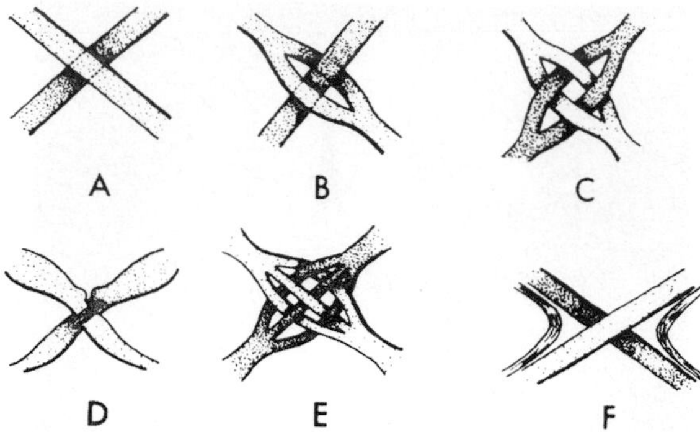

Fig. 9.9A–F. The chiasm of vertebrates, according to Pirlot (1969). In fish, the optic nerves form the chiasm either by simple overlaying (**A**) or by passing one through the other (**B**). In reptiles, a dissociation of optic fascicles and a complete crossing-over are observed (**C–E**). In mammals, a new arrangement is presented, comprising crossed and uncrossed components (**F**) in relation to the apparition of a stereoscopic vision

Biometric studies have been made possible due to the definition of cephalic reference planes permitting a comparison of the slices obtained in humans and animals. In living animals, the neuro-ocular plane (NOP) (Cabanis et al. 1981a,b, 1982) has been used (Saban et al. 1983–1985, 1987, 1989). In formalin-fixed brains, in which neuro-ocular plane landmarks are lacking, it has been possible to use the CH-PC reference plane, defined in vivo using MR imaging (Tamraz et al. 1989, 1990, 1991a,b; Saban et al. 1990), close to the NOP and roughly oriented along the direction of the posterior visual pathways, as related to the temporal horn of the lateral ventricle.

C Elements of Teratology: The Spectrum of Cyclopia

Since the exhaustive preliminary works of both Geoffroy Saint-Hilaire (1822), the father of systematic teratology who defined cyclopia, ethmocephaly and cebocephaly, and his son Isidore (1832), the striking morphologic abnormalities associated with the spectrum of holoprosencephalic facies continue to fascinate researchers. The eyes and orbits are probably the most impressive of these craniofacial dysmorphisms and tend to be almost pathognomonic of holoprosencephaly.

We had the opportunity to noninvasively study, using MR imaging, several specimens of formalin-fixed monstrous fetuses, obtained from the historical collection of the Laboratory of Comparative Anatomy (J. Repérant) at the Museum National d'Histoire Naturelle, Paris (Tamraz 1991b).

The term holoprosencephaly was suggested by Demyer et al. (1964) to include the following conditions in order of the most to the least severe: cyclopia, ethmocephaly, cebocephaly, median cleft lip with orbital hypotelorism, premaxillary agenesis and philtrum-premaxillary anlage with orbital hypotelorism. Intermediate forms are common.

Cyclopia shows a median monophthalmia (Fig. 9.12) or synophthalmia (Fig. 9.13) or anophthalmia. But the sine qua non for the diagnosis is the presence of a single median orbit. Commonly, the face may show a proboscis, which may be single or double protruding from the glabella, just above the median eye, but which might also be absent. True cyclopia has complete arhinia with no nose, no nasal bones, but a homologue of a nose, the median proboscis. Patients with a proboscis lateralis and two orbits should not be considered as cyclopian and tend to survive. The incidence of cyclopia is estimated to average 1/40,000 births. The degree of facial dysmorphism is strongly correlated with the severity of brain malformation: "the face predicting the brain" (Demyer et al. 1964).

Ethmocephaly is characterized by hypoteloric separate eyes in two separate orbits and a median proboscis as a rudimentary nose, which may be displaced upward. The median facial bones are hypoplastic or absent as in cyclopia. Considered as a transitional form between cyclopia and cebocephaly, it seems to be the rarest type (Fig. 9.14).

Cebocephaly, defined by Saint-Hilaire (1832), designates a facies characterized by orbital hypotelorism with two separate eyes in separate orbits and a nose with a single nostril. Its single median canal ends blindly. Cebocephaly has an incidence of about 1/15 ,000 births.

Concerning prognosis, patients with cyclopia and ethmocephaly do not survive the neonatal period in most cases. Cebocephalic patients may survive for days, week or several months. Ultrasonography as well as in utero MR imaging as early as the 19th week of gestation may reveal the malformative facies.

Concerning the brain malformation in holoprosencephaly, one may distinguish three main categories: (1) alobar holoprosencephaly corresponding to an abnormally small forebrain vesicle with absence of cleavage in two cerebral hemispheres; (2) semi-lobar holoprosencephaly, which is an intermediate form, showing a single ventricle with rudimentary lobes and an incomplete interhemispheric fissure; (3) lobar holoprosencephaly, which includes a

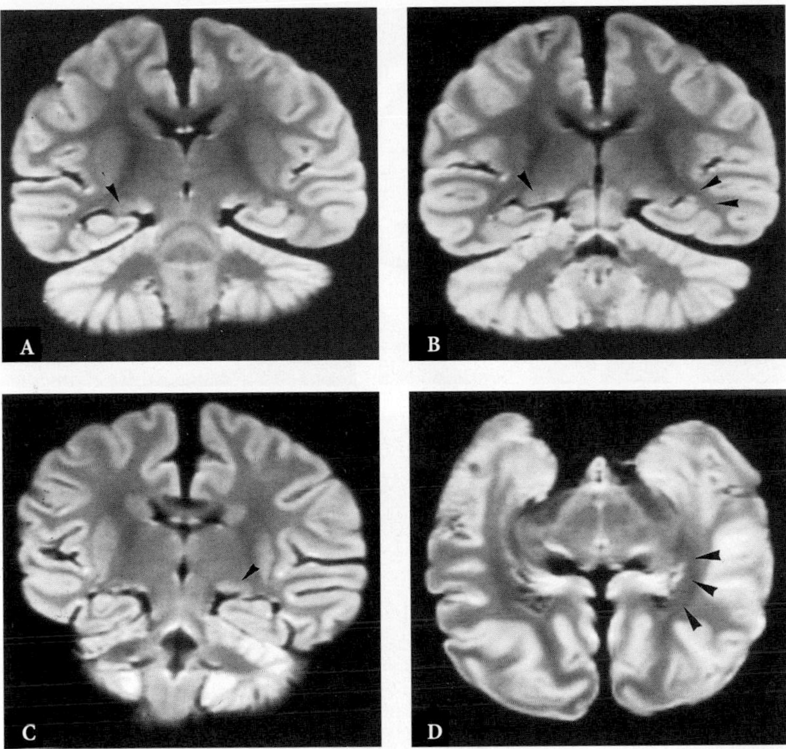

Fig. 9.10A–D. Magnetic resonance cuts of formalin brains (3 mm thick) showing the lateral geniculate bodies and the optic radiations of primates: Chimpanzee (**A,B** coronal) and orangutan (**C** coronal; **D** axial). The coronal cuts (**A–C**) are performed according to the commissural-obex (PC-OB) reference plane which includes in primates, as defined in humans, the lateral geniculate bodies (*arrow*). **D** An axial cut oriented in the chiasmatico-commissural plane showing the origin of the optic peduncles (*arrows*) from the lateral geniculate body. (Formalin specimen from the Museum National d'Histoire Naturelle, Laboratoire d'Anatomie Comparée, Paris; courtesy of R. Saban and J. Repérant; MR exams performed in the department of Neuroradiology, E.A. Cabanis, Quinze-Vingts National Hospital, Paris; from Tamraz 1991)

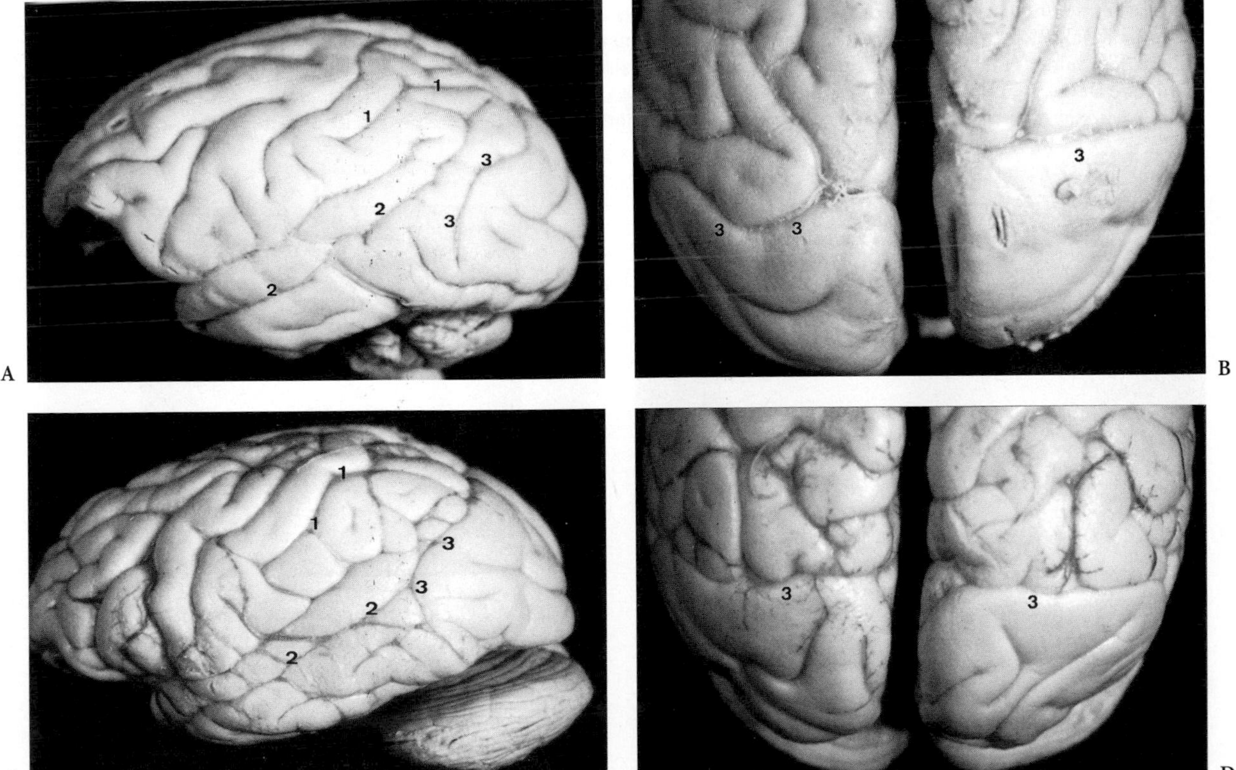

Fig. 9.11A–D. Lateral view of formalin brain of primates showing the sulcation (**A** *Papio*, **C** *Pan*) and posterior view of the hemisphere showing the occipital lobes (**B** *Papio*, **D** *Pan*). In catarrhinians, an increase in sulcation of the intraparietal (*1*), the parallel (*2*) and the lunate (*3*) sulci is observed. This is more marked in Anthropomorpha such as *Pan* than in Cynomorpha such as *Papio*. The lateral calcarine fissure is still observed in *Papio*. (Formalin specimen from the collection of the Museum National d'Histoire Naturelle, Laboratoire d'Anatomie Comparée, Paris; courtesy of R. Saban and J. Repérant)

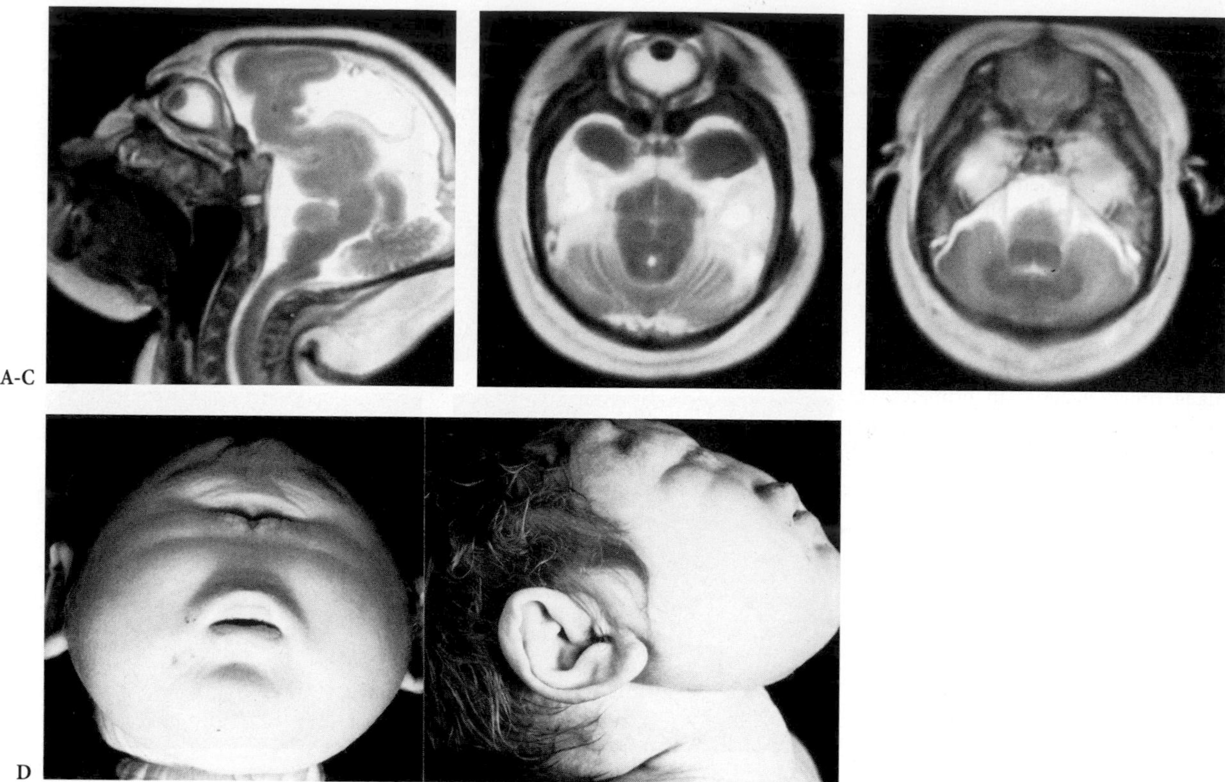

Fig. 9.12A–D. Cyclopia: the face (**D**) shows some typical clinical features comprising a single median aperture (hidden orbit), no nose but no proboscis, no philtrum and a mouth. MR shows in the sagittal (**A**) and axial (**B,C**) planes the single bony orbit, the optic canal, the median well-developed eye and the optic nerve. The associated cerebral malformation, which is an alobar holoprosencephaly with a tilted forward holotelencephaly, is also evidenced. (Formalin specimen from the Museum National d'Histoire Naturelle, Laboratoire d'Anatomie Comparée, Paris; courtesy of R. Saban and J. Repérant; MR exams performed in the department of Neuroradiology, E.A. Cabanis, Quinze-Vingts National Hospital, Paris; from Tamraz et al. 1991))

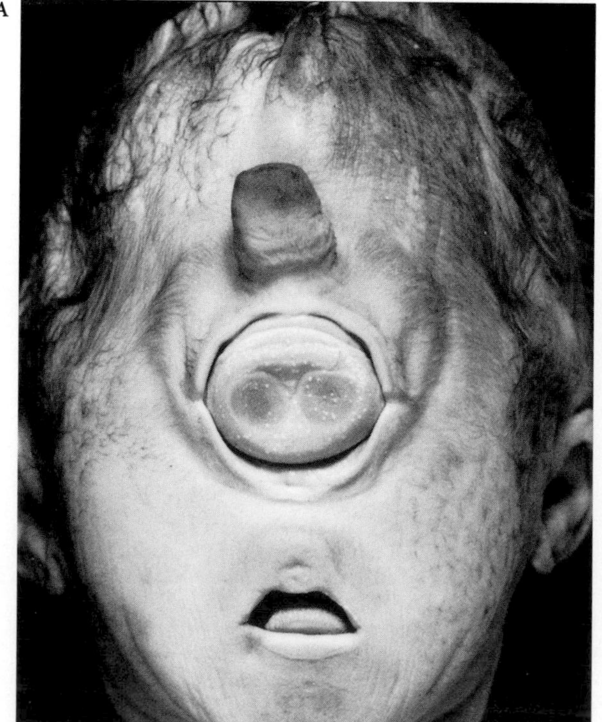

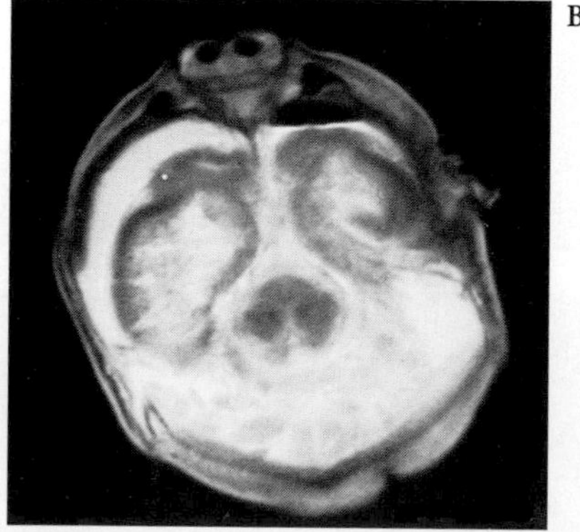

Fig. 9.13A,B. Cyclopia: The face (**A**) shows a single median orbit containing an eye with a partially doubled cornea and two lenses (synophthalmia). A median proboscis is clinically apparent protruding from the glabella above the eye. The mouth lack of philtrum. MR demonstrates the single bony orbit, the synophthalmia and the two lenses (**B**) as well as the absence of nasal bones. The median proboscis shows a single outer opening and a dead-end canal. (Formalin specimen from the collection of the Museum National d'Histoire Naturelle, Laboratoire d'Anatomie Comparée, Paris; courtesy of R. Saban and J. Repérant; MR exams performed in the department of Neuroradiology, EA Cabanis, Quinze-Vingts National Hospital, Paris; from Tamraz et al. 1991))

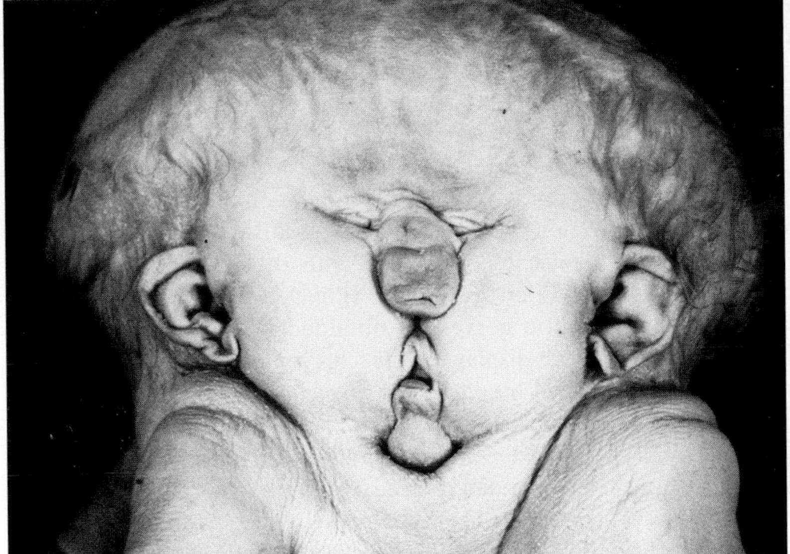
A

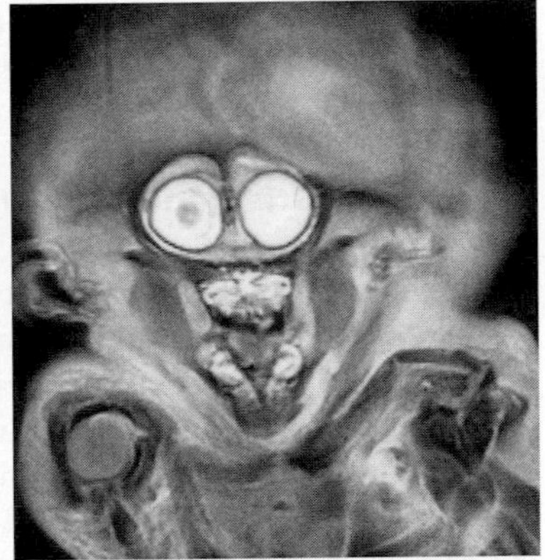
B

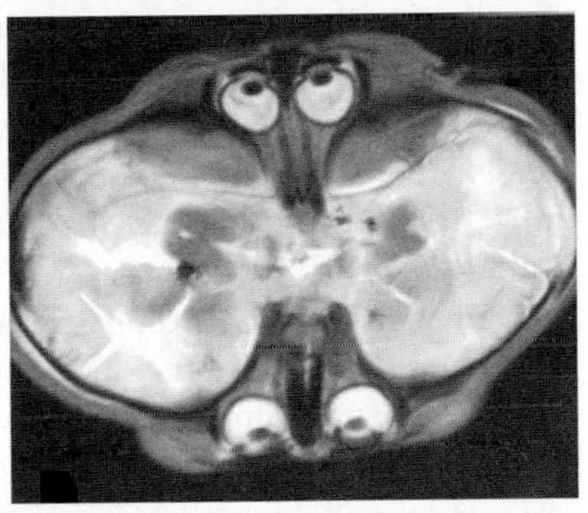
C

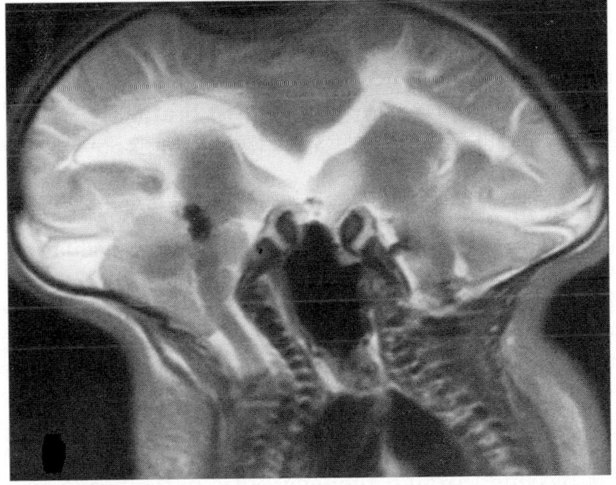
D

Fig. 9.14A–C. Monstrous fetus ("janiceps"): the face (**A**) shows the ethmocephalic facies with two separate palpebral fissures and hypoteloric orbits and a median proboscis between the two eyes). MR in the axial (**B**) and the coronal (**C**) planes shows an impressive arrangement of both orbits and both posterior fossa, facing each other in the axial NOP plane and crossed by both brainstems disposed on each side and oriented symmetrically in relation with the midsagittal plane, as shown on the coronal cut. (Formalin specimen from the Museum National d'Histoire Naturelle, Laboratoire d'Anatomie Comparée, Paris; courtesy of R. Saban and J. Repérant; MR exams performed in the department of Neuroradiology (EA Cabanis), Quinze-Vingts National Hospital, Paris; from Tamraz et al. 1991)

distinct interhemispheric fissure, with a possible midline cortical continuity mainly in the frontal lobes and a communication of the lateral ventricles due to the absence of the septum pellucidum.

Embryologically, holoprosencephaly is due to a failure of cleavage of the prosencephalon into cerebral and optic vesicles. The associated malformations of the brain and face, in humans and animals, may result from a primary defect in the prechordal mesoderm, which fails to produce the normal facial structures (the frontonasal prominence from which the median sector of the face derives) and causes abnormal brain development (Demyer and Zeman 1963). There is also evidence for related genetic causes (Réthoré 1977; Réthoré and Pinet 1987; Tamraz et al. 1987a; Cohen 1989; de Grouchy and Turleau 1982). Since the first reports concerning trisomy of a D group chromosome and deletion of the short arm of an E group chromosome, most of the available reports about phenotype-karyotype correlations concern trisomy 13 and monosomy 18p. To these may be added duplication of the distal short arm of chromosome 3 and deletion of the distal long arm of chromosome 7, among other syndromes.

IV Morphology and Functional Anatomy and Magnetic Resonance Imaging of the Visual System

A Cephalic Orientations and Visual Pathway

The interest shown by anatomists, anthropologists and neurosurgeons in anatomic and topographical correlations is widely documented in the scientific literature. Most of the reference works and atlases concerning the brain are based on an approach using the stereotaxic bicommissural line, as discussed in Chap. 2. Unfortunately such a cephalic orientation, roughly parallel to the orbitomeatal line, is much too oblique with respect to the visual pathways. This is why an accurate cephalic orientation becomes a necessity – in order to best visualize the optic pathways, either the optic nerves or the chiasm and the optic radiations.

Many authors have proposed reference planes and have tried to describe the different angulations with respect to the orbitomeatal line or according to an anthropologically based line (Van Damme et al. 1977; Hilal and Trokel 1977; Vining 1977; Cabanis et al. 1978; Salvolini et al. 1978; Unsold et al. 1980a–c; Tamraz et al. 1990, 1991a). The best compromise would be a reference plane suitable for exploration of both the optic pathways and the brain.

For this reason, the NOP, as the anatomophysiological cephalic reference plane, appears undoubtedly to be the most suitable for studying the visual pathway. It is, in our opinion, also efficient enough for evaluation of the retrochiasmatic pathways in routine practice.

1 The Neuro-ocular Plane

a Anatomical Imaging Correlations

From an anatomical point of view, the NOP is defined as passing through the lens, optic nerve heads and optic canals, with the patient maintaining primary gaze. Such an orientation provides the optimal condition for computerized tomography (CT) or MR exploration of the intraorbital structures, the partial volume effect on the optic nerves in particular being reduced to a minimum (Fig. 9.15). The mean angle between the NOP and the Frankfurt-Virchow plane (FVP) is about 7° (Cabanis et al. 1980, 1982a). The mean displacement of this plane from the anthropological plane is about 33 mm. The orbitomeatal plane, which is the classic radiologic reference plane (World Federation of Neurology 1961), is tilted at approximately 10° relative to the FVP. Fenart et al (1982), in an exhaustive work, described the relation of the orbital axis plane to several craniofacial reference lines, showing particularly its close parallelism to the prosthion-opisthion line (see Chap. 2).

It is interesting to note that the NOP provides a meridian cut through the globe and through the horizontal recti muscles, from the annulus of Zinn to their tendinous attachment on the eyeball. Cuts inferior and superior to the NOP show the vertical recti muscles (Fig. 9.16) with the MR correlation (Fig. 9.17). Coronal cuts (Fig. 9.24) perpendicular to the optic nerves, as obtained using NOP orientation, best display the muscles cone, showing the oculo-orbital muscles, and the related orbital intra- and extraconal spaces as well as the optic nerves.

In the chiasmal region, CT or the MR cut in the NOP is determined by the individual anatomy of this area, the height of the sella turcica and the type and obliquity of the chiasm. Considering the retrochiasmal visual pathways, these benefit from this cephalic orientation. In fact, the afferent visual paths in their entirety are oriented roughly parallel to the NOP successive cuts, depending on the slice thickness. However, some parts of the visual pathways depart somewhat from the ideal horizontal plane, for example, the chiasm, because of its variable position in the optic-chiasmatic cistern, the optic radiations, because they are thicker than a single cut, and the calcarine fissure, especially with its ascending portion.

Practically, the NOP is easily determined and allows rapid alignment of the head in the gantry. The line joining the centers of the pupils, which is precisely horizontal in the normal, determines the anterior portion of the plane. The second point is found about 33 mm above the tragion. External cutaneous landmarks, experimentally determined and visualized by an acanthomeatal line, close to Camper's line (see Chap. 2), are helpful in orienting the patient's head in the routine practice. Bony landmarks such as the prosthion-opisthion line may also be used in order to determine this plane on a scout view, as available with CT (Fig. 9.18).

b Oculo-orbital Topometry

The major advantage of the NOP orientation is the ability to perform several biometric measures that help in the evaluation of many normal, developmental or pathological conditions, as used, for example, in exophthalmometry (Fig. 9.19). Cabanis et al. (1980, 1982a,b) developed and reported using statistically validated, biometric, CT data, which include the following: (1) the external bicanthal plane (PBCE) constitutes the first reference line joining both external orbital rims in the NOP (average 97.5 mm ±4,4); (2)

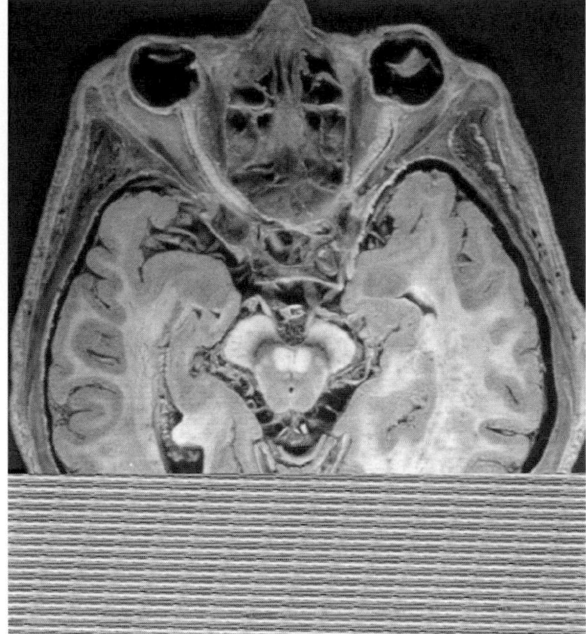

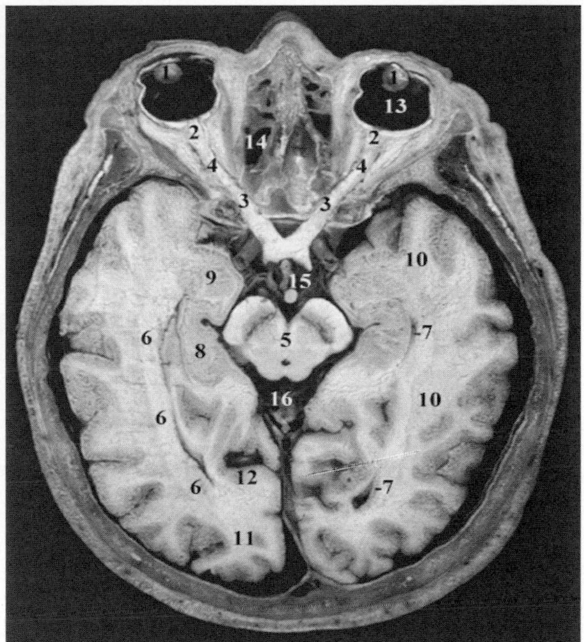

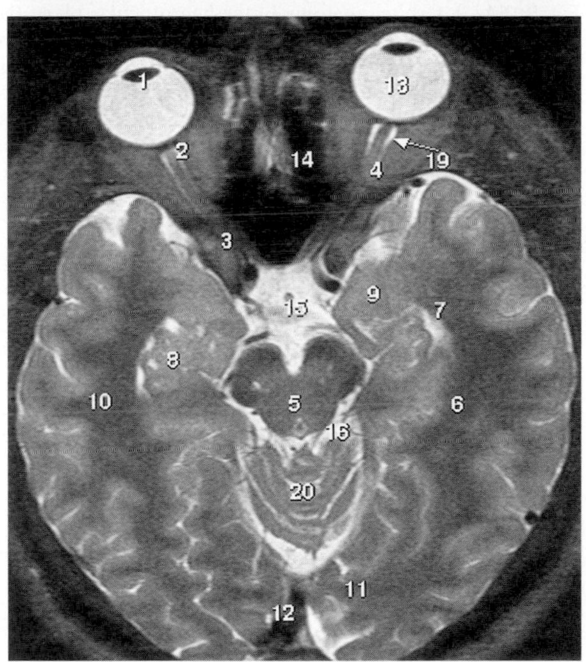

Fig. 9.15A–C. The neuro-ocular plane (NOP). Anatomic correlations showing the cephalic landmarks of this reference plane: the lenses, the optic cups and the optic canals. **A** Primary anatomical description, according to Cabanis 1978; **B** cut from the 3D cross-sectional anatomical atlas. (From Tamraz 1983; Cabanis et al. 1987). **B** is slightly more tilted caudad than A and passes through the upper part of the mesencephalon at the level of the superior colliculi and the red nuclei (**B**), the reference cut passing through the inferior collicular level and the decussation of the superior cerebellar peduncles and cutting through the entire length of the intraorbital optic nerves. **C** MR correlation using T2-w sequence. *1* Lens; *2* optic nerve head; *3* intracanalicular optic nerve; *4* intraorbital optic nerve; *5* midbrain; *6* optic radiation; *7* temporal horn of lateral ventricle; *8* hippocampus; *9* amygdala; *10* temporal lobe; *11* occipital lobe; *12* calcarine sulcus; *13* eyeball; *14* ethmoidal sinus; *15* chiasmal cistern; *16* ambient cistern; *17* cisternal optic nerve; *18* mamillary bodies; *19* perioptic subarachnoid spaces

the interocular distance (DIO) joining the center of both two lenses (average 63.7 mm±3.6); (3) the maximal interplanal distance (DIPM) separating the two internal orbital walls (average 28.7 mm±2.6 mm); (4) the maximal anteroposterior axial length of the eyeball (LAM) (average 24.1 mm±1 on the right as well as on the left side); (5) the pre-PBCE segment (ABCE) of the eyeball (average 16 mm±1.9); (6) the retro-PBCE segment (RBCE) of the eyeball, corresponding to the complementary of the last value; (7) the transverse diameter of the intraorbital optic nerve, measured at its middle portion (average 3.5 mm±0.5). Several indices are also proposed: (1) the neuro-ocular index (INO), corresponding to DNO/LAM (average 14,8±0,74); (2) the oculo-orbital index, or index of proptosis, corresponding to PBCE segment/LAM (average 65.44) and meaning that 65% of the eyeball in adults is located anterior to the

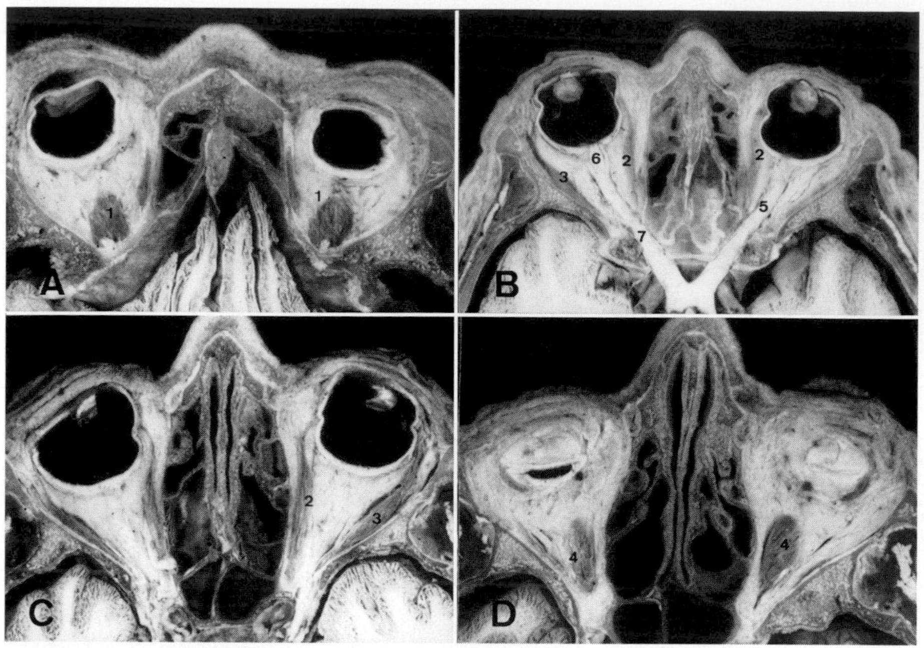

Fig. 9.16A–D. Orbital anatomy in the neuro-ocular plane (NOP). plane. The successive axial cuts display from superior to inferior the ocular muscles: the superior recti (**A**), the lateral recti (**B,C**), the inferior recti (**D**), well-displayed from their ocular attachment to the orbital apex. *1* Superior rectus muscle; *2* medial rectus muscle; *3* lateral rectus muscle; *4* inferior rectus muscle; *5* intraorbital optic nerve; *6* optic nerve head; *7* intra-canalicular optic nerve; *8* orbital fat; *9* lens; *10* eyeball; *11* ophthalmic artery (latero-optic loop); *12* intra-canalicular ophthalmic artery; *13* internal carotid artery (supra-clinoid segment); *14* anterior clinoid process; *15* superior oblique muscle (trochlea); *16* sphenoid sinus; *17* ethmoidal cells; *18* chiasmal cistern; *19* superior ophthalmic vein; *20* sella turcica; *21* lacrimal gland; *22* superior orbital fissure

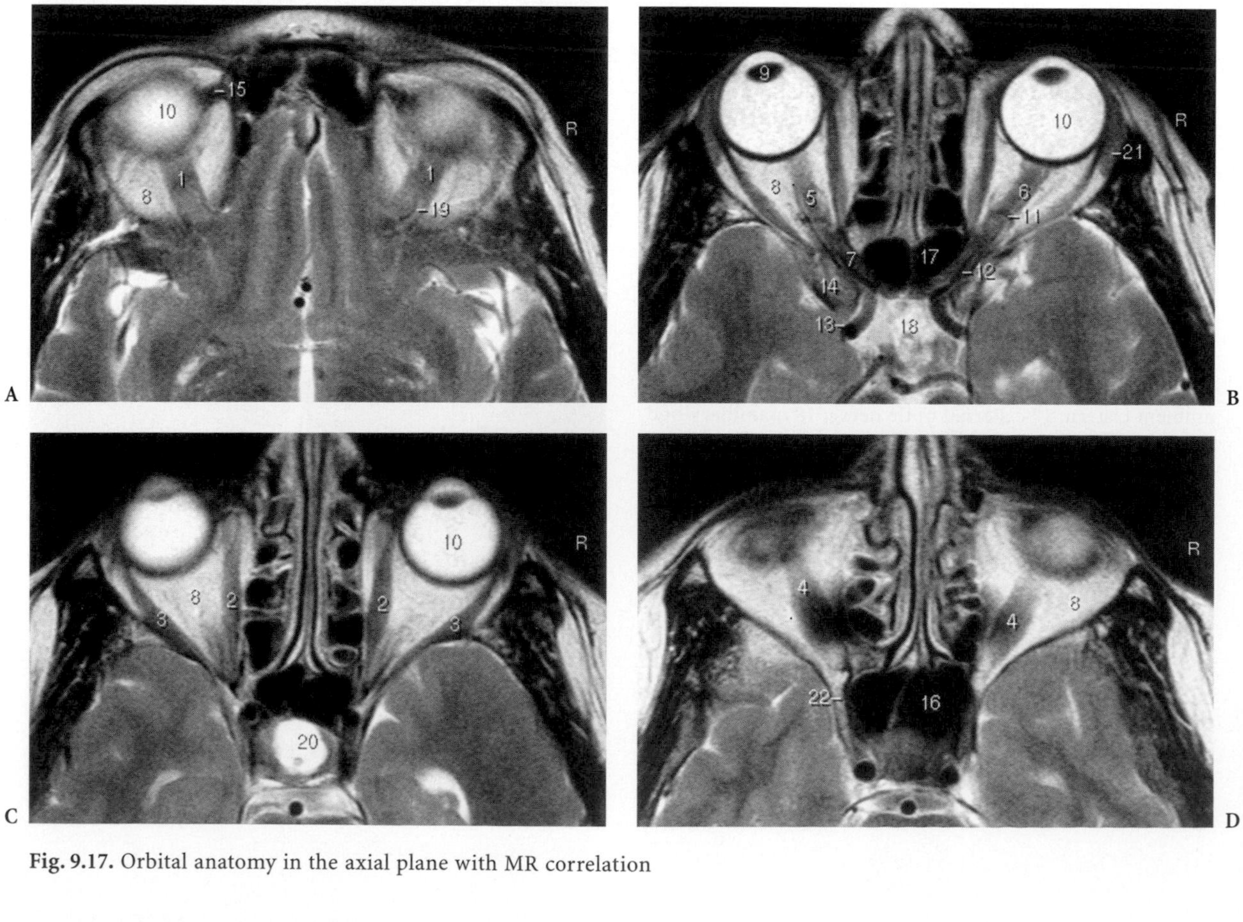

Fig. 9.17. Orbital anatomy in the axial plane with MR correlation

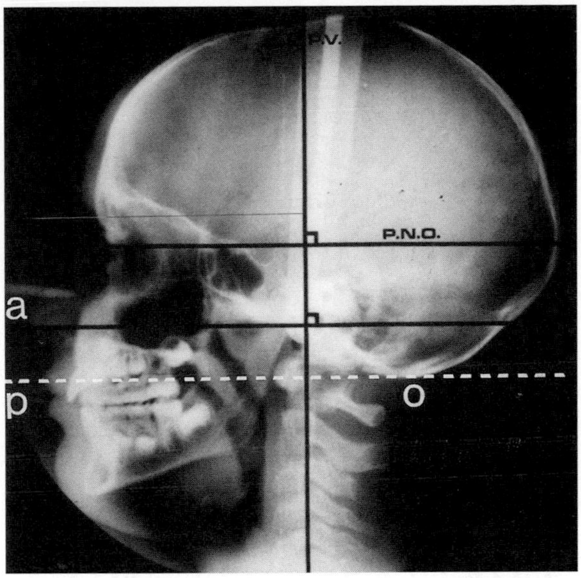

Fig. 9.18. Cutaneous and cranial landmarks of the neuro-ocular plane (NOP).. Teleradiography of the head showing the projection of the cutaneous "acanthomeatal" line on the skull and its parallelism to NOP orientation (Courtesy of E.A. Cabanis, Paris, modified), and the close parallelism of the prosthion-opisthion cranial reference line (from Fenart et al. 1982). *PNO,* neuro-ocular plane; *a,* acanthomeatal line (cutaneous landmarks); *po,* prosthion-opisthion line (cranial landmarks)

external bicanthal plane in normal conditions; (3) the interocular distance index (IDIO) corresponding to DIO/DBCE (average 65.3), indicating that the interpupillary distance corresponds to two thirds of the external intercanthal distance (DBCE). Other distances, indices and angular measures are also defined.

2 The Chiasmatico-Commissural Plane

In order to facilitate the neuro-anatomical approach and optimize topometric studies of the brain and, more particularly, the retrochiasmal visual pathways and the oculomotor system: the chiasmatico-commissural line (CH-PC line), defining a chiasmatico-commissural reference plane is used (Tamraz et al. 1990, 1991a,b, 1994). Its anatomical landmarks are: the chiasmal point (CH) anteriorly and the PC posteriorly, readily shown on a midsagittal MR scout view. The accuracy of these brain midline structures need not be demonstrated here, either from an anatomical or a phylogenetic point of view, being located at the meso-diencephalic junction. The orthogonality of this plane as to the long vertical axis of the brainstem, as defined by the PC-OB, and its close parallelism to the direction of the first temporal sulcus demonstrate its real horizontality and close relationship to the direction of the inferior horn of the lateral ventricle, as shown previously in Chap. 2.

These axial and coronal reference lines are therefore suitable for imaging the brainstem and cerebellum and may be used whenever anatomo-clinical correlations are needed. The reproducibility of the cuts oriented according to these landmarks and lines is also very helpful for follow-up of small lesions, as observed most interestingly in cases of oculomotor disturbances.

a Anatomic Correlations

These anatomic correlations, as shown by projection of the cross-reference on successive sagittal multislices, demonstrate the parallelism of the CH-PC reference line with the lateral fissure-posterior ramus plane, considered to be angled about 23°–25° to the AC-PC plane (Szikla et al. 1977). This explains the close relationship of the CH-PC line with the first temporal sulcus. Therefore, the temporal horn of the lateral ventricle and, hence, the optic radiations are studied according to their anteroposterior long axis. Moreover, the CH-PC horizontal line shows a constant topography at the midbrain-diencephalic junction, passing almost always through the ambient cistern between the inferior border of the splenium and the upper limit of the culmen to intersect, usually, the common stem of the parieto-occipital sulcus and the calcarine sulcus.

Thus, most of the calcarine fissure may reliably be found on the lower axial cuts, depending on the topography of the occipital lobes, which varies with respect to the cranial morphotype.

The other main anatomic result demonstrates the orthogonality of the CH-PC reference line with the great axis of the brainstem. Coronal cuts performed parallel to the PC-OB reference line very nicely display the geniculocalcarine tract and its temporal component originating from the lateral geniculate

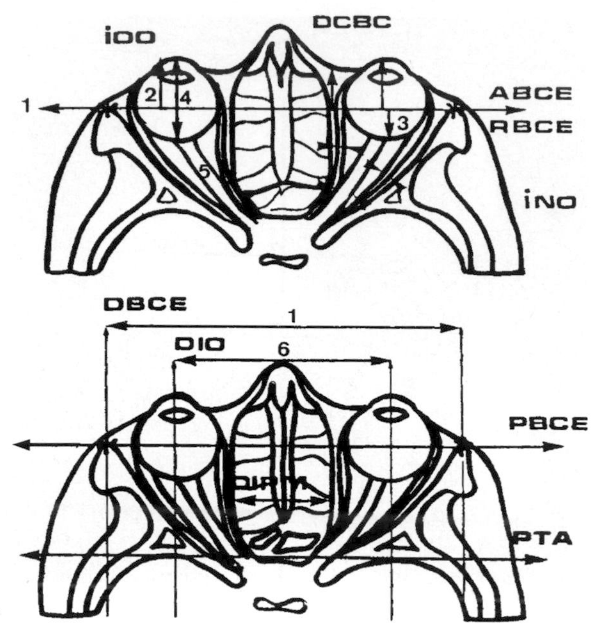

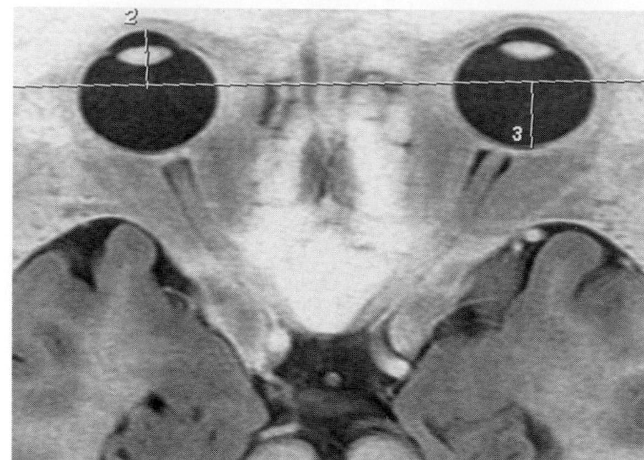

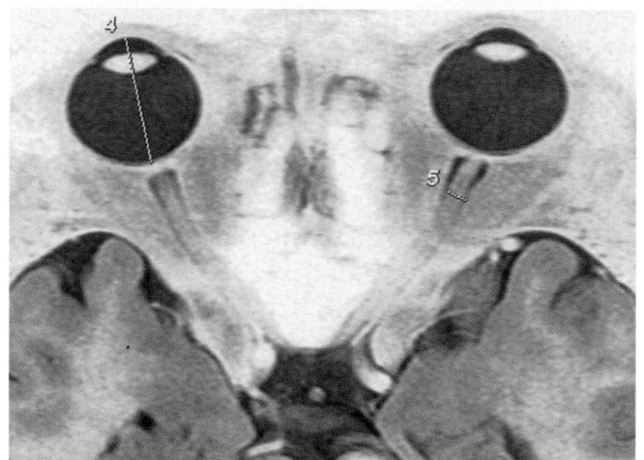

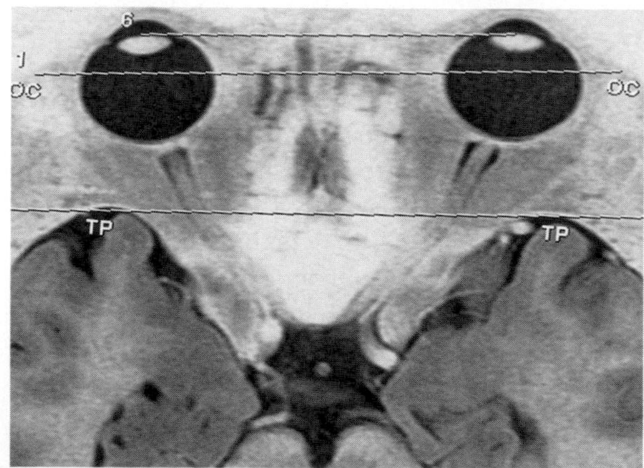

Fig. 9.19. Oculo-orbital biometry. The diagrams show the neuro-ocular plane (NOP), developing the oculo-orbital topometry and exophthalmometry, as routinely used for the evaluation of oculo-orbital diseases. Distances (as well as indices and angular values) are calculated in the NOP cut according to the external pre-bicanthal reference line, according to the methodology (diagram) proposed by Cabanis et al. (1982). MR correlation (in an enophthalmic subject, note the relative increase in the retrobicanthal segment with respect to the anterior bicanthal showing an inverse ratio as compared to the diagram): *1* PBCE, prebicanthal line and interbicanthal distance; *2* prebicanthal distance; *3* retrobicanthal distance; *4* axial diameter of eyeball; *5* optic nerve diameter; *6* interpupillary distance

bodies, beneath and lateral to the thalami and found at the PC-OB reference line itself.

The optic tracts and the cisternal and intracanalicular optic nerves are also well delineated and easily depicted in such coronal cuts, free of partial volume effect phenomena. This may also be explained by the close parallelism of the PC-OB plane to the cut passing through the anterior columns of the fornix, found roughly parallel to the anterior commissure-mamillary body (AC-CM) line, as demonstrated by Guiot (1959) (see Chap. 2). The chiasm may benefit also from this cephalic orientation despite its well known angular variations, being oriented in the adult along the CH-PC plane in most instances and displaying a characteristic X-shape in a single slice, including the cisternal optic nerves and the chiasm, and paralleling more characteristically the cisternal and pericrural optic tracts (Fig. 9.20).

In summary, the NOP remains the best cephalic orientation for investigation and biometric study and for follow-up of diseases of the eyes and the intraorbital optic nerves in the axial and coronal planes. Sagittal oblique cuts oriented along the optic nerve axis and/or the optic canal may be of great help in specific pathological conditions.

B The Eyes

Surface-coil MR imaging of the eye has greatly improved the anatomic resolution of images obtained from the eyeball (Langer et al. 1987). Spatial resolution of less than 1 mm is achieved. However, the major advantages of MR over CT are the lack of ionizing radiation, the absence of cataractogenic effect, direct multiplanar facility and, of course, a very high contrast discrimination, as shown in images of the lens in which the cortex and nucleus are well distinguished. The anterior and vitreous chambers and sclera are also readily seen. Additional information is provided by modifying the pulse sequences. The lens shows, for instance, a moderate T1 with a short T2, whereas the vitreous body, reflects the long T1 and T2 of its water content. The sclera is well identified on T2 weighted and proton density weighted (PD) sequences, exhibiting a low signal intensity due to its fibrous nature. The development of new surface coils to improve resolution with faster imaging pulse sequences to reduce eye movement artifacts have modified our anatomical approach to diseases of the eyes and the optic nerve head at the lamina cribrosa. Our knowledge of the anterior segment of the eye, and particularly the lens and the ciliary body, have already benefited from an evaluation of the blood ocular barrier, as demonstrated by contrast-enhanced MR (Fig. 9.21).

C The Optic Nerves

The optic nerve is about 50 mm long when measured from the eye to the chiasm. Four segments may be distinguished: intra-ocular, intraorbital, intracanalar, and intracranial.

1 The Intraocular Optic Nerve

The optic nerve head is about 1 mm long and 1.5 mm in diameter, slightly wider as it leaves the eye. Its anterior surface represents the clinically visible optic disc in the ocular fundus, with a diameter of 1.5–2 mm (Straatsma et al. 1969). Actually, the optic nerve heads are contained in the NOP itself, well-delimited by the uveoscleral rim. Well-oriented thin slices in the NOP or in the sagittal oblique plane through the optic nerves may help to evaluate its intraocular part more accurately within the low signal of the scleral canal (Fig. 9.22A,B).

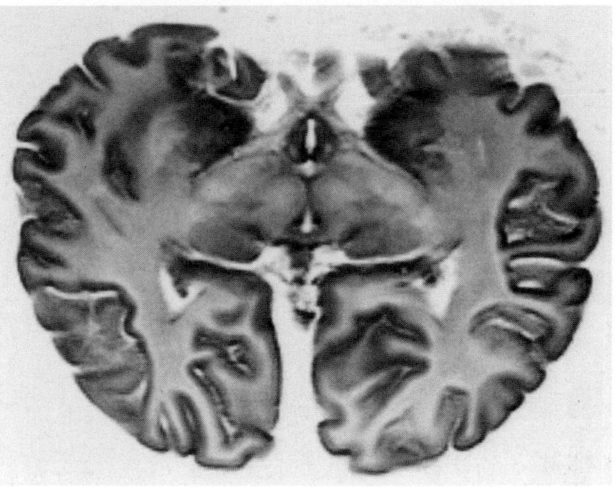

Fig. 9.20. The chiasmatico-commissural plane (CH-PC) more tilted (averaging −5° to −10°) than the neuro-ocular plane (NOP), displays the characteristic "X"-shape formed by the optic nerves and the chiasm and paralleling characteristically the cisternal and pericrural optic tracts, as observed when totally comprised in a single, thin, 3 mm MR slice in a formalin specimen. Note that the pericrural optic tracts are found at the midbrain diencephalic junction

2 The Intraorbital Optic Nerve

The orbital portion of the optic nerve begins as the optic nerve head exits from the sclera. Measuring about 20–30 mm in length, it extends from the posterior pole of the eyeball to the optic foramen (Fig. 9.23A). Its mean diameter in the orbit is 3.5 mm, much larger than the optic head diameter. The nerve is surrounded by the pia mater, the arachnoid and the dura, which is the outermost sheath. The dura fuses anteriorly with the sclera and posteriorly with the periorbita, passing through the optic foramen to join the intracranial dura. The optic nerve sheaths are therefore continuous with the leptomeninges of the brain, transmitting the cerebrospinal fluid. Arachnoidal villi have been shown in these sheaths (Shanthaveerappa and Bourne 1964). As the nerves leave the eyeballs they are surrounded by the posterior ciliary arteries, branches of the ophthalmic artery. The central retinal artery and vein penetrate the optic nerve from its inferior and medial aspect be-

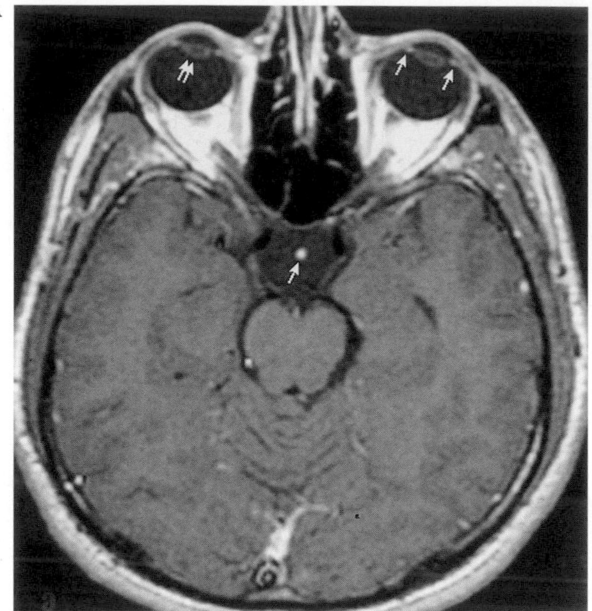

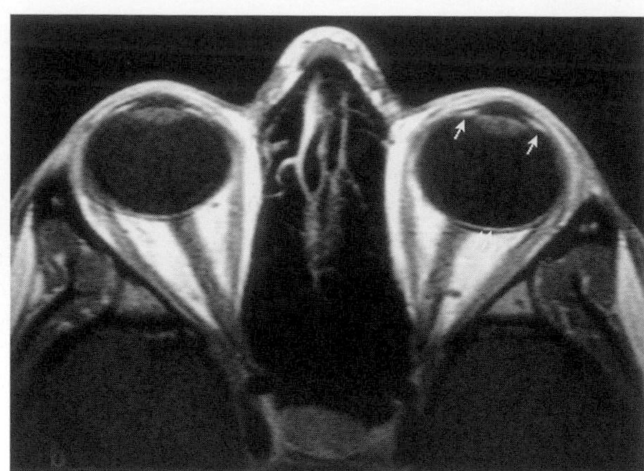

Fig. 9.21. A, B. Imaging of the eyes using a head coil (**A**) and a surface coil (**B**); contrast enhanced SE-T1-w axial cuts showing the enhancement of the ciliary bodies (*arrows*) and the intrinsic structure of the lens with differentiation of the cortical part and the internal nucleus (*double arrows*)

tween 5 and 15 mm behind the eye. The ophthalmic artery proceeds from the orbital apex to the midportion of the orbit along its inferolateral surface before it crosses over or under the optic nerve to project medially (Fig. 9.23B) Note that at the orbital apex the optic nerve is surrounded by the four rectus muscles arising from the Zinn circle, the medial and superior rectus muscles arising partly from the optic sheath (Whitnall 1932). The coronal cuts through the orbital regions display the intraorbital optic nerves and their surrounding sheaths as well as the orbital structures of the intraconal retrobulbar space (Fig. 9.24A–C).

Consisting of myelinated nerve fibers similar to the brain white matter, it becomes obvious that, on MR, the intraorbital optic nerve shows a signal intensity comparable to the cerebral white matter on T1 or T2 weighted (FSE or STIR) sequences. In proton density pulse sequences, there is no distinction between the optic nerve and its surrounding sheaths (Fig. 9.25), thus sometimes giving a false positive aspect of enlargement of the optic nerves with a grayish somewhat homogeneous appearance. The dense fibrous dural sheath is not distinguished from the CSF rim on the T1 weighted images but could be shown on high resolution, heavily T2 weighted pulse sequences. This appearance might not be confused with the artifactual images shown at the edge of the optic nerves when using a high-field system (1.5 T) and due to a chemical shift misregistration effect in the direction of the frequency-encoding gradient. This may become even more pronounced particularly when narrow bandwidths are used, giving an aspect of vertical doubling of the intraorbital optic nerve section in the coronal cuts.

Considering the topographical retinotopic and functional organization of the optic nerve, many reports estimate that each nerve comprises about one million myelinated fibers (Krause 1876; Arey and Bickel 1935; Kupfer et al. 1967). Axons from the papillomacular bundle occupy a wedge-shaped sector in the temporal portion of the nerve (Radius and Anderson 1979) and move centrally as it progresses toward the optic chiasm. Superior retinal fibers are observed in the upper part of the nerve and inferior ones below. The nasal and temporal fibers are found on their respective sides (Brouwer and Zeeman 1925, 1926). In fact, one can say that all the retinal fibers maintain their relative position throughout the visual pathways as reported for the optic nerves, except in the optic tracts and the lateral geniculate bodies in which the fibers undergo a rotation of 90°.

3 The Intracanalicular Optic Nerve

The intracanalicular portion of the optic nerve is very well demonstrated using MR because of the lack of signal from the outlining rim of cortical bone. A good knowledge of the shape and size of the optic canal helps in obtaining an accurate appreciation of any subtle pathological modification (Maniscalco and Habal 1978). The optic canal itself is comprised of the union of both roots of the lesser wing of the sphenoid bone. The dura is tightly adherent to the

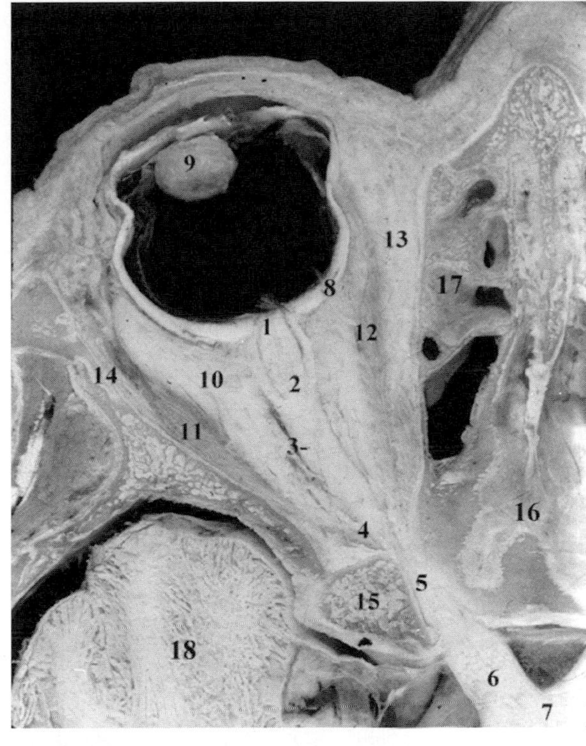

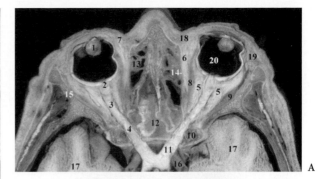

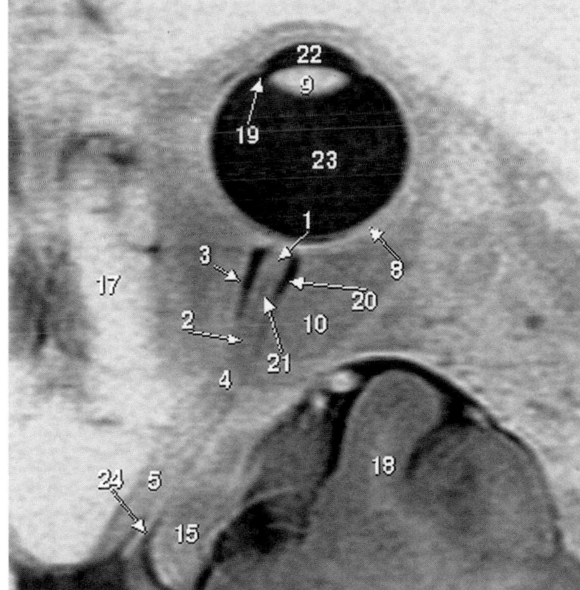

Fig. 9.22. A,B. Intra-ocular optic nerve (optic nerve head); anatomical MR correlation in the **A** axial plane (neuro-ocular plane, NOP) and **B** the sagittal oblique plane. *1* Optic nerve head; *2* intraorbital optic nerve; *3* dural sheath; *4* orbital apex; *5* intracanalicular optic nerve; *6* cisternal optic nerve; *7* optic chiasm; *8* sclera; *9* lens; *10* orbital fat; *11* lateral rectus muscle; *12* medial rectus muscle; *13* nasal extraconal space; *14* temporal extraconal space; *15* anterior clinoid process; *16* jugum sphenoidale; *17* ethmoidal cells; *18* temporal pole; *19* ciliary body; *20* perioptic subarachnoid space; *21* intra-optic vessels; *22* anterior chamber of eyeball; *23* vitreous body; *24* intracanalicular ophthalmic artery

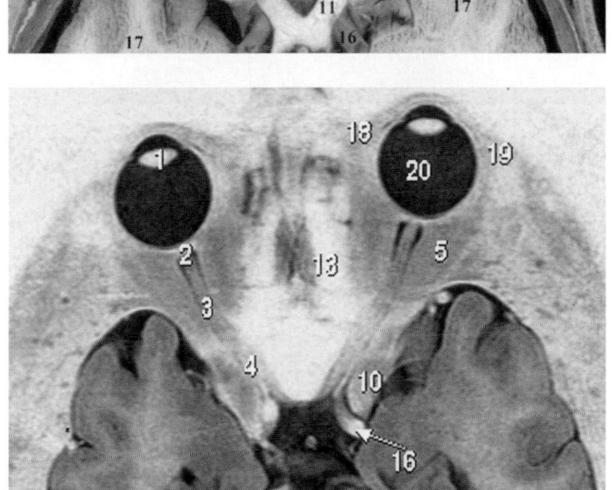

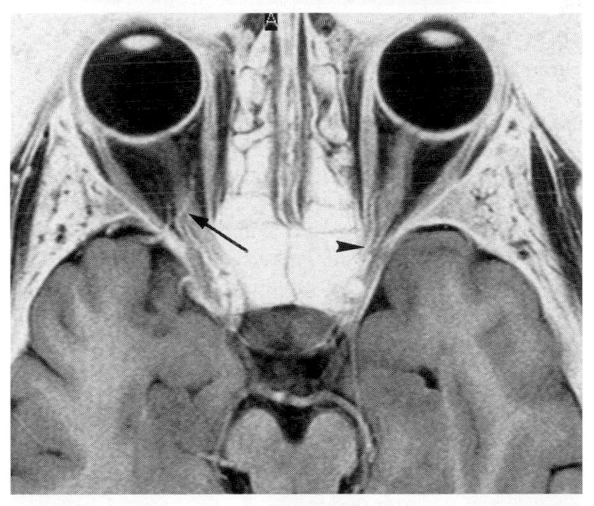

Fig. 9.23. A–C. The neuro-ocular plane **A**: investigation of the anterior optic pathways; anatomy and MR correlation **B,C**. *1* Lens; *2* optic nerve head; *3* intraorbital optic nerve; *4* intracanalicular optic nerve; *5* orbital fat (intraconal space); *6* extraconal (nasal) space; *7* preseptal region; *8* medial rectus muscle; *9* lateral rectus muscle; *10* anterior clinoid process; *11* cisternal optic nerve; *12* jugum sphenoidale; *13* ethmoidal cells; *14* lamina papyracea; *15* lateral orbital wall; *16* internal carotid artery; *17* temporal pole; *18* inner canthus; *19* outer canthus; *20* eyeball. **C** MR cut in the NOP showing the intracanalicular (*arrowhead*) and the intraorbital latero-optic (*arrow*) course of the ophthalmic artery

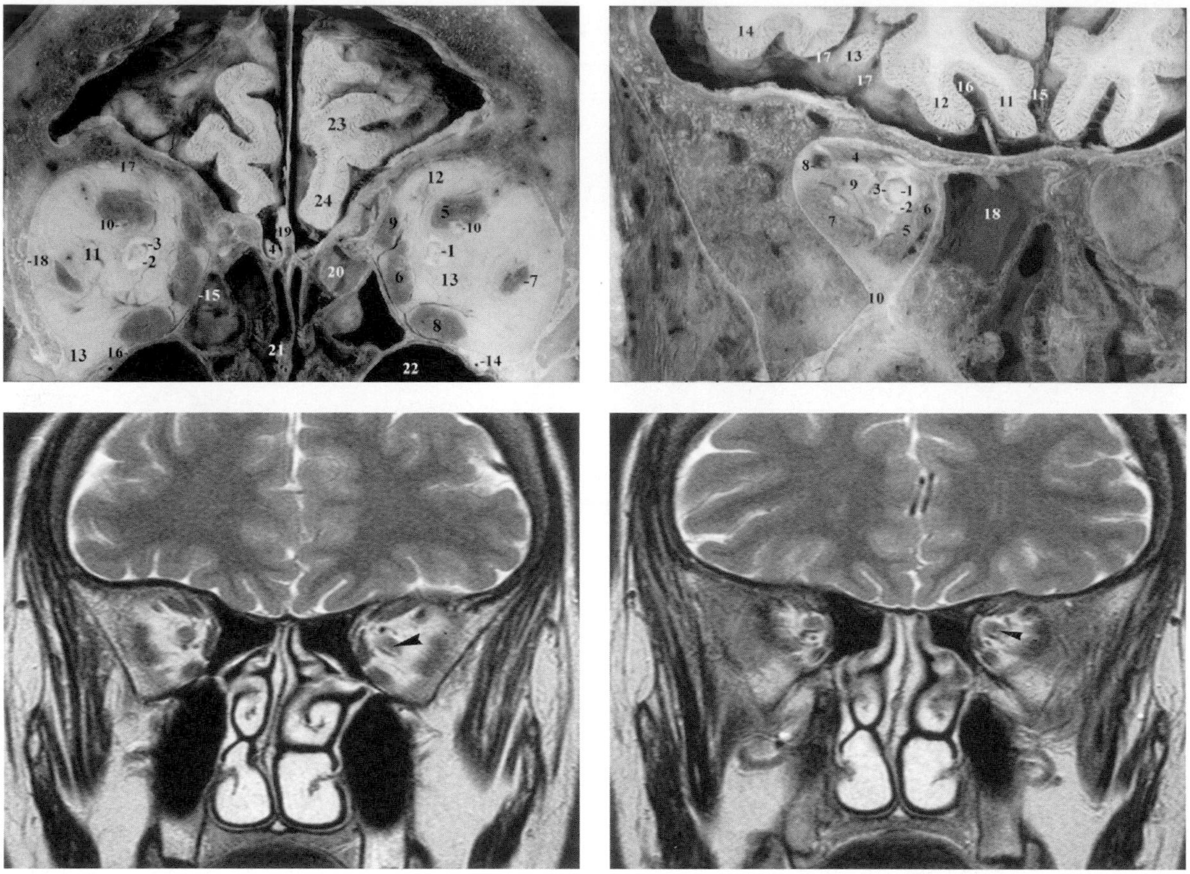

Fig. 9.24. **A** The intraorbital optic nerve, midorbital coronal anatomical cut. *1* Intraorbital optic nerve; *2* dural sheath; *3* perioptic subarachnoid space; *4* olfactory bulb; *5* superior rectus and levator palpebrae; *6* medial rectus muscle; *7* lateral rectus muscle; *8* inferior rectus muscle; *9* superior oblique muscle; *10* superior ophthalmic vein; *11* orbital fat; *12* superior extraconal space; *13* inferior orbital fissure; *14* infraorbital canal and nerve; *15* lamina papyracea; *16* floor of the orbit; *17* roof of the orbit; *18* lateral wall of the orbit; *19* crista galli; *20* ethmoidal sinus; *21* nasal septum; *22* maxillary sinus; *23* frontal pole; *24* gyrus rectus. **B** The intraorbital optic nerve, juxta-apexian coronal anatomical cut. *1,* intraorbital optic nerve; *2,* dural sheath; *3,* subarachnoid space; *4,* superior oblique muscle; *5,* inferior rectus muscle; *6,* medial rectus muscle; *7,* lateral rectus muscle; *8,* superior ophthalmic vein; *9,* orbital fat; *10,* inferior orbital fissure; *11,*rectus gyrus; *12,* medial orbital gyrus; *13,* posterior orbital gyrus; *14,* lateral orbital gyrus; *15,* interhemispheric fissure; *16,* olfactory sulcus; *17,* cruciform sulci (H orbital sulci); *18,* posterior ethmoidal sinus. **C** Intraorbital optic nerves and sheaths (*arrowhead*): MR correlations in the coronal plane at midorbital (*a*) and juxta-apexian (*b*) levels, showing the relation of the intraorbital optic nerves with the muscular cone

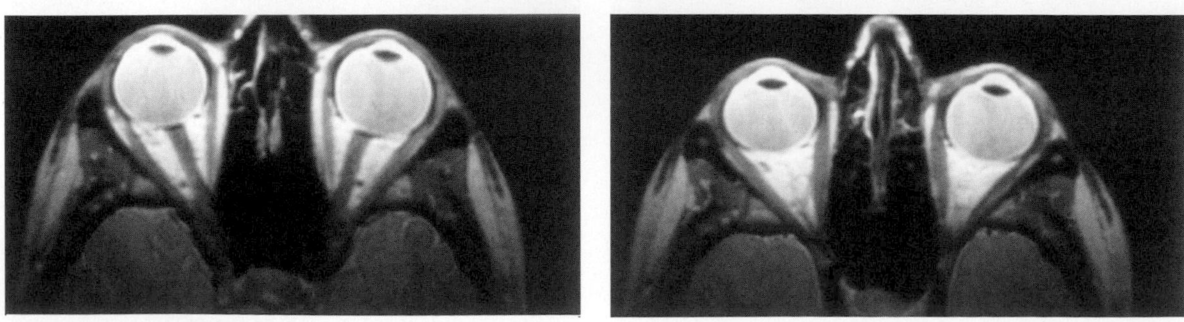

Fig. 9.25. Proton density images of the intraorbital optic nerves in the neuro-ocular plane (NOP) orientation showing no distinction between the optic nerve and its surrounding sheaths, including the subarachnoid spaces

bone within the optic canal and is not differentiated from it with MR (Fig. 9.26). Note that the optic nerve may be covered at its proximal portion by the dura exclusively, with an average length of 3 mm (Rhoton et al. 1977). Knowledge of the variations of thickness and structure of the optic canal walls is needed when decompressive procedures are attempted. The ophthalmic artery may be visualized within the optic canal, but may be missed or confused with the cortical bone because of its flow-void signal (Fig. 9.27).

The optic canals length averages 9 mm. Each canal is oriented posteriorly and medially and virtually meets its fellow at the center of the dorsum sellae. The angle between the axis of the optic canal and the median sagittal plane is about 40°. The angle between its axis and the Frankfurt-Virchow plane is about 15° in adults and 42° in newborns (Lang 1987) and, hence, about 25° as related to the canthomeatal line, i.e., roughly in the orientation of the CH-PC plane. Its anterior orbital opening or optic foramen is elliptical, with the widest diameter vertically oriented. It is located at a distance of about 50 mm from the supraorbital opening. The intracranial opening is also elliptical but with its largest diameter horizontally oriented (Fig. 9.28). This latter appearance should not be misinterpreted as optic nerve enlargement on axial MR slices. The distance separating both orbital openings is about 28 mm and the two cranial ones 15 mm.

The optic canal is separated from the superior orbital fissure by a bony ridge, which is sometimes misdiagnosed as the optic canal on inadequately oriented axial cuts. Accessory sinuses and various anomalies of the optic canal also have to be carefully evaluated when analyzing MR images. The relationships between the optic canals and the paranasal sinuses are variable and may become clinically important, accounting for visual loss when infected or when ballooned out, a condition named "pneumosinus dilatans." Whereas the intraorbital optic nerves move freely as the eyes move, the intracanalicular portion does not and thus permits accurate MR eval-

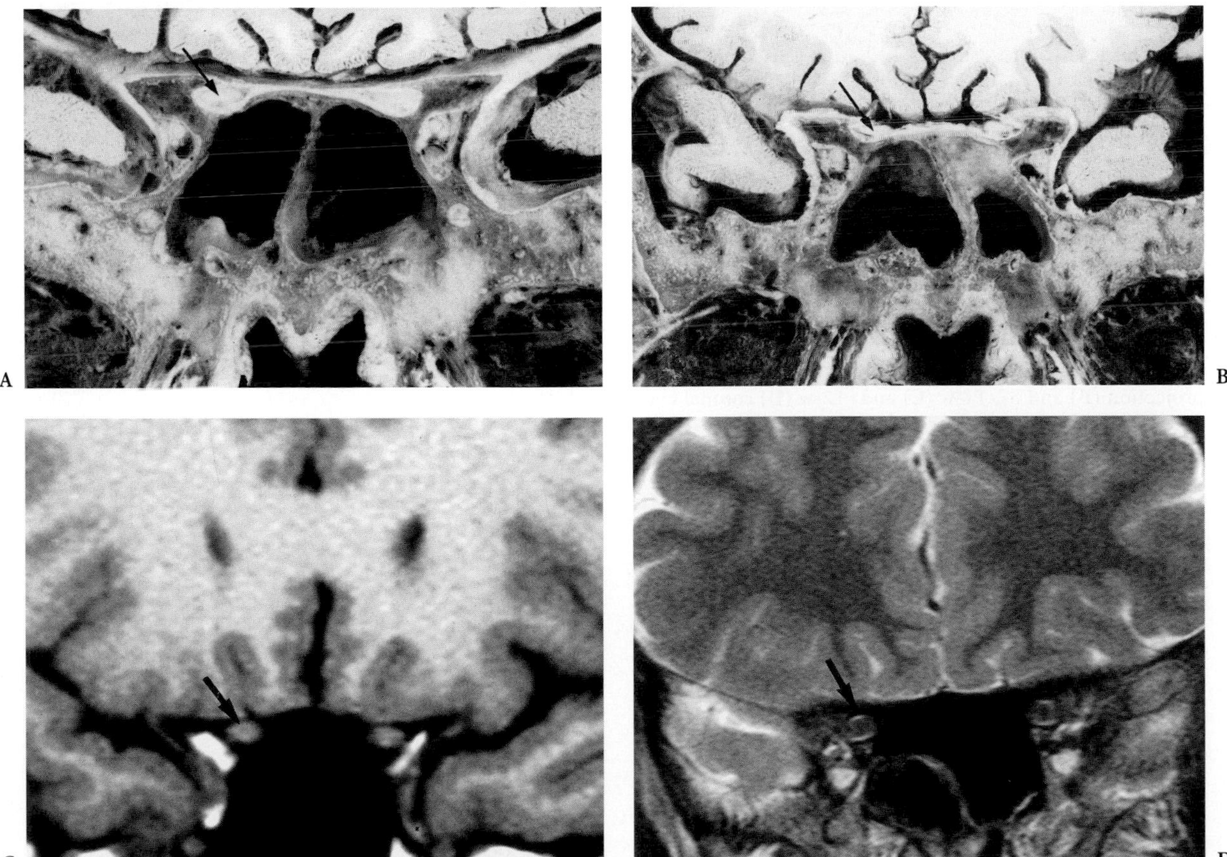

Fig. 9.26A–D. Intracanalicular optic nerve and sheaths (*arrow*). **A,B** Coronal anatomical cuts and MR correlations using SE-T1-w (**C**) and SE-T2-w (**D**) sequences in the coronal plane

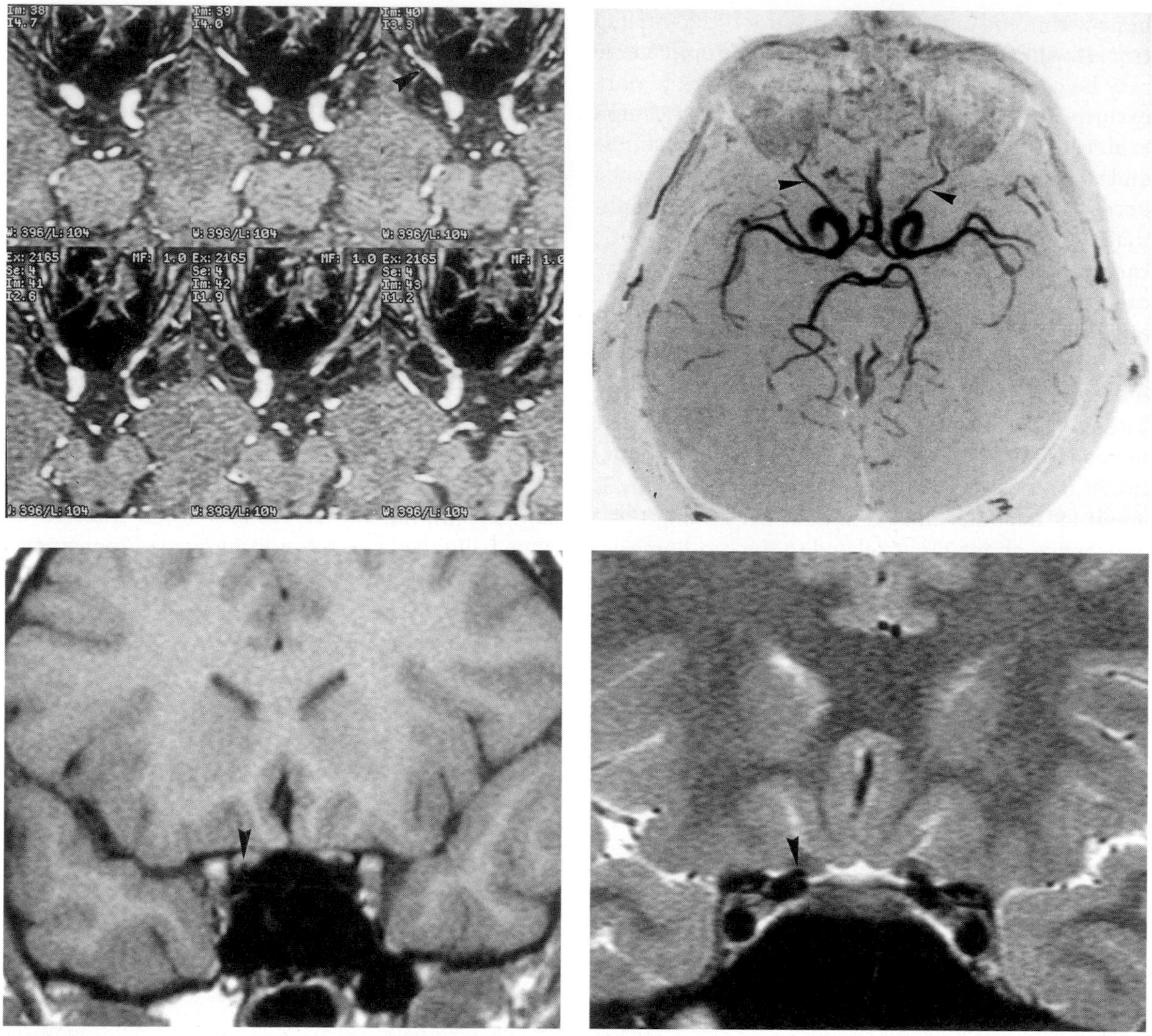

A B C D

Fig. 9.27 A–D. Magnetic resonance imaging of the ophthalmic artery (*arrowhead*) in relation to the cisternal artery at its origin and the intracanalicular portions of the optic nerve using 3D-TOF MR angio. Native cuts in the axial plane (**A**) and the axial projection (**B**) and SE-T1-w (**C**) and -T2-w (**D**) coronal cuts

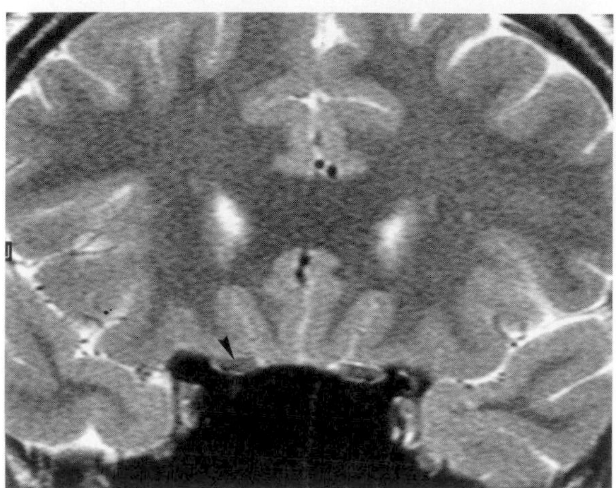

Fig. 9.28. SE-T2-w coronal cut through the intracranial opening of the optic canal and the origin of the cisternal optic nerves (*arrowhead*), laterally bounded by the anterior clinoid processes

uation, free from movement or bony artifacts, using contiguous thin slices and a small field of view.

Estimating the cross-sectional size of the intraosseous optic nerves and the adjacent cisternal portion remains difficult with MR and requires high resolution, thin (2 or 3 mm), coronal oblique cuts perpendicular to the axis of the optic canal (Fig. 9.29A) or, more easily, strictly oblique sagittal views (Fig. 9.29B) oriented along its anterior-posterior axis. Comparative slices are necessary for a better appreciation of optic nerve diameters, performed using T1 weighted (IR or SE) or heavily T2 weighted (FSE or STIR) pulse sequences, either in the coronal plane perpendicular to the CH-PC plane or, more efficiently, when possible in a single acquisition in coronal oblique cuts oriented perpendicular to each canal. To the morphologic data obtained it is necessary to add FSE-T2 weighted or STIR sequences, which are more sensitive to the detection of pathological conditions such as edema, gliosis or demyelination. In case of extrinsic processes or negative results on STIR sequence (T2 weighted) with no bright signal of the intracanalar optic nerve, one should administer an intravenous paramagnetic agent (Gd-DOTA or Gd-DTPA). Enhancement is usually best depicted on T1 weighted spin echo sequences, demonstrating the abnormal increased permeability of the blood brain barrier.

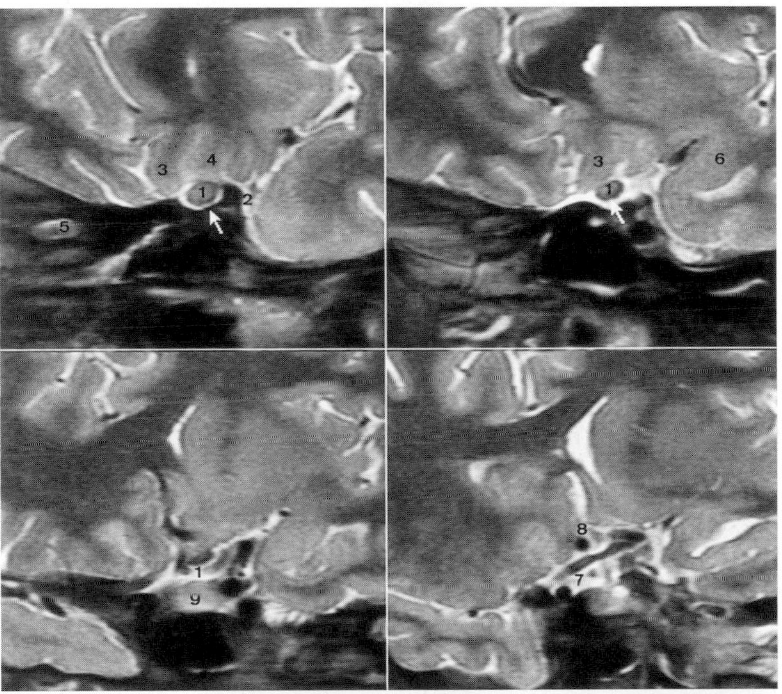

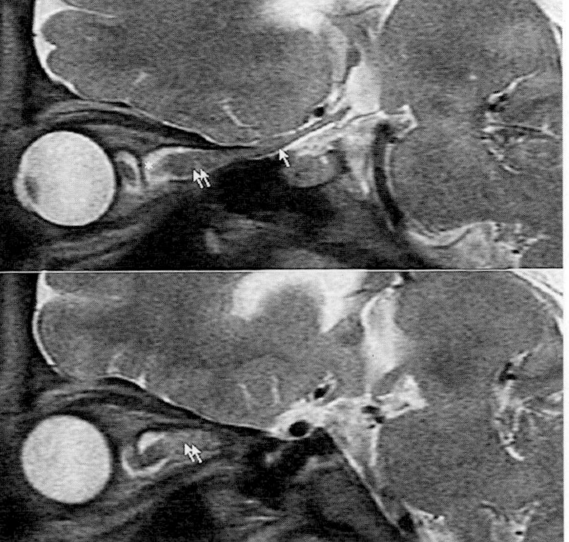

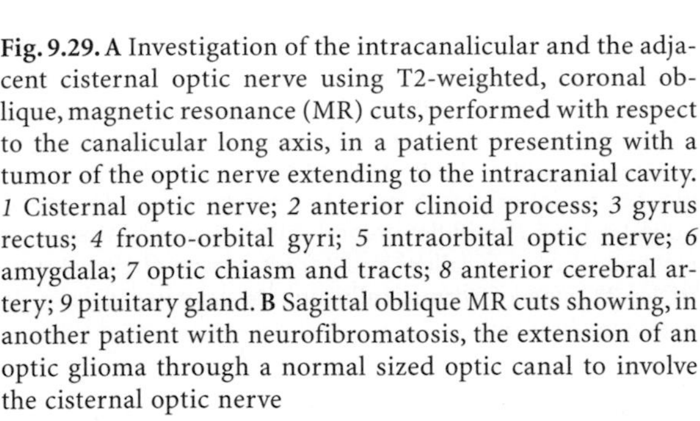

Fig. 9.29. A Investigation of the intracanalicular and the adjacent cisternal optic nerve using T2-weighted, coronal oblique, magnetic resonance (MR) cuts, performed with respect to the canalicular long axis, in a patient presenting with a tumor of the optic nerve extending to the intracranial cavity. *1* Cisternal optic nerve; *2* anterior clinoid process; *3* gyrus rectus; *4* fronto-orbital gyri; *5* intraorbital optic nerve; *6* amygdala; *7* optic chiasm and tracts; *8* anterior cerebral artery; *9* pituitary gland. **B** Sagittal oblique MR cuts showing, in another patient with neurofibromatosis, the extension of an optic glioma through a normal sized optic canal to involve the cisternal optic nerve

4 The Intracranial Optic Nerve

The intracranial portion of the optic nerve varies in length, from 3 mm to 16 mm with an average of 10 mm, being flattened in coronal sections and measuring about 4.5 mm at its greatest diameter. The cisternal optic nerve is covered by the inferior aspect of the posterior part of the frontal lobe, which is why great difficulty is encountered when evaluated in the axial plane even with MR. The coronal MR approach should be adopted to avoid partial volume effects and to evaluate both optic nerves, very nicely and comparatively outlined by the low (Figs. 9.30, 9.31) or the high signal intensity of the surrounding cisternal CSF on the SE-T1 or SE-T2 sequences, respectively (Fig. 9.32A,B). Above and laterally, the olfactory tracts are also well displayed.

Slices oriented parallel to the PC-OB reference line are optimal when using very thin contiguous slices (3 mm) to evaluate the shape and size of these nerves in case of relative atrophy or subtle enlargement. Using the brainstem reference plane (PC-OB line) provides the opportunity to obtain reproducible slices with certainty, due to the fact that the landmarks, the PC and the obex (OB) are distant from the optic nerves. The chiasm and the optic tracts benefit from the same orientation.

D The Optic Chiasm

The chiasm is a flattened, quadrilateral, commissural bundle of fibers located at the junction of the anterior wall of the third ventricle with its floor. It is formed by the fusion of both optic nerves with their partial decussation of the nasal retinal fibers crossing to the opposite optic tract. The chiasm averages 14 mm (10–20 mm) in its transverse diameter with an anteroposterior width of about 8 mm (4–13 mm) and a thickness of 3–5 mm (Whitnall 1932; Hoyt 1969). The chiasm is located in the chiasmatic cistern behind the tuberculum sellae and the chiasmatic sulcus, superior to the body of the sphenoid bone, but is rarely found in the chiasmatic sulcus (Schaeffer 1924). In fact, its position varies in relation to the sella turcica and the pituitary gland. In 79% of cases, the chiasm overlies the posterior two-thirds of the sella. In 12% of cases the chiasm is found over the

A

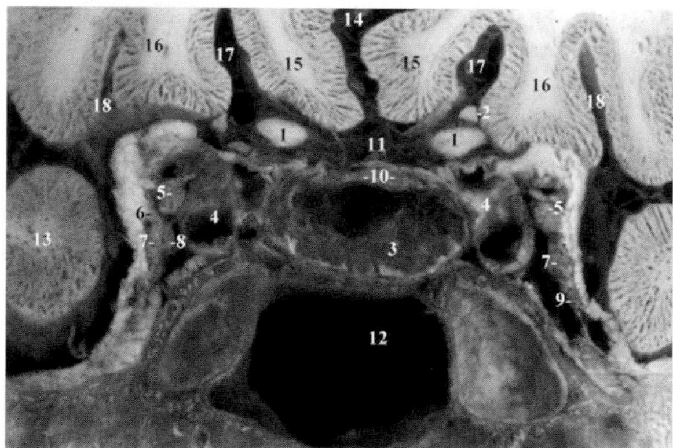

B

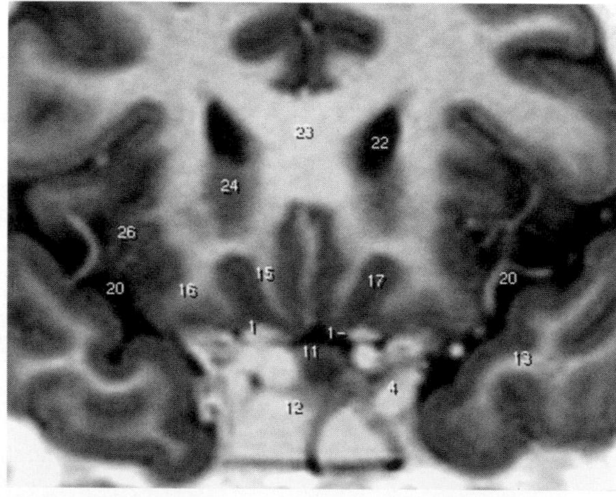

C

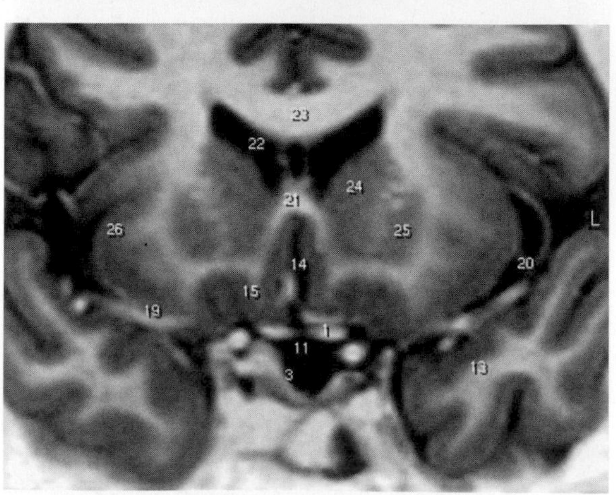

Fig. 9.30. The cisternal optic nerves: coronal anatomic cut with MR correlations using inversion recovery, T1 weighted sequence. *1* Cisternal optic nerve; *2* olfactory tract; *3* adenohypophysis; *4* intracavernous internal carotid artery; *5* oculomotor nerve (III); *6* trochlear nerve (IV); *7* ophthalmic nerve (V1); *8* abducens nerve (VI); *9* maxillary nerve (V2); *10* diaphragma sellae; *11* suprasellar cistern; *12* sphenoid sinus; *13* temporal pole; *14* interhemispheric fissure; *15* gyrus rectus; *16* medial orbital gyrus; *17* olfactory sulcus; *18* medial orbital sulcus; *19* middle cerebral artery; *20* lateral fissure; *21* rostrum of corpus callosum; *22* frontal horn of lateral ventricle; *23* genu of corpus callosum; *24* caudate nucleus; *25* putamen; *26* insula

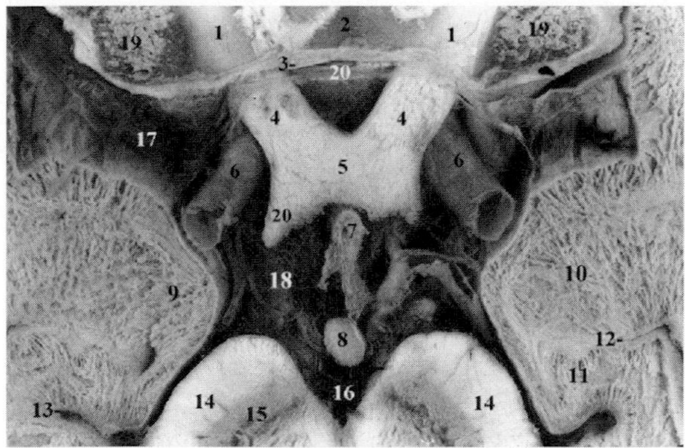

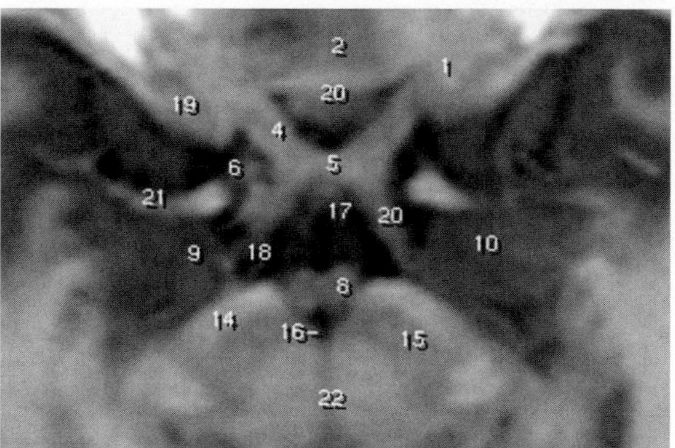

Fig. 9.31. The cisternal optic nerves: axial anatomical cut with MR correlation using inversion recovery T1 weighted sequence, 3 mm thick. *1* Intracanalicular optic nerve; *2* jugum sphenoidale; *3* dura mater; *4* cisternal optic nerve; *5* inferior aspect of the optic chiasm; *6* internal carotid artery; *7* lateral fissure; *8* mamillary body; *9* uncus; *10* amygdala; *11* hippocampus; *12* uncal recess of temporal horn; *13* hippocampal sulcus; *14* crus cerebri; *15* substantia nigra; *16* interpeduncular cistern; *17* pituitary stalk and infundibulum; *18* chiasmal cistern; *19* anterior clinoid process; *20* chiasmatic sulcus; *21* middle cerebral artery; *22* midbrain

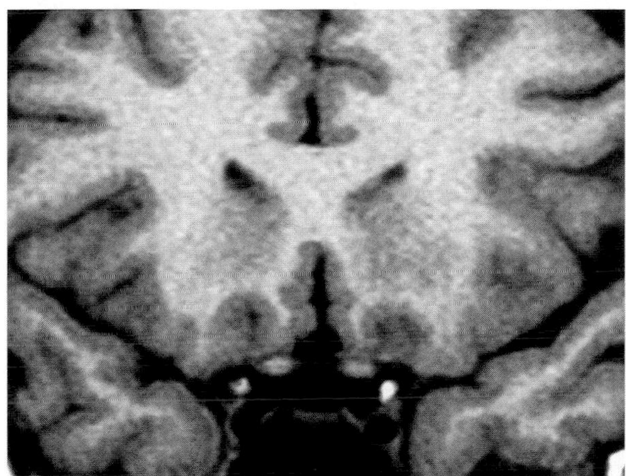

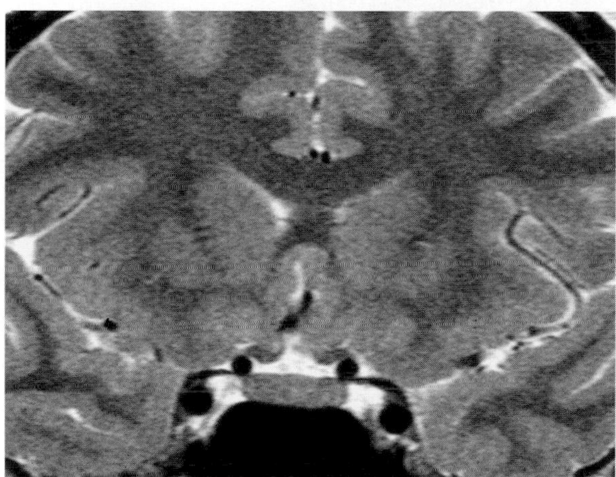

Fig. 9.32. A, B. Coronal magnetic resonance cuts of the cisternal optic nerves using **A** SE-T1-w and **B** SE-T2-w pulse sequences (3 mm thick)

diaphragma sellae. It lies over and behind the dorsum sellae in 4% of individuals and rests in the chiasmatic sulcus in only 5% (Schaeffer 1924; Bergland et al. 1968). The variable position of the chiasm and its prefixation or postfixation situation account for the variations in its appearance in the axial plane, as shown with CT or MR. Its usual X-shape, mainly comprising the cisternal optic tracts surrounding the MB and the crura cerebri, is nicely delineated in the CH-PC horizontal reference plane (Tamraz 1991).

Moreover, the position of the chiasm itself varies according to the shape of the skull and the cephalic index, being more rostral and dorsal in brachycephaly than in dolichocephaly. The distance between the lower margin of the chiasm and the nasotuberculum line is about 10.7 mm (Walker 1962). Thus, the actual position of the optic chiasm and its obliquity vary widely among normal persons. For that reason, additional sagittal MR sections are necessary to evaluate the location, shape, and thickness of the chiasm, the third ventricle and its optic recess superiorly, the internal carotid arteries on each side, the anterior cerebral arteries and the anterior communicating artery in front and posteriorly the tuber cinereum, the infundibular recess, and the pituitary stalk within the interpeduncular fossa (Fig. 9.33). The basal or suprasellar cistern separates the chiasm from the pituitary gland lying in the sella turcica. The optic chiasm is thus virtually circumscribed by CSF.

The relation of the chiasm and the adjacent part of the cisternal optic nerves and tracts, with the basal vessels of the circle of Willis, are of importance

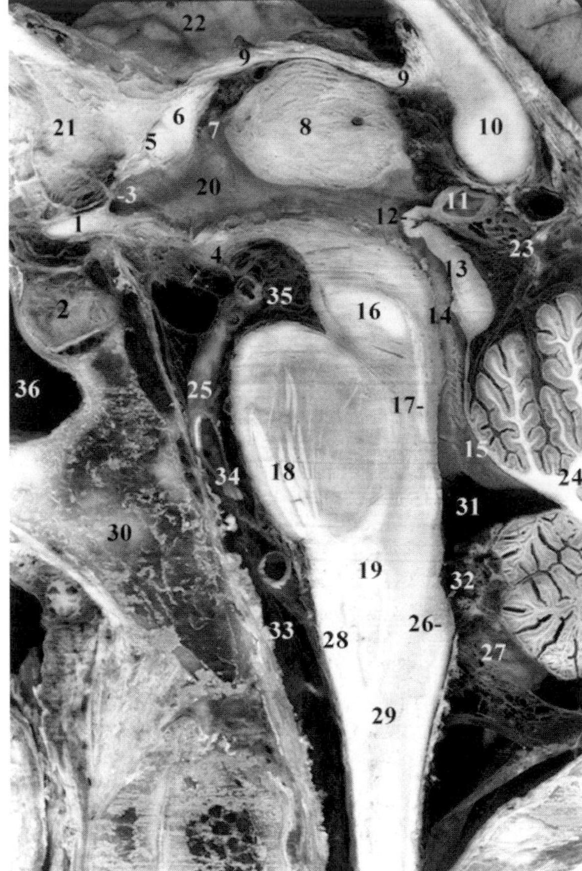

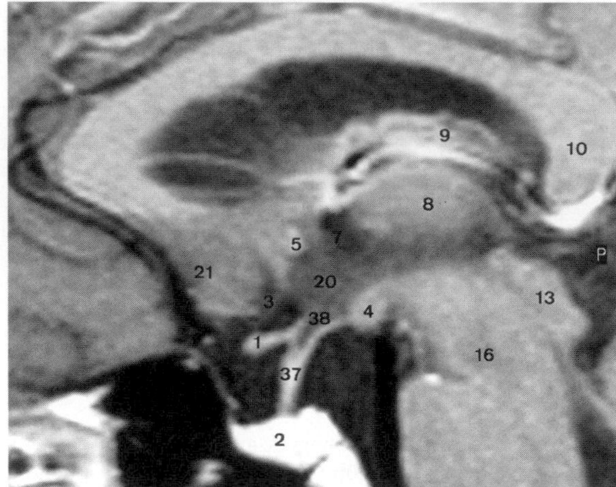

Fig. 9.33. The optic chiasm: midsagittal anatomic cut with MR correlations. *1* Optic chiasm; *2* pituitary gland; *3* lamina terminalis; *4* mamillary body; *5* anterior commissure; *6* anterior column of fornix; *7* interventricular foramen (Monro); *8* thalamus; *9* fornix; *10* splenium of corpus callosum; *11* epiphysis or pineal gland; *12* posterior commissure; *13* quadrigeminal plate; *14* cerebral aqueduct; *15* superior medullary velum; *16* decussation of superior cerebellar peduncles; *17* medial longitudinal fasciculus; *18* corticospinal tracts; *19* medulla oblongata; *20* third ventricle; *21* subcallosal region; *22* caudate nucleus; *23* ambient cistern; *24* vermis of cerebellum; *25* basilar artery; *26* obex; *27* cisterna magna; *28* pyramid; *29* spinal cord-medullary junction; *30* clivus; *31* fourth ventricle; *32* foramen of Magendie; *33* laterobulbar cistern; *34* prepontine cistern; *35* interpeduncular cistern; *36* sphenoid sinus

and thus ought to be described (Fig. 9.34A–F). In fact, this portion of the visual path may be injured by ectatic as well as arteriosclerotic dysplastic vessels. It is not uncommon to find a displaced chiasm or optic nerve by a dolichoectatic vessel, for example the tip of the basilar artery. Moreover, the circle of Willis is the most common site of aneurysm. It is therefore important to perform axial cuts in the NOP or in the CH-PC plane using the appropriate pulse sequence, which depicts the flow-void signal of these vessels as obtained with any of the PD or T2 weighted sequences. Angio-MR may be efficiently reformatted in this plane orientation in order to best display the basal vessels, the bifurcations and the middle cerebral arteries and their insular branches (see Chap. 2).

The topographical anatomy of the chiasmal fibers was extensively studied by many authors at the end of the nineteenth century. Major recent contributions were reported and improved our understanding of chiasmal visual defects (Ronne 1914; Hoyt and Luis 1963), due to the apparent similarities between the retina and retinotopic fiber anatomy of the monkey and humans. The most important feature of the optic chiasm is that the macular fibers, like the peripheral fibers, are crossed and uncrossed. The ventral peripheral crossed fibers remain ventral and loop in the prechiasmal part of the opposite nerve (Willbrand's knee) before entering the optic tract, the dorsal fibers penetrating the dorsomedial portion of the optic tract. The uncrossed fibers maintain their relative position at the lateral aspect of the chiasm progressing toward the ipsilateral tract. The association of fibers originating from corresponding points of the two retinas seems to begin in the posterior portion of the chiasm but is completed only in the posterior portion of the optic radiations.

E The Optic Tract and the Lateral Geniculate Body

The optic tract begins in the posterolateral angle of the chiasm, runs laterally and backward between the anterior perforated substance and the tuber cinereum (Fig. 9.35A,B), constitutes the anterolateral boundary of the interpeduncular fossa and then

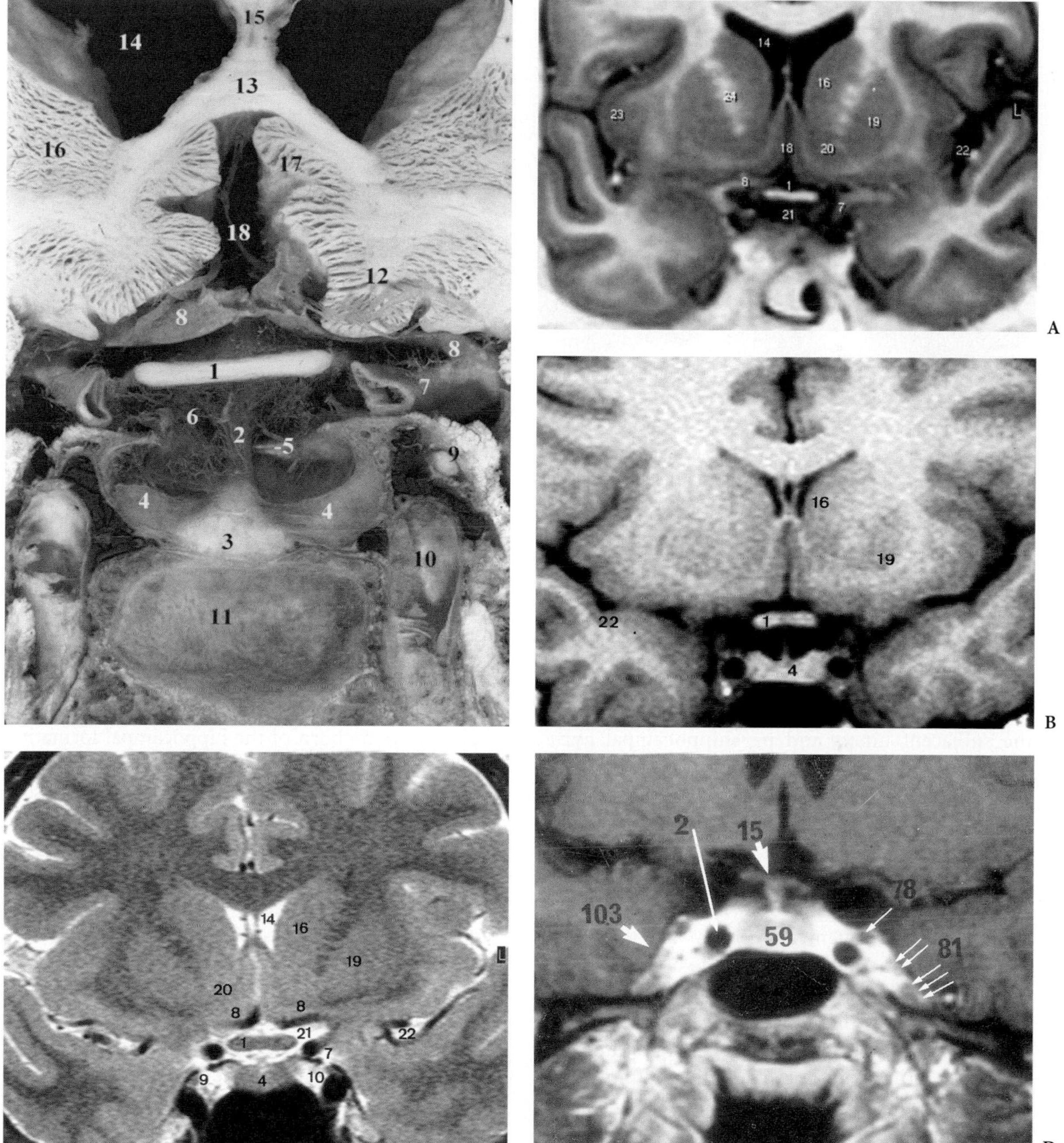

Fig. 9.34A–D. The optic chiasm: coronal cut with MR correlations, using inversion recovery T1-w (**A**) SE-T1-w (**B**) and T2-w (**C**) sequences, and T1-w after gadolinium infusion showing the intracavernous cranial nerves (**D**), 3 mm thick. *1* Optic chiasm; *2* pituitary stalk; *3* neurohypophysis (posterior pituitary gland); *4* adenohypophysis (anterior pituitary gland); *5* diaphragma sellae; *6* suprasellar cistern; *7* supraclinoid internal carotid artery; *8* proximal segment of anterior cerebral artery; *9* oculomotor nerve (III); *10* intracavernous internal carotid artery; *11* sphenoid sinus; *12* gyrus rectus; *13* rostrum of corpus callosum; *14* frontal horn of lateral ventricle; *15* septum lucidum; *16* head of caudate nucleus; *17* subcallosal area; *18* cistern of lamina terminalis; *19* putamen; *20* nucleus accumbens; *21* chiasmal cistern; *22* lateral fissure; *23* insula; *24* internal capsule anterior limb. **D** *2* Intracavernous segment of the internal carotid artery; *15* optic chiasm and adjacent optic tract; *59* pituitary gland; *103* cavernous sinus; *78* oculomotor nerve (III); *81* trochlear nerve (IV) and, mesially, in the intracavernous space adjacent to the carotid, the abducens nerve (VI); *81* trigeminal nerve, ophthalmic root. Note the enhancement of the venous sinuses in the intracavernous space and the delimitation of the pituitary gland laterally in the normal state

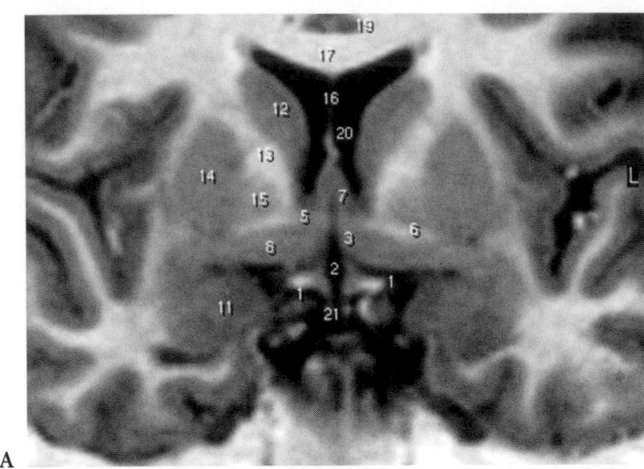

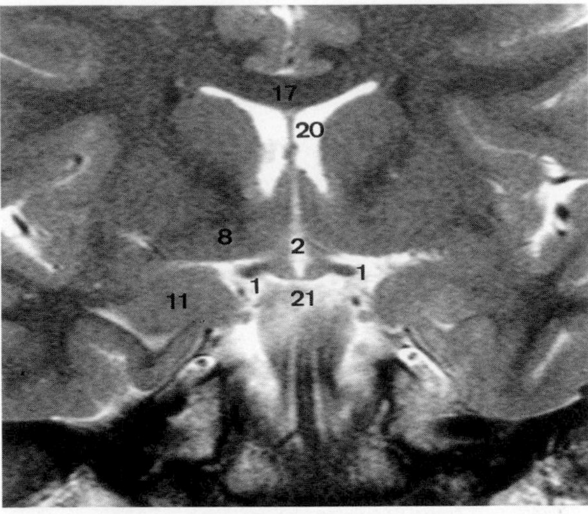

Fig. 9.35A,B. The cisternal optic tract: coronal anatomic cut with MR correlations using inversion recovery T1 weighted (**A**) and FSE T2 weighted (**B**) MR slices, 3 mm thick. *1* Cisternal optic tract (*arrow*); *2* third ventricle; *3* hypothalamus; *4* floor of the third ventricle (tuberal region); *5* anterior commissure; *6* anterior commissure, lateral limb; *7* anterior columns of fornix; *8* substantia innominata; *9* olfactory tubercle; *10* ansa peduncularis; *11* uncus (amygdala); *12* head of caudate nucleus; *13* internal capsule (anterior limb); *14* putamen; *15* pallidum; *16* septum lucidum; *17* corpus callosum; *18* cingulate gyrus; *19* callosal sulcus; *20* frontal horn of lateral ventricle; *21* chiasmal cistern

sweeps around the upper part of the cerebral peduncles, to which it adheres (Fig. 9.36, 9.37A,B). Along this portion of its route, each optic tract is hidden by the subjacent uncus and parahippocampal gyrus. The optic tracts run in close association and directly above the posterior cerebral arteries along their perimesencephalic route and end in the lateral geniculate bodies at the posterolateral aspect of the thalamus. The tracts divide at the level of the lateral geniculate body into two roots, the lateral one penetrating the lateral geniculate body and the medial root entering the medial geniculate body.

The visual fibers, both crossed and uncrossed, corresponding to the entire contralateral hemifield converge in each tract. The fibers originating from the upper retinas run dorsolaterally and those from the lower retinas run ventrolaterally. The macular fibers are found dorsolaterally.

Highly developed in primates, the lateral geniculate body is a small, ovoid, cap-shaped mass of gray and white matter located on the posterior and lateral aspects of the pulvinar thalami (Fig. 9.38) with an anterior pole blending with the optic tract, as observed on a parasagittal anatomic cut (Fig. 9.39). It is found above the lateral recess of the ambient cistern, well displayed on coronal MR cuts oriented parallel to the PC-OB reference line. Perimesencephalic optic tracts, the corpus geniculatum laterale and the optic peduncle necessitate high resolution and contrast images in order to be well-depicted, as obtained with T1 weighted IR or T2 weighted STIR sequences in the coronal PC-OB reference plane (Fig. 9.40) or in the parasagittal planes through the hippocampus.

The Ammon's horn of the hippocampal formation and the fimbria are also shown across the cisterna ambiens. Each lateral geniculate body receives nearly 80% of the fibers from the corresponding optic tract. Some of the fibers do not end in it, but pass over it to reach the superior colliculus. The lateral geniculate bodies are the end-stations for the anterior visual pathways and the origins of the optic radiations, through which they are connected to the calcarine cortex.

The lateral geniculate body is divided into a ventral phylogenetically older part and a dorsal nucleus. The latter became increasingly important during the course of evolution and projects to the occipital primary visual cortex by way of the optic radiations. The ventral nucleus retains, in humans, connections with the midbrain. From a histological point of view, the lateral geniculate body consists of six alternating layers of gray and white matter, numbered from ventral to dorsal. In the macaque, crossed fibers terminate in layers 1, 4, 6 while the uncrossed fibers end in layers 2, 3, 5 (Minkowski 1913; Von Noorden and Middleditch 1975). In humans, the ultrastructure of the lateral geniculate body with its laminar constitution seems more variable and is more often found in the posterior half of the nucleus, according to Hickey and Guillery (1979), while the anterior portion of the nucleus frequently shows irregular interdigitations.

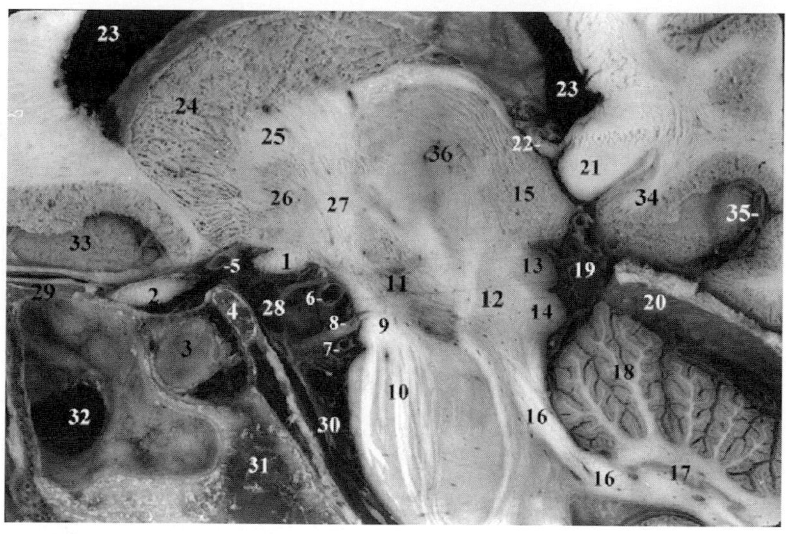

Fig. 9.36. The cisternal optic tract: parasagittal anatomic cut with MR correlation. *1* Optic tract; *2* cisternal optic nerve; *3* hypophysis; *4* dorsum sellae; *5* proximal segment of anterior cerebral artery; *6* proximal segment of posterior cerebral artery; *7* superior cerebellar artery; *8* oculomotor nerve (III); *9* cerebral peduncle (crus cerebri); *10* corticospinal tract in the pons; *11* substantia nigra; *12* midbrain tegmentum; *13* superior colliculus; *14* inferior colliculus; *15* pulvinar thalami; *16* superior cerebellar peduncle; *17* dentate nucleus; *18* culmen vermis; *19* ambient cistern; *20* tentorium cerebelli; *21* splenium of corpus callosum; *22* fornix; *23* lateral ventricle, body; *24* caudate nucleus; *25* corona radiata; *26* lentiform nucleus; *27* internal capsule; *28* interpeduncular cistern; *29* jugum sphenoidale; *30* prepontine cistern; *31* clivus; *32* sphenoid sinus; *33* gyrus rectus; *34* isthmus; *35* parieto-occipital-calcarine common stem; *36* thalamus

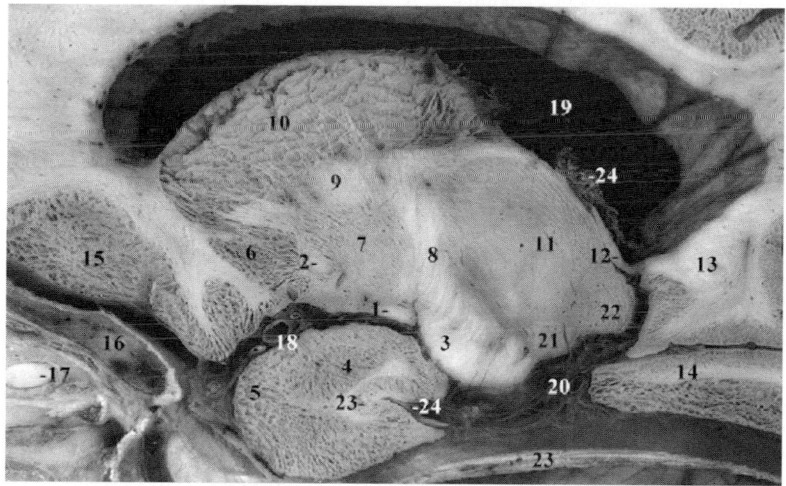

Fig. 9.37. The pericrural optic tract: parasagittal uncal cut with MR correlation. *1* Optic tract; *2* anterior commissure; *3* cerebral peduncle (crus cerebri); *4* amygdala; *5* uncus; *6* putamen; *7* pallidum; *8* internal capsule; *9* corona radiata; *10* caudate nucleus; *11* thalamus; *12* posterior column of the fornix; *13* isthmus; *14* lingual gyrus; *15* orbitofrontal lobe; *16* anterior clinoid process; *17* intraorbital optic nerve; *18* middle cerebral artery; *19* lateral ventricle; *20* ambient (perimesencephalic) cistern; *21* medial geniculate body; *22* pulvinar thalami; *23* tentorium cerebelli; *24* uncal sulcus

F The Geniculocalcarine Tract or Optic Radiation

The anterior visual fibers are relayed to the occipital cortex as the optic radiation (of Gratiolet), which extends from the lateral geniculate body (Fig. 9.41) to the striate cortex. The geniculocalcarine tract leaves the lateral geniculate body as the optic peduncle, well-shown on MR parasagittal cuts (Fig. 9.42). It forms a prominent ribbon-like lamina about 2 cm wide in the temporal, parietal and occipital lobes. Its fibers are grouped into fiber bundles arranged in parallel, with a definite topographic origin from the lateral geniculate body, and end on the visual cortex. The optic radiation then divides into three main anatomic-functional bundles which occupy the external sagittal stratum. These can be discerned mainly on coronal slices using either the FSE-PDw (Fig. 9.43B) or the STIR pulse sequences (Fig. 9.43C,D), performed perpendicular to the long axis of the temporo-occipital lobe – as obtained with the PC-OB reference line – due to their relationship to the inferior horn of the lateral ventricle (Fig. 9.43A).

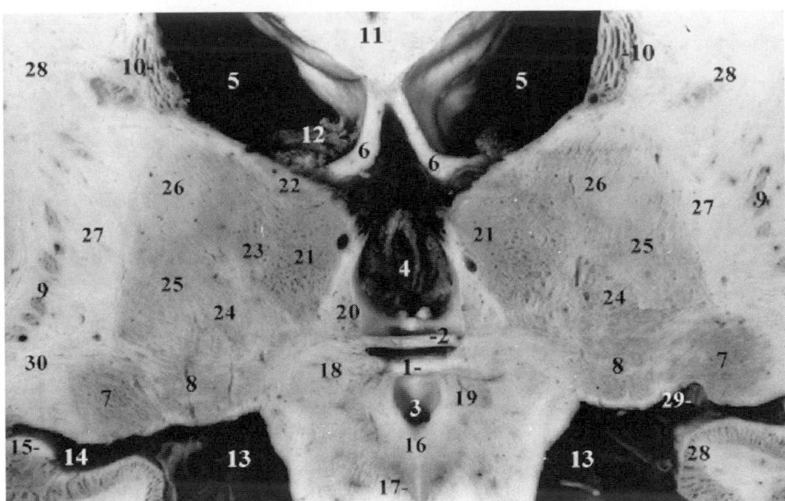

Fig. 9.38. The lateral geniculate bodies: coronal anatomic cut showing that the lateral geniculate bodies are actually included in the commissural-obex (PC-OB) reference plane. *1* Posterior commissure (upper landmark of PC-OB reference plane); *2* habenular commissure; *3* cerebral aqueduct (superior aperture); *4* third ventricle; *5* lateral ventricle; *6* posterior columns of fornix; *7* lateral geniculate body (constant structures in the reference plane); *8* medial geniculate body; *9* posterior border of putamen; *10* caudate nucleus body; *11* corpus callosum; *12* choroid plexus of lateral ventricle; *13* lateromesencephalic cistern (transverse fissure); *14* choroidal fissure (transverse fissure); *15* fimbria of hippocampus; *16* periaqueductal gray matter; *17* oculomotor nuclear complex (V-shape); *18* pretectal nucleus; *19* nucleus of posterior commissure; *20* habenular nuclei; *21* dorsomedian nucleus of thalamus; *22* lateral dorsal nucleus of thalamus; *23* centromedian nucleus of thalamus; *24* ventral posteromedial nucleus of thalamus; *25* ventral posterolateral nucleus of thalamus; *26* ventral lateral nucleus of thalamus; *27* internal capsule (posterior extremity of posterior limb); *28* corona radiata; *29* posterior cerebral artery; *30* internal capsule, retrolenticular part

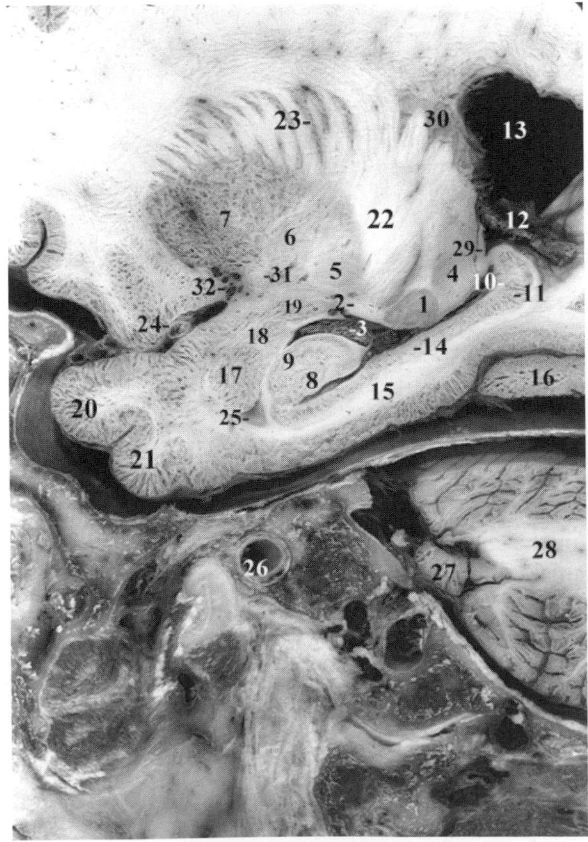

Fig. 9.39. The lateral geniculate body: parasagittal anatomic cut passing through the hippocampus and amygdala, showing the terminal segment of the optic tract which abuts the anterior aspect of the cap-shaped lateral geniculate body with its internal specific lamination. *1* Lateral geniculate body; *2* optic tract; *3* temporal horn of the lateral ventricle (and choroid plexus); *4* pulvinar thalami; *5* medial pallidum; *6* lateral pallidum; *7* putamen; *8* hippocampal head, gyrus dentatus; *9* hippocampal head, Ammon's horn; *10* hippocampal tail, gyrus dentatus; *11* hippocampal tail, Ammon's horn; *12* choroid plexus of lateral ventricle; *13* atrium of lateral ventricle; *14* subiculum; *15* parahippocampal gyrus; *16* fusiform gyrus; *17* amygdala, lateral nucleus; *18* amygdala, basal nucleus; *19* amygdala; *20* superior temporal gyrus; *21* middle temporal gyrus; *22* internal capsule; *23* lenticular caudate bridges of gray matter; *24* middle cerebral artery; *25* temporal horn of lateral ventricle; *26* internal carotid artery (carotid canal); *27* flocculus; *28* cerebellar white matter; *29* posterior column of fornix; *30* caudate nucleus, body; *31* anterior commissure; *32* anterior perforated substance

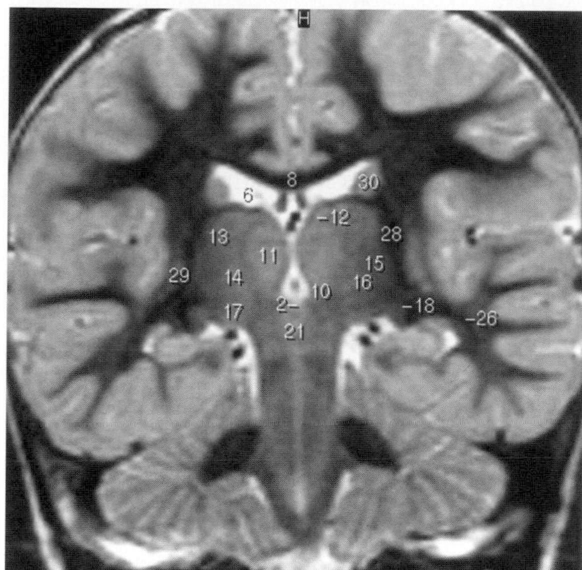

Fig. 9.40. The lateral geniculate bodies. Coronal MR cut passing through the lateral geniculate bodies (*18*) which are constantly found throughout the cut and contained in the cross-section corresponding to the commissural-obex (PC-OB) reference line, and bounded laterally by the relative low signal of the white bundles constituting the triangular area of Wernicke. Laterally, in the temporal lobes the geniculo-calcarine tracts (Meyer's loop, 26) are displayed, well depicted on STIR (or proton density or diffusion weighted) MR sequences

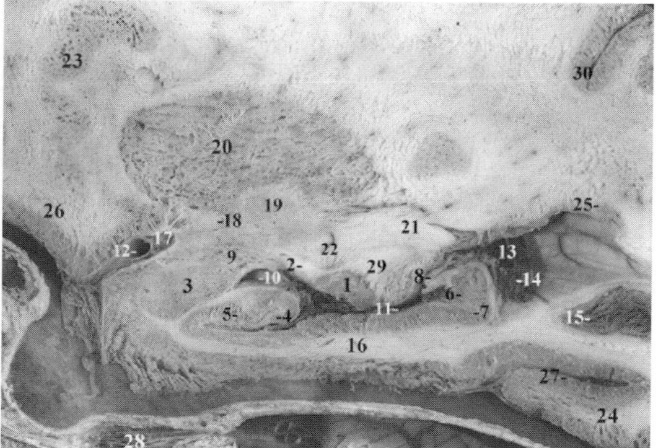

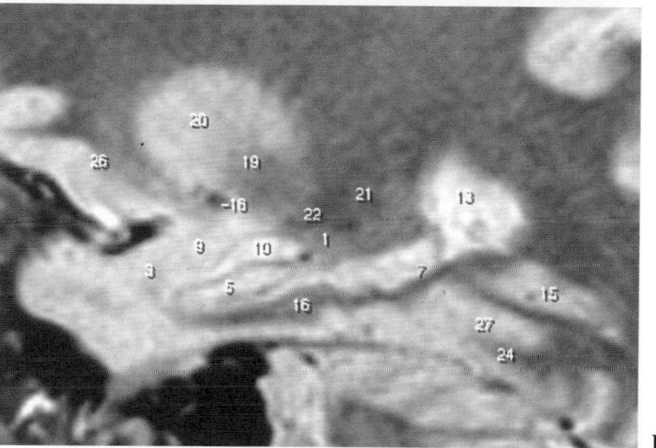

Fig. 9.41A,B. The optic peduncle and the geniculocalcarine tract: parasagittal anatomic cut with MR correlation, using STIR pulse sequence, 3 mm thick. *1* Lateral geniculate body; *2* optic tract; *3* amygdala, basal nucleus; *4* hippocampal head, dentate gyrus; *5* hippocampal head, Ammon's horn; *6* hippocampal tail, dentate gyrus; *7* hippocampal tail, Ammon's horn; *8* fimbria; *9* amygdala, medial nucleus; *10* temporal horn of lateral ventricle; *11* perimesencephalic cistern; *12* lateral fissure; *13* atrium of lateral ventricle; *14* choroid plexus of lateral ventricle; *15* anterior calcarine sulcus; *16* parahippocampal gyrus; *17* limen insulae; *18* anterior commissure; *19* pallidum; *20* putamen; *21* retrolenticular portion of internal capsule; *22* sublenticular portion of internal capsule; *23* anterior insular cortex; *24* fusiform gyrus; *25* tail of caudate nucleus; *26* orbitofrontal gyrus; *27* collateral sulcus; *28* trigeminal cave; *29* triangular area of Wernicke; *30* intraparietal sulcus

The dorsal and lateral bundles spread directly posteriorly through the posterior temporal and parietal lobes. The ventral bundle makes a loop into the temporal lobe anteriorly and laterally, above and around the temporal horn of the lateral ventricle, before it spreads backward to reach the striate cortex, just like the other two bundles. The anterior deviation of the inferior optic radiation, known as Meyer's loop (Meyer 1907), is about 0.5–1 cm lateral to the tip of the inferior horn of the lateral ventricle, providing that the visual fibers are not encountered, as far as is known, in the first 5 cm from the temporal pole. The optic radiations and the intracranial optic pathways are very well shown on the meticulous dissections of Klingler (1948; Fig. 9.44).

Considering their MR correlation and signal appearance, the optic radiations are easily depicted under normal conditions – are well as in pathologic states, dissected, for instance, by vasogenic edema – in both the coronal and axial planes on accurate T2 weighted sequences showing the low signal intensity of the bulky fibers along the temporo-occipital horn of the ventricle.

The relatively lower signal of the optic radiations, as compared to the rest of the loosely organized white matter core of the hemispheres, could be due to the orientational dependence of T2 relaxation of the tracts on the static magnetic field direction (Bo). This would cause, at least partly, a relative shortening of the T2 relaxation of the radiations, which are roughly orthogonal to the coronal cuts parallel to the PC-OB line. The latter may become oriented in the Bo direction in routine positioning of the patient's

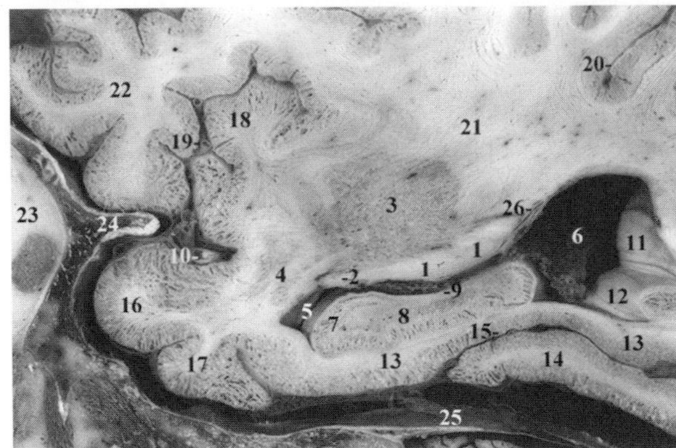

A

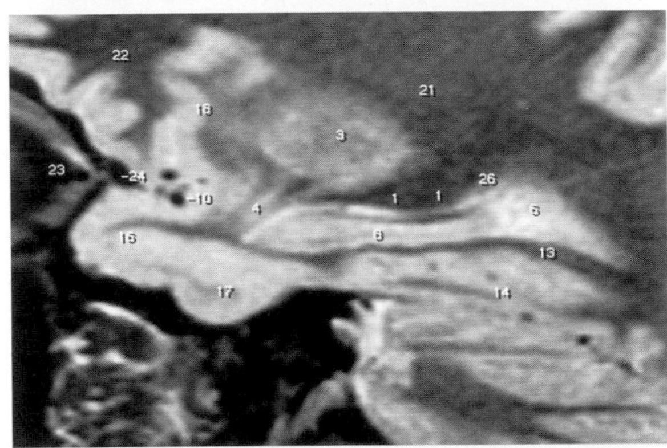

B

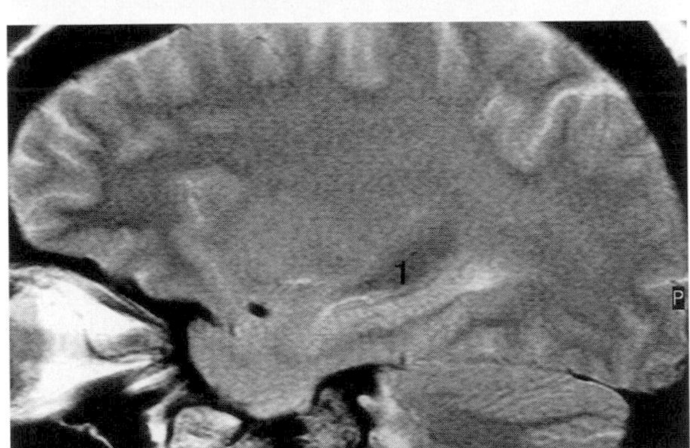

C

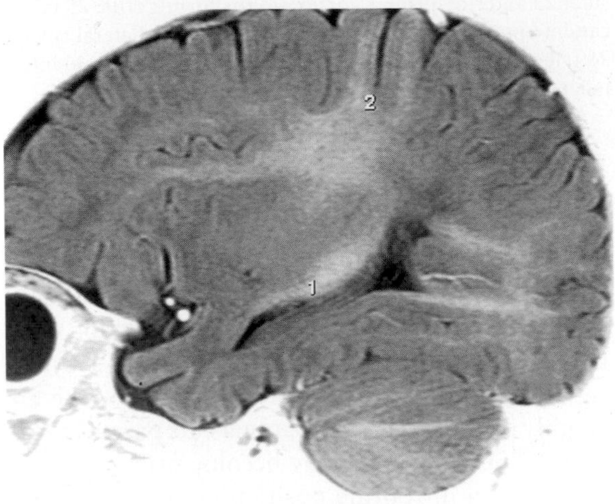

D

head in the magnet bore (Fullerton and Cameron 1988).

Considering the functional aspect:

- The vertical or lateral bundle, comprising more than half of the optic radiation, corresponds to the macular fibers originating from both homonymous hemimaculas. The upper half of the segment represents the upper quadrants and the lower half the lower quadrants. These fibers supply the striate cortex over the pole of the occipital lobe.
- The dorsal bundle includes fibers originating from the medial part of the lateral geniculate body and corresponding to the upper extramacular portions of both homonymous hemiretinas. This bundle projects to the upper lip of the calcarine fissure.
- The ventral horizontal bundle includes fibers originating from the external part of the lateral geniculate body and corresponding to the lower extramacular or peripheral portions of the homonymous hemiretinas. This bundle projects to the lower lip of the calcarine fissure.

G The Striate Visual Cortex (Area 17)

The striate or visual cortex, also referred to as area 17 of Brodmann, occupies the superior and inferior lips of the calcarine sulcus. It is limited posteriorly by the lunate sulcus, when present, and may extend beyond the occipital pole of the hemisphere for a distance of 1–1.5 cm. This extension onto the medial posterior aspect of the occipital pole shows important individual variations. The cortex of the visual sensory area is striate and identified histologically by a white line, the line of Gennari, which is a layer of myelinated terminals of optic radiations fibers, not visible at

Fig. 9.42A–D. The geniculocalcarine tract or optic radiations: parasagittal anatomic cut (**A**) with MR correlations using STIR sequence (**B**), FSE-T2-w. sequence (**C**) and STIR sequence with inverse video display, in an infant (**D**). *1* Optic radiations (geniculocalcarine tract); *2* optic peduncle; *3* putamen; *4* temporal stem; *5* inferior horn of lateral ventricle; *6* atrium of lateral ventricle and choroid plexus; *7* hippocampal body, Ammon's horn; *8* hippocampal body, dentate gyrus; *9* fimbria; *10* middle cerebral artery; *11* calcar avis; *12* calcar avis; *13* parahippocampal gyrus; *14* fusiform gyrus; *15* collateral sulcus; *16* superior temporal gyrus; *17* middle temporal gyrus; *18* insular cortex; *19* circular sulcus of the insula; *20* intraparietal sulcus; *21* centrum semi-ovale; *22* frontal lobe; *23* orbit; *24* pterion; *25* tentorium cerebelli; *26* tail of caudate nucleus

present on routine MR imaging using a standard head coil. The parieto-occipital sulcus limits the striate cortex anteriorly. An average of 67% of the visual cortex is buried in the depth of the calcarine fissure and its branches (Zuckerkandel 1906; Hines 1942; Stensaas et al. 1974).

The extent of the calcarine fissure is variable, usually restricted to the medial surface of the hemisphere, well delineated on the MR parasagittal cut (Fig. 9.45). It begins near the occipital pole, then runs anteriorly with a slightly curved course before it joins the parieto-occipital sulcus. The area of the striate cortex is greater below than above the calcarine fissure, extending about 2 cm more anteriorly. Moreover, the floor of the calcarine fissure is sometimes crossed by buried gyri, such as the anterior and posterior cuneolingual gyri of Déjerine, evidenced on the parasagittal cuts. The anterior part of the calcarine is a limiting sulcus producing an elevation in the medial wall of the posterior horn of the lateral ventricle (Lazorthes and Poulhes 1948), named the calcar avis (Fig. 9.42). The striate cortex is relatively thin, averaging 2.2 mm according to Von Economo and Koskinas (1925). The visual radiations constitute the afferent connections of the striate cortex and terminate in area 17 after coursing in the stripe of Gennari (Bailey and Von Bonin 1951).

The striate cortex is situated between the cuneus, a wedge-shaped area located above the calcarine sulcus whose surface is generally indented by one or two small sulci, and the lingual gyrus lying below, between the calcarine sulcus superiorly and the collateral sulcus inferiorly (Fig. 9.46). Note that the collateral sulcus begins near the occipital pole and extends anteriorly, roughly parallel to the calcarine sulcus.

Considering the functional and anatomic aspects of the visual cortex, there, is at least partly, general agreement regarding Holmes' (1919, 1931) conception of cortical representation, i.e., the upper half of each retina covering the dorsal part of the occipital striate cortex and the lower half the ventral part. Regarding the disposition of the macular fibers, Holmes considered it to be located on the tip of the posterior pole of the cerebral hemisphere, while according to Von Monakow (1896, 1914) and Polyak (1958) a wide distribution of these fibers along the calcarine fissure is observed. Hubel and Wiesel (1968, 1969, 1972; Hubel et al. 1976, 1977), working on the macaque, provided a major contribution to the modus operandi of the striate visuosensory cortex and the functions of the striate cortical cells.

H The Parastriate (Area 18) and Peristriate (Area 19) Cortex

The striate cortex (area 17) is intimately related to the parastriate cortex (area 18) which lies in a portion of the occipital lobe contiguous to the latter. The Gennari band is not found in this area. The peristriate area (area 19) is much larger than area 18, lying on the lateral aspect of the cerebral hemisphere and extending beyond the medial aspect of the hemisphere to surround the parastriate area from above and below. Most of the peristriate area lies in the posterior part of the parietal lobe. It extends inferomedially to the posterior portion of the temporal lobe.

Considering the lateral aspect of the occipital lobe, major variations in the sulcal patterns have been reported by numerous authors, as discussed in Chap. 3, and need further investigation.

Both area 18 and area 19 are concerned with visuointegrative functions with respect to area 17, which is specifically concerned with visual sensations. Lesions affecting this prestriate visuomotor cortex cause disturbances in visual orientation and visual agnosia as well as loss of topographic memory and the inability to estimate distances. Zeki (1969, 1971, 1973,1978a,b) showed, in the rhesus monkey, the presence of fibers projections from the striate cortex to the prestriate cortex (areas 18 and 19). In mammals, Zeki (1977) demonstrated the presence of an anatomical region, the V-4 or fourth visual area, which is believed to be concerned with color information analysis. In fact, two subregions are identified in the rhesus monkey, the first situated in the anterior lip of the lunate sulcus and the other in the lateral aspect of the posterior bank of the superior temporal sulcus. Clinical and functional MR data tend to confirm such results in humans.

I The Superior Colliculi as Related to the Visual System

The superior colliculi are found in the midbrain tectum caudal to the posterior commissure and the pineal body and at the same level as the red nuclei on axial cuts. Part of the quadrigeminal plate, the superior colliculi are observed inferior to the splenium, partly overlapped on each side by the pulvinar thalami, as displayed on coronal anatomic and MR views or the parasagittal cuts (see Chap. 8). From a functional point of view, the superior colliculi as well as

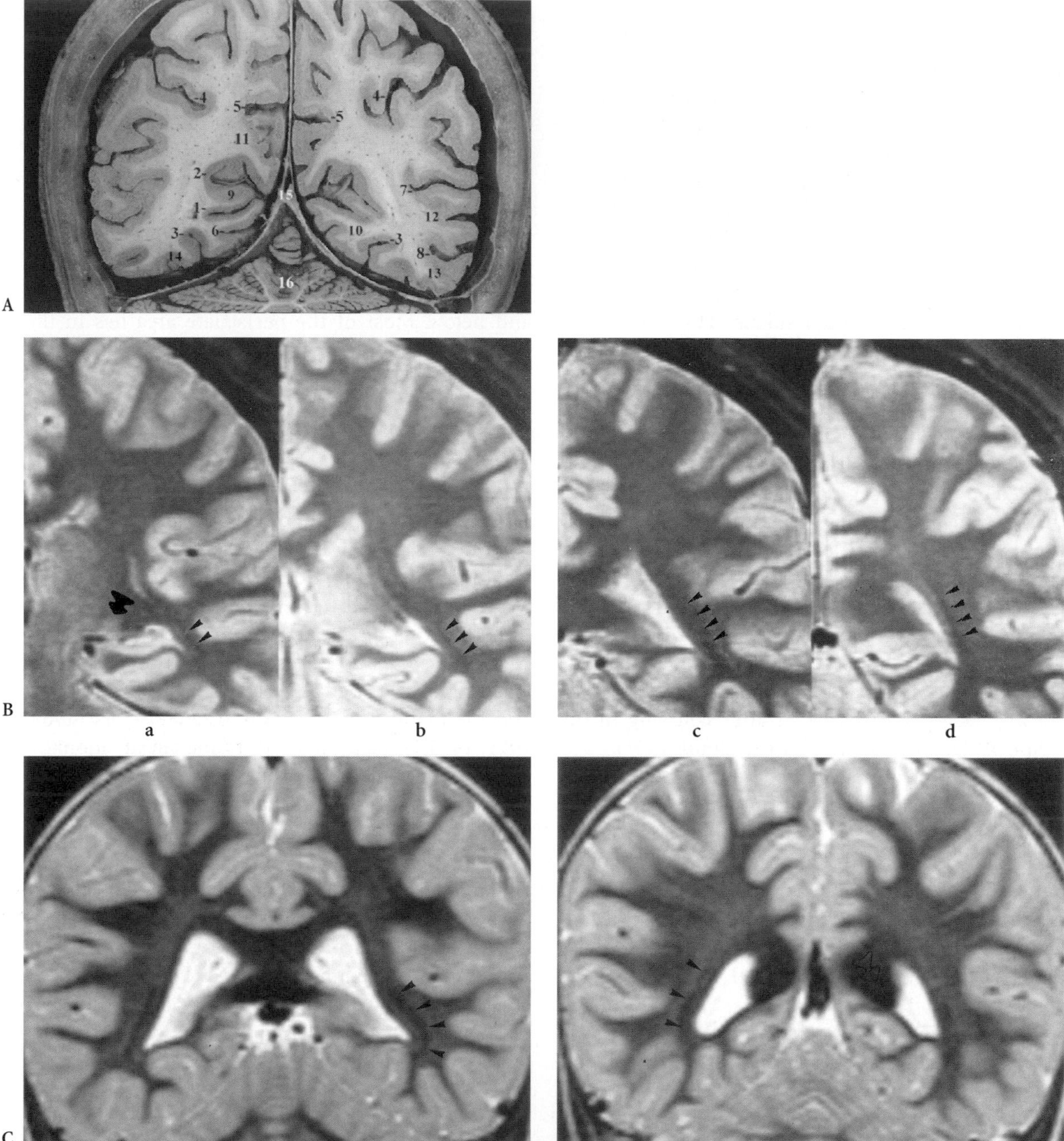

Fig. 9.43. A The calcarine sulcus: coronal anatomic cut. *1* Calcarine sulcus; *2* parieto-occipital sulcus; *3* collateral sulcus; *4* intraparietal sulcus; *5* subparietal sulcus; *6* lingual sulcus; *7* superior temporal (parallel) sulcus; *8* inferior temporal sulcus; *9* cuneus; *10* lingual gyrus; *11* precuneus; *12* superior temporal gyrus; *13* lateral occipito-temporal gyrus; *14* medial occipitotemporal gyrus; *15* gyrus rectus; *16* cerebellum; *17* tentorium cerebelli; *18* lateral sinus. **B,C** The optic radiations (*arrowheads*): coronal MR cuts showing the geniculocalcarine tracts (*arrowheads*), using proton density (**B**) and STIR pulse sequences, in an adult (**C**); at the level of the lateral geniculate bodies (**a,** *black arrow*), in the PC-OB reference plane; at the level of the pulvinar thalami (**b**); lateral to the atrium of the lateral ventricles (**c**); lateral and in close relation to the occipital horns of the lateral ventricles (**d**). **D,E** The optic radiations (*arrow*): coronal MR cuts in the commissural-obex reference plane (PC-OB) orientation, showing the early myelinated geniculocalcarine tracts in two infants, 4 months (**D**) and 6 months (**E**), explored using STIR sequences and displayed with inverse video. **D** *1* Lateral geniculate body; *2* optic radiation; *3* corticospinal tract; *4* calcarine fissure; *5* cerebral peduncle; *6* superior cerebellar peduncle; *7* middle cerebellar peduncle; *8* inferior colliculi; *9* atrium of lateral ventricle; *10* pulvinar thalami. **E** *1* Thalamus; *2* lateral geniculate body; *3* optic radiations; *4* corticospinal tract; *5* album cerebelli; *6* ambient cistern and tectal plate; *7* splenium of corpus callosum; *8* atrium; *9* splenium; *10* lateral fissure; *11* calcarine sulcus; *12* parieto-occipital sulcus

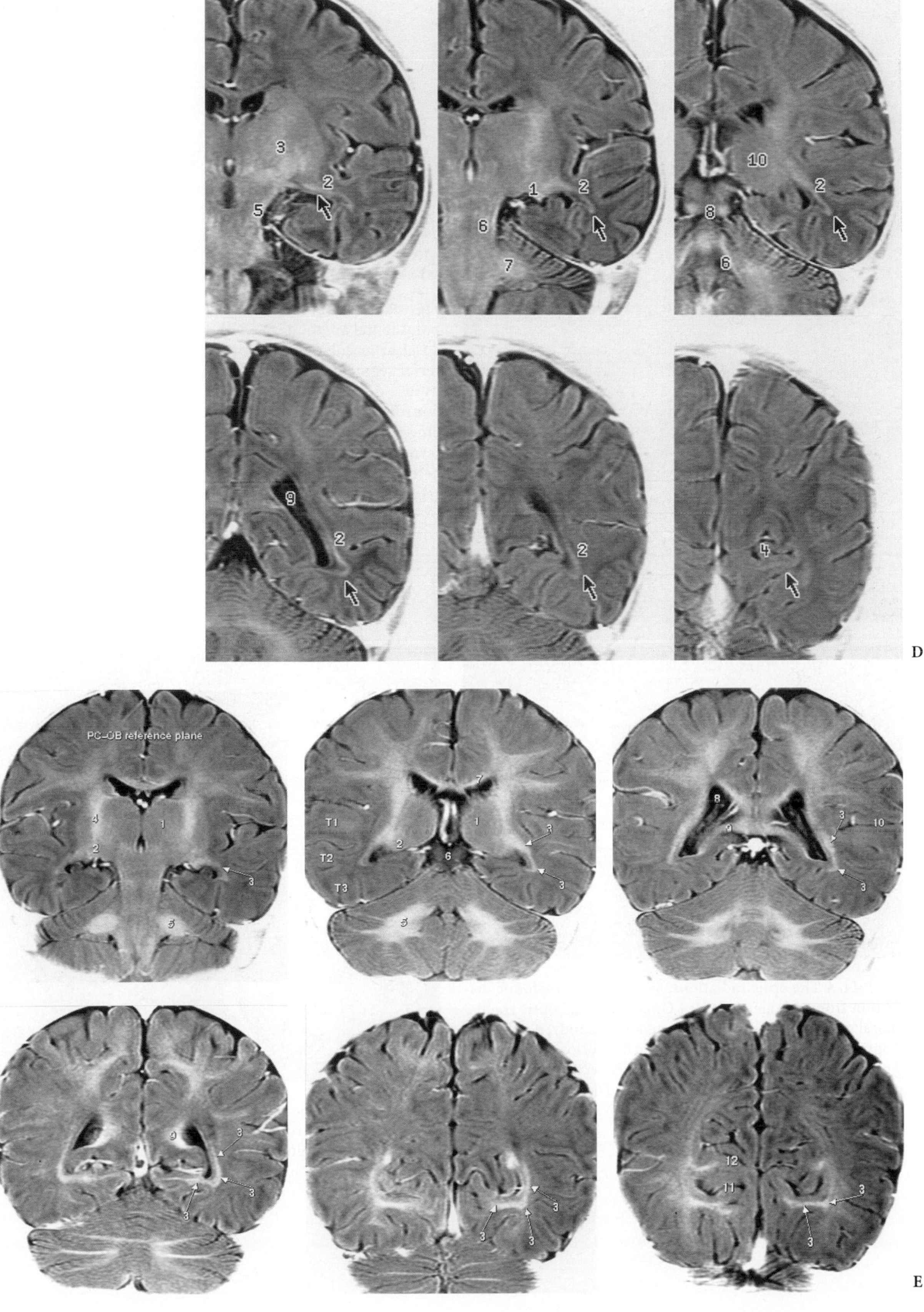
3
2
5
1
2
6
7
10
2
8
6
9
2
2
4
D
PC-OB reference plane
4
1
2
3
5
7
T1
1
3
T2
2
6
T3
3
5
8
3
10
9
3
9
3
3
3
3
3
3
12
11
3
3
E

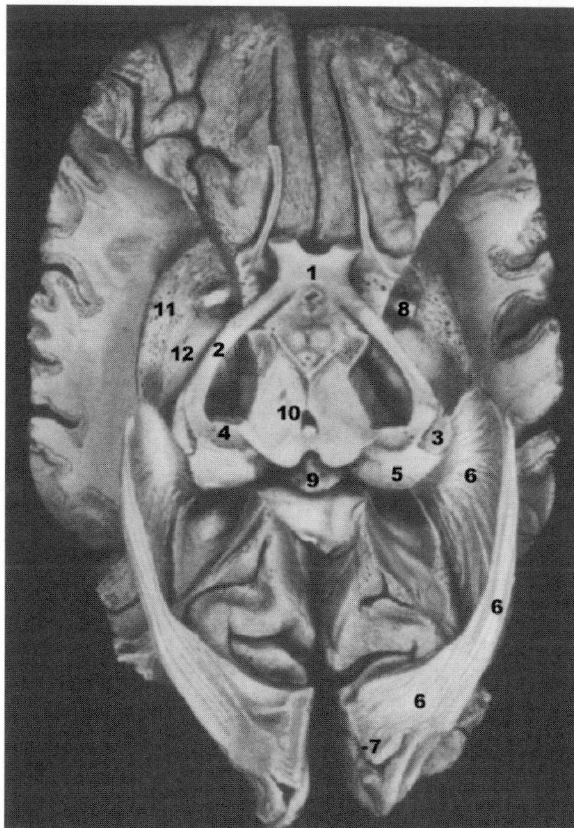

A

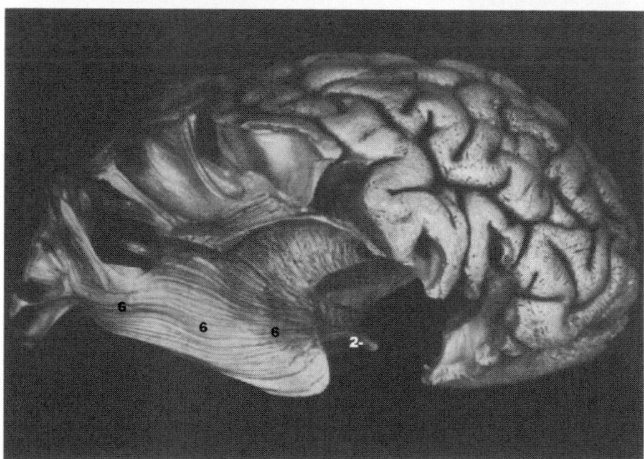

B

Fig. 9.44. A The optic radiations, inferior view. Anatomic dissection from Klingler (1948): *1* Optic chiasm; *2* optic tract; *3* lateral geniculate body; *4* medial geniculate body; *5* pulvinar; *6* optic radiations; *7* calcarine sulcus; *8* anterior commissure; *9* pineal body; *10* section of midbrain; *11* section of the putamen; *12* section of the globus pallidus. **B** The optic radiations, lateral view. Anatomic dissections from Klingler (1948); *2* optic tract; *6* optic radiations

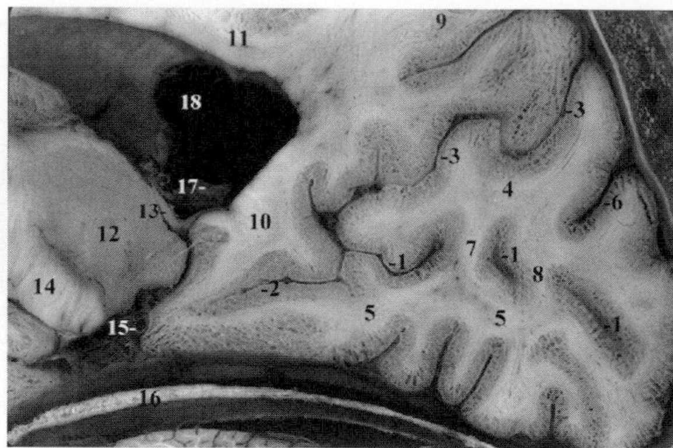

Fig. 9.45. The calcarine and parieto-occipital sulci: parasagittal anatomic cut with MR correlation (see Chap. 3): *1* Calcarine sulcus, posterior segment; *2* calcarine sulcus, anterior segment; *3* parieto-occipital sulcus; *4* cuneus; *5* lingual gyrus; *6* sulcus cunei; *7* cuneolingual gyrus, anterior; *8* cuneolingual gyrus, posterior; *9* precuneus; *10* isthmus; *11* cingulum; *12* thalamus; *13* posterior column of fornix; *14* internal capsule; *15* posterior cerebral artery; *16* tentorium cerebelli; *17* choroid plexus of lateral ventricle; *18* lateral ventricle, body

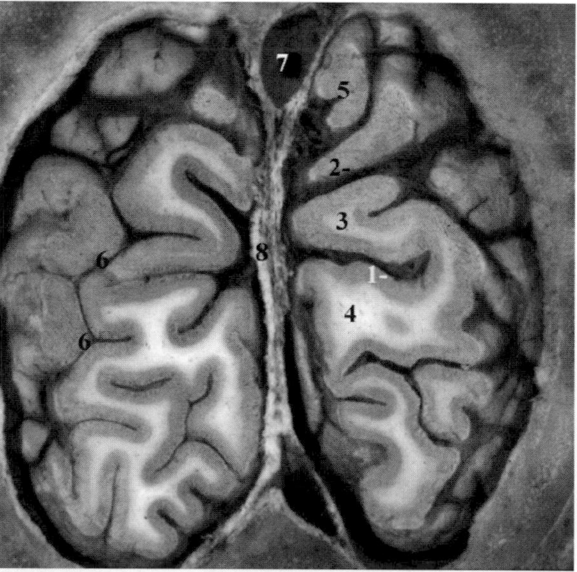

Fig. 9.46. The calcarine and parieto-occipital sulci; coronal anatomic cut. *1* Retrocalcarine sulcus; *2* parieto-occipital sulcus; *3* cuneus; *4* lingual gyrus; *5* precuneus; *6* occipital sulcus; *7* superior sagittal sinus; *8* falx cerebri

the pretectum are mainly concerned with pupillary functions and ocular motility. Clinical observations show that the superior colliculi are also involved in the ability to localize stimuli, a function presumably mediated through a retinotectal pathway (Zihl and Von Cramon 1979a,b).

J Vascular Supply to the Visual Pathway

The vascularization of the very long visual pathways is supplied by different pedicles originating from the carotid and basilar systems and the anastomotic circle of Willis. Anteriorly, the ophthalmic artery supplies the intraocular and the intraorbital portions of the orbital optic nerve. An additional contribution is frequently observed from the external carotid system through the middle meningeal artery. The intracanalicular portion of the optic nerve is vascularized mainly by pial vessels originating from the internal carotid arteries, and rarely by collateral pedicles arising from the ophthalmic arteries (Hayreh 1962a,b).

Vasular supply of the intracranial portion of the optic nerves depends on small pedicles arising from the internal carotid arteries, the anterior communicating artery and the proximal A1 segments of the anterior cerebral arteries (Perlmutter and Rhoton 1976; Rhoton et al. 1977). Anatomical variations are noted depending on the length of the cisternal optic nerve.

The blood supply to the dorsal optic chiasm is primarily through the A1 segment of the anterior cerebral arteries, with variable contributions from the internal carotid arteries and the anterior communicating artery (Bergland and Ray 1969; Wollschlaeger et al. 1971; Perlmutter and Rhoton 1976). The ventral optic chiasm is vascularized by branches originating from the posterior communicating artery, the posterior cerebral artery, and even the basilar artery, according to Bergland and Ray (1969). The major contribution is from the carotid arteries.

The optic tract receive its blood supply mainly from the anterior choroidal artery, a branch of the internal carotid, according to Carpenter et al. (1954). The lateral geniculate body is supplied laterally by the anterior choroidal artery and medially by the lateral posterior choroidal artery (Abbie 1933; François et al. 1956).

Considering the posterior optic pathways along their intracerebral route, the middle cerebral artery supplies the upper portion of the optic radiations while the inferior portion is vascularized by branches of the posterior cerebral artery. The vascular supply to the striate cortex is mainly via the posterior cerebral artery and its branches (Zeal and Rhoton 1978). At the occipital pole, Beauvieux and Ristich-Goelmino (1926) pointed out the existence of an anastomotic network between branches of the posterior cerebral artery and middle cerebral artery.

V Magnetic Resonance Approach to Neuro-ophthalmological Disorders

Because of the close anatomical relationship between the eyes and brain, one should be aware that neuro-ophthalmological signs or symptoms are diagnostic and of localizing significance. Since more than half of patients with brain tumors present with some form of impairment of the visual pathways or the ocular motor system, one must realize the importance of the conjugate responsibility of the neuro-opththalmologist and the neuroradiologist in discovering minute brain pathologies as early as possible. An MR examination strategy depends very closely on the clinical and the paraclinical neuro-ophthalmological data, mainly visual acuity, ocular fundus, visual field, and evoked potentials (Walsh 1947; Guillaumat 1959; Cogan 1966; Walsh and Hoyt 1969; Bregeat 1973; Duke Elder 1973; Jones and Jakobiec 1979; Leigh and Zee 1983; Glaser 1990; Burde et al. 1992; Miller and Newman 1997).

In most cases, the positive diagnosis will depend upon an accurate anatomic and clinical correlation with respect to the neuroradio-ophthalmological results. Regarding imaging (Tamraz et al. 1988; Tamraz 1994) three main anatomic and functional areas along the visual pathways can be distinguished: the orbits, the opticochiasmatic region and the optic radiations.

A The Orbital Region

There is no doubt concerning the accuracy of the NOP as the cephalic orientation of choice in the examination of the intraorbital optic nerves. Coronal cuts perpendicular to the NOP will best show and help to evaluate any discreet modification in size or signal intensity involving the intraorbital segment or the perioptic sheaths. Sagittal oblique slices oriented in the long axis of the optic canals best evaluate, if needed, the intracanalicular and the cisternal optic nerve, in case of doubt about possible extension of a gliomatous process, from the orbit to the cranial cavity. Partial volume effect phenomena and false enlargements, due to wide variations in the size and shape of the optic canal itself or the adjacent spheno-ethmoidal sinuses, may therefore be avoided. Thin slices (3 mm average) and high resolution images are recommended in all cases. Oblique coronal cuts perpendicular to the NOP may be necessary if a perioptic infiltrating process is suspected. In such cases a trail of contrast infusion is recommended and thin, T1 weighted, contiguous slices with fat suppression (3 mm) are mandatory using small fields of view and a surface coil.

B The Chiasmal Region

Imaging of the opticochiasmatic region, including the chiasm and the adjacent cisternal optic nerves and optic tracts, has greatly benefited from MR sagittal and coronal approaches (Tamraz et al. 1987c). Using CT in the axial plane, the first step in diagnosing a suspected lesion in this area was based on analysis and shape recognition of the chiasmatic cistern, which usually takes the aspect of a star. The shape of the chiasm itself varies according to its position which is known to change with the cephalic index and with aging. MR modified the examination algorithms by using the primary sagittal approach, which permits both a direct appreciation of the possible existence of a lesion in or about the chiasm and an efficient evaluation of its intrinsic or extrinsic nature. An increased thickness of the chiasm, disorganization and infiltration of the floor of the third ventricle, anterior and/or posterior extensions of the process along the optic pathways are all readily evidenced at a glance. Tumorous conditions of the sellar region or the jugum sphenoidale as well as other regional extrinsic processes arising from the sphenocavernous region or the clivus are hence differentiated.

The next step in MR or CT will be the coronal approach, using, for instance, the perpendicular to the NOP in extremely large lesions or the PC-OB brainstem reference line in small, mainly infiltrative lesions involving the pregeniculate anterior optic pathways and needing long-term follow-up. In optic gliomas, it is of interest to visualize the anterior-posterior extension of the infiltrating tumor, mainly on T2 weighted horizontal cuts, showing the highly characteristic "mustache" appearance of the enlarged optic tracts extending laterally from the chiasm and encircling the rostral mesencephalon on each side to reach the lateral geniculate bodies in a symmetric or asymmetric manner. But, optic tract enlargement, even if easily evidenced in the axial plane when the optic tract is tumorous, is better evaluated on coronal cuts when any modification of its perimesencephalic part is suspected. This is particularly true in the case of neurofibromatosis. Coronal cuts will best evaluate the superior and lateral extension of infiltrating gliomas arising from the chiasm, optic tracts or third ventricular walls. Hamartomas of the pallidum are very easily evidenced on these coronal T2 weighted cuts, lying above the AC, which characteristically separates them from the optic tracts and the sublenticular area (Tamraz et al. 1987b). Follow-up of patients with neurofibromatosis necessitates a strict reproducibility of the slices in order to depict as early as possible any modification of the extent or signal intensity of the hamartomatous lesions.

The lateral geniculate bodies and the adjacent part of the optic tract show an important relation to the pulvinar and the crura cerebri and are best depicted on the coronal cut parallel to the PC-OB reference line. The lateral geniculate bodies are found anterior to this plane in most instances, depending on slice thickness.

Parasagittal cuts contribute greatly in showing the lateral geniculate body above the hippocampal formation. Coronal multislices, oriented according to the PC-OB line and extending from the tectal plate to the genu of the corpus callosum, allow reliable and efficient investigation of the anterior intracranial optic pathways, from the optic canal to the origin of the geniculocalcarine tracts.

Imaging the lateral geniculate bodies in the sagittal plane also permits a perpendicular evaluation of the bulky optic peduncle as it spreads laterally above the inferior horn of the lateral ventricle. Axial and coronal cuts, if performed according to the previously discussed reference lines, will be most helpful in evaluating the temporal, parietal, and occipital lateroventricular route of the geniculocalcarine tract. Vertical topographical correlations, as compared to perimetry, will best benefit from the coronal approach perpendicular to the long axis of the inferior ventricular horns, as obtained using the PC-OB reference line.

C The Striate Cortex

The calcarine fissures are readily shown on the midsagittal cut of the brain, which can easily be used to evaluate the medial aspect of the cerebral hemisphere. The striate cortex, lying in the depth of the fissure and forming its upper and lower lips, may also be depicted on coronal and axial cuts. Its close relationship to the occipital horns of the lateral ventricle, and the visibility of the optic radiations on PD weighted or STIR coronal cuts at its vicinity, may aid in its recognition. Actually, there is no ideal cephalic orientation for studying the calcarine fissure, as it is variable in shape among individuals. Note that the CH-PC reference line most frequently intersects the common stem of the parieto-occipital and calcarine sulci.

To conclude, one can state that the optic pathways are roughly axial and symmetrical, beginning at the retina and extending from anterior to posterior to end in the visual cortex in the occipital lobe. Efficient MR exploration largely depends on previously known, clinical neuro-ophthalmological data. Such data help in choosing the most accurate reference plane and examination algorithm in order to obtain results that are as precise and reproducible as possible. Proper choice of the cephalic reference plane and the orientation and thickness of the slices is of the utmost importance. The cuts should be accurately oriented in order to optimally disclose the morbid process, either intrinsic or extrinsic with respect to the visual path. Moreover, the cephalic reference plane used should allow reliable and reproducible follow-up of the lesion either in order to evaluate its natural history or to appreciate the effect of therapy. Finally, the imaging technique ought to be scrupulously adapted to obtain the best anatomic result, free of eye movements and flow artifacts, to detect even the most elusive abnormality in or about the optic path. At least for the eyes and optic pathways, MR imaging is the modality of choice in evaluating neuro-ophthalmological disorders, due to its well-known, noninvasive tridimensional approach and its high contrast resolution.

References

Abbie AA (1933) The blood supply of lateral geniculate body with note on morphology of choroidal arteries. J Anat 67:491–521

Arey LB, Bickel WH (1935) The fibers in the optic nerve. Anat Rec [Suppl]:61

Bailey P, Von Bonin G (1951) The isocortex of man. University of Illinois Press, Urbana

Beauvieux J, Ristich-Goelmino K (1926) De la vascularisation du centre cortical de la macula. Arch Ophthalmol (Paris) 43:5–20

Bembridge BA (1956) The problem of myelination in the central nervous system, with special reference to the optic nerve. Trans Ophthalmol Soc UK 76:311–322

Bergland R, Ray BS (1969) The arterial supply of the human optic chiasm. J Neurosurg 31:327–334

Bergland RM, Ray BS, Torack RM (1968) Anatomical variations in the pituitary gland and adjacent structures in 225 human autopsy cases. J Neurosurg 28:93–99

Bregeat P (1973) Les syndromes opto-chiasmatiques. Masson, Paris

Broca P (1862) Sur les projections de la tête, et sur le nouveau procédé de céphalométrie. Bull Soc Anthropol Paris, 31st series, pp 514–544

Broca P (1873) Sur le plan horizontal de la tête et sur la méthode trigonométrique. Bull Soc Anthropol 8:48–96

Brouwer G, Zeeman WPC (1925) Experimental anatomical investigations concerning the projection of the retina and the primary optic centers in apes. J Neurol Psychopathol 6:1–10

Brouwer B, Zeeman WPC (1926) The projection of the retina in the primary optic neuron in monkeys. Brain 49:1–35

Burdach K (1819–1826) Vom Baue und Leben des Gehirns. Leipzig

Burde RM, Savino PJ, Trobe JD (1992) Clinical decisions in neuroophthalmology. Mosby Year Book, St Louis

Cabanis EA, Salvolini U, Radallec A, Menichelli F, Pasquini U, Bonnin P (1978) Computed tomography of the optic nerve: part II Size and shape modifications in papilledema. J Comput Assist Tomogr 2:150–155

Cabanis EA, Haut J, Iba-Zizen MT (1980) Exopthtalmométrie tomodensitométrique et biométrie TDM oculo-orbitaire. Bull Soc Ophtalmol, 80:63–66

Cabanis EA, Iba-Zizen MT, Coin JL (1981a) Les voies visuelles un "nouveau" plan d'orientation de la tête (Plan Neuro-Oculaire). Bull Soc Ophtalmol 81:433–439

Cabanis EA, Iba-Zizen MT, Pineau H, Coin JL, Newman N, Salvolini U (1981b) CT scanning in the "neuro-ocular plane": the optic pathways as a "new" cephalic plane. Neuroophthalmology 1:237–251

Cabanis EA, Iba-Zizen MT, Pineau H, Tamraz J, et al. (1982a) Le plan neuro-oculaire (PNO) en tomodensitométrie (TDM ou scanner RX), détermination d'un "nouveau" plan horizontal de référence céphalique orienté selon les voies visuelles/The neuro-ocular plane (NOP) with CT: a new horizontal cephalic reference determined by the optic pathways. Biométrie Hum 17:21–48

Cabanis EA, Iba-Zizen MT, Tamraz J, Muzac S (1982b) Topométrie oculo-orbitaire: aspect dynamique normal et pathologique. In: Tomodensitométrie en pathologie oculo-orbitaire. Bull Soc Ophthalmol, Ann Rep 31–56

Cabanis EA, Iba-Zizen MT, Tamraz J, Stoffels C (1984) IRM de la tête et du cou orientée selon le plan neuro-oculaire (PNO): une condition d'efficacité anatomique. J Bioph Med Nucl 8:48–50

Cabanis EA Laugier A, Iba-Zizen MT, Tamraz J, Stoffels C (1985) Anatomie de la tête. Imagerie par Résonance Magnétique, Le concours médical, 107:3191–3197

Cabanis EA, Tamraz J, Iba-Zizen MT (1986) Imagerie par Résonance Magnétique (IRM) de la tête à 0,5 Tesla. Atlas de corrélations anatomiques normales dans 3 dimensions, selon l'orientation du Plan Neuro-Oculaire (PNO). Feuillets Radiol 26:308–416

Cabanis EA, Tamraz J, Iba-Zizen MT (1988) Corrélations anatomiques normales dans 3 dimensions, selon l'orientation du plan neuro-oculaire In: Atlas d'IRM de l'encéphale et de la moelle. Aspects normaux. Masson, Paris, pp 11–120

Carpenter MB, Norback CR, Moss ML (1954) The anterior choroidal artery, its origins, course, distribution, and variations. Arch Neurol Psychiatr 71:714–722

Cohen M (1989) Perspectives on holoprosencephaly. III. Spectra, distinctions, continuities and discontinuities. Am J Med Genet 34:271–288

Crescitelli F (1977) The visual system in vertebrates. Springer, Berlin Heidelberg New York

Da Vinci L (1911–1916) Quadrerni di anatomia Christiana. Vaugsten, Fonahn et Hopstock

Delattre A, Fenart R (1960) Cranio-cerebral topometry in man. Masson, Paris

Demyer W, Zeman W (1963) Alobar holoprosencephaly with median cleft lip and palate: clinical, nosologic and electroencephalographic consideration. Confin Neurol 23:1–36

Demyer W, Zeman W, Palmer C (1964) The face predicts the brain: diagnostic significance of medial facial anomalies for holoprosencephaly. Pediatrics 34:256–263

Descartes R (1966) L'Homme de René Descartes et un traité de la formation du foetus du même auteur Avec les remarques de Louys de la Forge sur le traité de l'Homme de René Descartes et sur les figures par lui inventées. Charles Angot, Paris

Duke-Elder S (1973) System of ophthalmology. Mosby, St Louis

Elliot Smith G (1903) The morphology of the retrocalcarine region of the cortex cerebri. Proc R Soc 73:59–65

Elliot Smith G (1904) The morphology of the occipital region of the cerebral hemisphere in man and the apes. Anat Anz 24:436–451

Elliot Smith G (1907) New studies on the folding of the visual cortex and the significance to the occipital sulci in the human brain. J Anat 41:198–207

Fenart R, Vincent H, Cabanis EA (1982) Le plan orbitaire chez l'adulte jeune, sa position relative à d'autres éléments architecturaux de la tête Etude vestibulaire. Bull Mém Soc Anthropol 9:29–40

Flechsig PE (1896) Gehirn und Seele. Veit, Leipzig

Flechsig PE (1900) Meine myelogenetische Hirnlehre. Berlin

Francois J, Neetens A, Collette JM (1956) Vascularization of the optic pathways: IV. Optic tract and external geniculate body. Br J Ophthalmol 40:341–354

Fullerton GD, Cameron IL (1988) Relaxation of biological tissues. In: Wehrli FW, Shaw D, Kneelan JB (eds) Biomedical magnetic resonance imaging. VCH, New York

Galen C (131-201) De usu partium de corporis hymani De nervorum dissections and Tyroxes De anatomicis administrationebus

Geoffroy Saint-Hilaire E (1822) Des monstruosités humaines. In "Philosophie anatomique." Imp de Rignoux, Paris, tome II

Geoffroy Saint-Hilaire I (1832) Histoire générale et particulière des anomalies de l'organisation chez l'homme et les animaux. Baillière, Paris, vol II

Glaser JS (1990) Neuroophthalmology. Lippincott, Philadelphia

Gratiolet P (1854) Mémoire sur les plis cérébraux de l'Homme et des Primates. Bertrand, Paris

Grouchy J de, Turleau C (1982) Atlas des maladies chromosomiques, 2nd edn. Expansion Scientifique Française, Paris

Guillaumat L, Morax PV, Offret G (1959) Neuro-ophtalmologie, Masson, Paris

Hamilton WJ, Boyd JD, Mossman HW (1962) Human embryology. Williams and Wilkins, Baltimore

Hayreh SS (1962a) Arteries of the orbit in the human being. Br J Surg 50:938–953

Hayreh SS (1962b) The ophthalmic artery. Br J Ophthalmol 46:212–247

Hickey TL, Guillery RW (1979) Variability of laminar patterns in the human lateral geniculate nucleus. J Comp Neurol 183:221–246

Hilal SK, Trokel SL (1977) Computerized tomography of the orbit using thin sections. Semin Roentgenol 12:137–147

Hines M (1942) Recent contributions to localization of vision in the central nervous system. Arch Ophthalmol (Chicago) 28:913–937

Hirschberg J (1985) The history of ophthalmology The . Wayenbergh, Bonn

Holmes G (1919) The cortical localization of vision. Br Med J 2:193–199

Holmes G (1931) A contribution to the cortical representation of vision. Brain 54:470–479

Hoyt WF, Luis O (1963) The primate chiasm: details of visual fiber organization studied by silver impregnation techniques. Arch Ophthalmol 70:69–85

Hoyt WF (1969) Correlative functional anatomy of the optic chiasm. Clin Neurosurg 17:189–208

Hubel DH, Wiesel TN (1968) Receptive fields and functional architecture of monkey striate cortex. J Physiol (Lond) 195:215–243

Hubel DH, Wiesel TN (1969) Anatomical demonstration of columns in the monkey striate cortex. Nature 221:747–750

Hubel DH, Wiesel TN (1972) Laminar and columnar distribution of geniculocortical fibers in the macaque monkey. J Comp Neurol 146:421--450

Hubel DH, Wiesel TN (1977) Functional architecture of macaque monkey visual cortex. Proc R Soc Lond (Biol) 198:1–59

Hubel DH, Wiesel TN, Le Vay S (1976) Functional architecture of area 17 in normal and monocularly deprived macaque monkeys. Cold Spring Harbor Symp Quant Biol 40:581–589

Jones IS, Jakobiec F (1979) Diseases of the orbit. Harper and Row, Hagerstown

Klingler J (1948) Die makroskopische Anatomie der Ammonsformation: Denkschriften der schweizerischen naturforschenden Gesellschaft. Fretz, Zürich, vol 78 (1)

Krause W (1876) Allgemeine und microscopische Anatomie. Handbuch der menschlichen Anatomie, vol 1. p 165

Kupfer C, Chumbley L, Downer J de C (1967) Quantitative histology of optic nerve, optic tract and lateral geniculate nucleus of man. J Anat 101:393–401

Lang J (1987) Clinical anatomy of the head neurocranium, orbit, cranio-cervical region. Springer, Berlin Heidelberg New York

Langer BG, Mafee MF, Pollack S, Spigos DG, Gyi B (1987) MRI of the normal orbit and optic pathway. In: Mafee MF (ed) Imaging in ophthalmology, part I. Saunders, Philadelphia

Lansizi JM (1717) Tabulae anatomicae clarissimi vizi Bartholomaei Eustachii quas e tenebri tandem vindicatas et Clementis XI pontif. maxim. prefatione, notis que illustravit. Coloniae Allobrogum, Cramer et Perachon

Lazorthes G, Poulhes J (1948) Les variations de la scissure calcarine et de la corne occipitale des ventricules latéraux .CR Ass Anat:210–218

Leigh RJ, Zee DS (1983) The neurology of eye movements. Davis, Philadelphia

Le Gros Clark WE (1941) The laminar organization and cell content of the lateral geniculate body in the monkey. J Anat 75:419–433

Ludwig E, Klingler J (1956) Atlas cerebri humani. Karger, Basel

Magoon EH, Robb RM (1981) Development of myelin in human optic nerve and tract. Arch Ophthalmol 99:655–659

Maniscalco JE, Habal MB (1978) Microanatomy of the optic canal. J Neurosurg 48:402–406

Mann I (1964) Development of the human eye, 3rd edn. Grune and Stratton, New York

Meyer A (1907) The connections of the occipital lobes and the present status of the cerebral visual affections. Trans Assoc Am Physicians 22:7–15

Meynert T (1869) Med Zeitung, Vienna, T14, 107–115

Minkowski M (1913) Experimentelle Untersuchungen uber die Beziehungen der Grosshirnrinde und der Netzhaut zu den primaren optischen Zentren, besonders zum Corpus geniculatum externum. Arb Hirnanat Inst Zurich 7:255–362

Osman Hill WC (1953–1974) Primates comparative anatomy. Univ Edinburgh Press

Perlmutter D, Rhoton AL (1976) Microsurgical anatomy of the anterior cerebral anterior communicating recurrent artery complex. J Neurosurg 45:259–272

Polyak S (1957) The vertebrate visual system. University of Chicago Press, Chicago

Polyak SL (1958) The vertebrate system. In: Kluver H (ed) University of Chicago Press, Chicago

Pirlot P (1969) Morphogénèse évolutive des chordes. Press Univ Montréal

Radius RL, Anderson DL (1979) The course of axons through the retina and optic nerve head. Arch Ophthalmol 97:1154–1158

Repérant J, Saban R (1986) Anatomie comparée du système visuel primaire chez les Mammifères In: Hamard H, Chevaleraud J, Rondot P (eds) Neuropathies optiques. Masson, Paris, pp 43–94

Repérant J, Micelli D, Vesselkin NP, Molotchnikoff S (1989) The centrifugal visual system of vertebrates: a century-old search reviewed. Int Rev Cytol 118:115–171

Rethore MO (1977) Chromosome deletions and ring chromosome syndromes. In: Vinken PJ, Bruyn GW (eds) Handbook of Clinical Neurology, vol 31. North Holland, Amsterdam, pp 549–620

Rethore MO, Pinet J (1987) New deletion and ring chromosome syndromes. In: Vinken PJ, Bruyn GW (eds) Handbook of Clinical Neurology, vol 6. Elsevier, Amsterdam, pp 577–597

Rhoton AL, Harris FS, Renn WH (1977) Microsurgical anatomy of the sellar region and cavernous sinus. In: Smith JL (ed) Neuro-ophthalmology. Mosby, St Louis

Rochon Duvigneaud A (1943) Les yeux et la vision des vertébrés. Masson, Paris

Ronne H (1914) Ueber doppelseitige Hemianopsie mit erhaltener Makula. Klin Monatsbl Augenheilkd 53:470–487

Saban R, Iba-Zizen M T, Rinjard J, Christov K, Strazielle L, Cabanis EA (1983) Tomodensitométrie céphalique in vivo chez Macaca irus. I. Geof dans le plan neuro-oculaire: comparaison avec l'Homme. CR Acad Sci Paris III 297:131–136

Saban R, Cabanis EA, Iba-Zizen MT, Rinjard J, Villiers PA, Meuge C, Strazielle L, Dupuis R (1984) Tomodensitométrie céphalique in vivo chez Hylobates lar lar L 1771, (Catarhini, Anthropomorpha) dans le plan neuro-oculaire. C R Acad Sci Paris, III, 299:151–156

Saban R, Cabanis EA, Iba-Zizen MT, Rinjard J, Villiers PA Meuge C, Strazielle L, Dupuis R (1985) Tomodensitométrie céphalique in vivo chez Pan troglodytes L (Catarhini, Anthropomorpha) dans le plan neuro-oculaire. C R Acad Sci Paris, 300:341–346

Saban R, Cabanis EA, Iba-Zizen MT, Rinjard J, Leclerc-Cassan M, Villiers PA, Christov C, Hugues F, Boitard A (1987) Tomodensitométrie céphalique in vivo du Lion (Felis léo L Fissipeda) dans le plan neuro-oculaire. C R Acad Sci Paris, 305:355–361

Saban R, Cabanis EA, Iba-Zizen MT, Rinjard J, Leclerc-Cassan M, Villiers PA, Lopez A (1989) Biométrie in vivo de la cavité orbitaire des Catarhiniens en tomodensitométrie. Cah Anthropol Biom Hum 7:81–108

Salamon G (1971) Atlas of the arteries of the human brain. Sandoz, Paris

Salamon G, Huang Y (1976) Radiologic tomography of the brain. Springer, New York Berlin Heidelberg

Salvolini U, Cabanis EA, Rodallec A (1978) Computed tomography of the optic nerve. I. Normal results. J Comput Assist Tomogr 2:141–149

Schaeffer JP (1924) Some points in the regional anatomy of the optic pathway with special reference to tumors of the hypophysis cerebri and resulting ocular changes. Anat Rec 28:243–279

Schaltenbrand G, Bailey P (1959) Introduction to stereotaxis with an atlas of human brain, vols I-II. Thieme, Stuttgart

Shanthaveerappa TR, Bourne GH (1964), Arachnoid villi in the optic nerve of man and monkey. Exp Eye Res 3:31–35

Stensaas SS, Eddington DK, Dobelle WH (1974) The topography and variability of the primary visual cortex in man. J Neurosurg 40:747–755

Straatsma BR, Foos RY, Spencer LM (1969) The retina – topography and clinical correlations. Trans New Orleans Acad Ophthalmol. Mosby, St Louis

Szikla G, Bouvier G, Hori T, Petrov V, Cabanis EA, Farnarier P, Iba-Zizen MT (1977) Angiography of the human brain cortex. Springer, Berlin Heidelberg New York, pp 239–259

Talairach J, Ajuriaguerra J de David M (1952) Etudes stéréotaxiques des structures encéphaliques profondes chez l'homme. Presse Med 28:605–609

Talairach J, Szikla F (1967) Atlas stéréotaxique du télencéphale. Masson, Paris

Talairach J, Tournoux P (1988) Co-planar stereotaxic atlas of the human brain. Thieme, Stuttgart

Tamraz J (1983) Atlas d'anatomie céphalique dans le plan neuro-oculaire (PNO). MD Thesis, Paris

Tamraz J, Iba-Zizen MT, Cabanis EA (1984) Atlas d'anatomie céphalique dans le plan neuro-oculaire (PNO). J Fr Ophtalmol 7:371–379

Tamraz J, Iba-Zizen MT, Atiyeh M, Cabanis EA (1985) Atlas d'anatomie céphalique dans le plan neuro-oculaire (PNO). Bull Soc Fr Ophtalmol 8–9, 85:853–857

Tamraz J (1986) Atlas d'anatomie céphalique dans le plan neuro-oculaire. Schering, Paris

Tamraz J, Rethore MO, Iba-Zizen MT, Lejeune J, Cabanis EA (1987a) Contribution of magnetic resonance imaging to the knowledge of CNS malformations related to chromosomal aberrations. Hum Genet 76:265–273

Tamraz J, Iba-Zizen M T, Veres C, Cabanis EA, Godde-Jolly D, Braun M, Cosnard G, Laval-Jantet M (1987b) IRM et forme centrale de la neuro-fibromatose de Von Recklinghausen. J Neuroradiol 14:365–382

Tamraz J, Iba-Zizen MT, Cabanis EA (1987c) Exploration neuroradiologique du chiasma et des bandelettes optiques. In: Encyclopédie médico-chirurgicale, opthtalmologie. EMC Editor, Paris, 3-C, 1-21008 A20, 1-2

Tamraz J, Iba-Zizen MT, Cabanis EA (1988) Magnetic resonance imaging of the eyes and the optic pathways In: Gouaze A, Salamon G (eds) Brain anatomy and magnetic resonance imaging Springer, Berlin Heidelberg New York, pp 71–83

Tamraz J, Saban R, Cabanis EA, Reperant J, Iba-Zizen MT (1990) Définition d'un plan de référence céphalique en Imagerie par Résonance Magnétique: le plan chiasmato-commissural. CR Acad Sci Paris, 311, III:115–121

Tamraz J, Saban R, Reperant J, Cabanis EA (1991) A new cephalic reference plane for use with magnetic resonance imaging: the chiasmato-commissural plane. Surg Radiol Anat 13:197–201

Tamraz J (1991) Morphométrie de l'encéphale par résonance magnétique: applications à la pathologie chromosomique humaine, à l'anatomie comparée et à la tératologie Thèse Doctorat ès-Sciences, Paris

Tamraz J (1994), Neuroradiologic investigation of the visual system using magnetic resonance imaging. J Clin Neurophysiol 11:500–518

Unsold R, Newton TH, Hoyt (1980a) CT examination technique of the optic nerve. J Comput Ass 4:560–563

Unsold R, De Grott J, Newton TH (1980b) Images of the optic nerve; anatomic-CT correlation. Am J Neurorad 1:317–323

Unsold R, De Grott J, Newton TH (1980c) Images of the optic nerve: anatomic-CT correlation. Am J Roentgenol 135:767–773

Van Damme W, Kosman P, Wackenheim C (1977) A standard method for computed tomography of orbits. Neuroradiology 13:139–140

Varoli C (1591) Anatomiae sive de resolutione corporis.. De nervi opticis no nullisque aliis preter communem opinionem in humano capite observatis wechelum, Fischerum, Francofurti, 184 p

Vesali A (1543) Humani corporis fabrica libri septem Joannem Oporium, Basileae

Vicq D'Azyr F (1786) Traité d'Anatomie et de Physiologie avec des planches coloriées représentant au naturel les divers organes de l'Homme et des animaux, vol 1, Anatomie du cerveau. Amb Didot l'aîné, Paris

Vining DQ (1977) Computed tomography in ophthalmology. In: Smith L (ed) Neuro-ophthalmology update. Masson, New York, pp 271–279

Von Economo CF, Koskinas GN (1925) Die Cytoarchitektonik der Hirnrinde des Erwachsenen. Springer, Vienna

Von Monakow C (1896) Discussion on paper of Flechsig. Versamml Naturforsch Arzte Frankfurt 68:1003–1004

Von Monakow C (1914) Die Lokalisation im Grosshirn und der Abbau der Function durch kortikale Herde. Bergmann, Wiesbaden

Von Noorden GK, Middleditch PR (1975) Histological observations in the normal monkey lateral geniculate nucleus. Invest Ophthalmol Vis Sci 14:55–58

Walker AE (1962) The neurosurgical evaluation of the chiasmal syndromes. Am J Ophthalmol 54:563–581

Whitnall SE (1932) An anatomy of the human orbit and accessory organs of vision, 2nd edn. Oxford University Press, London

Willis T (1664) Cerebri anatome cui accessit nervorum descriptio et usus. Flescher, Martyn, Allestry, Pauli, Londini

Wollschlaeger P, Wollschlaeger G, Ide C, Hart W (1971) Arterial blood supply of the human optic chiasm and surrounding structures. Ann Ophthalmol 3:862–869

World Federation of Neurology (1962) Problem Commission of Neuroradiology: study meeting on projections and nomenclature, held in Milan 1961. Br J Radiol 35:501–503

Zeal AA, Rhoton AL (1978) Microsurgical anatomy of the posterior cerebral artery. J Neurosurg 48:534–559

Zeki SM (1969) Representation of central visual fields in prestriate cortex of monkey. Brain Res 14:271–291

Zeki SM (1971) Cortical projections from two prestriate areas in the monkey. Brain Res 34:19–35

Zeki SM (1973) Colour coding in rhesus monkey prestriate cortex. Brain Res 53:422–427

Zeki SM (1977) Colour coding in the superior temporal sulcus of rhesus monkey visual cortex. Proc R Soc Lond Biol 197:195–223

Zeki SM (1978a) The third visual complex of rhesus monkey prestriate cortex. J Physiol 277:245–272

Zeki SM (1978b) Uniformity and diversity of structure and function in rhesus monkey prestriate visual cortex. J Physiol 277:273–290

Zihl J, Von Cramon D (1979a) The contribution of the "second" visual system to directed visual attention in man. Brain 102:835–856

Zihl J, Von Cramon D (1979b) Collicular function in human vision. Exp Brain Res 35:419–424

Zuckerkandl E (1906) Zur Anatomie der Fissura calcarina. Arb Neurol Inst Univ Wien 13:25–61

10 Atlas of Cross-Sectional Anatomy of the Brain

I Atlas of Cross-Sectional Anatomy Using the Commissural-Obex Reference Plane (Figs. 10.1, 10.2)

This high resolution atlas of thin cut cross sections of the human brain is compiled from 3D SPGR-T1 weighted pulse sequence. It is presented in 3 mm contiguous slices, made along the long axis of the brainstem, as obtained using the PC-OB reference line.

This coronal cephalic orientation of the cuts is, in our opinion, the most natural and efficient imaging approach to brain structures and is similar to the neuropathological method of sectioning. It is also the most anatomic orientation to adopt when considering that the PC-OB reference line is parallel to the brainstem vertical long axis and, in addition, almost perpendicular to the parallel sulcus and the sylvian fissure planes, as obtained in the CH-PC reference orientation. Based on such references , the anatomic cuts respect the exact topography of the anatomic structures, with their rostrocaudal and dorsoventral relationships scrupulously preserved.

The first atlas can be divided into five sections. Each section can be individually accessed and studied, depending on the pathology or structure under investigation.

A From the Frontal Pole to the Genu of the Corpus Callosum (Figs. 10.3–10.10)

This first slab includes cuts involving the entire frontal lobes proceeding from the frontal pole to the temporal poles posteriorly. The coronal cuts display the cortical mantle and the subcortical white matter exclusively. These successive anterior frontal cuts permit the evaluation of the basal frontal lobes, most efficiently displaying, from medial to lateral, the olfactory sulcus and the orbital cruciform sulci, which

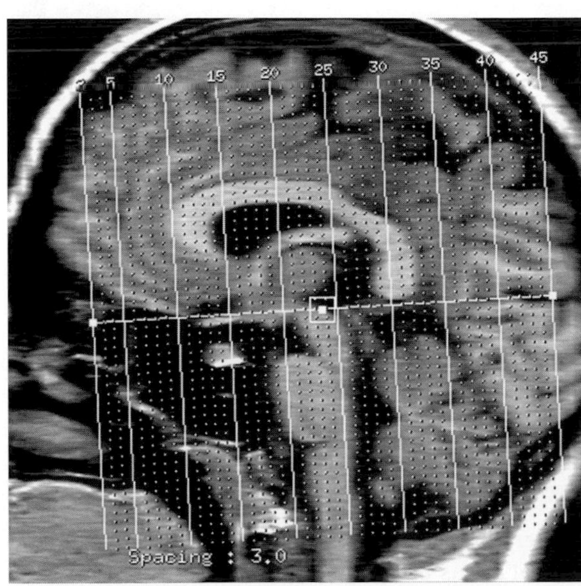

Fig. 10.1. Images for cross reference

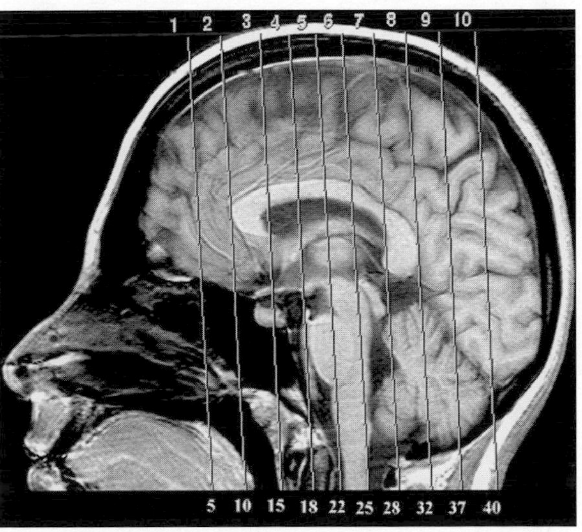

Fig. 10.2. Ten major parallelisms to the PC-OB reference plane and their correspondence with the cross-reference images

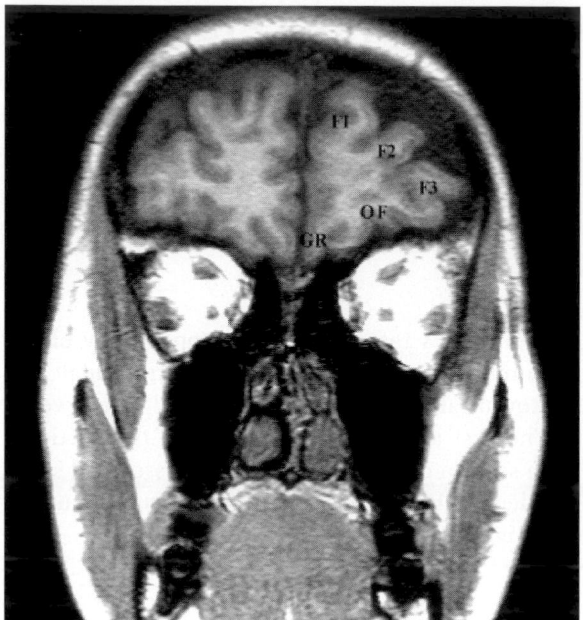

Fig. 10.3.

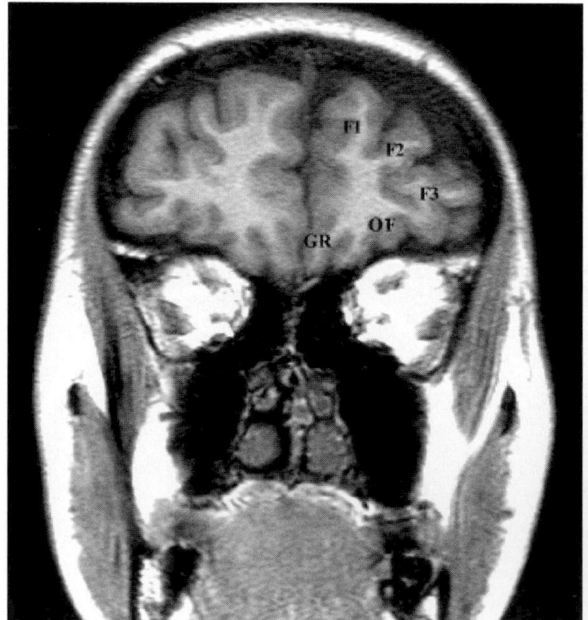

Fig. 10.4.

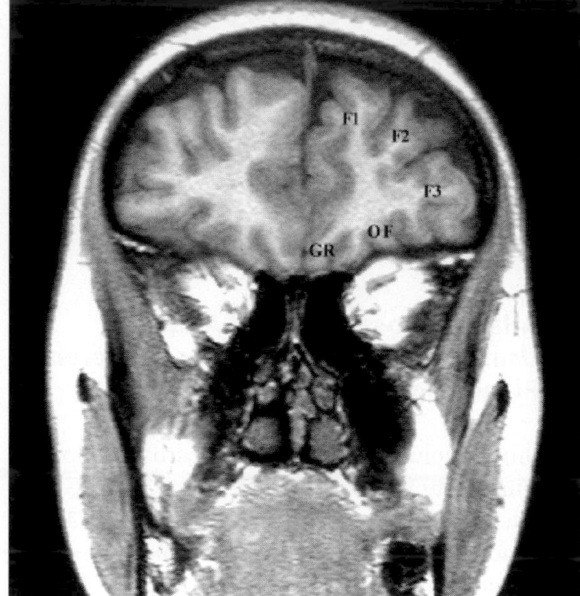

Fig. 10.5.

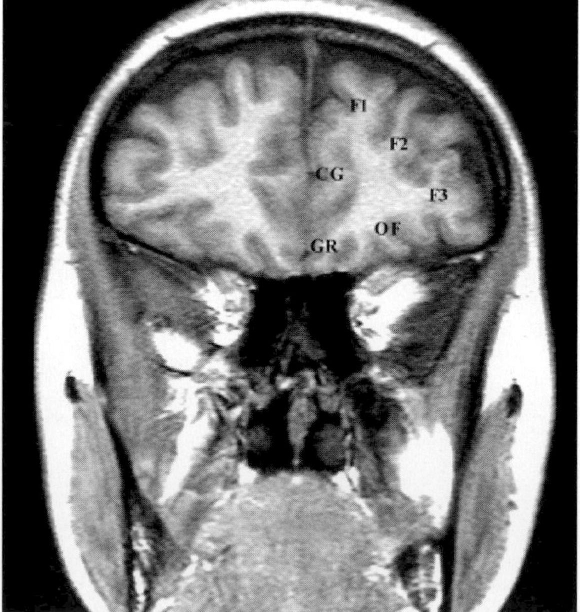

Fig. 10.6.

delimit the rectus gyrus medial to the olfactory sulcus and the orbital gyri lateral to the orbital sulcus, respectively. The optic bulbs and tracts are well depicted beneath the olfactory sulci, coursing from front to back above the cribriform plate. The white matter core does not involve the anterior tips of the frontal horns of the lateral ventricles. The posterior cut is found at the level of the orbital apex and orbital opening of the optic canal.

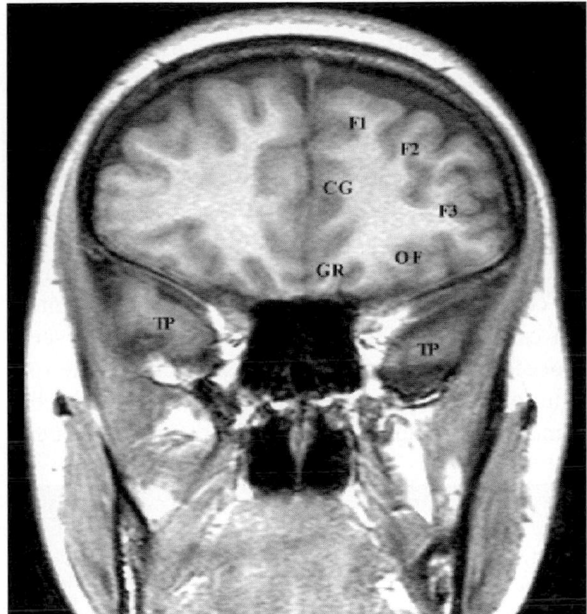

Fig. 10.7.

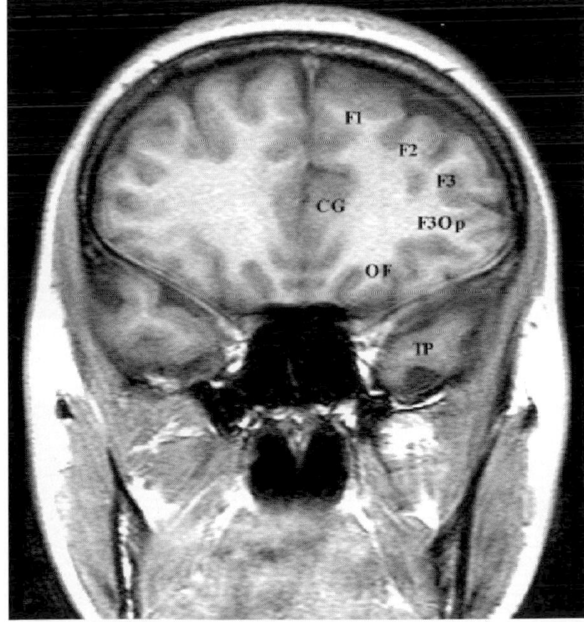

Fig. 10.8.

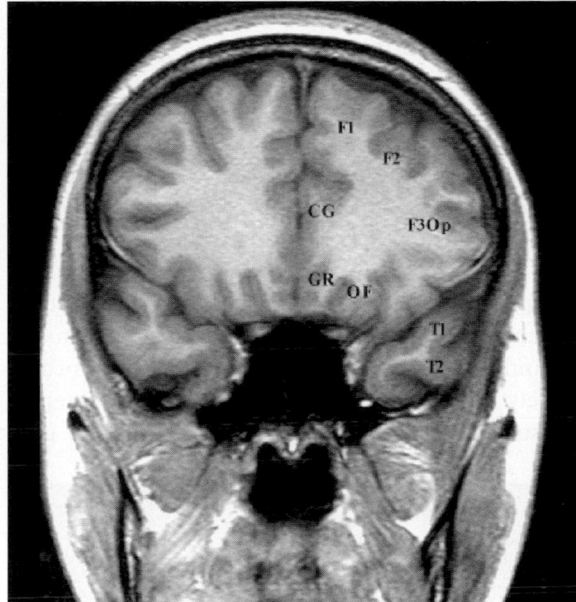

Fig. 10.9.

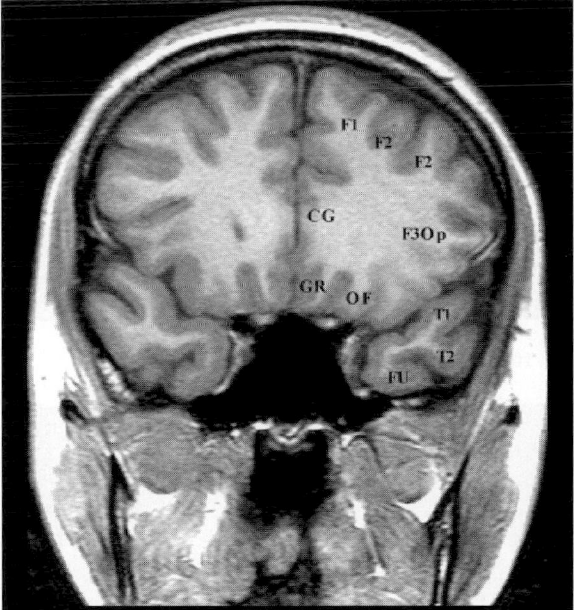

Fig. 10.10.

B From the Genu of the Corpus Callosum to the Anterior Commissure (Figs. 10.11–10.16)

The coronal cuts are both frontal and temporal polar. The central region of the slices are occupied by the transverse white matter fibers of the genu of the corpus callosum, overlying the frontal horns of the lateral ventricle. The intrinsic core brain structures comprising the anterior striatum, which consists of the anterior aspects of the head of the caudate nucleus and the putamen, are shown. These are incompletely cleaved by the anterior limb of the internal capsules and linked by the striatal bridges of gray matter. The caudate nucleus and the putamen, which form a single entity named the striatum, meet ventrally at the level of the accumbens nucleus or the nucleus leaning against the septum. Beneath the frontal horns are displayed the septal area and the diagonal band of Broca, extending posteriorly to the level of the AC and bordering the medial aspect of the hemispheres. Inferiorly and laterally, the limen insulae is reached with the ending of the rostrum of the corpus callosum, and the bifurcation of the internal carotid arteries. The temporal poles are seen. Proceeding from the posterior extremity of the rostrum of the corpus callosum, the temporal poles become linked to the frontal lobes by the temporal stem.

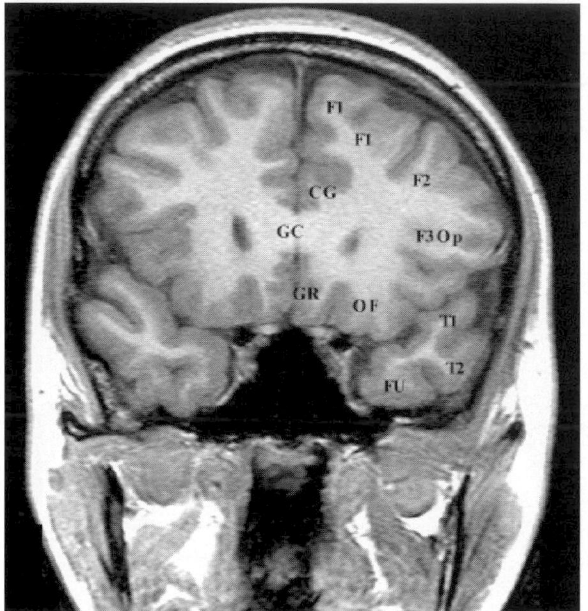

Fig. 10.11.

Fig. 10.12.

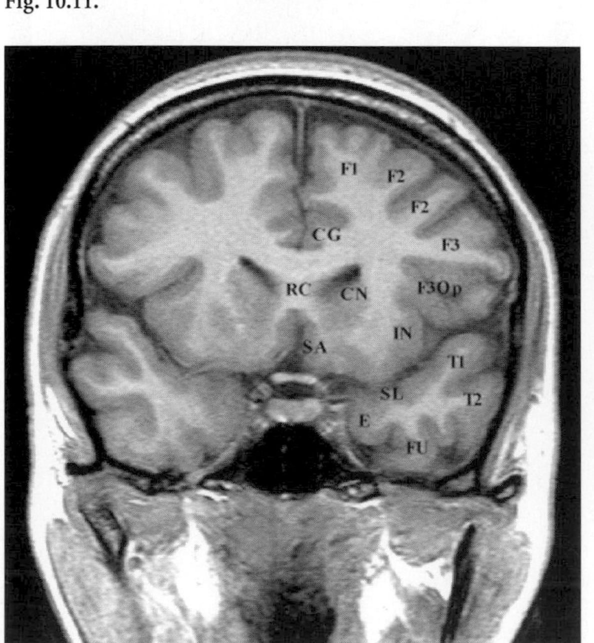

A

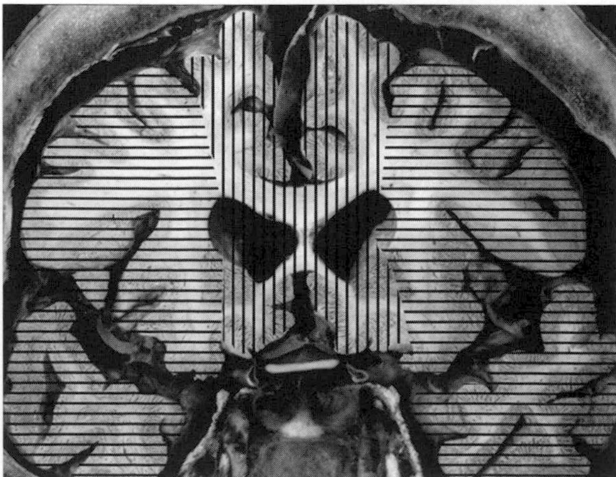

B

Fig. 10.13A. B Supplementary image describing the vascular territories in the coronal plane (A and B same cuts from different brain specimens)

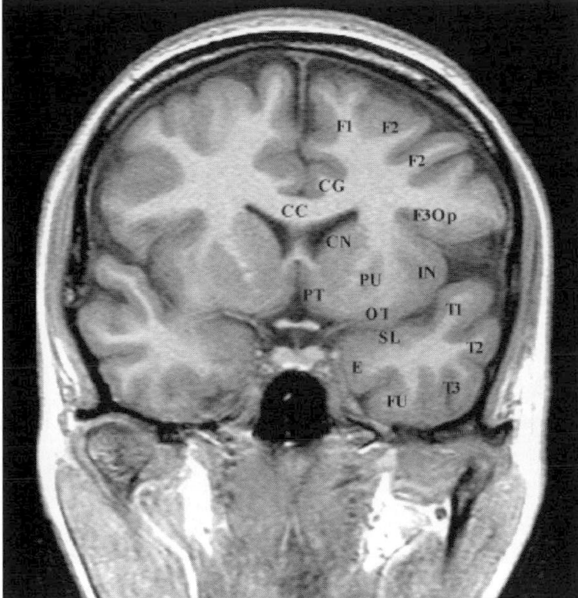

Fig. 10.14.

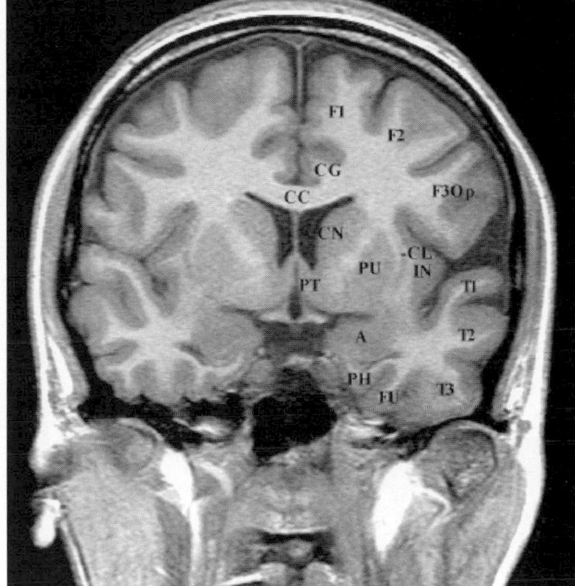

Fig. 10.16.

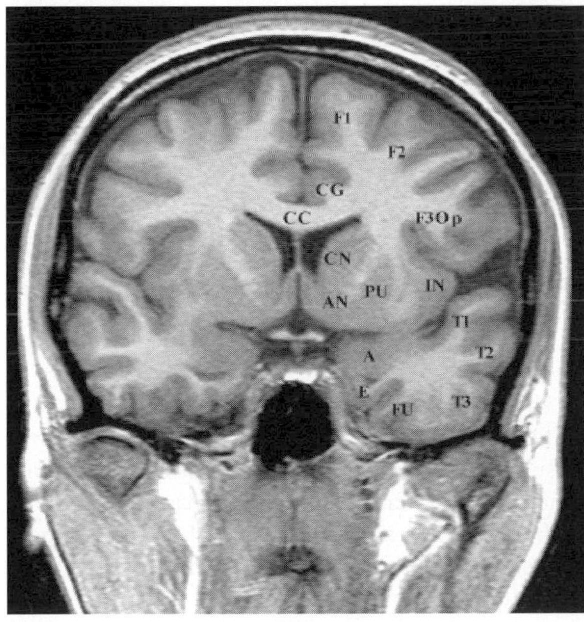

Fig. 10.15.

C From the Anterior Commissure to the Commissural-Obex Reference Plane (Figs. 10.17–10.24)

The anterior coronal cuts display the AC, which separates a broader superior region from the inferior basal region. Superior to the AC are found the lentiform nuclei, with their individual subdivisions into an external putamen and an internal pallidum, divided itself into a lateral and a medial part. Both laterally limit the internal capsule. The infra-commissural region involves the substantia innominata including the ventral striatum. This basal region abuts the hypothalamic preoptic region medially and extends laterally toward the anterior perforated substance, following the lateral wings of the AC, and meeting with the dorsal aspect of the amygdala. Note the inverted coma-shape of the amygdaloid complex and its dorsomedial extension into the substantia innominata of. The slice passing through the AC usually involves the tubero-infundibular portion of the floor of the third ventricle.

The retrocommissural slice displays the columns of the fornix medially projecting downward through the hypothalamic nuclei toward the mamillary bodies. At this level, the amygdala overhangs the anterior extremity of the hippocampal head, which shows a number of characteristic dorsal incisures. The hippocampal head is separated from the amygdaloid

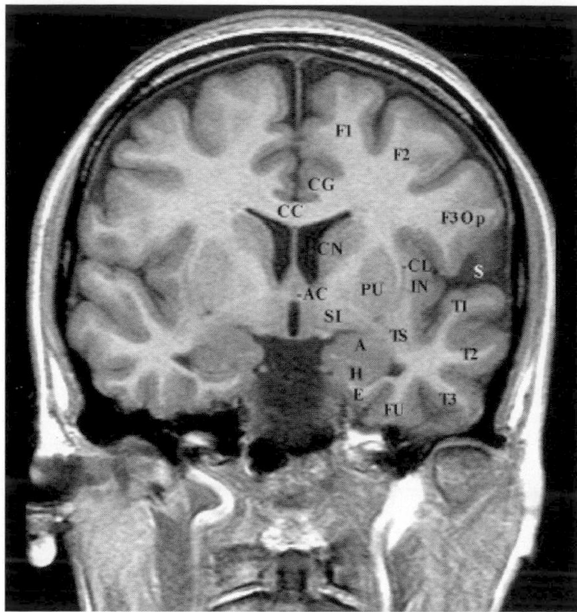

Fig. 10.17.

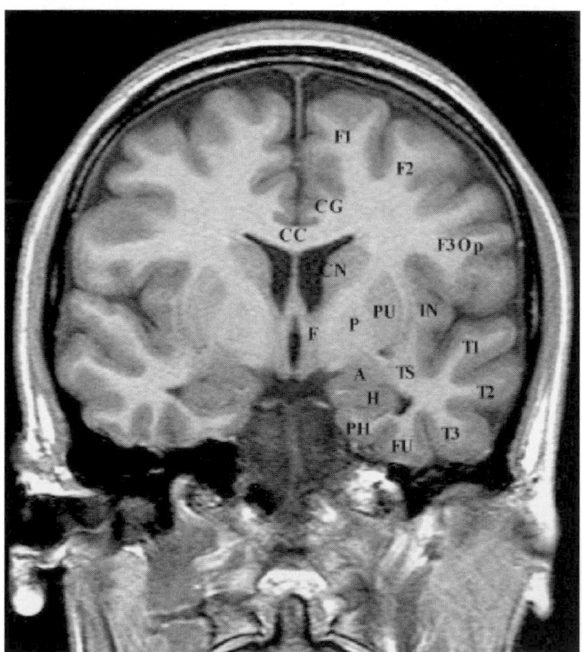

Fig. 10.18.

nuclear complex by the uncal recess of the temporal horn of the lateral ventricle.

The basal ganglia formed by the head of the caudate nuclei and the lenticular nuclei are separated by the white matter tracts of the internal capsule. Lateral to the putamen, the claustrum separates the external capsule from the extreme capsule, which is covered by the insular cortex.

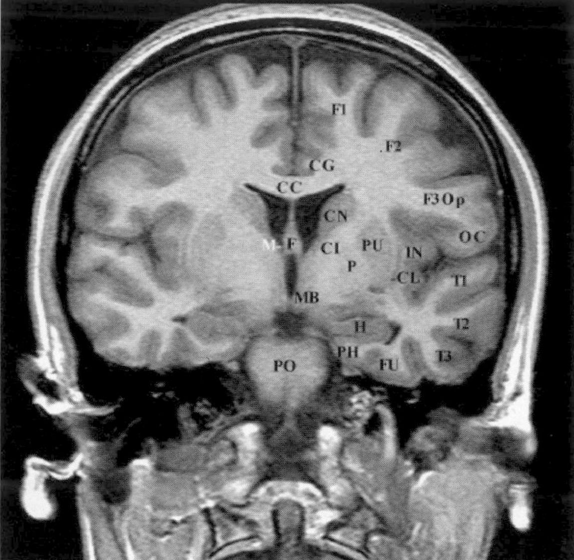

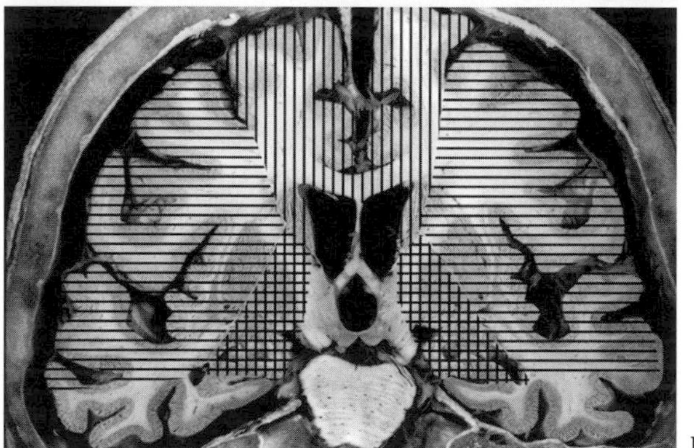

Fig. 10.19A. B Supplementary image describing the vascular territories in the coronal plane (A and B same cuts from different brain specimens)

The cortex of the frontal and temporal lobes, separated by the sylvian fissure, shows the major parallel sulci of the anterior portion of the cerebral hemispheres. In the temporal lobes, inferior and parallel to the posterior ramus of the lateral fissure, the parallel sulcus is found , separating the superior from the middle temporal gyri and, less conspicuously due to common interruptions, the inferior temporal sulcus separates the middle temporal gyrus from the inferior temporal gyrus found at the inferolateral border of the lateral aspect of the temporal lobe.

The inferior aspect of the temporal lobe is traversed laterally by the lateral temporo-occipital sulcus and medially by the rhinal sulcus, separating the inferior temporal gyrus from the fusiform laterally, and the fusiform from the parahippocampal gyrus medially.

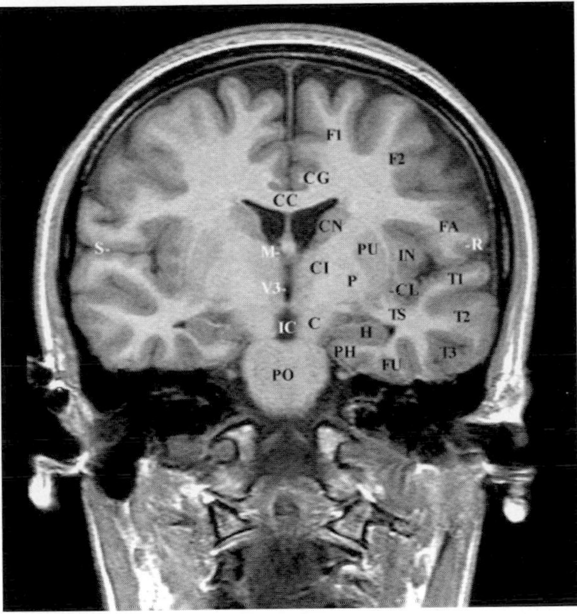

Fig. 10.20.

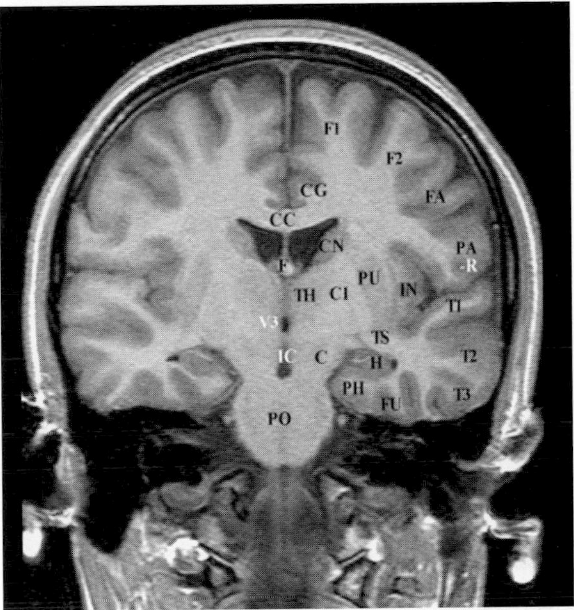

A

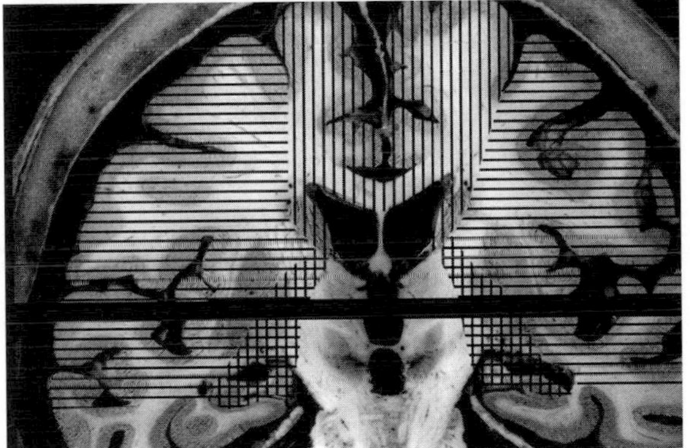

B

Fig. 10.21 A. B Supplementary image describing the vascular territories in the coronal plane (A and B same cuts from different brain specimens)

The frontal lobe superior to the lateral fissure displays two major sulci: the first one named the inferior frontal sulcus superiorly limits the inferior frontal gyrus and is recognized as the first deep sulcus roughly parallel to the sylvian fissure and directed toward the superior border of the frontal horn reaching, at the depth of the white matter, the parasagittal cut tangent to the superior border of the insular circular sulcus. The inferior frontal sulcus separates the inferior frontal gyrus from the middle frontal gyrus on the lateral aspect of the frontal lobe. The middle frontal gyrus is limited superomedially by the second deep sagittally oriented sulcus, roughly parallel to the interhemispheric fissure which corresponds to the superior frontal sulcus.

At the level of the interventricular foramen, the coronal slice passing through the MB involves the inferior end of the precentral gyrus. The interventricular-mamillary plane also reaches the anterior aspect of the thalamus, involving the posterior aspect of the hypothalamus, and roughly abuts the anterior aspect of the basis pontis. Then, the successive cuts display, rostrocaudally, the major diencephalic anatomic structures recognized as the central ovoid gray matter nuclei bounded by the genu and the posterior limb of the internal capsules on each side.

More laterally, the lentiform nuclei are followed rostrocaudally to their posterior limit, represented by the PC-OB plane. The internal capsules are displayed, extending on each side toward the midline to become the cerebral peduncles, bounding the subthalamic region laterally, and bounded medially by the substantia nigra. The latter together with its homologue displays on T2-w sequences a V-shaped configuration clearly seen on the brainstem coronal cut passing through the posterior border of the interpeduncular cistern and passing through the whole brainstem.

This coronal cut, parallel and anterior to the reference plane, passes through the upper extremity of the midbrain and shows the most prominent anatomic structures of the brainstem-diencephalon continuum. The major structures observed on this almost mid-coronal cerebral cut are: the thalamus, superior to the horizontal CH-PC plane and divided

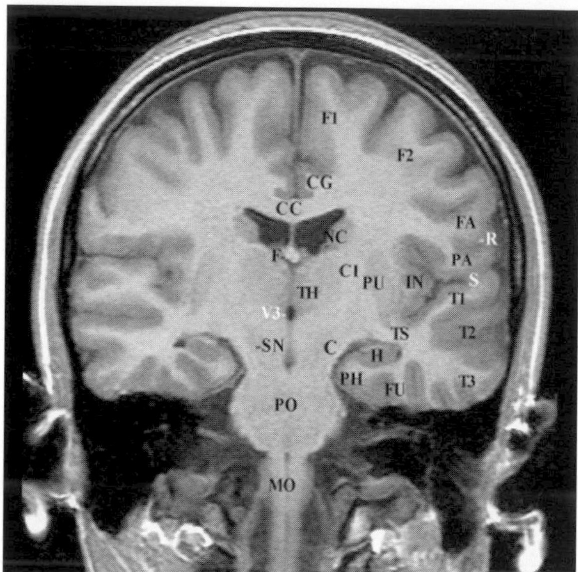

Fig. 10.22.

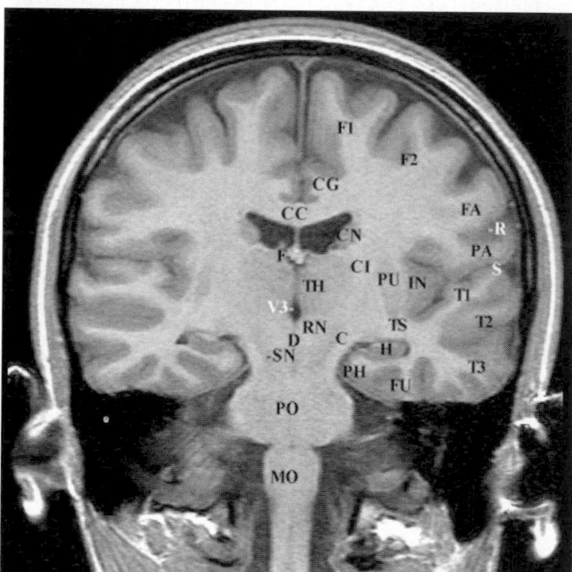

Fig. 10.23.

by the internal medullary laminae into anterior, medial, and lateral nuclear groups; the posterior limb of the internal capsule situated laterally, containing the corticospinal tract; the lentiform nucleus more laterally, divided into the external putamen and internal globus pallidus, which in turn is divided into its lateral and medial portions; and the external capsule, which laterally separates the claustrum from the extreme capsule covered by the insular cortex. The external capsule, the claustrum, the extreme capsule, and the insular cortex are cut in profile and show a

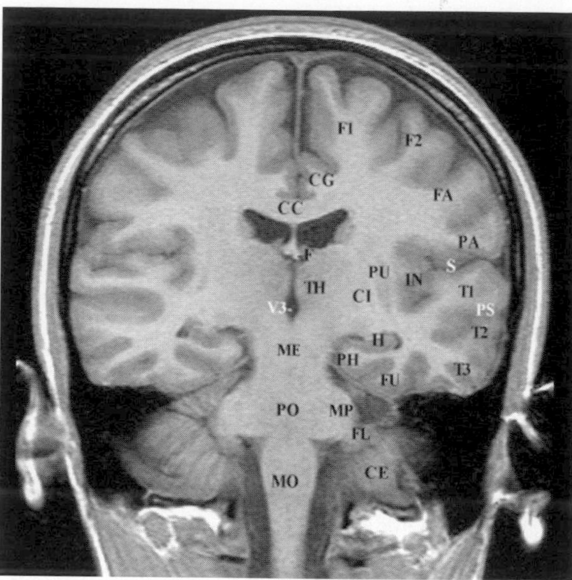

Fig. 10.24.

roughly parallel disposition tilted superomedially toward the ventricular roof.

The infra-CH-PC portion of the cut, roughly symmetrical in height to the upper portion, involves the whole brainstem, both the midbrain and the midbrain-diencephalic junction as well as the hindbrain structures. These structures are craniocaudally the subthalamic regions, the red nuclei, the substantia nigra, the cerebral peduncles, the basis pontis and the pyramids of the medulla oblongata. The corticospinal tracts are very nicely displayed from the corona radiata through the posterior limb of the internal capsule, to the level of their decussation at the spinal cord-medullary junction, along their route in the cerebral peduncles, the basal aspect of the pons, and the medullary pyramids, as seen on T2 weighted MR slices. Lateral to the cerebral peduncles, the body of the hippocampal formation is cut frontally almost perpendicular to the choroidal fissure, showing a close parallelism to the CH-PC plane.

D From the Commissural-Obex Plane to the Splenium of the Corpus Callosum (Figs. 10.25–10.32)

The cut represented by the PC-OB plane shows the main landmarks characterizing this reference plane, which are on the midline of the AC at the junction between midbrain and diencephalon. Superiorly and inferiorly, the plane passes through the lower extremity of the calamus, involving the floor of the

A

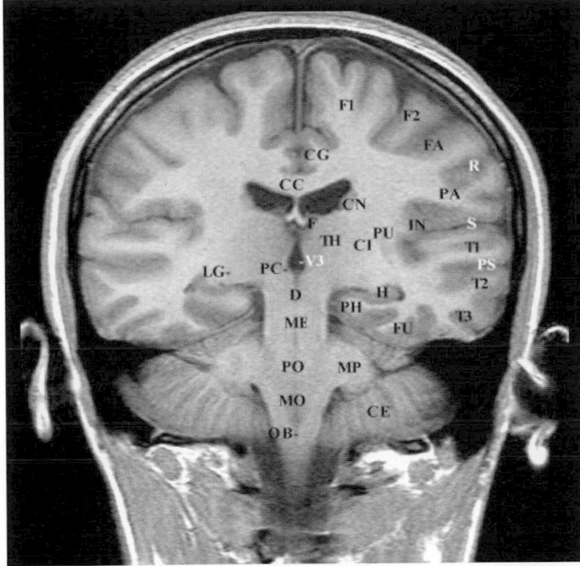

B

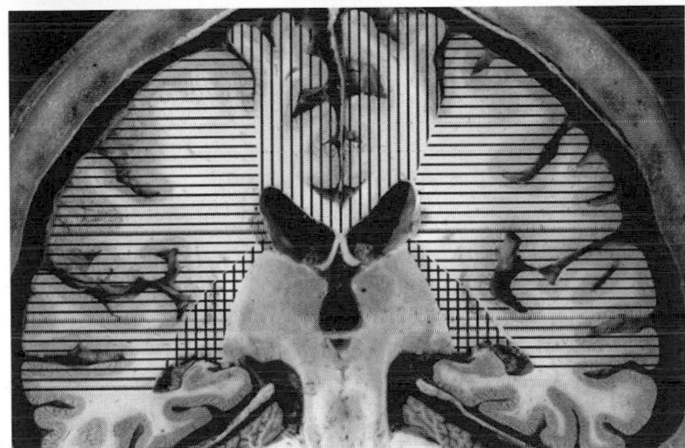

Fig. 10.25A. B Supplementary image describing the vascular territories in the coronal plane (A and B same cuts from different brain specimens)

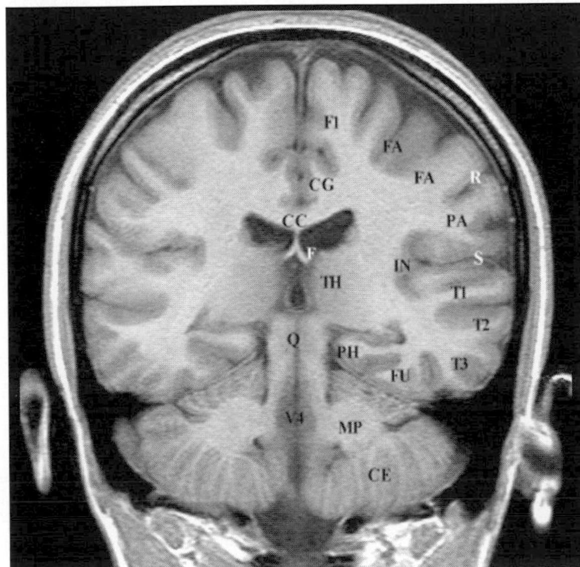

Fig. 10.26.

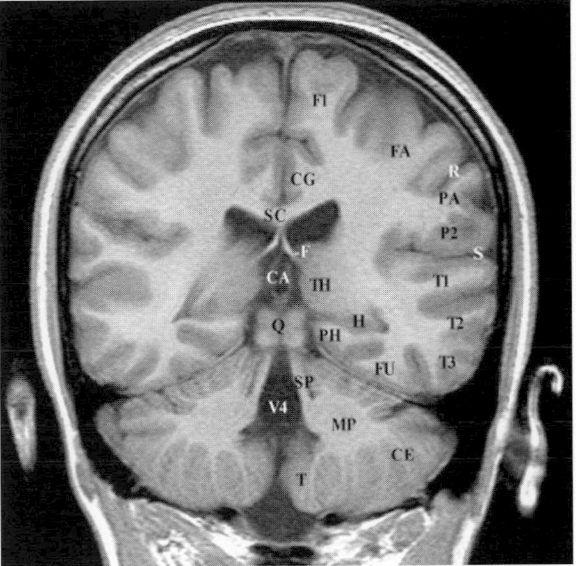

Fig. 10.27.

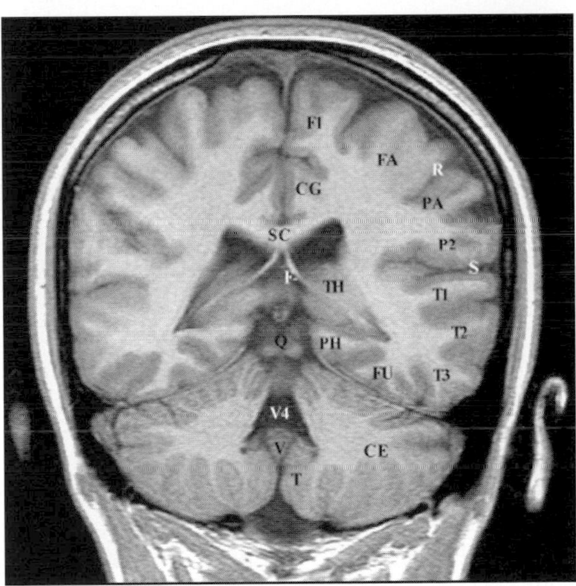

Fig. 10.28.

fourth ventricle and cutting through the posterior aspect of the midbrain tegmentum, in which the decussation of the superior cerebellar peduncles is shown. This cut roughly follows the direction of the medial longitudinal fasciculus, which is the most conspicuously observed tract on sagittal cuts of the brainstem.

Lateral to the midbrain-thalamic region, the cap-shaped lateral geniculate bodies are regularly displayed at the inferior lateral aspect of the thalamus on each side, at the level of the parallel sulci. The CH-

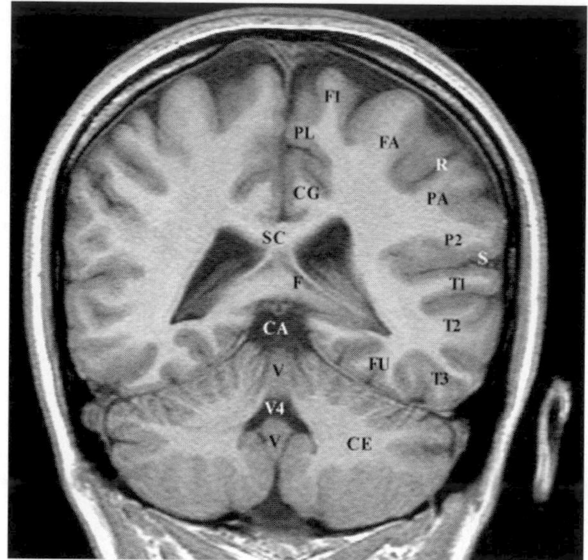

Fig. 10.29.

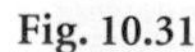

Fig. 10.31.

A

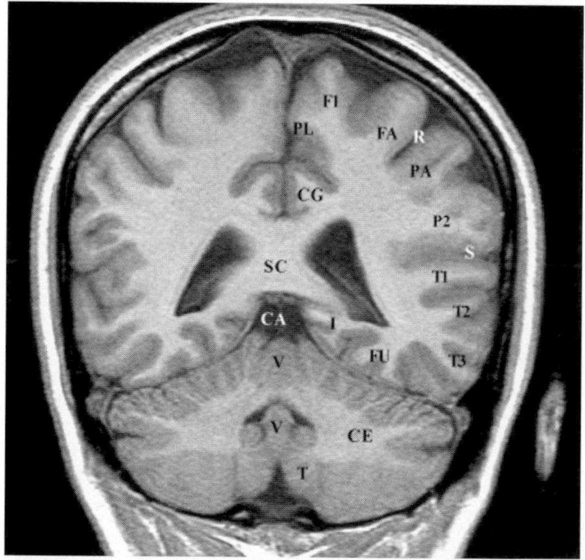

B

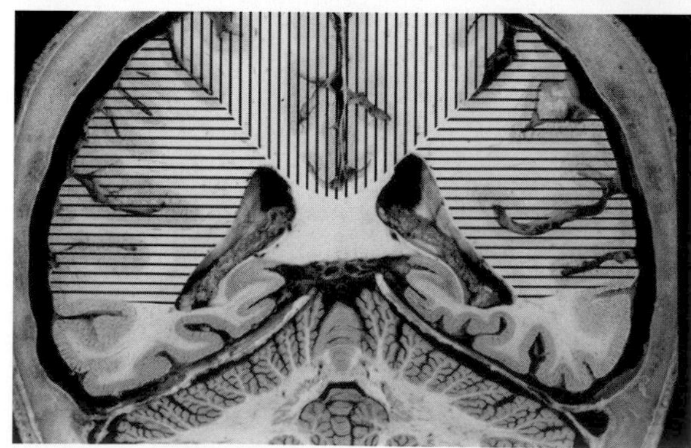

Fig. 10.30A. B Supplementary image describing the vascular territories in the coronal plane (A and B same cuts from different brain specimens)

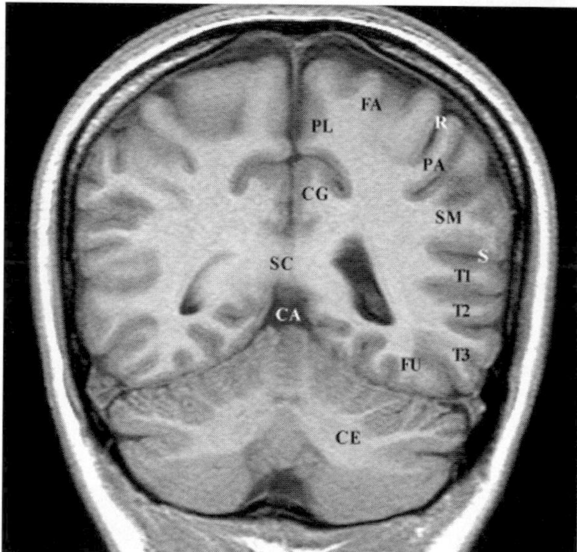

Fig. 10.32.

PC reference line, as projected on the coronal cut, is tangent to the superior border of the lateral geniculate bodies, which are topographically and topometrically constant. The upper portion of the cut involves most of the posterior thalamic nuclei and the subthalamic nuclei. Laterally, islands of gray matter are observed in the retrolenticular limb of the internal capsule, corresponding to the caudal pole of the putamen. Lateral to the geniculate body, and under these sheets of gray matter, are the lateral projections of the optic peduncle and the auditory radiation, projecting to Heschl's gyrus. Beneath, the tail of the caudate nucleus is shown in contact with the dorsal roof of the temporal horn. Inferiorly, the cut involves the middle cerebellar peduncles and passes through the anterior superior and the anterior inferior aspect of the cerebellar hemispheres separated by the anterior extent of the horizontal fissure of Vicq d'Azyr.

Posterior to this cut, the pulvinar nuclei of the thalamus are displayed bounded superiorly by the posterior central portions of the lateral ventricles and medially by the posterior columns of the fornix. The pulvinar laterally limits the ambient cistern in which the internal cerebral veins are shown. Inferior and medial to the pulvinar, the cuts involve the quadrigeminal plate, showing the superior and inferior colliculi cut almost completely along their rostrocaudal axis and overhanging the cavity of the fourth ventricle bounded by the superior cerebellar peduncles. Lateral and beneath the pulvinar are the hippocampal tails and, more posteriorly, the retrosplenial gyri.

At the level of the splenium on the posterior cuts, the diverging posterior columns of the fornix are well delineated, bounding the inner aspect of the atrium of the lateral ventricle. Inferiorly, the cuts pass through the corpus cerebelli, displaying the album cerebelli on each side. The last slice is tangent to the splenium of the corpus callosum and involves the culmen vermis.

E Posterior to the Splenium Toward the Occipital Pole (Figs. 10.33–10.45)

The cuts involve the isthmus and, more posteriorly, the occipital lobes from the junction of the parieto-occipital sulcus with the calcarine sulcus to the occipital pole; the number of slices vary with brain morphotype and the occipital descent. The cerebellar hemispheres are frontally cut from the level of the culmen vermis to the cerebellar horizontal fissure, posteriorly limiting the superior from the posterior inferior aspects of the cerebellum.

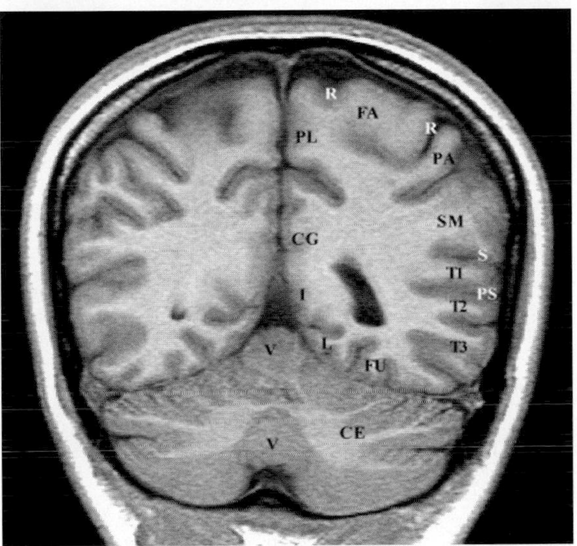

Fig. 10.33.

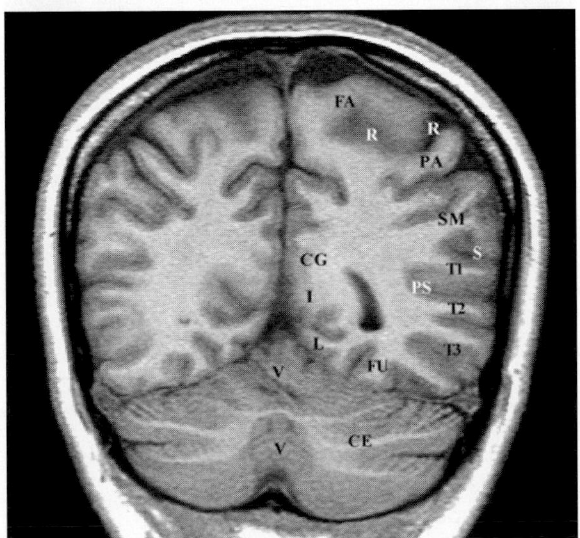

Fig. 10.34.

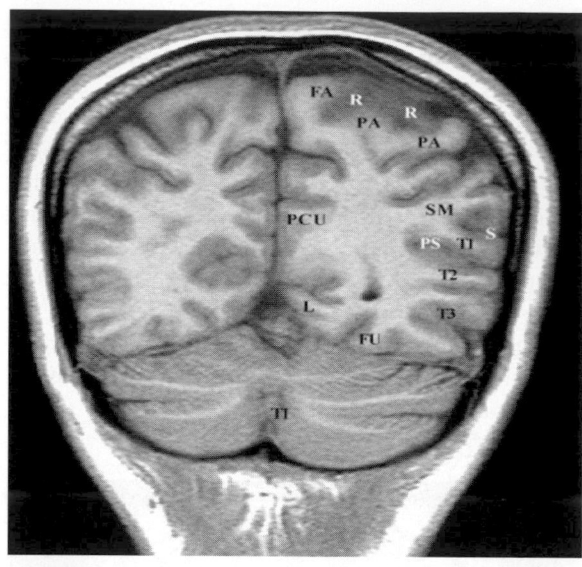

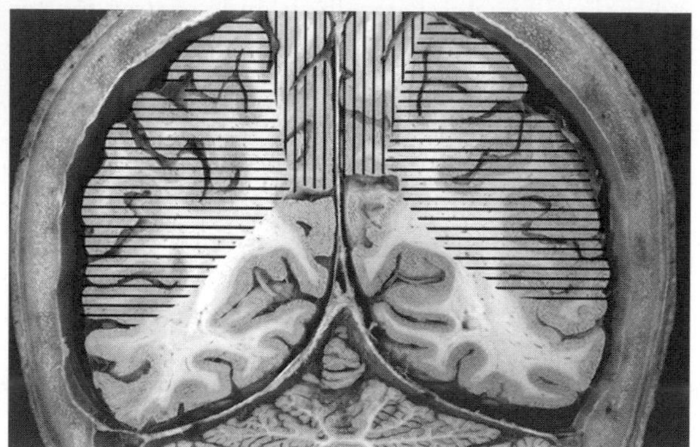

Fig. 10.35A. B Supplementary image describing the vascular territories in the coronal plane (A and B same cuts from different brain specimens)

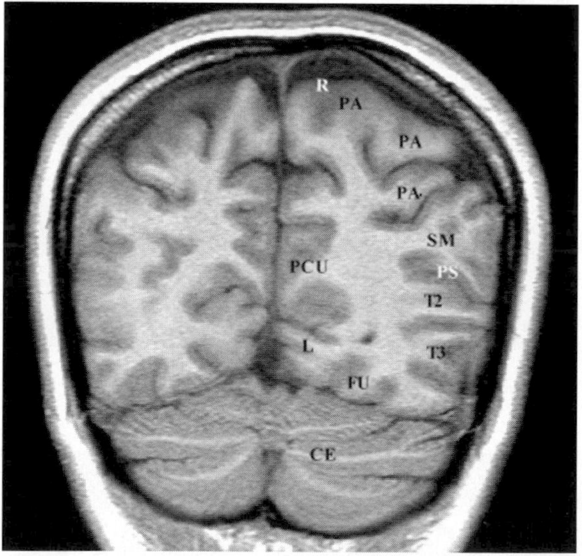

Fig. 10.36.

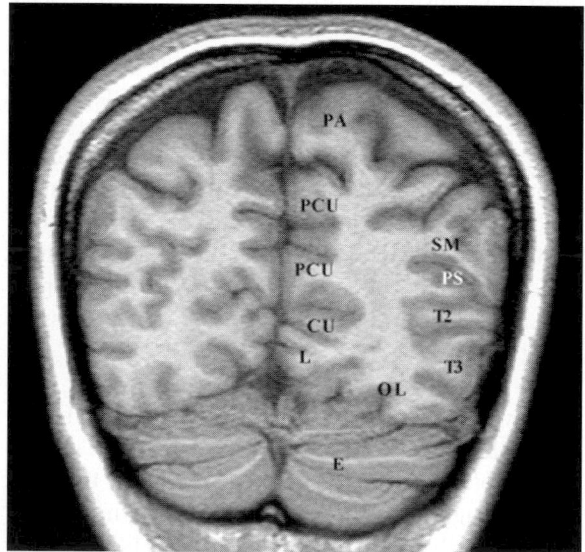

Fig. 10.37.

Abbreviations

A Amygdala
AC Anterior commissure
AF Fornix, anterior column
AG Angular gyrus
AN Accumbens nucleus
C Crus cerebri
CA Cisterna ambiens
CC Corpus callosum
CF Fornix, crus
CG Cingulate gyrus
CI Internal capsule
CN Caudate nucleus
CR Corpus callosum, rostrum
CS Calcarine sulcus
D Decussation of brachia conjunctiva
DN Dentate nucleus of cerebellum
F1 Superior frontal gyrus
F2 Middle frontal gyrus
F3 Inferior frontal gyrus
FA Precentral gyrus
FL Flocculus
FU Fusiform gyrus or lateral occipital gyrus

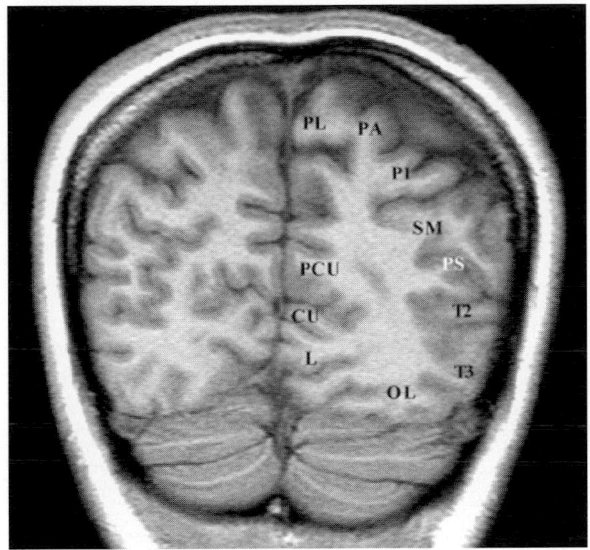

Fig. 10.38.

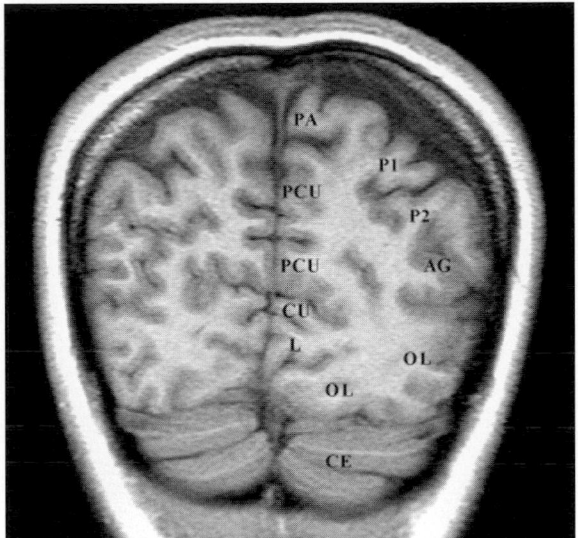

Fig. 10.39.

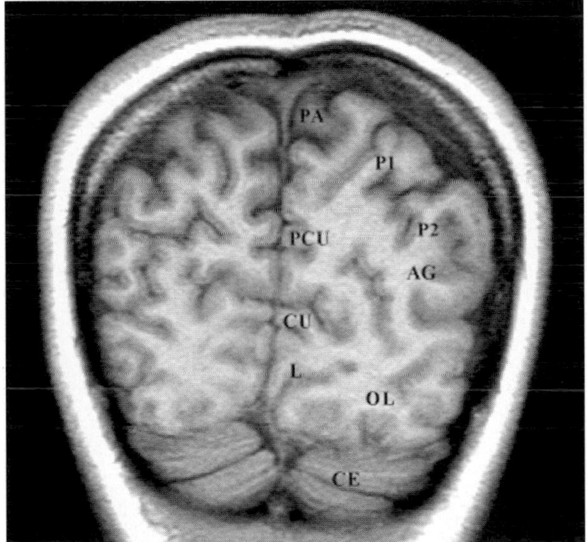

Fig. 10.40.

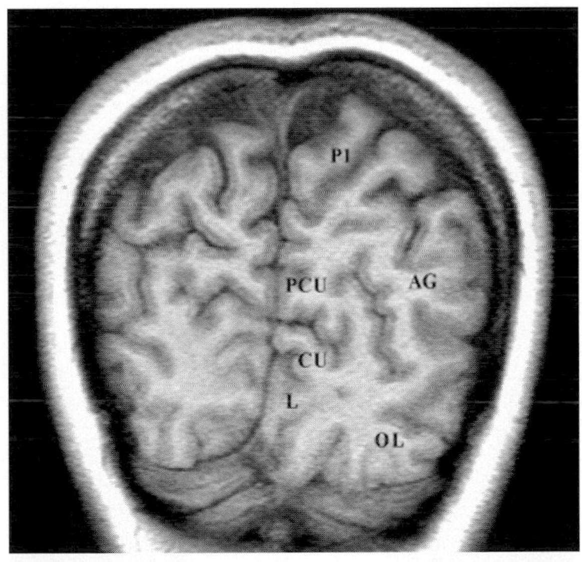

Fig. 10.41.

GC	Corpus callosum, genu
GE	Globus pallidus, lateral segment
GI	Globus pallidus, medial segment
GR	Gyrus rectus
H	Hippocampus
I	Isthmus of cingulate gyrus
IC	Interpeduncular cistern
IN	Insula
LG	Lateral geniculate body
M	Interventricular foramen of Monro
MB	Mamillary body
MP	Middle cerebellar peduncle
OB	Obex
OF	Orbitofrontal gyri
OL	Occipital lobe
OT	Optic tract
P1	Superior parietal gyrus
PA	Postcentral gyrus
PC	Posterior commissure
PH	Parahippocampal gyrus
PL	Paracentral lobule
PO	Pons
PS	Superior temporal sulcus or parallel sulcus
PU	Putamen

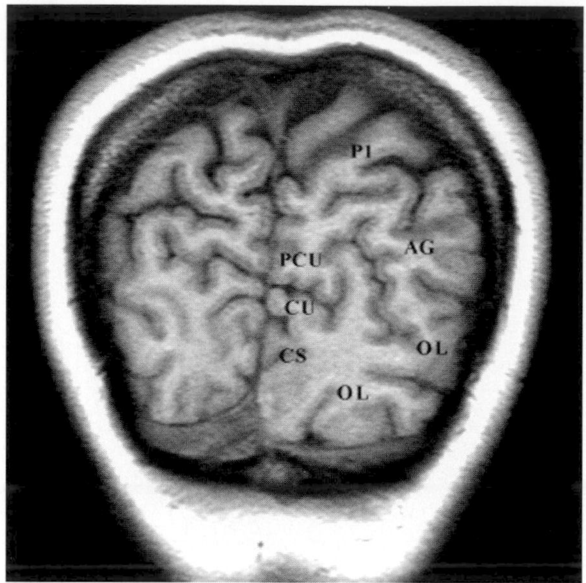

Fig. 10.42.

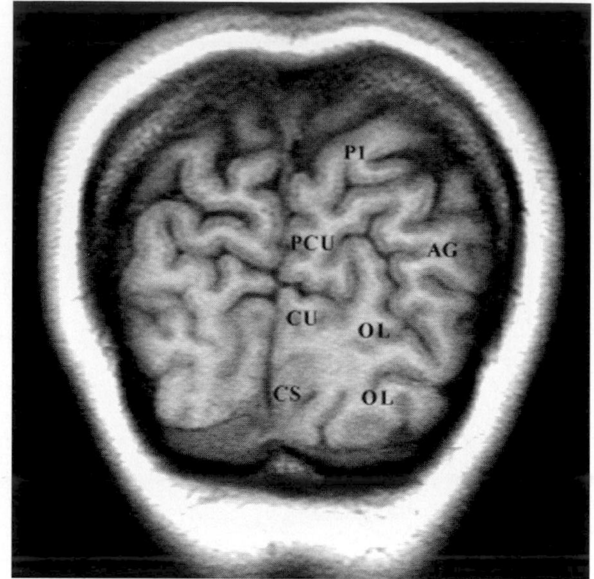

Fig. 10.43.

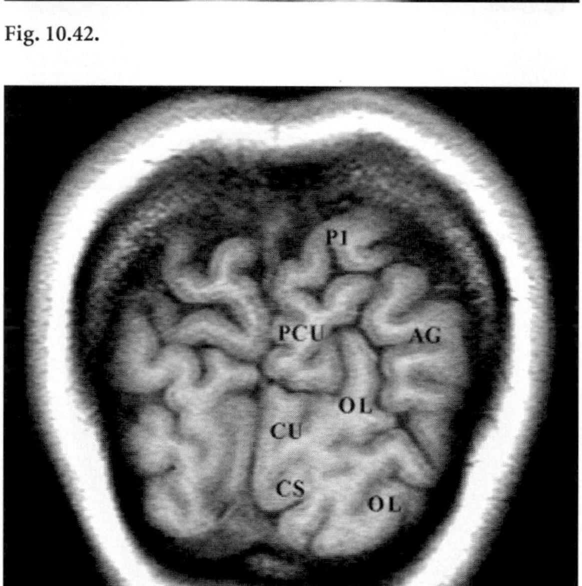

Fig. 10.44.

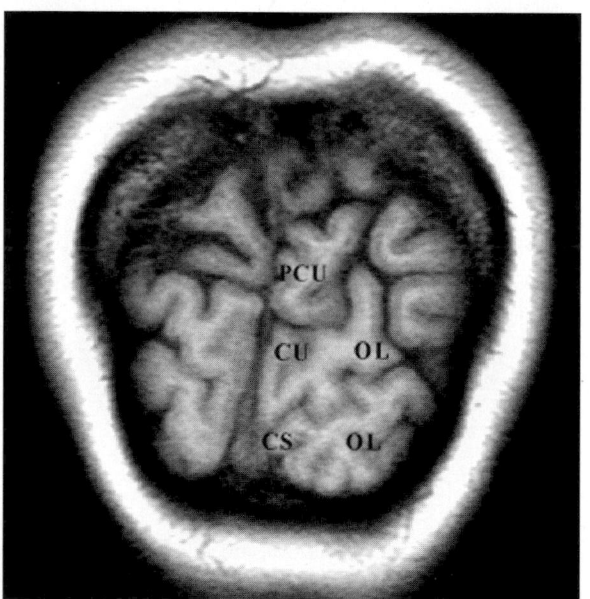

Fig. 10.45.

Q Tectal or quadrigeminal plate
R Central sulcus of Rolando
RN Red nucleus
S Lateral fissure of Sylvius
Sa Septal area
SC Splenium of corpus callosum
SI Substantia innominata
SM Supramarginal gyrus
SN Substantia nigra
SP Superior cerebellar peduncle
T Tonsil of cerebellum
T1 Superior temporal gyrus
T2 Middle temporal gyrus
T3 Inferior temporal gyrus
TG Transverse temporal gyrus of Heschl
TH Thalamus
TP Temporal pole
V Vermis of cerebellum
V3 Third ventricle
V4 Fourth ventricle

II Atlas of Cross-Sectional Anatomy Using MR Oriented According to the Ventricular Reference Plane (Figs. 10.46–10.59)

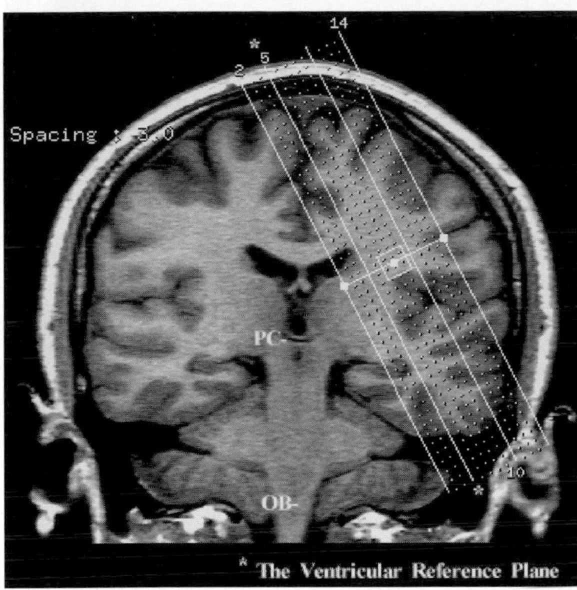

Fig. 10.46. Topogram of the MR oblique cuts (3 mm thick, contiguous) oriented according to the ventricular reference plane

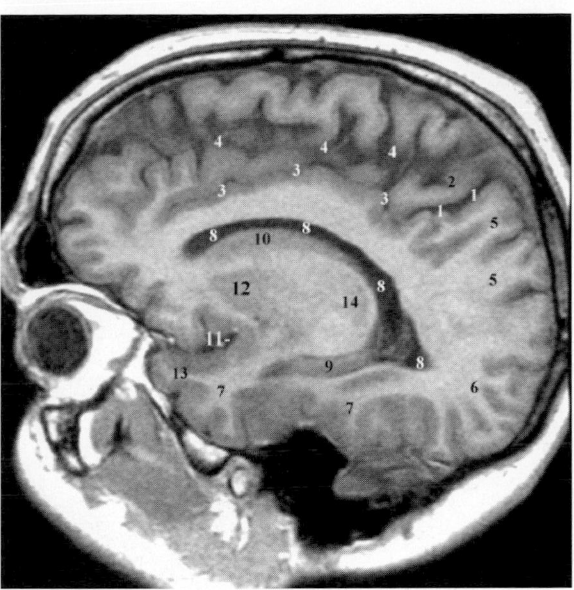

Fig. 10.48. *1*, Marginal ramus of cingulate sulcus; *2*, paracentral lobule; *3*, cingulate sulcus; *4*, interhemispheric fissure; *5*, precuneus; *6*, occipital lobe; *7*, temporal lobe; *8*, lateral ventricle; *9*, hippocampus; *10*, caudate nucleus; *11*, endorhinal sulcus; *12*, putamen; *13*, temporal pole; *14*, thalamus

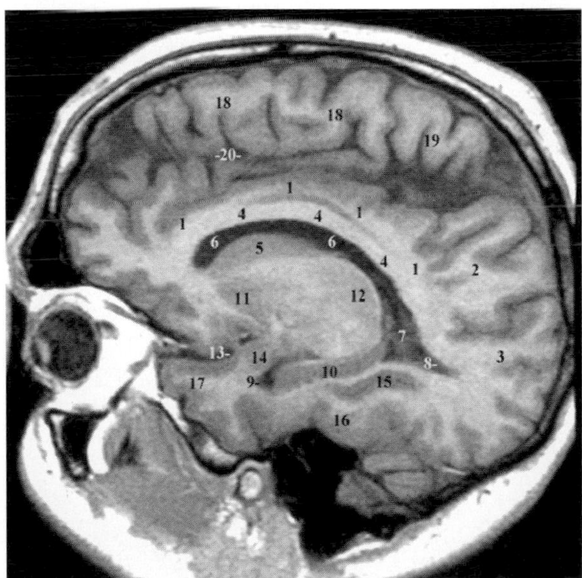

Fig. 10.47. *1*, Cingulate gyrus; *2*, precuneus; *3*, cuneus; *4*, corpus callosum; *5*, caudate nucleus; *6*, lateral ventricle; *7*, atrium of lateral ventricle; *8*, occipital horn of lateral ventricle; *9*, temporal horn of lateral ventricle; *10*, hippocampus; *11*, putamen; *12*, thalamus; *13*, endorhinal sulcus; *14*, amygdala; *15*, collateral sulcus; *16*, temporal lobe; *17*, temporal pole; *18*, medial frontal gyrus (contralateral); *19*, paracentral lobule (contralateral); *20*, interhemispheric fissure

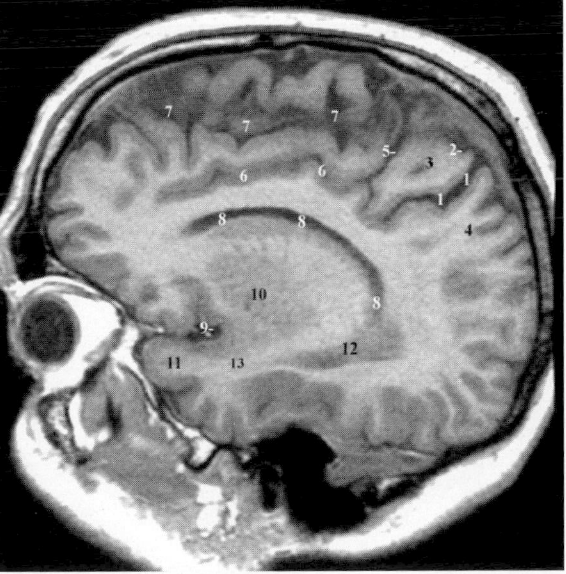

Fig. 10.49. *1*, Marginal ramus of cingulate sulcus; *2*, central sulcus; *3*, paracentral lobule; *4*, precuneus; *5*, paracentral sulcus; *6*, cingulate sulcus; *7*, interhemispheric fissure; *8*, lateral ventricle; *9*, falciform sulcus; *10*, putamen; *11*, temporal pole; *12*, hippocampus; *13*, temporal stem

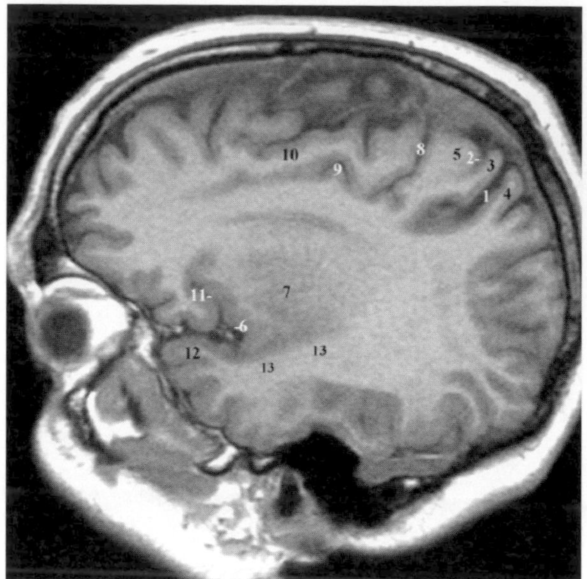

Fig. 10.50. *1*, Marginal ramus of cingulate sulcus; *2*, central sulcus; *3*, postcentral gyrus; *4*, precuneus; *5*, precentral gyrus; *6*, limen insulae; *7*, putamen; *8*, paracentral sulcus; *9*, cingulate sulcus; *10*, medial frontal gyrus; *11*, circular sulcus insulae; *12*, temporal pole; 13, temporal stem

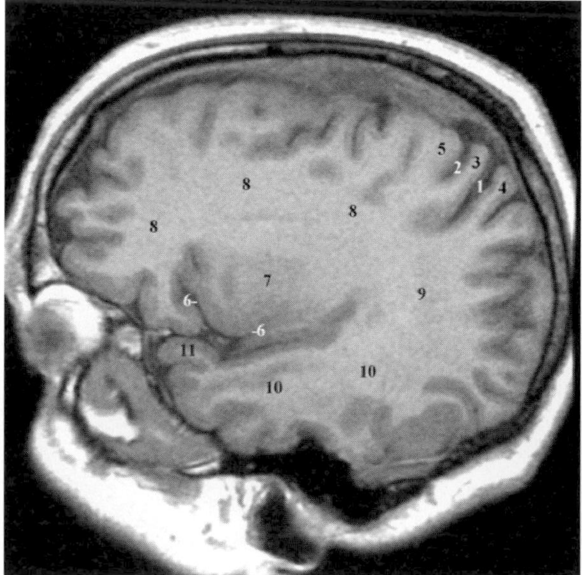

Fig. 10.51. *1*, Marginal ramus of cingulate sulcus; *2*, central sulcus; *3*, postcentral gyrus; *4*, precuneus; *5*, precentral gyrus; *6*, circular sulcus of insula; *7*, claustrum; *8*, frontal lobe white matter core; *9*, parietal lobe white matter core; *10*, temporal lobe white matter core; *11*, temporal pole

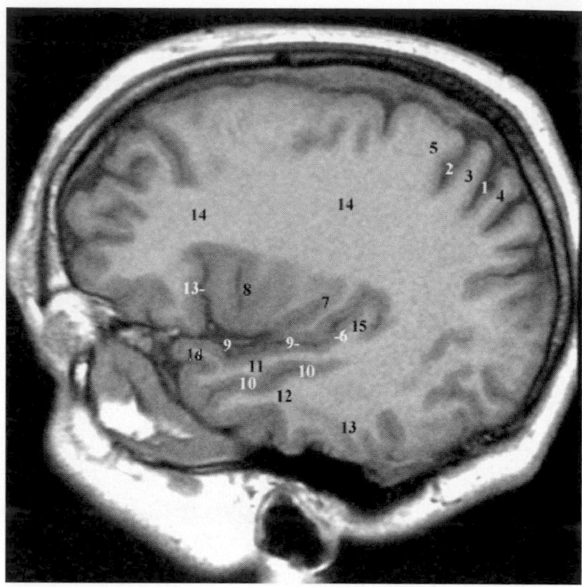

Fig. 10.52. *1*, Central sulcus; *2*, precentral sulcus; *3*, precentral gyrus; *4*, postcentral gyrus; *5*, transverse temporal gyrus; *6*, anterior transverse temporal sulcus; *7*, long gyri of insula; *8*, short gyri of insula; *9*, lateral fissure; *10*, parallel sulcus; *11*, superior temporal gyrus; *12*, middle temporal gyrus; *13*, circular sulcus insulae; *14*, temporal pole; *15*, Heschl gyrus; *16*, frontal white matter

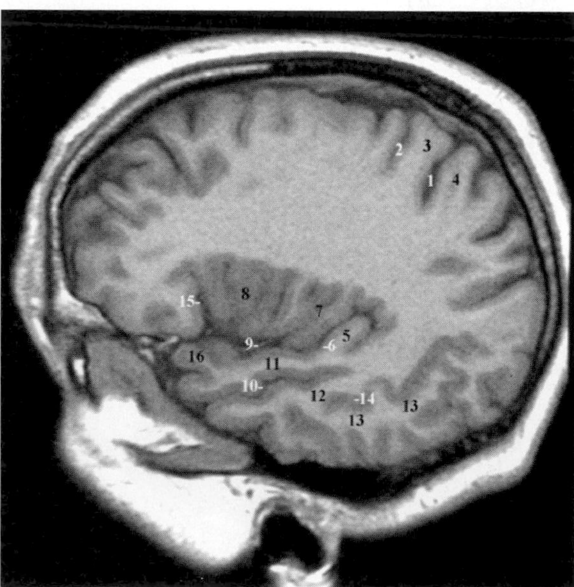

Fig. 10.53. *1*, Central sulcus; *2*, precentral sulcus; *3*, precentral gyrus; *4*, postcentral gyrus; *5*, transverse temporal gyrus; *6*, anterior transverse temporal sulcus; *7*, long gyri of insula; *8*, short gyri of insula; *9*, lateral fissure; *10*, parallel sulcus; *11*, superior temporal gyrus; *12*, middle temporal gyrus; *13*, inferior temporal gyrus; *14*, inferior temporal sulcus; *15*, circular sulcus insulae; *16*, temporal pole

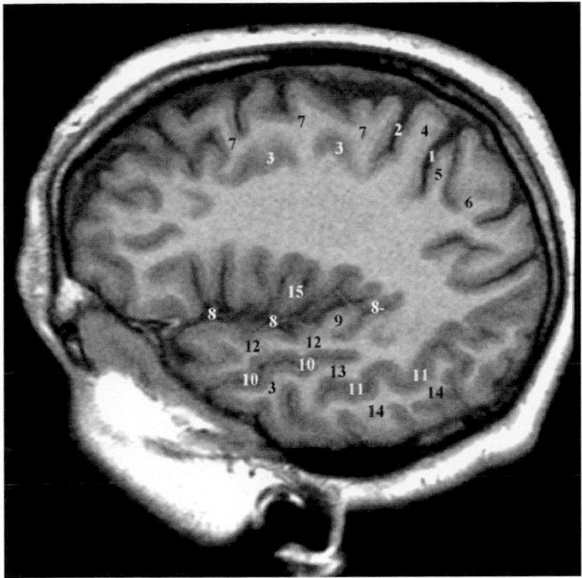

Fig. 10.54. *1*, Central sulcus; *2*, precentral sulcus; *3*, superior frontal sulcus; *4*, precentral gyrus; *5*, postcentral gyrus; *6*, superior parietal lobule; *7*, superior frontal gyrus; *8*, lateral fissure; *9*, transverse temporal gyrus; *10*, parallel sulcus; *11*, inferior temporal sulcus; *12*, superior temporal gyrus; *13*, middle temporal gyrus; *14*, inferior temporal gyrus; *15*, insula

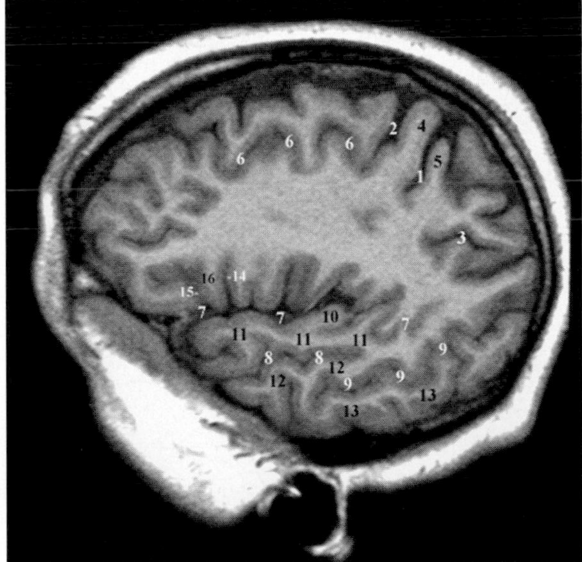

Fig. 10.55. *1*, Central sulcus; *2*, precentral sulcus; *3*, intraparietal sulcus; *4*, precentral gyrus; *5*, postcentral gyrus; *6*, superior frontal sulcus; *7*, lateral fissure; *8*, parallel sulcus; *9*, inferior temporal sulcus; *10*, transverse temporal gyrus; *11*, superior temporal gyrus; *12*, middle temporal gyrus; *13*, inferior temporal gyrus; *14*, vertical ramus of lateral fissure; *15*, horizontal ramus of lateral fissure; *16*, inferior frontal lobule, pars triangularis

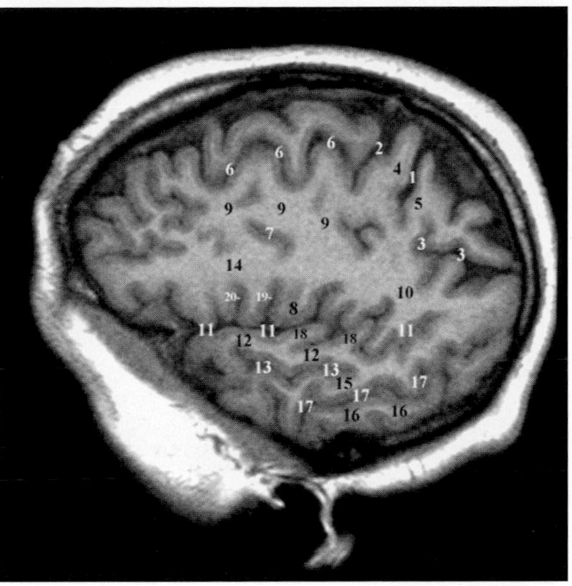

Fig. 10.56. *1*, Central sulcus; *2*, precentral sulcus; *3*, intraparietal / postcentral sulcus; *4*, precentral gyrus; *5*, postcentral gyrus; *6*, superior frontal sulcus; *7*, inferior frontal sulcus; *8*, central operculum; *9*, middle frontal gyrus; *10*, inferior parietal lobule; *11*, lateral fissure; *12*, superior temporal gyrus; *13*, parallel sulcus; *14*, inferior frontal gyrus; *15*, middle temporal gyrus; *16*, inferior temporal gyrus; *17*, inferior temporal sulcus; *18*, transverse temporal gyri; *19*, inferior precentral sulcus; *20*, vertical ramus of lateral fissure

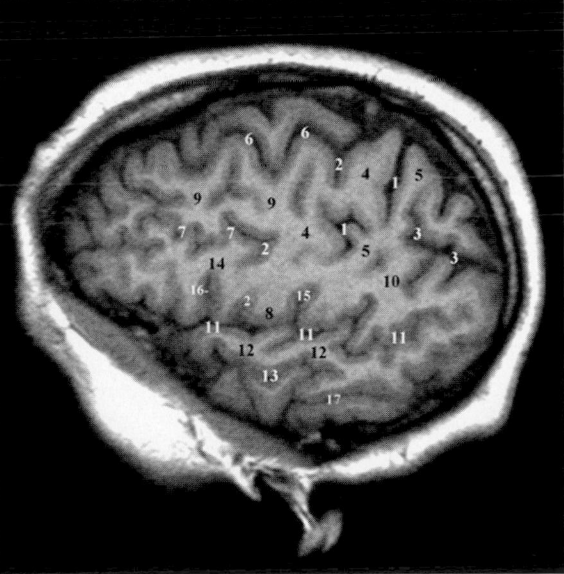

Fig. 10.57. *1*, Central sulcus; *2*, precentral sulcus; *3*, intraparietal / postcentral sulcus; *4*, precentral gyrus; *5*, postcentral gyrus; *6*, superior frontal sulcus; *7*, inferior frontal sulcus; *8*, central operculum; *9*, middle frontal gyrus; *10*, inferior parietal lobule; *11*, lateral fissure; *12*, superior temporal gyrus; *13*, parallel sulcus; *14*, inferior frontal gyrus; *15*, posterior subcentral sulcus; *16*, vertical ramus of lateral fissure; *17*, inferior temporal sulcus

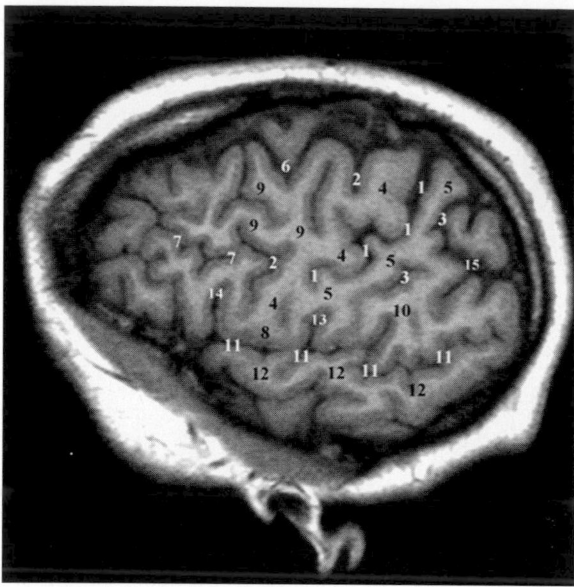

Fig. 10.58. *1*, Central sulcus; *2*, precentral sulcus; *3*, postcentral sulcus; *4*, precentral gyrus; *5*, postcentral gyrus; *6*, superior frontal sulcus; *7*, inferior frontal sulcus; 8, frontal operculum; 9, middle frontal gyrus; *10*, superior parietal lobule; *11*, lateral fissure; *12*, superior temporal gyrus; *13*, posterior subcentral sulcus; *14*, vertical ramus of lateral fissure; *15*, intraparietal sulcus

III Atlas of Cross-Sectional Anatomy Using the Forniceal Reference Plane (Figs. 10.60–10.89)

This atlas is based on MR oblique 2 mm contiguous cuts which are oriented in the „Forniceal plane" (Ff). Figure 10.60 is a topogram of the slices, as defined and projected on the coronal PC-OB reference plane; Figs. 10.61–10.81 are successive corresponding MR slices.

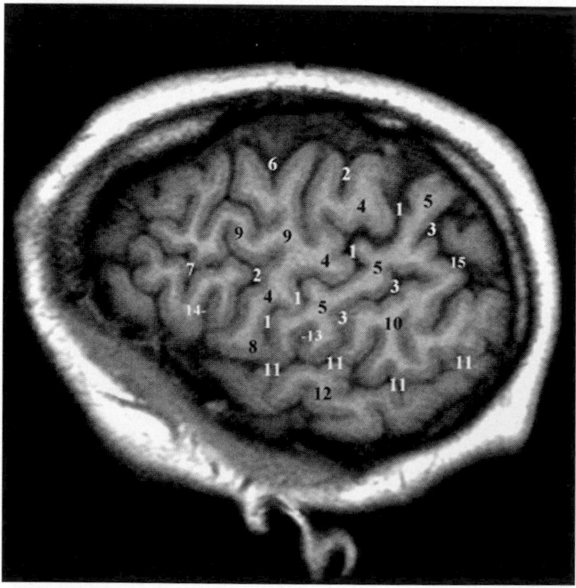

Fig. 10.59. *1*, Central sulcus; *2*, precentral sulcus; *3*, postcentral sulcus; *4*, precentral gyrus; *5*, postcentral gyrus; *6*, superior frontal sulcus; *7*, inferior frontal sulcus; *8*, frontal operculum; *9*, middle frontal gyrus; *10*, inferior parietal lobule; *11*, sylvian fissure; *12*, superior temporal gyrus; *13*, posterior subcentral sulcus; *14*, vertical ramus of lateral fissure; *15*, intraparietal sulcus

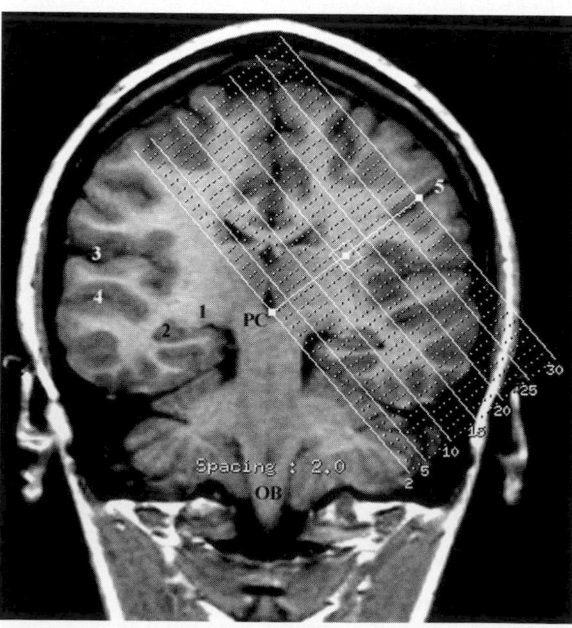

Fig. 10.60. MR topogram with the oblique cuts oriented according to the „fimbria-Fornix" reference plane. *1*, Lateral geniculate body; *2*, hippocampus; *3*, lateral fissure; *4*, parallel sulcus

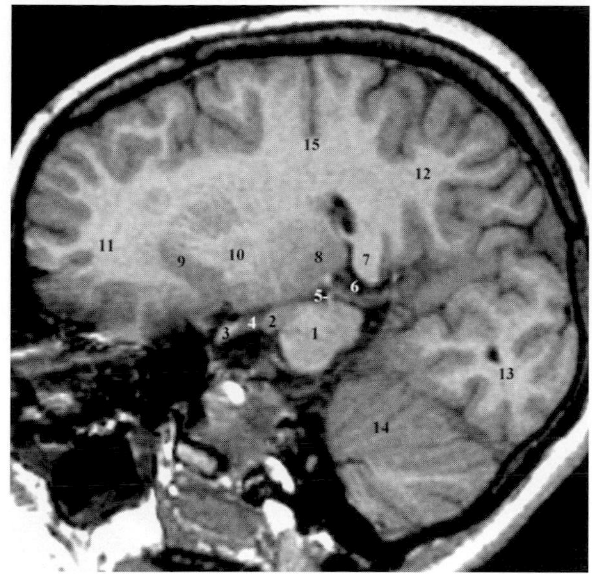

Fig. 10.61. *1*, Mesencephalon; *2*, mamillary body; *3*, chiasma; *4*, third ventricle; *5*, posterior commissure; *6*, ambient cistern; *7*, splenium of corpus callosum; *8*, thalamus; *9*, caudate nucleus; *10*, internal capsule; *11*, frontal lobe; *12*, parietal lobe; *13*, occipital lobe; *14*, cerebellar hemisphere; *15*, central sulcus

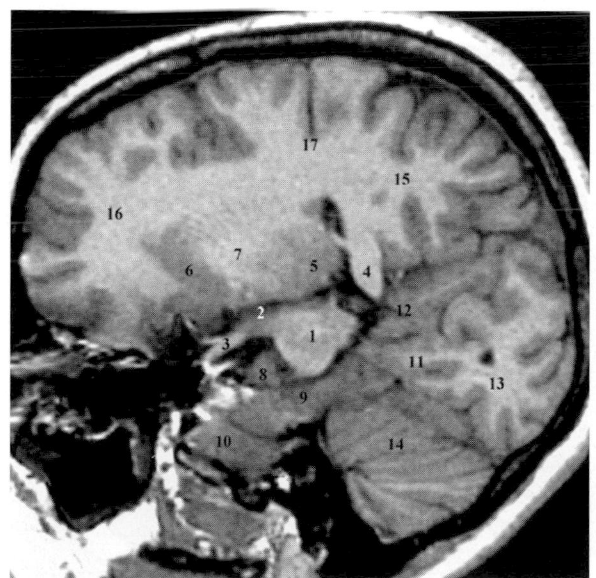

Fig. 10.62. *1*, Mesencephalon; *2*, third ventricle; *3*, chiasma; *4*, splenium of corpus callosum; *5*, thalamus; *6*, caudate nucleus; *7*, internal capsule; *8*, uncus; *9*, parahippocampal gyrus; *10*, fusiform gyrus; *11*, lingual gyrus; *12*, isthmus; *13*, occipital lobe; *14*, cerebellar hemisphere; *15*, parietal lobe; *16*, frontal lobe; *17*, central sulcus

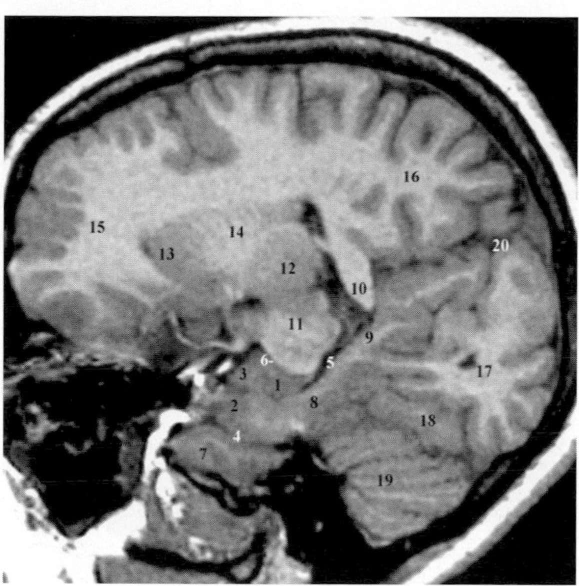

Fig. 10.63. *1*, Gyrus uncinatus; *2*, parahippocampal gyrus; *3*, semilunar gyrus (cortical nucleus of amygdala); *4*, rhinal sulcus; *5*, choroidal fissure; *6*, endorhinal sulcus; *7*, fusiform gyrus; *8*, parahippocampal gyrus; *9*, isthmus; *10*, splenium of corpus callosum; 11, mesodiencephalic region; *12*, thalamus; *13*, caudate nucleus; *14*, corona radiata and gray striatal bridges; *15*, frontal lobe; *16*, parietal lobe; *17*, occipital lobe; *18*, lingual gyrus; *19*, cerebellum; *20*, interhemispheric fissure

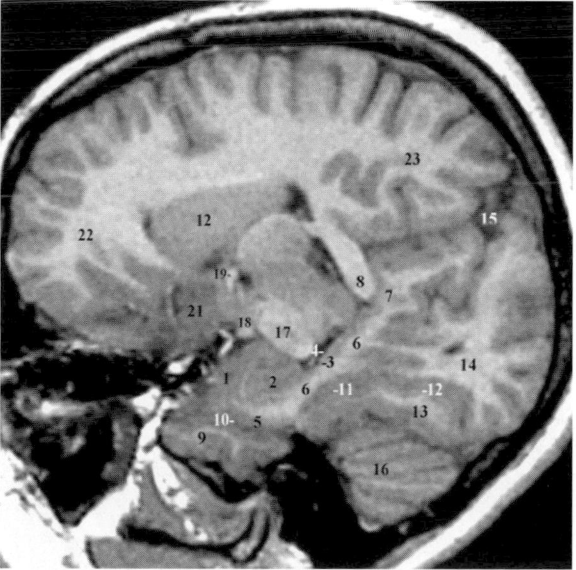

Fig. 10.64. *1*, Amygdala; *2*, hippocampal head; *3*, presubiculum; *4*, choroidal fissure; *5*, endorhinal cortex; *6*, parahippocampal gyrus; *7*, isthmus; *8*, splenium of corpus callosum; *9*, fusiform gyrus; *10*, rhinal sulcus; *11*, collateral sulcus; *12*, calcarine sulcus; *13*, lingual gyrus; *14*, cuneus; *15*, interhemispheric fissure; *16*, cerebellum; *17*, cerebral peduncle; *18*, optic tract; *19*, anterior commissure; *20*, caudate nucleus; *21*, subcallosal region; *22*, frontal lobe; *23*, parietal lobe

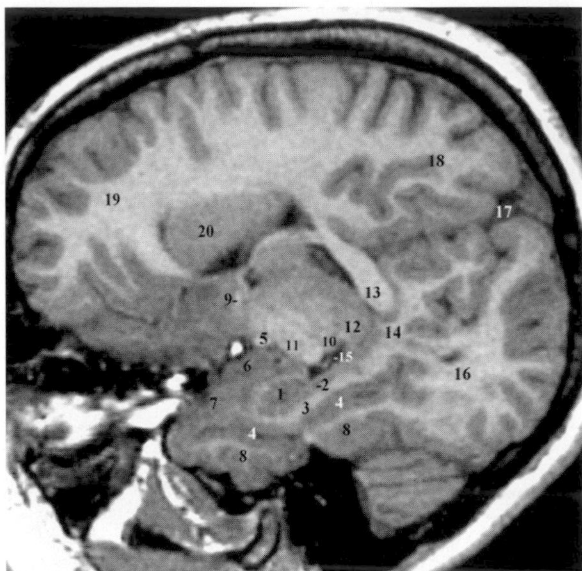

Fig. 10.65. *1*, Hippocampal head; *2*, subiculum; *3*, parahippocampal gyrus; *4*, collateral sulcus; *5*, optic tract; *6*, cortical nucleus of amygdala; *7*, gyrus ambiens (entorhinal cortex); *8*, fusiform gyrus; *9*, anterior commissure; *10*, lateral geniculate body; *11*, crus cerebri; *12*, thalamus (pulvinar); *13*, splenium of corpus callosum; *14*, isthmus; *15*, transverse fissure; *16*, occipital lobe; *17*, interhemispheric fissure; *18*, parietal lobe; *19*, frontal lobe; *20*, caudate nucleus; *21*, interhemispheric fissure

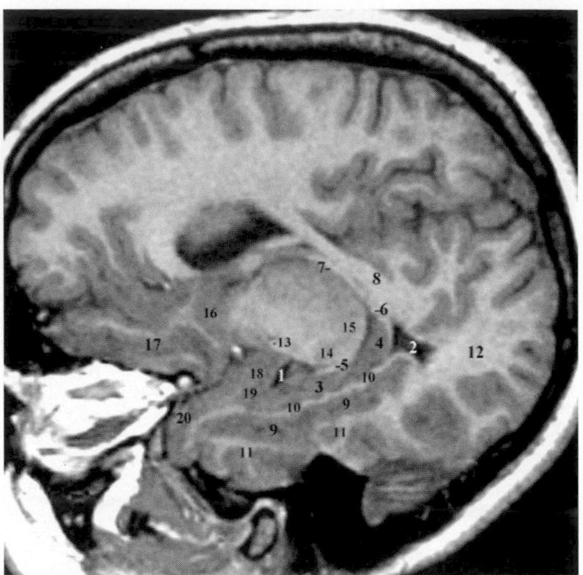

Fig. 10.67. *1*, Temporal horn of the lateral ventricle; *2*, atrium of the lateral ventricle; *3*, hippocampal body; *4*, hippocampal tail; *5*, fimbria; *6*, fornix, crus; *7*, fornix, body; *8*, splenium of corpus callosum; *9*, collateral sulcus; *10*, parahippocampal gyrus; *11*, fusiform gyrus; *12*, occipital lobe; *13*, optic tract; *14*, lateral geniculate body; *15*, pulvinar; *16*, putamen; *17*, rostral sulcus; *18*, basal nucleus of amygdala; *19*, hippocampal-amygdala junction; *20*, temporal polar cortex

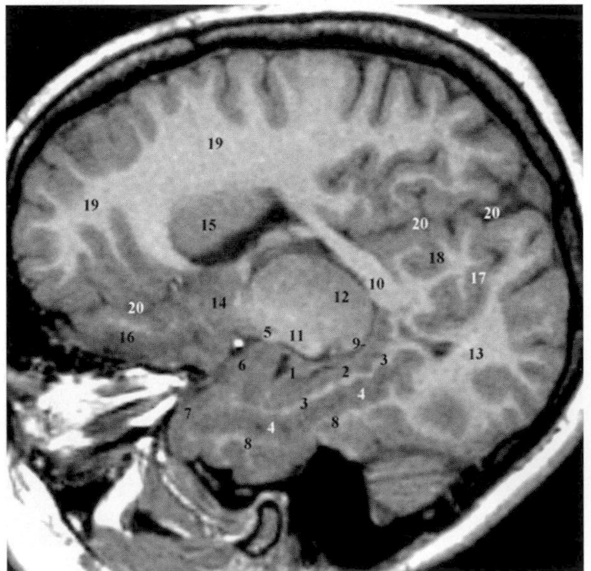

Fig. 10.66. *1*, Hippocampal head; *2*, subiculum; *3*, parahippocampal gyrus; *4*, collateral sulcus; *5*, optic tract; *6*, cortical nucleus of amygdala; *7*, gyrus ambiens (entorhinal cortex); *8*, fusiform gyrus; *9*, fimbria; *10*, splenium of corpus callosum; *11*, crus cerebri; *12*, thalamus (pulvinar); *13*, occipital lobe; *14*, septal area; *15*, caudate nucleus; *16*, orbitofrontal gyri; *17*, parieto-occipital sulcus; *18*, parietal lobe; *19*, frontal lobe; *20*, interhemispheric fissure

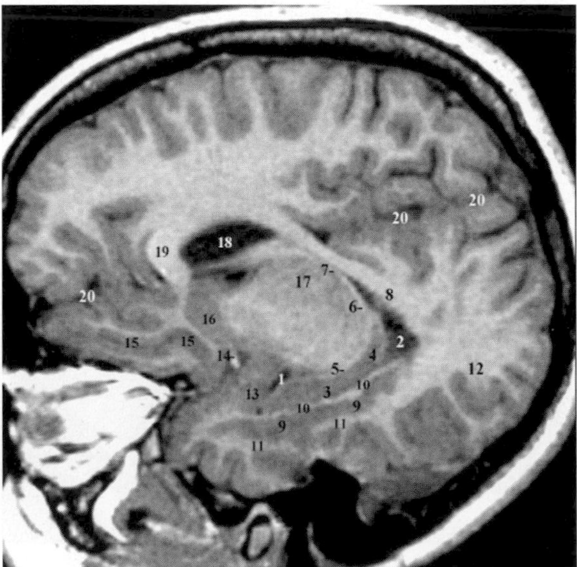

Fig. 10.68. *1*, Temporal horn of the lateral ventricle; *2*, atrium of the lateral ventricle; *3*, hippocampal body; *4*, hippocampal tail; *5*, fimbria; *6*, fornix, crus; *7*, fornix, body; *8*, splenium of corpus callosum; *9*, collateral sulcus; *10*, parahippocampal gyrus; *11*, fusiform gyrus; *12*, occipital lobe; *13*, lateral nucleus of amygdala; *14*, middle cerebral artery; *15*, rostral sulcus; *16*, putamen; *17*, thalamus; *18*, lateral ventricle; *19*, genu of corpus callosum; *20*, interhemispheric fissure

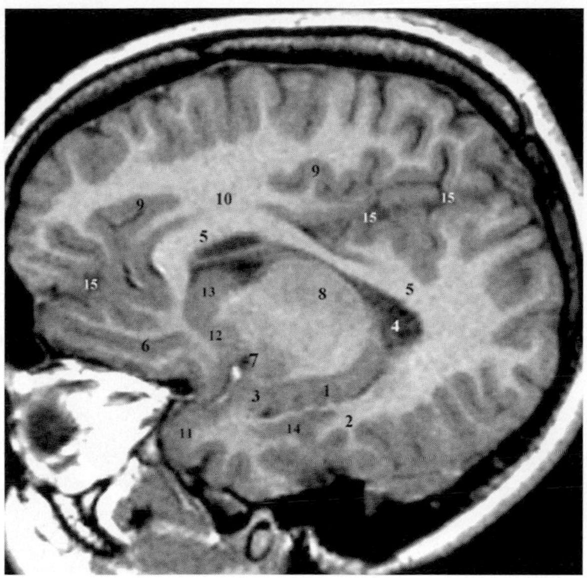

Fig. 10.69. *1*, Hippocampus; *2*, parahippocampal gyrus; *3*, lateral nucleus of amygdala; *4*, atrium; *5*, corpus callosum; *6*, rostral sulcus; *7*, endorhinal sulcus; *8*, thalamus; *9*, cingulate sulcus; *10*, cingulate gyrus; *11*, temporal pole; *12*, putamen; *13*, caudate nucleus; *14*, collateral sulcus; *15*, interhemispheric fissure

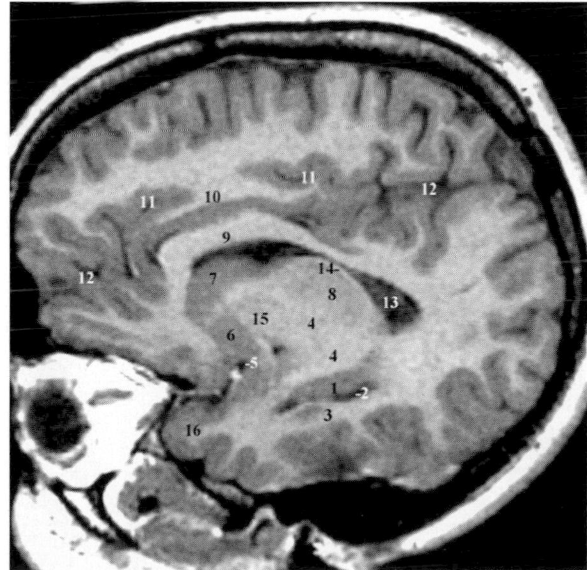

Fig. 10.70. *1*, Hippocampus; *2*, temporal horn of lateral ventricle; *3*, parahippocampal gyrus; *4*, internal capsule; *5*, endorhinal sulcus; *6*, putamen; *7*, caudate nucleus; *8*, thalamus; *9*, corpus callosum; *10*, cingulate gyrus; *11*, cingulate sulcus; *12*, interhemispheric fissure; *13*, lateral ventricle; *14*, fornix; *15*, internal capsule ; *16*, temporal pole

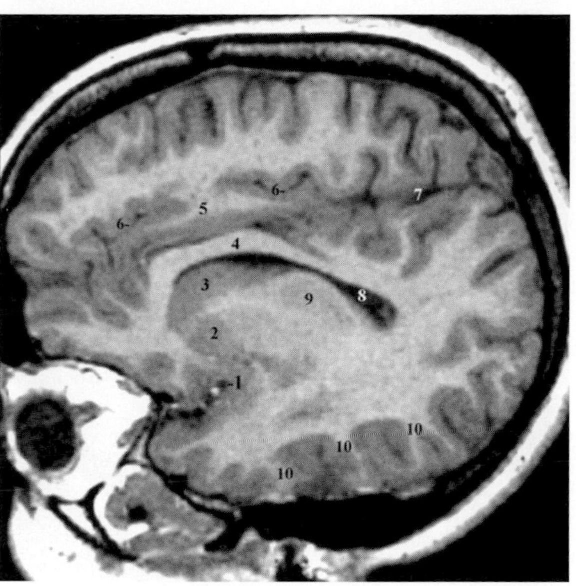

Fig. 10.71. *1*, Falciform sulcus of insula; *2*, putamen; *3*, caudate nucleus; *4*, corpus callosum; *5*, cingulate gyrus; *6*, cingulate sulcus; *7*, interhemispheric fissure; *8*, lateral ventricle; *9*, thalamus; *10*, inferior temporal gyrus

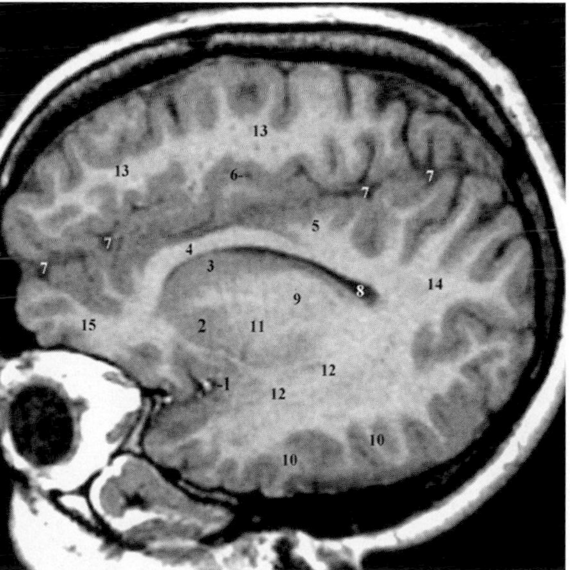

Fig. 10.72. *1*, Falciform sulcus; *2*, putamen; *3*, caudate nucleus; *4*, corpus callosum; *5*, cingulate gyrus; *6*, cingulate sulcus; *7*, interhemispheric fissure; *8*, lateral ventricle; *9*, thalamus, reticular nucleus; *10*, inferior temporal gyrus; *11*, internal capsule; *12*, temporal stem; *13*, frontal lobe; *14*, parietal lobe; *15*, orbitofrontal gyri

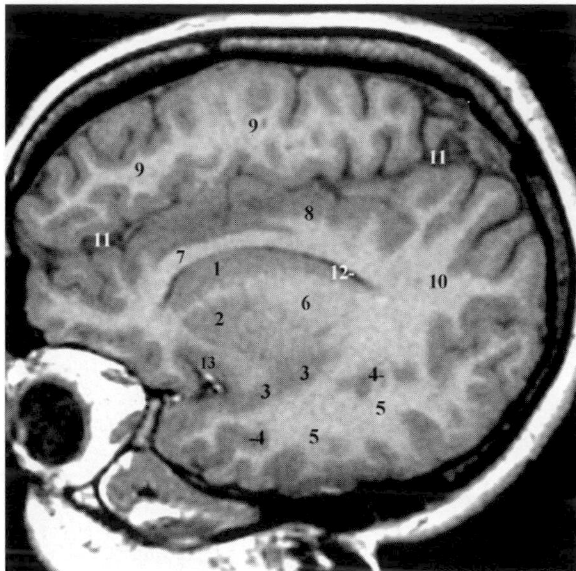

Fig. 10.73. *1*, Caudate nucleus; *2*, putamen; *3*, limen insulae (circular sulcus); *4*, parallel sulcus; *5*, middle temporal gyrus; *6*, internal capsule; *7*, temporal stem; *8*, cingulate gyrus; *9*, internal frontal gyrus; *10*, parietal lobe; *11*, interhemispheric fissure; *12*, lateral ventricle; *13*, anterior perforated substance

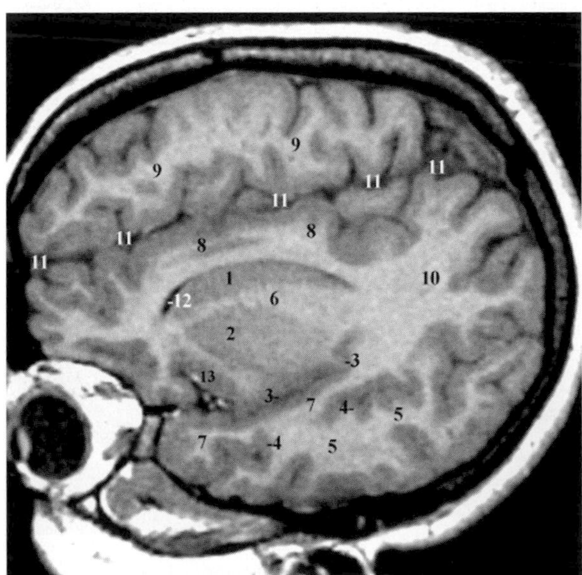

Fig. 10.74. *1*, Caudate nucleus; *2*, putamen; *3*, limen insulae (circular sulcus); *4*, parallel sulcus; *5*, middle temporal gyrus; *6*, corona radiata; *7*, superior temporal gyrus; *8*, cingulate gyrus; *9*, internal frontal gyrus; *10*, parietal lobe; *11*, interhemispheric fissure; *12*, lateral ventricle; *13*, anterior perforated substance

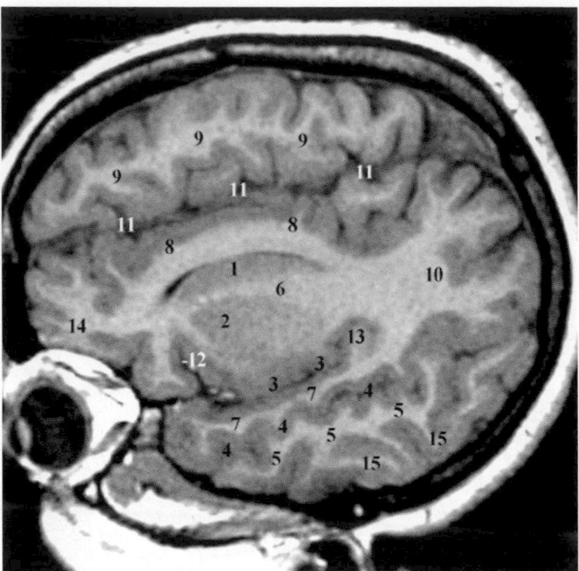

Fig. 10.75. *1*, Caudate nucleus; *2*, putamen; *3*, limen insulae (circular sulcus); *4*, parallel sulcus; *5*, middle temporal gyrus; *6*, corona radiata; *7*, superior temporal gyrus; *8*, cingulate gyrus; *9*, internal frontal gyrus; *10*, parietal lobe; *11*, interhemispheric fissure; *12*, circular sulcus insulae; *13*, transverse temporal gyrus and auditory path; *14*, orbitofrontal gyri; *15*, inferior temporal gyrus

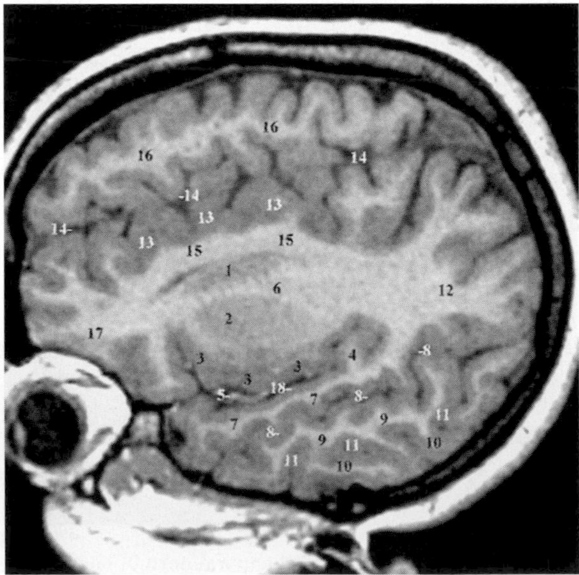

Fig. 10.76. *1*, Caudate nucleus; *2*, putamen; *3*, insular cortex; *4*, Heschl gyrus; *5*, middle cerebral artery; *6*, corona radiata; *7*, superior temporal gyrus; *8*, parallel sulcus; *9*, middle temporal gyrus; *10*, inferior temporal gyrus; *11*, inferior temporal sulcus; *12*, parietal lobe; *13*, cingulate sulcus; *14*, interhemispheric sulcus; *15*, cingulate gyrus; *16*, internal frontal gyrus; *17*, orbitofrontal gyrus; *18*, sylvian fissure, posterior ramus

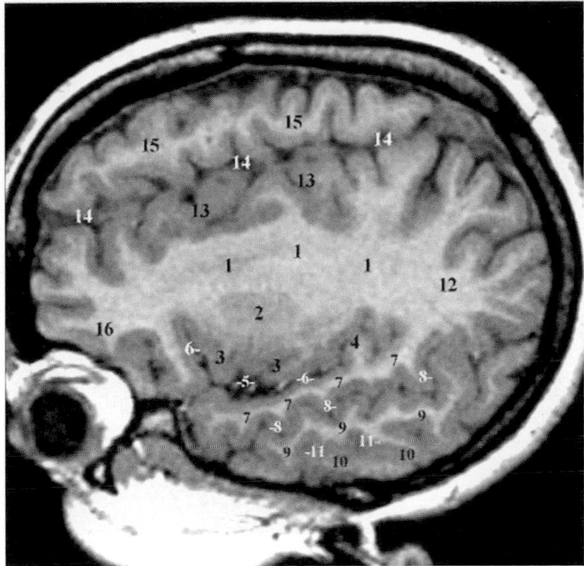

Fig. 10.77. *1*, Corona radiata; *2*, claustrum ; *3*, insular cortex; *4*, Heschl gyrus; *5*, middle cerebral artery, insular branches; *6*, circular sulcus insulae; *7*, superior temporal gyrus; *8*, parallel sulcus; *9*, middle temporal gyrus; *10*, inferior temporal gyrus; *11*, inferior temporal sulcus; *12*, parietal lobe; *13*, cingulate sulcus; *14*, interhemispheric sulcus; *15*, medial frontal gyrus; *16*, orbitofrontal gyri

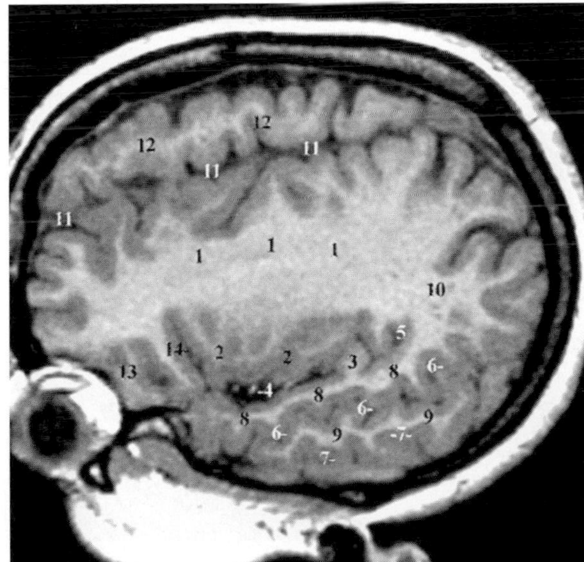

Fig. 10.78. *1*, Corona radiata; *2*, insular cortex; *3*, transverse temporal gyri; *4*, arterial branches of middle cerebral artery; *5*, terminal ascending branch of lateral fissure; *6*, parallel sulcus; *7*, inferior temporal sulcus; *8*, superior temporal gyrus; *9*, middle temporal gyrus; *10*, inferior parietal lobule; *11*, interhemispheric fissure; *12*, medial frontal gyrus; *13*, fronto-orbital gyri; *14*, circular sulcus insulae

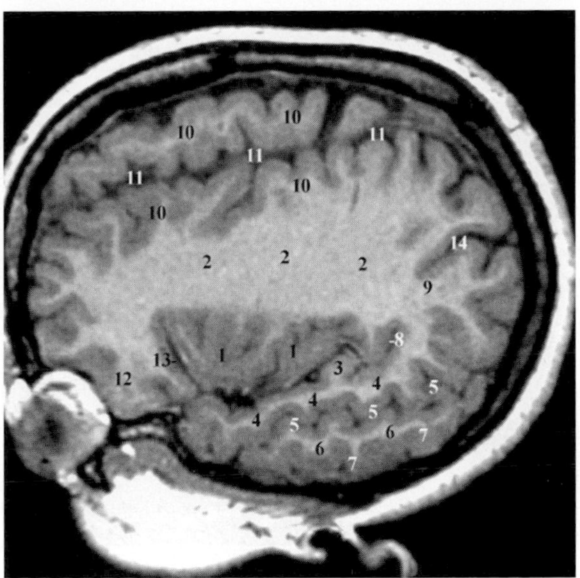

Fig. 10.79. *1*, Insula; *2*, corona radiata; *3*, transverse temporal gyrus; *4*, superior temporal gyrus; *5*, parallel sulcus; *6*, middle temporal gyrus; *7*, inferior temporal sulcus; *8*, terminal ascending branch of lateral fissure; *9*, inferior parietal lobule; *10*, medial frontal gyrus; *11*, interhemispheric fissure; *12*, fronto-orbital gyrus; *13*, circular sulcus; *14*, intraparietal sulcus

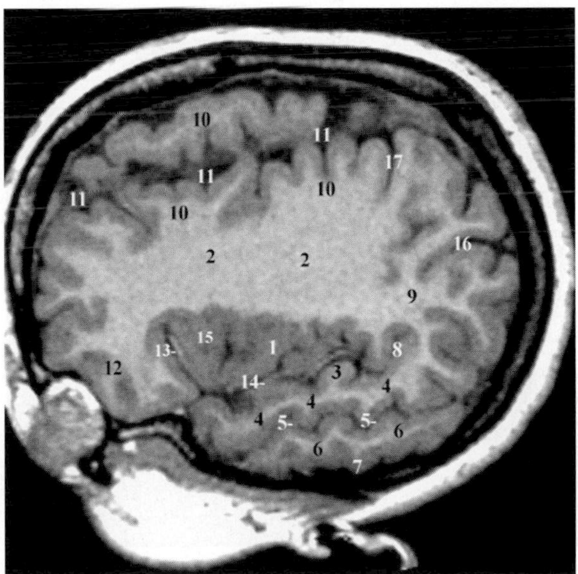

Fig. 10.80. *1*, Insula; *2*, corona radiata; *3*, transverse temporal gyrus; *4*, superior temporal gyrus; *5*, parallel sulcus; *6*, middle temporal gyrus; *7*, inferior temporal sulcus; *8*, terminal ascending branch of lateral fissure; *9*, inferior parietal lobule; *10*, medial frontal gyrus; *11*, interhemispheric fissure; *12*, fronto-orbital gyrus; *13*, circular sulcus of insula; *14*, lateral fissure, posterior ramus; *15*, short gyri of insula; *16*, intraparietal sulcus; *17*, central sulcus

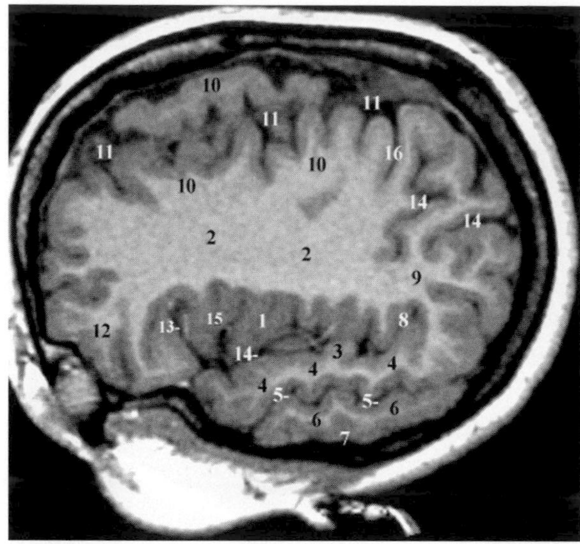

Fig. 10.81. *1*, Insula; *2*, corona radiata; *3*, transverse temporal gyrus; *4*, superior temporal gyrus; *5*, parallel sulcus; *6*, middle temporal gyrus; *7*, inferior temporal sulcus; *8*, terminal ascending branch of lateral fissure; *9*, inferior parietal lobule; *10*, medial frontal gyrus; *11*, interhemispheric fissure; *12*, fronto-orbital gyrus; *13*, circular sulcus insulae; *14*, intraparietal sulcus, ascending part; *15*, short gyri of insula; *16*, central sulcus

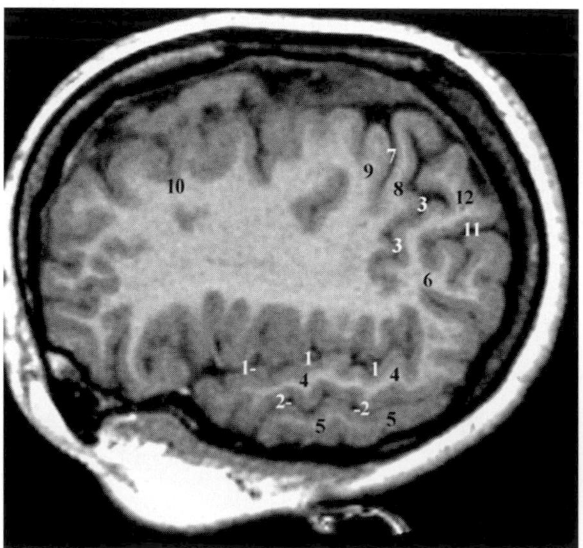

Fig. 10.82. *1*, Lateral fissure; *2*, parallel sulcus; *3*, intraparietal sulcus, ascending part; *4*, superior temporal gyrus; *5*, middle temporal gyrus; *6*, inferior parietal lobule; *7*, central sulcus; *8*, postcentral gyrus; *9*, precentral gyrus; *10*, frontal lobe; *11*, intraparietal sulcus, horizontal part; *12*, superior parietal lobule

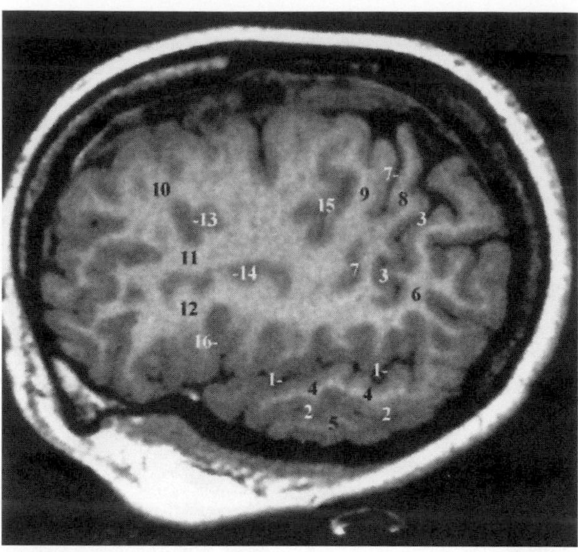

Fig. 10.83. *1*, Lateral fissure; *2*, parallel sulcus; *3*, intraparietal sulcus; *4*, superior temporal gyrus; *5*, middle temporal gyrus; *6*, inferior parietal lobule; *7*, central sulcus; *8*, postcentral gyrus; *9*, precentral gyrus; *10*, superior frontal gyrus; *11*, middle frontal gyrus; *12*, inferior frontal gyrus; *13*, superior frontal sulcus; *14*, inferior frontal sulcus; *15*, superior precentral sulcus; *16*, vertical ramus of lateral fissure

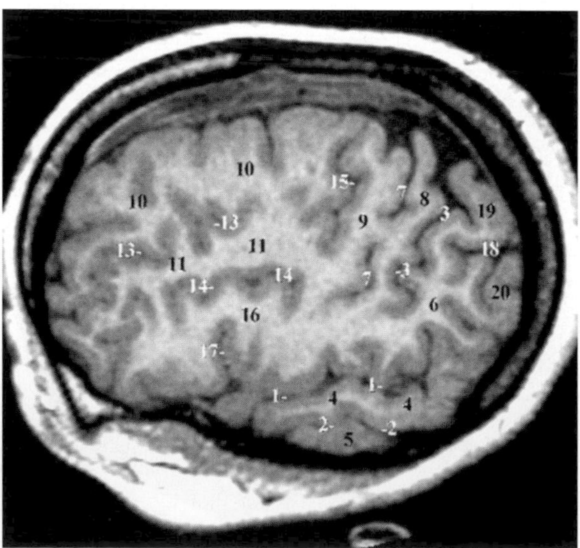

Fig. 10.84. *1*, Lateral fissure; *2*, parallel sulcus; *3*, intraparietal sulcus; *4*, superior temporal gyrus; *5*, middle temporal gyrus; *6*, inferior parietal lobule; *7*, central sulcus; *8*, postcentral gyrus; *9*, precentral gyrus; *10*, superior frontal gyrus; *11*, middle frontal gyrus; *12*, inferior frontal gyrus; *13*, superior frontal sulcus; *14*, inferior frontal sulcus; *15*, superior precentral sulcus; *16*, inferior frontal gyrus; *17*, vertical ramus of lateral fissure; *18*, intraparietal sulcus, horizontal part; *19*, superior parietal lobule; *20*, inferior parietal lobule

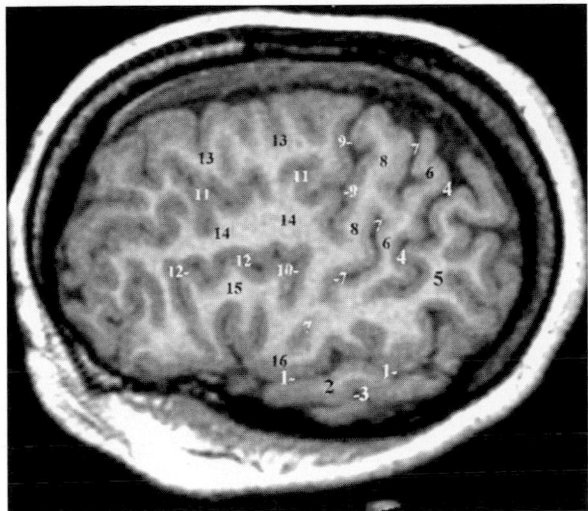

Fig. 10.85. *1*, Lateral fissure; *2*, superior temporal gyrus; *3*, parallel sulcus; *4*, intraparietal sulcus; *5*, inferior parietal lobule; *6*, postcentral gyrus; *7*, central sulcus; *8*, precentral gyrus; *9*, superior precentral sulcus; *10*, inferior precentral sulcus; *11*, superior frontal sulcus; *12*, inferior frontal sulcus; *13*, superior frontal gyrus; *14*, middle frontal gyrus; *15*, inferior frontal gyrus; *16*, frontoparietal operculum

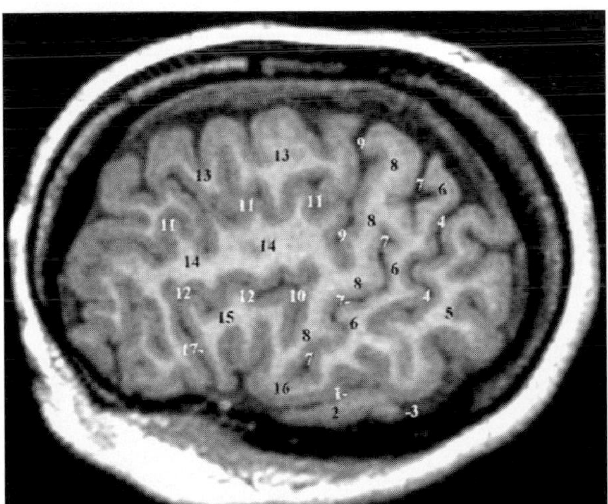

Fig. 10.86. *1*, Lateral fissure; *2*, superior temporal gyrus; *3*, parallel sulcus; *4*, intraparietal sulcus; *5*, inferior parietal lobule; *6*, postcentral gyrus; *7*, central sulcus; *8*, precentral gyrus; *9*, superior precentral sulcus; *10*, inferior precentral sulcus; *11*, superior frontal sulcus; *12*, inferior frontal sulcus; *13*, superior frontal gyrus; *14*, middle frontal gyrus; *15*, inferior frontal gyrus; *16*, frontoparietal operculum; *17*, lateral orbital sulcus

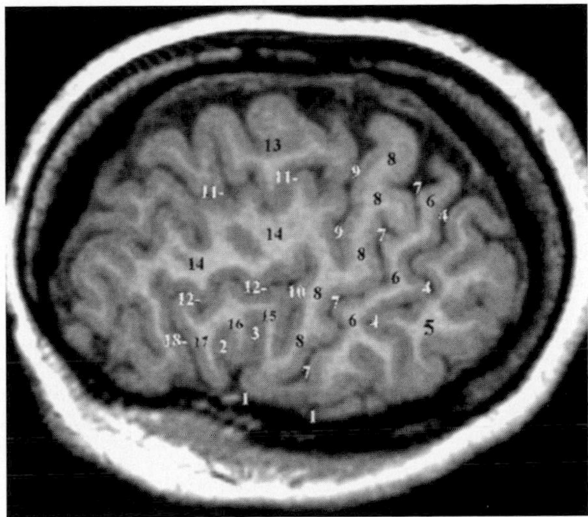

Fig. 10.87. *1*, Lateral fissure; *2*, horizontal ramus of lateral fissure; *3*, vertical ascending ramus of lateral fissure; *4*, intraparietal sulcus; *5*, inferior parietal lobule; *6*, postcentral gyrus; *7*, central sulcus; *8*, precentral gyrus; *9*, superior precentral sulcus; *10*, inferior precentral sulcus; *11*, superior frontal sulcus; *12*, inferior frontal sulcus; *13*, superior frontal gyrus; *14*, middle frontal gyrus; *15*, inferior frontal gyrus, opercular part; *16*, inferior frontal gyrus, triangular part; *17*, inferior frontal gyrus, orbital part

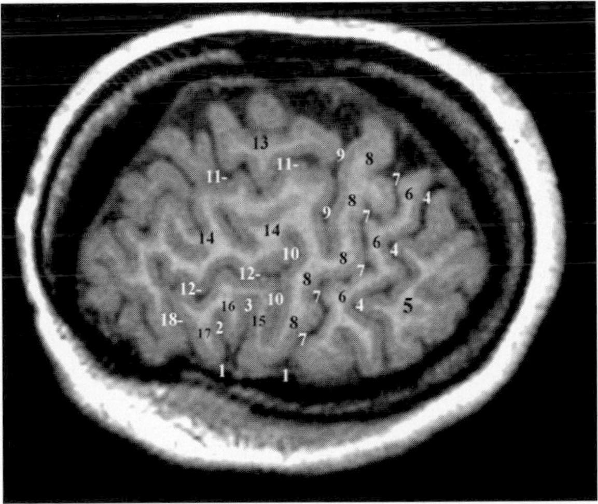

Fig. 10.88. *1*, Lateral fissure; *2*, horizontal ramus of lateral fissure; *3*, vertical ascending ramus of lateral fissure; *4*, intraparietal sulcus; *5*, inferior parietal lobule; *6*, postcentral gyrus; *7*, central sulcus; *8*, precentral gyrus; *9*, superior precentral sulcus; *10*, inferior precentral sulcus; *11*, superior frontal sulcus; *12*, inferior frontal sulcus; *13*, superior frontal gyrus; *14*, middle frontal gyrus; *15*, inferior frontal gyrus, opercular part; *16*, inferior frontal gyrus, triangular part; *17*, inferior frontal gyrus, orbital part; *18*, lateral orbital sulcus

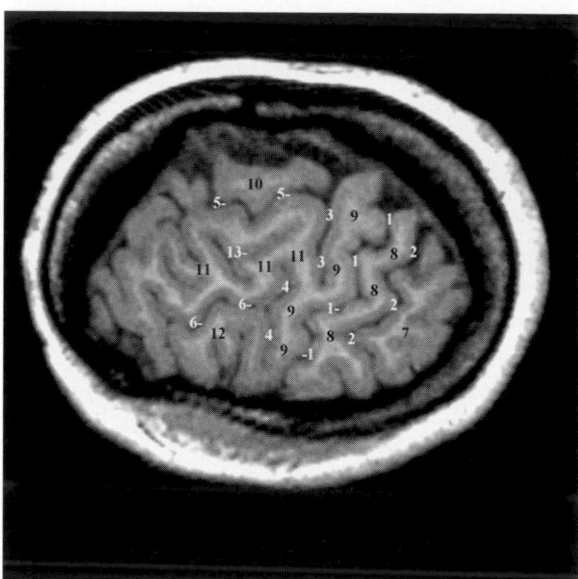

Fig. 10.89. *1*, Central sulcus; *2*, intraparietal sulcus, ascending segment; *3*, superior precentral sulcus; *4*, inferior precentral sulcus; *5*, superior frontal sulcus; *6*, inferior central sulcus; *7*, inferior parietal lobule; *8*, postcentral gyrus; *9*, precentral gyrus; *10*, superior frontal gyrus; *11*, middle frontal gyrus; *12*, inferior frontal gyrus; *13*, intermediate frontal sulcus

Subject Index